Little
Changes

The impossible adventure of a lifetime

By Priscilla Houliston

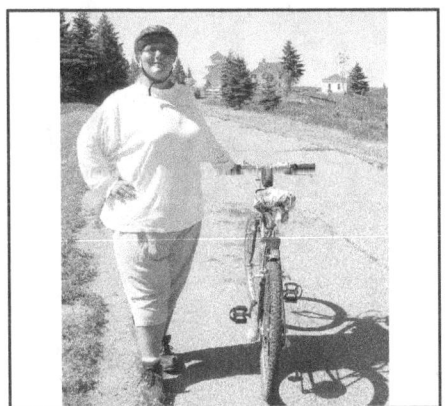

Priscilla Houliston in Quoddy Head, Maine after bicycling 3,013 miles : June 17, 2007
Weight 250 pounds

Copyright 2007

LITTLE CHANGES *The impossible adventure of a lifetime*

Dedications

This book is dedicated to all the people who helped make this journey happen,
everyone reading the book and getting a glimpse of inspiration & motivation.

To my daughter Sarah who provided endless tech support on the phone when I was lost,
to my son James who mapped out the adventure and to my husband Morton,
without whom the journey would have been quite impossible.

To my mother who found the strength to go on after a stroke that saved her life and mine.

Finally, to my grandson Alexander,
who is the answer to all the questions in my universe and my reason
to be as healthy as I can and stick around on this
wonderful gigantic planet for as long as possible.

All my love for all of time.

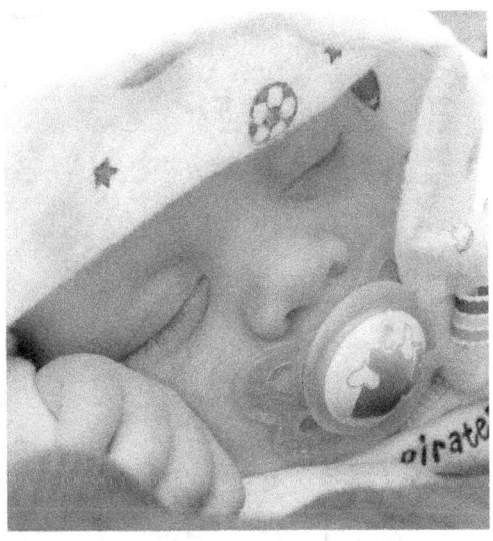

My first grandson, Alexander. My life.

Sponsors of the Journey

Our sponsors in Florida
Sugar Loaf Lodge MM 17
Sunshine Key RV Resort MM 39
Sea Dell Motel MM 50
The Jolly Roger MM 59
Kon Tiki Resort MM 81.2
Theater of the Sea MM 84.5
Pelican Cove Resort MM 84.5
Keys Wild Bird Center MM 93.6
Sunset Cove Beach Resort MM 99.5
Coral Castle *Homestead*
Holiday Inn *University of Miami*
Holiday Inn *Highland Beach*
Queen's Motor Lodge West *Palm Beach*
Jensen Beach Boat Rentals
Jonathan Dickinson State Park
River Tours : Cabins
Sebastian Inlet State Park
Beach House Motel *Indiatlantic*
Holiday Inn Express *Cocoa*
Luna Sea Motel *Cocoa Beach*
Riverside Inn *Titusville*
Ripley's Believe It Or Not Museum, Ghost Train, Sightseeing Train *St. Augustine*
Old St. Augustine Village
LaPentola *St. Augustine*
95 Cordova at Casa Monica Hote *St. Augustine*
The Agustin Inn *St. Augustine*
Holiday Inn   *St. Augustine Beach*

Our sponsors in Georgia
Guesthouse Inn & Suites *Brunswick*
Fort King George *Historic Darien*
Olde Harbour Inn *Savannah*
South Beach Ocean Rentals on *Tybee Island*
Clary's Cafe *Savannah*
Savannah Day Spa

Our sponsors in South Carolina
Court Capri *Myrtle Beach*
Pawleys Plantation Golf & Country Club
Brookgreen Gardens
Brookwood Inn *Murrell's Inlet*
Broad Street Guest House Kosher B&B *Charleston*
Wild Wing Cafe *Charleston*
Bubba Gumps Shrimp Company *Charleston*
Joe Pasta *Charleston*
Charleston Area Convention & Visitors Bureau
American Military Museum
The Charleston Museum
Edmondston - Alston House
Forever Charleston
Heyward - Washington House
IMAX
Joseph Manigault House
Nathaniel Russell House
Old Exchange & Provost Dungeon *Charleston*
Bulldog Tours - Haunted Jail Tour *Charleston*
Grayline Bus Tours *Charleston*
Palmetto Carriage Works
South Carolina Aquarium

Our sponsors in North Carolina
Shallotte/*Brunswick Beaches KOA*
Motel 6 *Wilmington*
Virginia Creek Campground *Hamstead*
Hampton Inn *Jacksonville*
Applebee's *Jacksonville*
Holiday Inn Express *Morehead City*
Village Marina *Hatteras*
Lighthouse View *Buxton*
Traveler's Inn Motor Lodge *Nags Head*

Our sponsors in Virginia
The Viking *Virginia Beach*
Super 8 *Norfolk*
The Cedars B&B *Williamsburg*
Seasons Restaurant *Williamsburg*

Our sponsors in Washington DC
The Watergate Hotel
Meiwah Restaurant

Our sponsors in Maryland
Baltimore Area Convention & Visitor Center
Phillips Seafood *Baltimore*
Country Inn & Suites *Annapolis*
Howard Johnson *Cheverly*
Best Western *Denton*
Best Western *Kent Narrows Inn*
Annapolis & Anne Arundel Co. Conference & Visitors Bureau

Our sponsors in Pennsylvania
Signs Now Hanover
Massage Therapy Associates *Camp Hill*
The Spa at Hotel Hershey
Carlisle Market Cross Pub
Churchtown Inn *Churchtown*
B F Hiestand House B&B*Marietta*
Intercourse Pretzel Factory
The Artist's Inn *Terre Hill*
Allimax Farm Carriage rides & horseback riding *Leola*
Zook's Motel *Leola*
Lititz House B&B *Lititz*
Lovelace Manor B&B *Lancaster*
Lost Treasure Golf *Lancaster*
Dutch Apple Dinner Theater
King's Cottage B&B *Lancaster*
Miller's Smorgasborg *Lancaster*
Dutch Wonderland
Walnut Lawn B&B *Lancaster*
Kromer's B&B *Ephrata*
Tree Top B&B *Ephrata*
The Keystone Inn B&B *Gettysburg*

Our sponsors in Delaware
Hotel Blue *Lewes*

Our sponsors in New Jersey
Caesars *Atlantic City*
Atlantic City Visitors Center
Phillips Seafood *Atlantic City*
Thank you to Carla, President of the Highlands Business Partnership
Nauvoo Cottages *Highlands*
Seastreak Ferry
The Palace Hotel of Cape May *Cape May*
Hershey Motel *Seaside Heights*

Our sponsors in New York
Hotel Pennsylvania *NYC*
Bubba Gumps Shrimp Comany *Times Square*
Hard Rock Cafe *Times Square*
Tasti D Lite *Frozen desserts that are good for you!*

Our sponsors in Connecticut
Hilton Mystic *Mystic*
Mystic Seaport *Mystic*
Mystic Aquarium *Mystic*
Seamen's Inne *Mystic*
S & P Oyster Company *Mystic*
RiverWalk Restaurant *Mystic*
Daniel Packer Inne *Mystic*
Mystic Chamber of Commerce

Our sponsors in Rhode Island
Shelter Harbor Inn *Westerly*
Narragansett Cafe *Jamestown*
Las Palmas Inn *Newport*
Rose Island Lighthouse *Newport*
Visitor & Convention Center *Newport*

Our sponsors in New Hampshire
Sise Inn *Portsmouth*

MBT Shoes - Worldwide

Our sponsors in Massachusetts
Lizzie Borden B&B *Fall River*
Boston Visitor & Convention Center *Boston*
The Red Hat B&B *Martha's Vineyard*
Craig's Bicycles *Martha's Vineyard*
Oak Bluffs Inn *Martha's Vineyard*
Nautilus Motor Inn *Woods Hole*
Pie In The Sky *Woods Hole*
Ridgewood Motel & Cottages *South Orleans*
Little Capistrano Bike Shop *Eastham*
Ship's Knees Inn *Orleans*
Sandbars *Truro*
The Inn at Cook Street *Provincetown*
Sandollar B&B *Sagamore Beach*
Omni Parker House *Boston*
HI Boston *A great hostel*
Rosewood Motel *East Wareham*
The Salem Inn *Salem*
Captain Haskell's Octagon House B&B *New Bedford*
Rosewood Motel *East Wareham*

Our sponsors in Maine
Dixon's Campground *Cape Neddick*
Maine Motel *South Portland*
Captain Lord Mansion *Kennebunkport*
Frontier Energy *East China*
Primrose Inn *A Bar Harbor*
Treasure *Bar Harbor*
Bar Harbor Chamber of Commerce
Oli's Trolley *Bar Harbor*
Mt. Desert Narrows RV & camground *MDI*
Comfort Inn *Brunswick*
Comfort Inn *Augusta*
Comfort Inn *Belfast*
Bucksport Motor Inn *Bucksport*
Quoddy Head Station *Quoddy Head*

Our sponsors in Wyoming
Howdy Pardner B&B *Cheyenne*
Cheyenne Visitors Center
Rubyjuice on 17th *Cheyenne*
Synergy Cafe *Cheyenne*
Bentwood Inn B&B *Jackson Hole*

Our sponsors in Oregon
Britannia at Terwilliger Vista B&B *West Hills of Portland*
The Lion & The Rose B&B *Portland*
Portland Classical Chinese Garden
Japanese Garden Portland

Our medical sponsors
Legacy Good Samaritan Hospital in Portland, Oregon
Dr. Andy Mones an incredible doctor who arranged for the hospital and his practice, *Northwest Acute Care Specialists, PC,* to see and treat my leg at no cost.

Thank you to everyone who allowed us to sleep in your homes, churches, yards and other little nooks and crannies we managed to call home for one night along the way.

Thank you to all of the members of the press who interviewed us, filmed us, photographed us and helped spread the news of the journey to the entire world.

Thank you to everyone who stopped us as we were bicycling to wish us well, offer us a drink and committed a random act of kindness to perfect strangers.

Thank you to everyone on the internet who followed this journey online. Stick around, the best is yet to come.

Priscilla

Chapters

Sitting in the small space, my arms touching the steel grey walls, I wondered how it was that I came to be trapped here. My face was just inches from the door in front of me and even though I could open the lock, I had no hope of getting out. Escape was physically impossible. Not knowing to laugh or cry, sitting back for a moment of reflection was what seemed the only logical thing to do. My husband Morton would be waiting for me outside. What would he do when I didn't show up at the spot we agreed to meet? He would wait I guessed, below the bronze statue of the big ram or maybe it's a goat, that sits in the middle of the double roads in this storybook little town. There are plenty of them here in Scotland. But none of that mattered right now. I wasn't going anywhere.

The hallway that led me into this prison seemed wide enough. It was a close call when I first entered the building and the man who was sitting in the booth collecting the money, a silver ten pence piece, didn't bat an eye when I pushed nonchalantly through the gate intended for wheelchairs and strollers. The turnstile would have never accommodated my girth. Never.

Finding my way to this room by following the signs on the wall, Morton had came in right before me, heading another direction. This was one of those quaint old stone buildings that Scotland has so many of, built a long time ago to be a town meeting hall or perhaps a corn exchange building and it now served a multitude of functions.

The small town we are in, Moffet, is in the Scottish Borders. Just a stones throw away from the English border and I'm sure that there were loads of prisons here in the olden days to keep ruffians in. But I'm not a ruffian. I'm just a 440 pound American woman, trapped in a toilet.

Looking at the angle of the door I wondered how I ever squeezed in here. Was this a special toilet for children only and I missed the sign? Surely I had been in this same facility a few years ago when we spent a glorious Saturday looking around the shops of the town. Morton led me into his favorite candy store in Scotland that held hundreds of jars of sugar goodness that you could buy by the piece. They were a bit more expensive now then his childhood days where he could spend his pocket money and have enough candy to last him a week if he rationed it.

We were in this very same building, using the facilities and I did fit. I knew I had put weight on living in Scotland, but I never imagined enough to get stuck in a toilet.

My eyes were swelling up and my mind was thinking back to some other horrible fat stories that my family history holds. I had a great aunt who had died from a fire in her apartment because she was too big to fit out the window. My mother had described how horrible it was that she was screaming and on fire and could go nowhere. My mom was just a child when it happened and the great aunt, who I of course had never met, was over 300 pounds. A hundred pounds lighter than I am sitting on this toilet today, going no where.

Hearing someone come in the room I think about asking for help. It will be one of those red face moments when the fire brigade has to take a wall down to get me out of here. Maybe, if I look at the hinges, I could just pop the door off. But they are on the outside.

The crawl space under the stall is only six inches off the floor. There wouldn't be room for me to get my big body down on the floor in here, let alone under my prison wall.The walls run right up to the ceiling, so climbing up on the porcelain throne and over isn't an option either. I'm doomed to just sit here.

Opening my cell phone, or mobile phone as they call it here in the United Kingdom, I contemplate calling Morton. "Hey honey, I'm not feeling too good. Do you suppose you can come and take the bathroom door off the hinges and get me outta here?!" But I couldn't bring myself to do it.

I hide my problem of being so massively heavy that my life is ruined from my husband. I hide it well. He must know how big I am, but I lie to myself and the world. I'm an expert at it.

Fifteen minutes have gone by inside this public bathroom prison.

How on earth did I ever get this fat? That is a question I have been asking myself for almost thirty years, each year passing, the question should get bigger, since I am. This is almost my fifth full year of living in Scotland and since moving here my scales have moved up at least a hundred pounds. I hate myself. Completely and utterly hate myself. Maybe I deserve to die in this toilet, or at least die of embarrassment when they have to rescue me out of here.

Thinking of how I know that I am the fattest person on this island, I try to think of anyone fatter than me. I don't know anyone, personally. Occasionally I see a show on television, some huge beast of a person, laying in a bed, ordering fish and chip suppers by the dozen and thinking they have a thyroid problem. It's easy for me to look and watch, knowing without a doubt, that they are in denial. Soothing myself with the fact that I'm not THAT fat, after all, I am a great liar. Proving it by eating that last piece of cheesecake lurking in the fridge, that was a whole cheesecake just a few short hours ago, I contemplate just when I will go on a diet.

Lying to myself is far worse than any lie I have ever told someone else. It is worse because I know the horrible truth, I just don't want to admit it. Come to think of it, I can admit it, I just can't be bothered doing anything about it.

My husband doesn't say anything about my weight, but he has to notice. How could he not? Telling myself that he must love me, after all, he married me fat, I again delude myself with the thought that there is always someone out there fatter. It soothes me thinking that I'm not the only person with this compulsion to eat myself to death.

But now, sitting trapped in a toilet in Moffet, I wonder. Do I have a life threatening problem? Four hundred plus pounds is a lot for any frame to carry. I'm only five foot eight, not eight foot five. I distract myself from my desperate situation by turning my mind to the only other person I know, somewhat related, that topped the scale at four hundred pounds.

This was a man who married the niece of an uncle, by marriage, who lived down south in America. He was a big man. Not tall, just five foot six inches. But his weight was over 400 pounds. He really was rounder than he was tall and he was divided in the middle, in the only photo I ever saw of him, by a big black leather belt. It had to have been custom made. It had holsters on it for his pistols and his tan police uniform was stretched over his rolls of fat to the point of looking almost like a cartoon.

Standing beside him in this photo that lived in my aunt's house, was a tiny blonde woman. She weighed 99 pounds, or so said my aunt. Her blonde hair was teased, then combed up in a flip on the bottom. This was the early 70's and she looked like a smaller version of Samantha from Bewitched. She looked like a tiny child beside this big fat man, who was her husband.

The story was never told to me how they wound up together, but they did. Little and large. Make that little and XXXXXtra-large.

The story now takes a really sad turn. Again, I only have pictures and the stories of my aunt to go by, but these two people have made a lasting impression on me, even though I haven't seen their photograph for decades. They had a baby, though I never saw any photos of her in this album my aunt would get out for morbid entertainment. A little girl, a perfect little blonde darling to this young couple of opposites. My aunt would begin by telling myself and her two daughters, all sitting at her fat dimpled knees, that the young wife had a hard life. She cooked mountains of food of course, cleaned and had to put up with the drinking exploits and temper of the fat man.

My aunt would keep the photo album shut, her fat fingers marking the spot, as she took us back through time with her voice. Though she had never even met the fat man, she knew just what his voice sounded like. Deep, growling, a distinct Southern drawl that would make the hair on the back of my neck stand up when she impersonated him. My aunt was a big woman herself and would sometimes stand up, hulking over, arms dangling and yell at us in that scary story voice that she wanted dinner. Once in a while she would slam a fist on her glass topped coffee table for effect. It worked. My two cousins and I sat still, terrified and still wanting more, even though we knew what would happen.

We would hear about all the things this little light-weight lady had to do, but the worst, without a doubt, was wiping the butt of the four-hundred pound man who was her husband. He was too fat and his arms were too short to reach around the bulk of his expansive backside. Did she know about this before she married him I wondered?

My aunt would stand and mimic the monster of a man trying to wipe his own backside. This was the only comic relief in her tale she told us as the smells of the south would drift in the windows, magnolia, orange blossoms and jasmine, depending on what time of the year we were hearing the story of woe.

The dreaded day had finally came. My aunt would continue slowly, dropping her voice for effect. He came home from work, hungry as usual. The young little mother had a rough day. Maybe her baby had cried all day and she had to walk her. Maybe she had gotten lost in front of the television dreaming of a happier life, trying to escape in the tube. Who knows what made it happen, but all we knew was, dinner was not cooked.

The police report said that a semi-frozen chicken, a whole chicken, was sitting beside the stove where a pan of water was boiling away when they entered the home that had become a crime scene.

Their friend and co-worker, fatty in a cop suit, had called them crying like a baby. His lovely young bride had an accident. She was reaching up to get down a big three pound can of coffee. The little stool she was on slipped. The can struck her on the head. She ended up on the floor in a puddle of blood, while the chicken-less water boiled on.

The baby was in the room next door, sleeping through the entire commotion. The four-hundred pound father didn't want to bring up baby on his own. Besides, her face reminded him too much of his beloved wife, he told relatives. He shipped the baby south to my aunt and uncle. She was now sitting beside me, listening to her pretend-mother, my own aunt, relive this horrible series of events.

If you think this picture can't get any worse, look away now. My aunt, who really was a wonderful woman, just had rather odd choices for stories to tell, would then flip the dark green faux-alligator skinned photo book back open. All the previous pages remained a mystery. It was only the last page in the book we ever saw.

She would show us the Polaroid picture of a bruised and beaten face, dark eyelashes resting on a snow white cheek. A tiny bow in the hair made you wonder if this was a little doll in a horrible scene. It was the young wife.

It seems the coffee can had broken her nose, three of her ribs, broke both her wrists and left it oddly bruised marks like hand prints, that you could plainly see on various parts of her skin, as she was lying there, dead hands folded around the stem of a rose.

Her nose was smashed almost flat on her face, more bruise marks around her neck looked like the hand marks that were on her pale wrists. My aunt would go on to describe what we couldn't see below the white satin sheet that covered my pretend-cousin's mother.

What became of the fat man? He stayed in his Southern town, wearing his uniform and never remarried. I guess not, who would want to sign up for that? A life of wiping his butt and then getting hit on the head with a coffee can would certainly not appeal to most women.

Four-hundred pounds of fat, trapping me in this stall. At least I can still take care of myself in the toilet. I always did have longish arms. But now, how do I get out of here?

Standing up, one leg wedged on either side of the toilet forgetting about germs, I backed up as far as I could go. Pulling the door open and towards me, it seemed physically impossible for me to have ever gotten in here in the first place. There was only a four inch gap between my stomach and the door and my body which touched both sides of this prison that had to only be three foot across. Time and space dimensions didn't add up. This must be some sort of a black hole in the universe toilet.

Then the light went on over my head. My butt must have been able to squeeze by the door. My big belly wouldn't. I shut the door then took a good five minutes to turn around. If there would have been a hidden camera in this place the film would have won an award for the funniest or saddest thing you have ever seen. Depending on your sense of humor of course.

Finally finished with my maneuver and very red in the face, I stood huffing and puffing. Straddling the toilet, I was now going to attempt to go out backwards. It had to work.

The joy of breaking out was so great, I didn't even mind the two ladies who snickered at me as I stumbled backwards towards the sinks upon escape. I kept my mouth shut so they wouldn't know I was a fat American, but I'm sure they could tell. There is a certain look that an American travels with, fat or thin. Outside Morton was standing in the sunlight, smiling as I waddled towards him, still traumatized. *"I thought you fell in!"* he joked. *"There was a huge line."* I lied.
Morton took my hand and led me down the street to the candy shop.

You would think that something like that hideous ordeal I suffered would have been a wake up call for me, but it wasn't.

We walked into the sweet smelling shop and I squeezed down the aisles to select goodies that should last a week, but would be lucky if they made the forty minute car ride back to our house.

Two : A Body Built By Lies

When did your weight problem begin? This is something that perfect strangers seem fine about asking me. It doesn't bother me. Neither do my feathers get flustered when a perfect stranger will ask me how much I weigh now. Putting myself out there to the public, I not only expect this, it actually feels good to finally tell the truth when it comes to my weight. I try to think of creative excuses for reporters on just when my weight started dashing above the normal scale, even though I know the answer. I can't tell them. After all, I'm a professional liar, being schooled in it from an early age up, this woman knows how to not only lie, but also how to keep secrets.

My siblings are pretty much all normal size. My mom and her mom were heavy. I never really thought of them as obese, but they were. My older sisters worked at keeping their figures, but me, when I hit the seventh grade, I really let myself go.

Things were odd in my house. We have a few skeletons, as does every family, plus a few tragedies, as do most families and one or two really bad eggs that I seriously doubt if any family in the history of the world have ever had. With six children, my parents had their hands full. There were problems with one of my older siblings in school that made my parents want to put me and a younger brother into a private Christian school. They thought this would protect us from the evils of the drug filled world of the early 1970's.

We dressed in red, white and blue uniforms and left the rigors of a public education to go to a big classroom in the concrete block basement of a church. There were about thirty kids there, all different ages. It suited me just fine. I was sick of public school, gym and most of all, the dreaded twice-yearly, weigh in.

I was tall and growing faster than the other kids. My body could not have been called fat in the sixth grade, but when you get weighed on a scale, in front of all the other kids, with the nurse calling out your weight to the teacher, who was sitting at a desk six feet away, I felt like a baby hippo.

In the spring of 1974 was the second heaviest in the class in sixth grade. It didn't matter that I was the tallest girl. I was the heaviest. All the ammunition needed to make recess an extra fun time for me. Fair game for getting all the fat jokes, I smiled through it, thinking of punch lines before my fellow students could and beating them to it was a favorite pastime of mine.

But the veil of the private school held up a secret treasure for me that would become my pitfall. There was no physical education whatsoever in that basement school house. We would do work related to the Bible and I think we must have done math and science, but I really just remember the memorizing verses, working on different chapters of the good book and getting the feeling that I was in a snug and safe cocoon.

My blue vest got tighter as my lunch was always packed, usually by myself, of rather odd things. Bad things. Packs of cookies, chips, peanut butter & margarine sandwiches, candy bars. All bad things.

The two years I spent at this private school were the most traumatic, without a doubt, of my child-hood. My oldest brother died, I was molested by a family member and I gained 80 pounds. For someone in the seventh grade, this is a whole other book. These facts are something I have pushed to the furthest points in my mind to just try to function.

It should have been a time of talking, getting help, treatment and counseling, but none of these things happened. Instead I buried these events with food and bad behavior. Running away became my secret pastime, with over fifty flights before I was sixteen.

Secretly I think I must have wanted to die. My self-esteem was non-existent and I always felt like a bad person. Food, though I acted like it was comforting, was trying to kill me, even back then. My parents went through many sleepless nights not knowing if I was dead or alive. My mother got angry with me and my father gave me the belt a time or two, but I just kept running. The furthest I got was California, hitchhiking from Pennsylvania, at the age of sixteen. I spent a missing month on the road, and was lucky to be alive before bumping into my older sister just a few miles from my home, who convinced me to come home and live with her. With a family of her own, my sister offered to have me move in to here house. It was a time that I foolishly gave up high school completely and started going down a path of lies and abusing food almost daily.Living with my sister settled me down for a bit. Perhaps I blamed my mother, but then don't we all, for the sexual abuse that had happened to me. It is a mother's job to protect their children, but we always seems to fail.

For whatever reason, I hated my mom at that time in my life. I just wanted to be as far away from my family as possible and forget the emotional pain I had burning inside my body.

I just wanted normal, but there was none of it on offer for me. Turning in to all the things my mom accused me of being, I hated myself. Liar, slut, thief. This life wasn't what I wanted. At seventeen I felt like I had lived a hundred years and had looked into the eyes of death more than once. Normal was something that I didn't even have a clue of how it looked or felt.

Then comes love, like a thunderbolt of goodness out of the blue.

My first real love was a prisoner. He was decades older, a bank robber and shared a prison with a family member who was kind enough to hook me up with him. We wrote, I accepted collect calls on my sister's phone from him and one day I knew that we would be together. It didn't matter that he was still married, had kids older than I was or was still serving time...this was love. After all, I was seventeen and knew everything.

The fact that my relationship with this inmate kept me from running away nearly every weekend made it alright with my family. Normal almost.

My weight was about 170 pounds and I thought I was so fat. Little did I know there would be a time that I would long to weigh just 170 pounds. The man, who I loved madly, thought I was fat and told me so. He told me what foods I should be eating. He also told me what foods I should pack and bring up to the prison to have picnics with him in the romantic prison yard that trustees got to take their visits in.

Working a job, living with my sister, my wages would go on gas to go to the prison once a week, food to take to the prison, clothes to wear to the prison and of course, stamps to write my prisoner each and every day. Imagine my surprise when I showed up one week to find him in the arms of his wife, sitting at a picnic table with his kids, eating someone else's homemade cookies. It was tough to have my teenage heart crushed in front of all those people that had watched me swooning over this bad man masquerading as a bad boy. Now though, I thank my lucky stars that it happened that way.

As I drove away from the prison in tears, I made a vow to marry the first man who asked. Love had nothing to do with it, timing was everything. I would show him. I would marry someone else, have someone else's children and live happily ever after without a second thought of prisoner K-36… whatever his inmate number was. Fate is a beautiful thing in our lives. We can blame it, be thrilled with it and sometimes just sit back and look over our lives and wonder what on earth was happening. It has danced through my life in ways that I could never begin to explain or comprehend.

Meeting my future husband and father of my children over a lost car key was just one of the odd things that have happened. The next few years were fate-filled and flawed, but it did yield two incredible children that have made my life worth living.

Married at seventeen (it didn't take long to get proposed to) then giving birth to my daughter at eighteen, my son at nineteen and a divorce when I was twenty, was indeed a lot of living packed into a small period. My kids and I grew up together, though they now have passed me up on being mature. The whole time my weight would rise and fall. If I was with a man, it would climb. When I was single, I would not eat and it would fall. It never really dipped back down into the hundreds again, but held mostly around 220 for my "light" weight and about 280 for my "fat" weight.

After many failed relationships, marriages and romances, I thought I was finally happily married. All was going right in my life. Married, good business, nice house, kids nearly grown and then it happened. I got the phone call from my husband of the moment, telling me that we were NOT happily married. He, in fact, had found real love on the internet with a woman he had never met in person.

As my world went spinning out of control, my weight fell without effort. Maybe heartbreak is the secret to being thin. This time it was really tough. I always did the leaving in the past. Three years was the longest I could stay in a relationship, don't ask me why. It might have been them, but it was probably me. Even though I laughed, remember, I hated myself. Lying to my family, they were convinced that I was a fat and jolly person. Divorce number 76 (it felt like that many anyway) was the last one. I would swear off marriage, men, romance, hope of anything other than lonely nights and working on the computer. My nights were spent sleeping on a couch we called "big blue" though my daughter still swears it was green. I couldn't stand going into my bedroom. Lies that floated in the air of the house really hit me the hardest in the bedroom, alone at night It felt like the last three years of my life were wasted, and the worst thing was, I wasn't the ones telling the lies. I was the woman scorned, the last to know and my self-esteem was beyond repair.

But alas, I have these incredible, resilient, remarkable kids. My daughter encouraged me to get right back on the love pony. Surely there was someone waiting just for me. Why not look online? I didn't have to chat to anyone local, try Scotland. Didn't I love the country when I visited last summer? My friend fate was waiting that night as I logged on. My daughter steered me to a Scottish chat room, telling me that I needed to talk to someone. It had been months since my break-up and she wanted me to get on with my life. Five hours ahead in Scotland, Morton sat on the computer. He was the first person I spoke to in the Scottish chat room.

For the first few weeks, I didn't even know if Morton was a man or a woman. We talked about the castles, the city, the country, the weather, then about our spouses. We gave each other free therapy, no strings attached. We were great friends, nothing more and could lose ourselves for hours online. We both thought that was all that would ever happen. The winter and spring flew by with my new Scottish online pal. I smiled easy and looked better than I had done in years. Divorce was finally starting to agree with me. Come summer, a friend in London asked if I would come over and housesit for her. She was off for five weeks to Milan, Italy. Single, semi-attractive and with a new sense of adventure, this was just what I needed. Booking the airline ticket to London, my daughter drove me and my large suitcase to the airport under cloudy

Pennsylvania skies. As I waited in line and then for the plane to board, the announcements were made. All the flights were cancelled because of severe storms. No one was going anywhere. Bugger! My daughter came back to the airport and collected me, taking me back the next day for a repeat performance thanks to the weather. On the third day I was told I could fly, if I wanted to go to Glasgow. This would work. I could take a train to London, or better yet, ride back with my friend who happened to be in Scotland that weekend for a wedding. I placed my first phone call to Morton to tell him the news. He knew that I was coming over and we had planned to have him come down to London for a weekend. We wanted to see some sights together and have lunch or dinner. Romance wasn't in the air or on offer, but adventure and friendship was.

It was tough understanding him. He has a really strong Scottish accent and he sounded mean and gruff on the phone. The only photo I had seen of him was one of him dressed as Jake Blues, at least I think he was Jake. He was the short half of the Blues Brothers for a fancy dress party and his tall friend was the other half. Morton was smiling behind those dark shades looking a lot like the famous Belushi. We talked quick, I only had three minutes. He offered to come and pick me up at the airport and take me to the train station. That was all she wrote. Meeting him I finally understood how life should be. Normal was finally within reach. He met me with flowers, a rare smile and within a few hours I had met everyone in his family and several of his closest friends. We both felt as though we had known each other forever and have gotten on like a house on fire ever since. I did make it to London, but just for one week. My friend had her brother move in, just a few weeks before she was set to go away, so it wasn't vital that I was there. I had lost my heart in Edinburgh and ended up staying in Scotland for the next six years.

Three : Roll Over and Wake Up

Morton is a great cook no matter how many times I tell you about the hideous things he throws together and calls food. True, he has made some of the worst food I have ever tasted, but most of the time he is spot on. He also makes way too much and growing up as a member of the "clean plate club" I would always finish all of it.

We both started working crazy schedules. Morton left his job of twenty years to help with a hobby job I had created with an arts and crafts gallery. It was growing like a monster, with me running it like a friendship rather than a business. We sunk all we had into it, even money we didn't have and it was dying slowly. Worse than that, it was taking me down with it.

My health was failing. I had a number of problems, all could be linked back to just being too damned fat. My knees were swollen all the time. My feet and ankles were as hard as rocks at the end of my twelve or fourteen hour days. In three years, we had two weeks off and that was to fly back to the States for a funeral. Art, or the pursuit of art, was putting me into an early grave.

We knew we had to do something so we bailed. We left too ashamed to really say goodbye to people. What do you really have to say though when a business fails? It was just one of those things that get out of control, slowly, then seem like there is no way out, other than running away. It is something I always have been good at and this time there really didn't seem to be any other way out.

I had talked Morton into the glamour job of working in a laundry. We would be washing sheets and gear from campgrounds around Europe. The great thing about this is that we would be living in France, having four days off in a row...together and getting paid in British pounds sterling. The company provides a house in the French countryside. I was planning on going on a diet as soon as we got there, but look out...here comes fate.

All the years I had been living in Scotland I had longed to make the short trip across the water and go see the tulip bulb fields blooming in Holland. We were always too busy to do this. With spring in the air, we decided it was now or never. Spring had a real feeling of change in the air. It motivated us on. We put the car with our gear for going to France on a ferry, sail away to Europe and then have a tour on a budget before washing all those never-ending sheets.

This was some of the best and worst weeks of my life. My weight stopped me from doing so many things I would need a whole other book just to tell you about that. From stairs leading up castle towers in Germany that I couldn't fit through to not riding in a gondola for fear of tipping it or sinking it in Venice, this European adventure was seriously lacking because I was just too fat.

My mind kept thinking, "the diet starts when you get to France" which might be the worst place in the world to think about dieting in. Diets and exercise are both words that had been stricken from my vocabulary for most of my life. I told myself I would learn the French words for these, then do them every day.

We were in France for just two days when my daughter called me. My mother in Pennsylvania had a stroke. She couldn't talk, walk, sit up or even grasp a hand. It looked very bad and I better get a flight to America as soon as I could. Morton and I had a hard time just leaving so fast. My daughter was married and living in Scotland. My son was in America and engaged to a girl from Scotland. He was with my dad, who was lost without my mother at home. We knew we just had to get there and we did both feel very helpless. What could we really do? My mom was still in the hospital when we arrived. It was a week after her stroke. My son picked us up at the airport and it felt great to hug him. We went right to the hospital on my forty-third birthday. Mom tried to smile when she saw me. She cried and called me Sarah, my daughter's name. We held hands and I stroked her hair back. It looked wild and felt like straw, needing washed and brushed. This was one of the rare times I saw my dad worried. They had been married for nearly 56 years and seeing her like this was really tough on him.

The stroke happened in the blink of an eye, like they do. Mom was sitting with a cigarette and her crocheting at her big kitchen table. She told me later how she felt like she just couldn't get this one stitch right. She was trying to answer my dad who had asked her a question and the words just wouldn't come. Everything changed for her forever at that moment. They moved my mom into a rehab center. My dad and I made it our home for the next several weeks. My weight, about 420 pounds, was just too heavy for me to function on a normal level. The rehab center was not just what my mom needed, it was what I needed too.

Mom couldn't really move around on her own. The nurses would come in and use the sheet to move her around on the bed. As I stood watching, trying to learn how to take care of her, I finally understood about health and weight. Health is the most important thing in our lives, hands down. We all know this but most of us ignore this. Seeing this procedure, strangers washing and wiping my mother, I finally realized that if I didn't take care of myself, someone else would have to. This thought terrified me.

My bad body image had me afraid of anyone seeing me without clothes on, let alone several people at a time. What if my daughter and son had to learn how to wash me because I got too fat? What if Morton had to wipe my butt because I got to fat to reach it? How can I get off this crazy ride of obesity and self-destruction? The words "I would do anything to have her body" have come out of my mouth at least a thousand times in my lifetime. It was always a lie. I wouldn't do anything and I didn't do anything, That is how I got to weigh over 400 pounds. Now I knew I had to do something, I just didn't know what.

Fear grabbed me as I started worrying about my own health failing while I was taking care of my mom. What if I'm too out of shape to do everything they are showing me to do to take care of her? Calling my daughter in Scotland, I broke down on the phone. Between gasps and streams of tears I told her all my fears. I don't want to die fat. I don't want to be a burden on you or your brother. I want to be healthy. How do I do it?

We talked about all sorts of things. Surgery, diets, crazy plans like getting my jaw wired shut to just shutting myself in a room for a few years with limited amounts of food, while the unwanted pounds would release me from my fat prison. These were all things that wouldn't work for me. I had to really work this one out this time and do it right. Failure wasn't an option with my life at stake. I wanted to live for the first time since I was twelve years old.

Four : Taking That First Step

Every journey, no matter how long, has to start somewhere. Mine began on the day I put on my cheap sneakers with a hole on the side and went for a walk out my parents driveway on the mile loop.

A combination of paved road, dirt road and loose stones was what I had to contend with. Even though a mile is not that far, for me it was like running the Boston Marathon. When you are so out of shape, even the three wooden steps to get off their porch was an effort.

With a beet red face, I huffed and puffed around this mile. After a solid week of working at this mile every day, I felt like losing weight was finally going to happen. I discovered the magic pill called exercise.

Over the next few weeks I made it a point to walk each and every day. It cleaned out my mind and made me feel more alive than I had since childhood. This was the secret ingredient that I had been looking for my whole life. Why hadn't anyone told me about this earlier?

My mother would spend three days a week at a Gettysburg rehab center learning how to speak, move and do simple tasks. I was her transportation to and from these sessions and I would walk back and forth in the parking lot or down the street while she was with her therapists doing her inside work.

On one hot summer day when my pace had really picked up and I was breathing better than I had in ages, this idea hit me like a bolt of summer lightening. If I didn't know about this exercise business, maybe the other millions of people around the world that struggle with their weight didn't know either. I needed to tell the world about this simple little trick that really works!

Exercise is the secret ingredient, the magic pill and the things that the infomercials WISH they could bottle and sell. The fire inside me was lit and I felt like I could walk to the moon if there was only a road there. Think of it, this four-hundred pound fatty actually getting up and walking somewhere BIG. Where could it be? The Appalachian Trail came to mind, but I knew I couldn't lose the almost 300 pounds I had to shed by the time the trail would end. Then the idea hit me, walk AROUND America. Not across it, not up and down it, but around it. The coastlines and borders would do the trick. Doing a bit of research on the Internet I learned that the trip would be about 16,000 miles. This would work. It would take two years and at the end I would be fit. Hopefully people all around the world would hear about the trip and start taking their own health into their own hands. I wanted to inspire anyone who didn't know about this thing called "movement" and change the way we take care of ourselves. Now I just had the task of breaking this new ambition in life to my husband.

Morton is the worst pessimist that I have ever met. He always looks for the downside to everything. It is my balance though because I'm the ultimate optimist. Anything is possible. Something that I always told my children, but never really believed inside. After all, it isn't possible for ME to lose weight…right?

Winning Morton over to support me on this journey was going to be tough. How could I do it? I hadn't even thought about the logistics of living on the road and being away from home for two years. He was going to fire this dream right out of the water.

My daughter and son-in-law had moved over from Scotland shortly after my mothers' stroke. Since my daughter had been so helpful with me really sinking my teeth into getting serious about weight loss, I decided to share my idea with her husband first. He has a real common sense that is so refreshing, I figured I would test it on him and if he thought it was a good idea, then I would clue Morton in.

At first I had this idea of me just walking alone. But as I sat in a car with my son-in-law, explaining that I wanted to really share this common secret and inspire others, I included not just him and my daughter on the journey, I bumped it up to my parents and my son and his future wife. It would be easier if there were more people around for help and support, right? Safety in numbers and all that other good stuff. One of my biggest surprises came at my wise son-in-law's reply. He thought about what I had just said in my twenty minute excited babble. He had to have felt the passion and importance this journey held for me. He offered me some great advice and after a talk with his wife, they agreed to go along on this adventure of a lifetime. Before I knew it, everyone was on board. Even Morton. My dad, who was 82 at the time was the most skeptical at first, but after talking as a group he looked at me and said, "You know, if you plan this right, it just might work!"

The idea of living on the road with family for two years was something that was a bit scary. My daughter-in-law to be was a nurse in Scotland, so she could help with my mom. My dad was a natural born camper, so he and my son could take care of the base camp and my daughter and I would do all the walking. Morton and my son-in-law would ride bicycles and act as support on our daily treks around the coastline. It would work like a charm. Three generations getting healthy. Surely we could find some corporate support to make it happen, if not, we could all pull together to pull it off.

My daughter has always had back pain and discovered these amazing shoes in the UK called MBT's. She said we could contact them, since we will be going through a lot of shoes and sure enough, they became our very first sponsor. Their help with shoes would prove invaluable to us and I'll most likely never wear another brand after falling in love with how they make my whole body feel.

When the company sent me my first pair, I'll never forget the thrill of putting on "real" shoes and walking. It really did feel like I was lighter than air and it even took away my knee and ankle pain I would normally feel on the daily walk. These miracle shoes gave me the feeling I hadn't had since childhood, a spring in my step and the feeling that I could actually walk around the whole world.

The next few months sailed by as we mapped out the journey, contacted people to help sponsor this trip and got involved with lots of local organized charity walks.

Our first walk that was with the *American Heart Association* was in Gettysburg in September 2006. My daughter and I were signed up for it eager to get out there.

We even hoped to do some press at it. The local press would play a big role in getting me prepared for what was in store for me in the upcoming months of microphones, photographers and riding in a circle just one more time for the cameras.

Fate reared it's sometimes ugly head though. As we were all on top of the world, my father passed away on a hot September Sunday morning. It was the hardest loss I have ever suffered and trust me when I say, I have lost more than my share of people close to me. Our parents should live forever and I never even thought of my dad as old, let alone ready to leave this world. But we all do, the really only thing we are ever certain of. No one really does get out of here alive. Sometimes I think if we all realized how short our lives are, even when you get 82 years, we would all follow our dreams a lot faster and a lot more honestly. The day after the funeral was the first scheduled walk. How could I go? How could I walk anywhere now? Everything and every dream that I had felt like it had died with my father. My heart hurt so very bad it wouldn't be able to take the exercise and the pain of loss.

Families can be truly golden at times and thank goodness, parts of mine are. My sister, niece and daughter all said they would walk with me. Of course Morton would as well, his faith and devotion to me is really the stuff that fairytales are made out of. It was a really hot day when we did that walk, three miles I think, in historic Gettysburg. Just a few weeks before we had arrived to my mom's therapy an hour too early and I had driven my parents around the battlefields, the same route we were now walking. All my thoughts were on my dad this autumn day.

The night before he passed away, my laptop was sitting on the kitchen table with me in front of it, route planning. I was up in Montana and there was this lovely picture that came up of a cabin at a campground that was overlooking a lake. I'm not sure why, but something made me point this out to my dad. It must have been the fishing report that was shown on the web site. Dad sat down beside me and we spent an hour on the computer. Dad didn't like computers. He never used them and would only really read over my mom's shoulder when she would be showing him an email from a far away family member. Tonight however, dad was glued to it. After looking for a few minutes, he looked across the table at my mom and said, *"Did you know all this stuff was on here?"* We all had a laugh and I feel like for that little moment, Dad was on the trip with us.

Five : Eight Become Two

With losing dad, we had an impromptu front porch group meeting about the journey. We decided that mom would stay home, with my son and daughter-in-law and there would just be the four of us going.

The next few months Sarah and I walked in organized walks in New York City, Baltimore and all points in between. We did interviews, learned that you are usually always misquoted and got use to telling strangers what our weight was. We did a walk in Washington D.C. that was really special. We met a lot of helpful people there, strangers who all were so supportive of our journey and had a fantastic weekend. It was also my first day of being followed around by a television camera all day. Little did I realize, events were happening that would be tangled in fate. Once again the face of the journey changed and our family in our nations capitol where little seems to ever change. It was just a little over a month away for our kick off in Key West to happen. We had decided it would be easier if we were just all on foot, so our expenses would become next to nothing. Just our daily food and water, a few clothes here and there and that would be that. Thanks to MBT we had our foot wear sorted. Sarah called me just before an interview I was getting ready to do and told me she had some good news and bad news for me. Any parent can relate to this sort of phone call. Your gut knots up and you are hoping that the giddy sound in her voice is joy, not tears that are ready to pop out at any moment. The bad news was, they were not coming with us. The good news was, I was going to be a grandmother. I was over the moon about the baby and when I did the interview, I actually said something to the reporter about it. This was my first lesson in "private things" that I would learn over the next year or so. The story ran in a paper and on television and the next day I get a call from my daughter. She had gotten so many calls from friends and business associates wishing her well. She started our conversation with a question, "Did you tell a reporter I was pregnant?" Of course I had, not thinking that they might want to announce this in their own time and own way. Since my daughter is an angel on earth, she wasn't mad at me. It was a lesson well taught and has helped me with future interviews and remembering to respect the privacy of others. Sort of.

Six : Heading South

Since we were living in Pennsylvania, Morton and I had the dilemma of getting 1000 miles south for our New Year's Day start. Our gear was massive. Two backpacks, a tent, sleeping bags, a laptop, a wheelchair to carry my backpack since I was still too fat to do it myself and our website that I had been doing since

June 2006, www.LittleChanges.com came in to play. It seems that a lady who was following along with our journey had a husband who was driving south. He was going to be able to pick us up in Baltimore and carry us all the way to my sister's house, near Daytona Beach, Florida. Morton had real and serious fears about jumping in a car with a stranger and most of all, he wondered what we would do when we stopped for the bathroom. The guy might drive off with all our possessions!

Morton didn't really know my history that could be summed up in a movie titled, *"I Was A Teenage Runaway"* and that strangers have never really scared me. Even though later in our journey, they would, at the moment, I was blissfully unaware that anything bad could happen when you are carrying around such good intentions in your heart.

The man pulled up in a Mercedes SUV that made Morton feel a bit better. When he introduced himself, we learned that he was a heart surgeon and one of the nicest people we ever met. He was fascinated with what we were about to do and was thrilled that I was taking control of my own health and being responsible for losing weight. We chatted for a while before he asked if I wouldn't mind driving, he could get some work done on his laptop.

The day melted away as I drove and he worked, talking to patients, discussing issues with other doctors and Morton had no fear at all when our first gas stop happened and this trusting man jumped out, leaving his laptop, car and wallet sitting on the dashboard, with the keys dangling in the ignition with me behind the wheel. I pointed them out to Morton without a word. Just raising my eyebrow let my husband know what I was thinking. The world isn't a horrible place.

It was late at night as we met my sister at the exit near her house. She helped us get our gear inside and then we discovered that Morton had left his jacket in the backseat of the SUV. We called our new found friend who had gone another 150 miles south and he said he would post it to us. People are good and helpful, never forget this. Morton's jacket arrived and I made a mental note to always check for things when we are breaking down our camp in the future. Morton is forgetful and I don't want this to be a regular habit over the next two years.

Seven : The First Day of My Life

Since we had been doing all our recent training walks in the cold Pennsylvania winter, it felt like paradise to be in t-shirts and shorts in the Florida warmth. "This was going to make it so much easier" I thought, the first of many mistakes and misjudgments I would make over the next few months.

The trip to Key West was with my sister who was going down for New Years. Sitting in the back seat I was sorry that it had gotten dark when we got to the Florida Keys. I wanted to look at the side of the roads, especially when we were going over bridges, to help get mentally ready to cross them on foot.

Unpacking all the gear from the trunk, the feeling that we were really going to do this was still not 100% certain in my head. I thought about everything other than the journey on the car ride to the Keys. Perhaps I was still lying to myself.

If we thought it was warm in Daytona, Key West was like an oven. We spent two days getting all our last minute things (like sunscreen) and then came the fateful morning. New Years Day, 2007 and I was ready to make the biggest resolution of my life.

It was early, still reasonably cool, when my sister drove us for one last time to the big concrete marker that sits at the southern most point in America. There were a few people there to see us off, but not the turnout that I had thought of. I pictured crowds of people wanting to walk with us and start the new year off right. Maybe they would catch up with us along the way. Many people here in paradise were still sleeping off the fun of seeing the old year out the night before. My sister hugged me goodbye and drove away. She had to go pack and face the long ride back up 95 north. Now it was starting to feel real. I was gripped with fear but couldn't tell Morton. This would be the start of several months of facing my fears because I had no other option. Bravery had nothing to do with it.

The phone rang and I did a telephone interview with Channel 8, WGAL in Lancaster, Pennsylvania, the NBC affiliate via telephone. The reporter, Carrie Fairchild had covered a story on us earlier and wanted an update. There were a few other calls and interviews and then we were off. It was enough to chase off my fear of being alone in the world and on the road. The journey officially began at 8:20 am on January 1, 2007. What a way to start a year! I highly recommend doing something that feels like it should be a dream, but just remember that it IS real and be prepared.

I wasn't. I don't know what I had been thinking as we started off with three gallons of water and food for three days. With just a bit over $100. in our pockets, we not only looked homeless, we really were. The sun got hot fast. The nice thing though, being between that crystal blue Atlantic Ocean and the Gulf of Mexico on the other side of the road, we had a salty breeze on us the entire day. A warm salty breeze.

After an hour or so, I had drank so much water that I was in dire need of a bathroom. It occurred to me, for the first time, that the next two years of my life was going to be spent using public toilets or the woods. Since there wasn't a palm tree fat enough to hide me, I was thrilled to see a restroom coming up ahead on the beach. As I was inside, Morton waited with our gear. Again, it hadn't crossed our minds that we wouldn't be able to go inside anywhere together anymore. We had to stand guard over our clothes, camping gear, laptop and camera. When I came back, Morton was chatting away with someone. As I approached them, the man got up and said, "Priscilla, it is great to meet you, I thought I missed you!" and gave me a hug. He had been following along on our website, and better still, was inspired to get out there and start walking. He had missed us at 8 am and had been driving up and down the route we were taking, waiting to say hello. This man, Rock, was just the person I needed to meet today. After the pressure of trying to find a bathroom I was close to calling my sister and asking her to come around and get us. I was thinking about calling off the whole journey before it had really even began. The fear of the whole idea of the trip was really getting to me even though we hadn't even made it through our first morning.

But here in the flesh was a person who told me this incredibly personal story about why he had gotten inspiration from what we were doing. He was a stranger to me and this was why I wanted to walk. It works and I wanted to pass this feeling on!

We headed off after just a few minutes of chatting, then Morton made a discovery that there are coconuts all over the place. He drilled into one with his handy pocket knife his brother in Scotland had gotten him. It took a few attempts, but he finally made it through. He smiled and drank the juice, delighted and commenting that you would never be able to do this in Scotland, even though palm trees do grow on the west coast, there are "nae coconuts" to be had.

Before long we had crossed a bridge that took us off our first key. It was a dream come true. I was lost in taking photographs, shooting video and just breathing. That was until reality set in and our water ran out. Morton had gone in to a store and found that water was over $2.00 for a bottle so small we drank it in two gulps. We were in serious trouble. Even though the place looked like paradise and we were surrounded with water, we were wilting under the hot sun. My heart was pounding in my face and all I could hear were the words of the doctor who had given us the ride, "Listen to your body, rest when you are tired." So we did. Right beside the road, right before another bridge to another sun-soaked island of a Key, I eased myself down to the ground in a soaking heap. I'm not going to lie to you and say I did this gracefully, I let gravity take over and just plopped. Spreading out the plastic tarp to protect me from fire ants and other insects, I was nearly asleep before my head hit the ground. I could hear myself snoring, my face shielded in the shade of the wheelchair. I must be insane. Morton sat up, dozing beside me. It was a scene that must have made every motorist passing us either pity us or hate us.

When I woke up after an hour or so, I was so thirsty. Consulting the little tourist map we had I tried to figure out where we were and when the next patch of businesses would be around us. I was ready to spend all the money we had on water. We crossed another bridge, cars whizzing by as we were walking against traffic. The free tourist map showed a restaurant coming up. We could get water there, perhaps from their kitchen and for free. It was just a half a mile up the road.

Since this was January and the first day of the year, we didn't think that things would be closed, but this place was. It really looked like it was closed for good or perhaps just the season. There were no outside water faucets, so our plastic bottles that we were saving had to just stay empty.

I tried to remember the rules on drinking salt water. How much could a person drink without getting sick? There were just no houses or businesses around and we couldn't understand that. The cars that passed us had no clue as to how thirsty we were.

Then one car heading north, on the other side of the road, started honking it's horn. That had happened a lot. Some people would wave, some would scream mean things and some would even call me "fatty" not very creative, but there you go.

This car however, was familiar. It crossed the road when southbound traffic was clear and pulled in beside us. It was my sister. She had one more look in a few shops in Key West and was just now, many hours later, heading home. She had also bought us a case of water.

If I could bottle up this feeling that we had just then, it would make me a millionaire a billion times over. Easily. These lifesaving bottles were treasured, drank and as she drove off my husband and I both agreed that she had been another miracle that happened. We felt as if we were the luckiest and richest people on the planet. To have water and extra water, we were able to squeeze several more miles of walking out.

The First Night of My Life

Since we didn't have anything planned, we were literally just making it up as we went along. I knew that each day I hoped we could get a shower. Each day we would hopefully have food to eat and water to drink and hopefully, people that were visiting our website would buy LittleChanges t-shirts and support our journey, with us getting two dollars for each shirt that was sold. All of these things though were really left to chance.

Come the end of our first day, after being more tired than I had been after two days of labor and child-birth, we needed a place to pitch our tent. When I knocked on a strangers door and asked if we could pitch the tent, we were told they were just renting it for the week and weren't allowed to have a tent. They wished us well but seemed a bit nervous. We did look as rough as a pair of grizzly bears, sweaty and wearing clothing I suppose. This happened another several times before we decided that we just needed to keep walking and hopefully come across a campground. Miles go slow when you are walking and pushing your worldly possessions around in a wheelchair. It was dusk and then dark came faster then I have ever seen it. We were breaking our own first rule. *Rule number 1: Never be out after dark.*

This was the time that we could get hit by a car, mugged, murdered or anything else. Bad things happen at night, or so we are all taught to believe.

There was a little grouping of houses coming up. There was a light on an American flag and I almost jumped out of my MBT's with joy when I saw it was a fire station. Hooray…they would surely let us pitch the tent on their lush green grass. We knocked for ages and after trying several doors, a lady finally came to one on the side where we had began our knocking campaign. I explained what we were doing, what we needed (a seven by seven foot bit of ground) and asked if we could pitch the tent.

Now in my mind, though I didn't tell Morton, I pictured the fire fighters inviting us in, giving us dinner and letting us take a shower. I was glad I hadn't voiced this. She told me she couldn't let us camp on their grass. If she did, she explained, the next night they would have 500 tents set up. After all, there was a really bad homeless problem in the Florida Keys. Since this was my very first night, I was timid, scared and starting to panic a bit. Was I going to have to just walk 24 hours a day for the next 16,000 miles? "What should we do?" I squeaked. She told us to just set up the tent by the water. I pointed out that there were signs all over the place telling you that you would be in serious trouble for doing this and you would get a $500. fine for camping. This was more that we wanted to spend in a whole month, let alone one evening illegally in a tent. She gave us these sage words of wisdom, "Just be careful and try to not let anyone see you." Fair enough. What else could we do?

We walked, looking in the dark for a stealth campsite. All I could imagine were mounds of fire ants and pits of snakes waiting for us in the dark. And the spiders. Did I mention how big they are there? HUGE…and taking a look at me, they could feast for a few decades on my massive 300 plus pound body. A bridge ahead didn't hold the same hope for me that it held in the daylight when it felt like anything could be just on the other side. I could see there was nothing over it. Nothing with lights anyway. It was going to be hard to cross at night too. We are big and we do stand out, but we don't have the night time gear. Me swinging Morton's wind up flashlight really doesn't cut it when it comes to nighttime safety. There was a billboard off to our left and a boat launch of sorts. It was very dark. The billboard was not lit and we had to shine our flashlights around to make sure we weren't about to pitch the tent on a fire ant hill, a snake, a gator or any other sort of thing that might hurt the tent or us. Burning up in a state of sweat and humidity that you can really only experience in the tropics, we settled inside the tent. It went up smoothly, Morton being quite the pro. This was a two person operation and I stayed inside as Morton handed our gear in. Having already donated a fair amount of blood to the mosquitoes, I would only open the mesh on the tent wide enough to take hold of whatever Morton was unloading. After what seemed like my toughest move ever, our gear was finally in the tent. We laid back, sweating, steaming up the tent from lack of ventilation and Morton killed a mosquito. "Do you hate me?" I asked. He chuckled. Actually not a chuckle, it might have been a sarcastic laugh come to think of it. Reaching out, he took my sweaty hand and I pulled mine away and said, "Don't touch me, I'm too hot!" At that, we both laughed and then fell almost instantly asleep.

Two a.m. I sat straight up, wide awake. A car pulled in right beside the tent. It had music going and was probably loaded with killers. My heart was pounding in my throat as I pushed Morton awake. Whispering to him I told him what I heard. He asked if I wanted him to look outside. Was he CRAZY? You never look outside! His answer to it all was to start snoring again. "Now they'll know we're in here" I thought. Nudging Morton again I asked him where our hatchet was that he used to drive the tent pegs in to the sand below us. He told me that it was laying outside the tent and my heart sank. Our first night out and we are going to get chopped to bits by our very own hatchet. About 4 am I was satisfied that there were no footsteps approaching to do away with us. My heart had settled back down and the music had long ago ceased. I found a sweaty sleep again for what seemed like a few seconds before the sun was beating in on the tent and heating it up fast for our wake up call.

Morning came and our campsite looked like it was suppose to be there. The billboard provided a clothes line for us to dry our fly sheet for our tent on. Morton and I both reckoned we had lost weight overnight with sleeping in the sauna that was the tent. Everything looked less scary in the light of day. Even the car of the night time killer in the morning light showed us that the killer was just a fellow traveler, only with wheels, that had gotten too tired to go another mile. The man was sitting behind the wheel with his head leaned back and snoring so loud he should have woken himself up. I had to resist the urge to go over and nudge him awake telling him he had scared the life out of me. No time for that though, there is a long road ahead with our names on it.

Priscilla's Journal

Day 2 : January 2, 2007 - Big Coppit Key to *Sugar Loaf Lodge,* Sugar Loaf Key FL

The first day walking taught us both more than we had learned in our combined lifetimes. We are not going to be able to do twenty miles in a day right now. Ten, yes. twenty, no way. There are things that we didn't think about, that are so simple, like getting the wheelchair up and down curbs, taking a LOT more rests than normal due to the heat, speaking with people along the way, searching for places to camp. All time consuming factors that will eat into my estimation of being able to walk twenty miles each and every day. We did factor in the set up and tear down of our tent each day. The walking, the computer, the other things that we knew the time of. Keep in mind though, this journey, though we do know the route we are taking (basically) is all unknown. We don't have a camera crew with us on a regular basis. We are doing all the work and walking ourselves. It also might be a few days between updates on our website, depending on internet connections, power and other important things that make the world go 'round. All things that we must have thought of in the planning stages, somehow we just never really thought about them.

Walking without a shower is horrible. Coming out of the tent and not being able to jump in the water was a hard thing to do. It turns out it wasn't a beach area. What looked like a dock that we had camped beside was really a concrete bank that an old boat was wrecked against. Not quite paradise.

So we walked, glad that we were outside, with just a little face wash bath with some water we had put into empty plastic bottles we filled in a bathroom.The next couple bridges yielded nothing. No houses or business. Just wilderness. As beautiful as the scenery is the heat is almost unbearable for both of us. Morton is suffering from a skin condition he was born with and I suffering from being buried under a mountain of fat that I grew myself. On day one when I laid down in the shade for the hottest part of the day, I instantly went to sleep. Today, when I did the same, I only rested. My body must be getting use to it after just twenty four hours of torture.

Speaking to all positive people today we met a really nice mosquito inspector who is walking this year and getting back into the shape of his former self, we met a lovely lady, Stephanie, who owns a great store - Halfway Home Convenience Store located at mile marker 14 1/2, where she was kind enough to give us water and Gatorade AND a map!

Walking on further we saw these HUGE and I mean HUGE lizards in the trees. They had striped tails and were at least two feet long. They jumped on things below them, but hopefully not us. We figure they only eat insects and smaller lizards. Reptiles and me have never really mixed. Thinking back to a time in Port St. John's Florida and I was about 10, home sick from school and a little lizard jumped off the curtain and down my pj top, I shiver a little. If one of these jumped down your shirt, you would know it. Though that lizard from long ago caused me to jump out of bed and feel a lot better, I really don't want to mix it up with anything scaly on this journey.

We kept a close eye on the time and when it was approaching 4 pm we were just closing in on Sugar Loaf Lodge. It looked like it might be a good place to pitch up for the night. Who knows, we might even be able to take a shower if they have an outdoor pool and shower area. Our budget has no money in for a room at night, so we were hoping only for a tent spot.

The lovely owner of the *Sugar Loaf Lodge* not only let us have showers, she let us have a room for the evening. Her business is fantastic, our room is spotless and it looks right out over the Gulf of Mexico. As I'm writing this, our sliding door is open and we are only 15 feet away from the water. Talk about a difference between our first and second night. No comparison at all.

Morton was kind enough to let me have my shower first. I had no hot water on at all, simply had the cold tap running and was loving it. The heat from the day had really worn me out and we had to do a lot more resting than our first day. I think mentally with the no shower and sleeping sort of disturbed, in the tent, day two was harder than day one. The shower was without a doubt, the best shower I have had in 43 years of living. The pressure was just perfect. Hard enough to be effective yet gentle enough to not take your skin off. Even though there was a beach and the Gulf of Mexico was just a stone's throw away, I had no real energy or desire to leave the lovely room.

Morton showered, I updated the website and my stomach started to growl for the first time since we started walking. I also felt hungry for the first time too. We went to the restaurant at the Sugar Loaf Lodge and were treated to authentic Florida delights. Conch (pronounced CONK) chowder, coconut shrimp with pineapple (the shrimp were huge and so very fresh) and we each had a fish sandwich. The buns were so soft and tasty, fresh lettuce and tomato garnished the lovely grilled fish and the whole thing stuffed us so much we couldn't even split a piece of Key Lime pie at the end, though I wanted to!

Now I hear what you're thinking. "Lady, you have almost 300 pounds to lose, why in the world do you want to eat Key Lime pie?" It's all about moderation and the secret of burning more calories than you eat. That, we are doing! I also said I wanted to split a piece of pie, not eat the whole thing. The big key to losing and maintaining weight is MODERATION and MOVEMENT. These are the lifestyle changes you hear people speaking about. Feeling refreshed and full, Morton and I walked back in the air that felt sweeter now, not so hot and humid to a real bed. In the cool of the evening I went to sleep much happier, much more optimistic and wanted to ask Morton how he was feeling, but his snoring told me all I needed to know.

Day 3 : January 3, 2007 - *Sugar Loaf Lodge,*Sugar Loaf Key to Summerland Key FL

Leaving the lovely Sugar Loaf Lodge we got a late start. Our goal of 6 am was missed by several hours when I made the mistake of checking my email. It was full of well wishes from the web site visitors and questions from reporters and before we knew it, we were leaving at 9:30 am. This was our first mistake of the day. Don't worry, we had a goal of making at least ten mistakes every day and they are easily met.

The sun gets so hot here, so fast, that you really have to just get your walk on before it has a chance to broil you. You feel like some sort of seafood that has landed in a pan here. The sand dances and glistens with heat bouncing up from it. We said goodbye to the owner of *Sugar Loaf Lodge*, Miriam (originally from Philadelphia) and thanked her for her kindness. We promised to keep in touch and see her again in three and a half years (more or less at this rate) and look a lot different when we do.

As we headed north on US 1 with a good nights sleep behind us, I felt like we could maybe hit our 10 miles that we hoped for. We had food for energy, breakfast bar, loads of water and clean clothes on. All the makings of a great day. Walking was harder this day. We thought it might get easier each and every day, but with our late start, it really made us feel it. The weather wasn't helping either. With no thermometer, we could only use our bodies to feel the heat climbing as we walked north. Though our clothes started out dry and clean, within minutes my t-shirt was soaking wet and clinging to me. Not a pretty sight. Looking out for shady spots that have a bench, rock, street light with concrete base or anything to sit on for 10 minutes in the shade became my priority. Crossing bridge after bridge we were overcome by the heat, the surroundings and the sun and just had to find a place to spread our tarp and sit a bit. Today we didn't take any naps. Just talked about how crazy we must be for doing this. It is a lot of walking for people who are so unfit (me especially) and I wonder if we will survive the heat. Morton seems happy enough to be along, but I can't help but feel that I'm really ruining his life. Since our first night of waiting so late to tent, we have made a new walking rule. Always be camping by 4 pm. No if's and's or but's...it must happen. We walk and discuss that we should start looking for a good spot beside the bridge that is going to be coming at the end of Summerland Key. Then we hear a shout from across the road.

There is a man standing on his deck that looks out on the Atlantic ocean. He waves and is saying something about would we like a drink of water. This man is clearly on the right track! Morton crosses the street taking along a bottle that we have emptied earlier. We know now that we can not afford to buy water, we have to refill our containers anywhere we can. Once Morton crosses the road he is out of my earshot, but I watch what is happening. There he chats away to this kind man who gives him a bottle of ice water. Before I know it, Morton is waving me over across the busy road. Captain Steven was inviting us to pitch our tent in his lovely back garden, sitting right beside a canal. We were so happy with just the use of the space and busily getting stuck in to getting it erected, we both had giant grins on our sweaty faces. Before you can say "human kindness" our home-like feeling was there as quick as we could manage and we were thinking about going to sleep, even though it was still daylight out.

Captain Steven and his wife Jennifer came outside to invite us to use their shower. They were so very kind and generous, Morton and I were ready to cry. Actually, I was ready to cry, Morton was just really grateful. When I got out of the shower, they asked if we'd like to have dinner with them. Could it get any better than this? Yes, and I'll tell you about it. It seems it was Captain Steven's birthday. He and his wife have a charter boat business with three boats and we spent a true enchanted evening on their deck, eating a delicious home-made meal with conversation that was second to none. Feeling very nostalgic and missing my father who passed away in September, Captain Steven told us stories about the sea and how they met.

It felt like we were all old friends that had gotten together for the evening, not strangers that had just met. The moon was full and the stars were bright, and we could have really talked all night. My mind kept thinking about my dad and the questions he would have asked the Captain. Are the fish running? Where are they biting now? What are you using for bait? Are they good eating? It felt like dad was right there with us. But all good things have to come to an end, so we said our goodnights about 10:30 and walked off their deck with an amazing view over the Atlantic ocean and the moon showed us the way to our tent.

Inside we talked about how delightful the evening was and about the high standard that was just set for all the nights in the future we will be spending with strangers. We both fell asleep quickly and though they had left their door open for us to go to the bathroom during the night, we both managed to sleep through the night without the need of a potty call. Perhaps it's all the walking or my head telling my bladder to behave, but my trips to the bathroom at night don't happen anymore.

The next morning we got up before the sun and the moon had slid across the sky with a group of silvery clouds. While tearing our camp down quietly, Morton and I both looked upwards. There was a cloud the shape of a dolphin jumping right over the moon. A good day was coming, we could just feel it.

Day 4 : January 4, 2007 - Summerland Key to Big Pine Key MM 39 *Sunshine Key RV Resort*

We tried to sneak out of Captain Steven's and Jennifer's yard without making a peep. Beating the sun to the road was our goal. The Captain was up early though and came out to bring us more ice water and hugs and handshakes goodbye. We all really feel that our paths crossed for a reason, and we will see them when we come back through.

Setting off at 7 am with the sun just peeking up, we made our best time yet. We had walked nearly 9 miles by 1 pm. The scenery was breathtaking and so many people were now honking and waving at us. It was going to be a red letter day...we could just tell. My camera and video equipment got the usual workout for the day, with images from this journey a vital part of what I want to capture. No souvenirs, just lots of pictures. Stopping in to a local radio station for a few minutes as we passed, the days seem so very different. I was worried that they might seem similar, but there isn't any of that. We never know what is around the corner, where we will be staying or what is waiting on us. We also really never know what we will be eating. A lot of that depends on the people we meet. Since our budget is so low, and our facility for cooking is nonexistent, we rely on people offering us food or eating out of our food bag. This can be in many different forms. We are not picky eaters at all. When a place gives us a free meal we will tell you about it, give you their details and ASK that you use them! Until then, we eat trail mix, nuts, fruit and jerky for a few more days.

Funny thing is, now that I don't eat whatever I want, when I want, everything tastes so good. It is really nice to eat when you are truly hungry and ready for it, rather then just eating because it's a habit. Walking is fast becoming my new and favorite habit. It's one I intend to keep until the end and never stop now that I've started. It's really good medicine for me. My outlook is so great with the exercise, my attitude is that I can do anything, and though my legs are a bit sore, I feel fantastic. As we made our way onto the Key that the Key Deer live on, it was approaching HOT TIME. Today we were going to try something different. We were going to go into a cafe and have a lunch that we would split, drink as much water as they could stand giving us, and I would work on the computer if possible.

When we went in to the cool, dark establishment, I approached the person who worked there. He was a bit ran off his feet because his help hadn't came in. (That brought back a few horrible memories for me from Scotland) He wasn't mean, but he wasn't in a great mood. I figured I wouldn't push it with the computer, just eat, rest and leave. This was a formula that worked. Going back into the hot air I looked at the sky hoping to see a few black clouds. No luck. Bright blue and big fluffy white floating cotton candy giants. We looked into the fences that were suppose to hold the timid, rare, deer back, but no luck. We just had to keep walking. Our destination was mile marker, MM, 37 to a state park. We were at MM 31 when we split our calzone. Six miles in the heat after already doing nine miles...it was going to be tough and close. Now let me explain about mileage. I say we left 22 and went to 31 and you think, nine miles. But we put on a lot more miles than just what the mile markers say. We cross roads to get shade, water, bathrooms, paths and many other reasons. We take loads of steps during the day that we log on the pedometer. So for the purist reading, we aren't breaking them all down...we are just walking.

The deer sanctuary was tough. It was blazing hot, no shade anywhere and no real place to sit and rest. We trudged on and I ignored what my body was telling me. Not a smart or safe thing to do, but we had a destination and we thought, reservations. Imagine the horror on my face as we approached 37 and our camp for the night and they said they were full. The man at the gate had no sympathy that we have no car, had been walking since 7 am (it was now 5:30 pm) and there was not even one little 7x7 foot section we could pitch in. No houses to be seen and I thought the Seven Mile Bridge was right in front of us. Earlier in the day I had called the camping reservation number and was assured they had plenty of spots and at a price that we could afford. After the long push, the hard push, the not-listening-to-my-body push, to be told "NO" was making me physically sick. Morton asked if there was anywhere around to camp. "Two miles up the road." the ranger replied and fired off the phone number to us. I sat for the first time in three hours on a rock to get out the phone and make the call.

Night was coming and we were in the wide open of the emptiness that is found in the Keys. I can't speak for Morton, but I was terrified. The voice that answered the phone was a lovely Southern accent. Kind and gentle, I could tell in a second. I related our fate for the day. Somehow, wires crossed, we had no were to stay in an area that we had no way out of, except for walking.

After listening, she asked me to hold on a minute. I looked up at Morton who was looking worried and around at the park. I know what he was thinking, we are in a tent, not a 40 foot motor home, surely we could pitch up somewhere here. Jobsworth is the term they use in Scotland for people like that park ranger. The voice of our angel came back on the line. The manager, Marlene, had said we could camp with them. Free, and for two nights. We needed a days rest after our hard days push and I had to catch up on the computer. Talk about a fantastic port in a storm. The kind lady told us to be careful getting here. I think she must have heard the panic in my voice. Walking fast on my sore feet and legs, we huffed and puffed up the road. Two miles. We were averaging 1.2 miles an hour. It would be dark soon. We passed the next mile marker and just had one to go. Dark was here, the cars all had their lights on. We had nothing reflective but our MBT shoes and only had about 3 feet of the edge of the road to walk on. Being as strong person of a person as I could, I was trying to hold back my fears and tears. Earlier we had passed a church that had a lot of people in the parking lot. Mentioning to Morton that we should maybe camp there for the night he came back with, "I thought you wanted to make the park?" I did, so we walked past it. Now I was wondering if it was a divine mistake.

If you have never driven down here, you won't understand. It's scary as it gets dark and you have wild growth off on each side of the road, no lights and no way to get out except walk. We had been seeing loads of iguanas and all I could think of was the movie, "Night of the Iguana" an old film that I've never seen, so I don't know if they ate people, took over the world or what, just that the two and three footers we were seeing looked daunting up in the trees, pouncing down upon their prey.

More frightening than reptiles of all sorts are the road dangers. Getting hit by a car, getting killed by someone that wants our heavy backpacks full of sweaty laundry, here we were, night walking...the thing we promised ourselves we were not going to do again.

It all got to me. The exhaustion from the day, the panic of being again out on the road at dark and the fear of the unknown. Bursting into tears Morton tried to comfort me. I didn't want a break, I didn't want a drink, I didn't want anything. Why didn't we camp back at the church was the only real thing that I could get out to him. After just a few seconds of venting all my fears though I felt a bit better.

Wiping my face with the small towel that had kept me cooler during the day, I blinked and saw a pick up truck pulling over. Great, now we are going to get mugged, killed or worse. Maybe a giant iguana was driving, after all, it was night.

First impressions mean so very much. Here was a guy, who with one look, we knew was going to help us. Though we just had under a mile to go, it was a dangerous mile. Our knight in shining armor was a professional truck driver who had been passing us for the last couple days. He asked if he could help. We took all of one second to say "Yes please!" Quickly Morton and the driver popped our wheelchair onto the back of the truck and Morton jumped up with the gear. I got to ride in the front and we were at Sunshine Key Campground in less than five minutes. It would have been another 40 minutes on foot, in the dangerous dark. We discovered that his wife is not only Scottish, but is from an area that is just 20 minutes from where Morton hails from. Near Edinburgh, but a small town. What a small world it is, on foot or in a pick up. When your walking however, the world is huge.

Once we came into the gate at Sunshine Key we were met by a man (our second knight in shining armor) in a golf cart who whisked us to our camp space. They had been wonderfully thoughtful and situated us near the bath house. Morton set up the tent in the moonlight as I tried not to cry. They would have been tears from joy this time, not fear and exhaustion. Instead I got out my shower kit, made sure he was fine on his own, and went to have a shower. The sure cure for the hard days walk. While Morton was having his shower I took some incredible pictures of the full moon, the palms swaying in the gentle night breeze and the paradise we were setting in to for the evening. The big blessing in disguise is, we are now two miles CLOSER to the Seven Mile Bridge. When we head off at 6 am, the day after tomorrow, to cross the monster bridge, we will be fresh and ready for it.

Day 5 : January 5, 2007 - MM 39 *Sunshine Key RV Resort*, Florida

Staying in one place for two nights has been odd. But it has allowed me to get caught up on the site, the email (there has been tons of it and I really want to be able to answer everyone) and our processing our photos & video. Last night when we got here I had the worst leg cramps in my life. It happened during the night and I kept waking Morton up and asking him what he thought was wrong. Tonight I found out, via my daughter-in-law Mari, who is an RN, that it was a combination including not enough water or eating enough food. Yikes, I'm already drinking about 1.5 gallons to 2 gallons daily.

Today we didn't really get to explore much. I started working on the pictures, the pages, the videos and the hundreds of emails we are getting and before I knew it, Morton was bringing me in an EVIL chocolate covered key lime coconut square. It was only 1.5 x 1.5 inches and was almost 200 calories. I ate it, liked it, but didn't want another. We had some sunflower seeds and the computer kept me busy until about 5 pm. We went to the pool where I put on my huge size 32W purple bathing suit with a pink glittery flower on it and jumped in to the nice warm water, and for the first time, when we got out, we felt cold! Chilly really, there was a breeze and we were wet. Oh what I would have given to have that feeling two days ago! After a swim we had a nice dinner at the outdoor tables by the pool. I had a really nice burger, water, pickle slice, French fries and half a piece of key lime pie. Not bad considering for breakfast I had 10 pieces of trail mix, 2 pieces of beef jerky and then the calorie filled coconut thing for lunch. My hunger has gone from that of a starving lion to that of a little wee bird. I put it down to the walking. Odd really, food isn't my priority anymore. I don't really think about it in the same light. It is gas for my engine and I look at what it's going to do for me if I put it in my body. We have to get to bed early tonight. I can't upload the video until I get somewhere wireless, frustrating. As I fall asleep I'm hoping that we can start our cross on the Seven Mile Bridge at 7 am tomorrow!

Lost & Found

While we are walking around America, you can believe we will find some STRANGE things. We expected this, but here you go...we have an AMAZING lucky streak going with what we find. Chance, good luck, guardian angels, fate, destiny...call it what you will but something has been really taking care of us. First, our wheelchair pulls to one side because the road slants. This caused Morton to say we should pick up a cord, strap, or something, that would allow me to pull it straight, while he pushed. Lo and behold, a few miles later, we find an orange strap, with a hook on one end. Not only perfect, but it's our color!

Second, our wheelchair lost a bolt on the first or second day. Morton replaced it with a bolt from the brake and made the shocking discovery that the little tool kit included with the chair to make repairs, didn't include a wrench that would fit. To our amazement, the next day we find two bolts with their nuts on them, two pair of pliers that will work for the wrench and a green small tool box to keep it all in. Third, learning as we are going about packing the wheelchair, Morton rigged the tent to hang under the seat. A flexible jug that holds about 2.5 gallons of water rides on top. Both of these, Morton secured with string, but we promised ourselves to splurge on two bungee cords at the next store we could get them cheap. Within a mile after setting out that day we found not one, but two black bungee cords. Different lengths. Both the perfect length for their job. We have also found pens, 58 cents and a lighter that works. All things we needed. Now, I've saved the oddest for last.

On the third day, you may have read about we were talking about fishing and I was really thinking about my dad and missing him. I still can't believe he's not here anymore. On the morning of the fourth day, Morton and I got the early start. It was almost chilly. We both wished we had a thermometer to take the temperature reading on. The contrast in the variation during the day would be shocking.

Coming to our first bridge, we both stopped to see a six inch round thermometer that was leaning up against the concrete wall. The big numbers on it made me think of my dad. He would always comment about being able to see the numbers from inside on an outside thermometer. This lightweight object was made for us. Picking it up, I looked at the back first, making sure it wasn't broken. Turning it over, and reading "63", I got chills. This was the year I was born. It wasn't due to the temperature though. The words, "Made in USA" were almost as large as the numbers and written across the bottom. Everyone who knew my dad knew that he always searched high and low to buy the things that he needed that were made in the USA.
It seemed to me that even though he's not here, he might be helping us from somewhere.

Day 6 : January 6, 2007 - *Sunshine Key RV Resort* MM39 to *Sea Dell Motel* MM50

Breaking camp early and fast were the first two things Morton and I wanted to do. Waking up at 5:45 we moved as fast as we could. Rolling the bags, putting everything where it goes on the wheelchair, making sure our water bottles were full and allowing room for adjustments, we missed our 6:30 am start I wanted.

As we were leaving the Sunshine Key RV Resort we had a little pre-bridge to walk over before we got to the big one. People were out walking in the early morning sunshine. Smiling and waving we asked how they were doing and didn't even miss a step. We had places to go and bridges to cross.

For weeks, maybe months, I've been letting my mind NOT think about the big Seven Mile Bridge. The total length of the bridge is actually 35,862 ft (10,931 m) or 6.79 miles (10.93 km). I have driven over it before, enjoyed the view and once even sat in a traffic jam on it. Today I was going to walk it. The impossible was happening in this fat girls life.

Let me take you back a year. My husband and I were living in Scotland. My weight had risen so much I was becoming a prisoner in my own body. I couldn't even tie my own shoes. My knees hurt all the time, it was hard getting up and down from the chairs, I couldn't climb the stairs without stopping to catch my breath several times. That was one year ago today.

Today I was thinking about the old me as I headed for the bridge. This bridge is lovely. It hangs, as if by magic (or big concrete pillars) over some of the prettiest water that dazzles you with various greens and blues. There are a few scattered islands or keys, that float off to the left and right and every where you look is sky, water and not a lot more. The old me would not have done this. Drive over it, yes, walk it, never. But then I had a serious wake up call. Now I was desperate with knowledge. I learned just how short life can be, and I was making mine even shorter by what I was eating and not getting any exercise.

Taking the bridge early was the key for getting over it. Morton and I had both agreed on this. About noon it gets too hot for us to walk, so we have to make good time. Either that, or set up shady little shelters on the bridge. That wasn't an option. We didn't want to cause any trouble on the bridge, just get to the other side safely.

Walking and walking, I spied the hump rising in the distance. Morton asked if we had to walk that, since the two bridges, old and new, run beside each other he was a bit confused. I told him that unless we wanted to jump over the side and swim, we had to climb the little summit that is 65 feet tall on the bridge. Poor Morton, pushing the wheelchair and carrying his backpack. He is the best husband in the history of the business of husbands. Speaking of the backpack, I could never carry mine right now. Between my extra 200 plus pounds of body fat I'm carrying around, my knee surgery and my other knee that is a bit iffy, pushing the backpack in the wheelchair will have to happen until I lose about 100 pounds. Plus the heat really does zap your energy. So Morton carries his own pack and pushes mine. Did I mention I have a fantastic husband? Up the bridge we stopped at the summit. Morton took his pack off for a moment and the thought just hit me.

When I strap my pack on, my body will be 100 pounds lighter. When will that be?

Right now time doesn't matter. I didn't even realize it was Saturday until I called my daughter to have her post our time and place on the site. I was surprised she was in bed and not at work. I asked if she wasn't working today, then her husband told me it was Saturday. My mind had been so focused on the walk, the bridge and drinking water, I didn't realize we were nearing the end of our first week.

Finishing the bridge by 11:30 Morton and I were both equally smiling. We shot a short video with our thoughts of the moment, babbling how we felt at this high point of our journey. People looked on as Morton belted out, "You take the high road and I'll take the low road" to my camera.

Giving each other hugs and pats on the backs, we got back to reality. I was almost running to find a bathroom. We had drank about a gallon of water each. Entering the first gas station we came to, I used the cleanest bathroom and found my first seat since 7 am.

The cold air conditioning made my head start to pound and leaned against the cool white tiles of the toilet, hoping that I wasn't going to have a heart attack right here and now. I hurried back outside wanting to collapse in the shade with the heat hitting me hard in the face, asking Morton to get us a Gatorade to split.

When he came out of the shop, we continued walking. We needed to find somewhere to sit down for a bit. Shade and a seat. Not really looking for food, since we were both still really overheated from the fast walking, we didn't have a lot of luck. I wanted to sit and savor the cold drink in the shade. What we needed was a shady bench FAST! There were loads of businesses, just none with benches out. Then we looked to the right and saw a cute little wooden bench shaded on either side with a coconut palm. We parked the wheel-chair, sat down and a loud speaker on the edge of the building piped Jimmy Buffett in our ears. Paradise found again.

We have a campsite lined up for Sunday night, but it's not until MM 58. We still needed to find a place near by to get to sleep early, wake up early, walk early and get to our next place with enough time to keep the site up-to-the-minute for the people following this journey online. The days are really busy for two homeless people. So we stopped at a lovely motel and asked for a room to use for the night. The kind and helpful young lady at the desk listened to who we were, why we were walking and made a call. Before we knew it, the lovely ladies at the *Sea Dell Motel* were giving us a room for the night. And not just ANY room. This is an incredible room with a big lovely bed, loveseat (that I'm using right now to work from!) and a kitchenette with lovely table and chairs. Did I mention the walk-in tiled shower that felt like a dip in a magical blue lagoon? So tonight we go to bed early, get up early, walk to beat the heat and see what we can see. A few more months of this and I'll be able to carry my own backpack!

Day 7 : January 7, 2007 - Sunday MM50 *Sea Dell Motel* to *The Jolly Roger Travel Park* MM59
Breaking News:
Morton types...6.45pm January typing two fingers and slow....unbelievable, I'm sitting at a picnic bench and it's probably still 70 degrees. Priscilla said it would be hot here but temperatures hitting the hundred mark in the sun and me walking in it, who would have thought, I used to take the car everywhere....not because I had to but because today it's too easy an option.

It's been an amazing starting week. Eating coconuts straight off the trees and seeing all the amazing plants, insects, iguanas (ABOUT TWO FEET LONG AND FAST!!!!!!), Lizards and fish. I'm not in Scotland any-more Toto. So far though no gators (phew) and unfortunately we didn't spot any key deer (only a stuffed one somewhere we ate, where we split an amazing calzone for lunch).

We have met and stayed with a lot of new and interesting people who have embraced us literally with open arms and wished us well with our journey and message we are passing on through our enormous walk. *Cheerio the now, Morton*

Priscilla: I'm surprised I got Morton to type at all. He was filling in the blanks as I took a million dollar shower. If you have ever wondered what a million dollar shower feels like, walk for six to eight hours a day in the scorching sun, then find a lovely campsite, like *The Jolly Roger* at MM59, and step in the shower. Pure lux-ury. After being sticky and hot all day to be cool and comfortable, worth all the money in the world actually. This morning we got off to a good start. We left the *Sea Dell Motel* about 7 am and were right on top of mile marker 50. The assistant manager, Janet, at *The Jolly Roger* had phoned me the day before to say we could have a free pitch for our tent on Sunday night. We knew where we were going, we just didn't know all the people and things we would see along the way. Remember, everyday is an adventure! As we set off the sky was a little overcast. We trusted the weather to hold true to what it has been doing and we left the tarp off. We have found a nifty way to store it under the chair with the tent, easy access. Making a pit stop in the grocery store we splurged on fresh bananas, six of them, and bought laundry detergent, trail mix bars and a bottle of lemon juice. We had a brilliant idea for the lemon juice.

The other night I suffered from really bad leg cramps. We weren't sure if it was from the mileage we walked that day or the fact that I didn't have enough salt in my system. My daughter-in-law recommended we make our own affordable power drink. Coming to our first resting area on the walk this morning I made a really dangerous mistake. I took the water bottles, all of the water bottles, and drank a little out of each. By this time we already had two or three empties, but the ones that still had water in them, I added a shot or two of the lemon. We tasted it, liked it and I proceeded to do this to all the bottles. NOT a good idea. We also put a pinch of salt in each of them. Again, not the best move.

The drink was great, is great, and we will be using this recipe along the way. The problem was I didn't leave any real water. Nothing, and I mean nothing, quenches my thirst like real water. Cold, warm or even the hot stuff that we've been drinking along the way. H_2O is the way to go. As we were walking up US1 our first person we spoke to for the day, other then the greeting of "Good Morning" to fellow walkers and bicyclists, was Gary. Gary approached us to talk, was very nice and told us how he had been told by some fellows down the road who happened to be prisoners, that there was a couple walking north. They didn't know who we were or where we were going, but they said a prayer for us. It was nice to be able to tell him about the walk, so he could take some of the worry they must have felt for us. They thought we might be homeless (which we are, besides our little tent!) and it was kind of them to care. After a few minutes of chatting, Gary invited us to come to his church that was just up the road. We knew that we had to walk to beat the heat, he understood and said a very nice prayer with us. When we come back in 3 plus years, we will perhaps take him up on the invitation.

We crossed to the left side of the road to try to find some shade, then back to the right. We settled on walking a bike path that runs where the old rail road line use to pass. It was shady and filled with very nice people. It's part of the Eastcoast Greenway, and if you haven't heard of it, you should look in it and walk or ride it with a bicycle. Spotting a shady bench, I sat down and my phone rang. It was Sarah, my daughter. I was be-having myself and not calling her too early on the Sunday morning. She still sounded sleepy and I got a bit homesick hearing her voice. While we were chatting, Morton started speaking to a lady who was preparing to go rollerblading. As we finished speaking, Morton introduced me to Kathleen, who is a nutritionist. She was talking about some great ways to lose weight and still stay healthy. Morton and I walked, and walked, and walked some more. We talked about how wonderful the path was. No cars to worry about. We both agreed that it is something that every road needs. We talked about the things we were seeing. Exotic plants and wildlife, a state park on our left. There were a few times I would hear a critter running or making noise in the bushes and hoped it wasn't something that bites. My son is so scared of spiders, but I think even he would have appreciated the lovely webs that hung over the top of the walk. Plus, the spiders were helping by catch-ing loads of mosquitoes and other flying critters. Some of the webs seemed big enough to even catch an iguana in.

The sun was getting really hot and my face was burning up. Morton and I both agreed it was time for a break that lasted longer than five minutes. Walking, we looked for a spot that would be good. Benches are on this trail, but one wasn't around when I needed it the most. After about twenty minutes we came to one of the big sturdy benches. They are made of concrete and are cool, almost cold, to the skin when your skin is so hot. Sitting down, Morton was taking off his backpack and going exploring across the walk. There was the Gulf of Mexico, or rather an inlet from it, and after all, he is a boy! He told me if we went over there we could sit on a coral ledge and dangle our feet in the water. He even took some pictures of shellfish that were growing on the coral. I passed. Tempting as it sounded, I knew we still had to make camp and had a few miles to go. If we were lured by the water, we might never walk on today. Reading our little maps, which are very lacking, we hoped being off the main road wouldn't have us walk right past *The Jolly Roger*. After all, there were no mile markers on the bike path.

We asked a few people in passing if they knew where it was, or where we were, and we got several fast answers that they were on holiday and didn't know the area. I think people might have thought we were homeless, which is still open to debate. So we walked. We figured that sooner or later the path would pop up and join up with US 1 again. Then we met Michael. The tall man was walking the opposite direction. He looked like he knew where he was going, and he might have even just came from *The Jolly Roger*. I whispered to Morton to ask him, people seem more inclined to speak to Morton with his Scottish accent then me with my Pennsylvania one. I think my hot, red face might put some folks off too!

We talked for ages with Michael about the walk, where the camp was (he knew!) and it was a very pleasant conversation. He was kind enough to get his picture taken with me and even put his arm on my sweaty shoulder for the picture. He then made a very kind donation to us, seeing our food budget through for several days, and was gone. Morton and I were standing on the trail saying how wonderful people are, generous with their time, with their stories and with help to total strangers.

Just then a biker (a bicycle, not in leather gear) came past us on the left, a lady followed by her husband. He stopped and said he just had to ask where we were going. They had seen us walking a few days ago. As we told them he said that he had commented to his wife that he thought I was too heavy to be out walking in this heat. Little did he know that I think the same thing several times each day. The thought goes through my mind almost daily, as I'm really having to work to walk, "WHY?"

Then I think about all the reasons that I'm here doing what we're doing. We need to walk, so you can watch. If I can move my 390 pound body into walking mode, so can you. Earlier I mentioned the big mistake I made with the water. It was just about noon when it hit me. The lemon water was good, but it wasn't water. My throat felt dry and tight. I needed a drink. I was ready to chance it on dark green canal water, but remembered the show the night before where it showed water like that filled with mosquito eggs and all sorts of nasty things. We left the bike trail to go back to US 1. There was civilization. People, cars and somewhere had to be water. We had several empty bottles we could ask someone to fill, if only we could find a place that didn't say, "No Trespassing". We spotted a little motel on the Atlantic side of the road and headed there. It was cool and shady, but not a soul was in sight. Morton walked around until he found a kind women who was cleaning the rooms. She not only gave us a drink, but filled the bottles with cold water. That combined with the shade around us at the moment, was the ultimate in living.

Staying on US 1 we were in the serious heat of the day. Feeling better with actual water and not just our lemon water, we kept walking. We would take little breaks when we need them. We were just 2 miles away. The quicker we got there, the faster we camp. But the Florida sun in the Keys was strong today. Very strong. Just one mile and we were wringing wet and bone tired. We had to find a place to rest. We were just able to see mile marker 58 coming up. Just one mile short of our goal, we were enticed by the ocean. The Atlantic glistened between the roots of some upturned trees from a past hurricane perhaps. Though there was no leaves on the trees, there was a strip of shade on the grass beside the road. Erosion had taken it's toll on the bank, and a little drop off filled with water that had pushed in from the ocean. Beyond this was the most amazing golden sandbar that fell away into ribbons of blues and greens that was gently lapping in.

Spreading out our tarp, we lounged and looked for about an hour. Drinking our water while it was still cool, we felt like the richest people in the world. Not money rich, experience rich...the best kind. When we decided to go for the last mile and a bit, we got up and went for it. Passing a variety of different signs and businesses, our eyes were peeled for *The Jolly Roger*. Finally we spotted it. Yo ho ho. Just ahead and on our left, situated on the Gulf of Mexico side. Walking into their entrance we were met by Norm, a great guy who introduced us to the assistant manager, Janet. We got our pictures taken with each of them, as well as with their wonderful sign on the door of their office, welcoming Little Changes! Janet got us set up with our space, was kind enough to let us do laundry and stopped by on her golf cart for a chat. Beneath the palm trees, where I'm writing this from, it would be very tempting to stay for a little, or a lot, longer. But in the morning we need to push off and walk. I almost forgot, as soon as we were on the site, Doctor Bob from next door brought us ice water and a lovely lady from across the road brought us bottles of water, nuts, fruit, little packs of crackers and treats and was so very kind. The world is full of beautiful strangers, you just need to get out their and meet them!

Day 8 : January 8, 2007 - Monday *Jolly Roger Travel Park* MM59 to MM67.5 *Long Key State Park*

Blustery day today. We had a lovely tour around *The Jolly Roger* in a golf cart by Janet and her little dog, Bruno. He's a lovely little dog (you know how I love them!) and I got to cuddle him as we rode around looking at what we had to walk away from. It was Janet's day off and she was going for a paddle in her kayak. She wanted to get a picture of us by her office, and then we were off. She is a lovely lady who will make you feel so welcome, we can't say THANK YOU enough to all the people at *The Jolly Roger*. But we did have to say our goodbyes and head up the road.

Getting in to our stride, we were talking about the bridges that we were going to be crossing. It's a real thrill to look at the map now and see how far we have come since we started. It's hard not to rush things along and enjoy the days and all the millions of moments, a real balancing act.

Something made us stop for a moment beside the road, maybe it was a drink of water since the sun was so hot and bright, but when we did, I turned around to see a sheet of black rain coming along the Atlantic side. I pointed and shouted to Morton that it was rain, but he's never been in a Florida storm before. Stuttering and almost jumping up and down, I grabbed the tarp below the wheelchair and told him to cover his pack. The sun shone so strong on us, he must have thought I was mad.

Maybe 45 seconds went by. We were both gazing almost frozen, as it came closer and closer. His pack was half covered when drops of rain the size of grapes, started hitting us. We worked together stretching our HUGE monster of a tarp over the chair, his pack which he gave up covering and pitched on top of the chair and finally pulling the tarp over us! Sitting on the guard rail that has become our dining table, sofa and even a thin bed, we huddled together and hoped we didn't hear any thunder.

We were sitting right in front of a huge bridge to cross. Just 15 minutes faster and the rain would have gotten us there, trapped on a bridge across the water. Good thing Janet and Bruno took us for a tour of *The Jolly Roger*! As the rain came pounding down, I pulled out the camera to make a video. What in the world were we thinking? Setting off without our things covered...not smart! But the sky was clear ahead. I had been away from Florida long enough to forget the golden rule that the rain can come anytime, from anywhere and leave almost faster than it appeared. The wind threatened to pull the tarp off of us and we used our feet to hold down the edges. The rain was bouncing so hard off the ground it was spraying us in the face from below the tarp. Even though it was so windy, underneath the tarp it was as hot as a furnace.

Pulling our chair to a safer spot by the road once the shower left us twenty minutes later, we got everything ready in case it happened again, of course...it didn't! The air smelled fresh as only a rain can make it and we were thankful that we didn't get our gear soaked. It was a lesson well learned. We met a man who was walking with the tiniest backpack I've ever seen, up to the Everglades. It strikes me as odd that people just set off on trips like this on their own, even though we are out here doing it. We strolled across a fishing bridge and before we knew it, our soaking wet clothes were hot and dry again.

We had hopes of making it to Fiesta Key and a swim on their beach, but when the rain came, though I tried to keep us all covered, my feet got wet. The worst way to discover you have a blister is when you are taking your sock off and part of your skin comes along with it. My ankle had been burning a little, but when I pulled the sock off to put dry ones on, it felt like someone had poured acid on my heel. Knowing we wouldn't make our goal with my foot like this and my walk turned to half a limp, we read our tourist books and decided to go for Long Key State Park. It was a smart, but scary move.

By the time we go to their gates my foot was keeping it's own heart beat with the one in my chest. Throbbing, I sat on a split rail fence while Morton went to see if they had any camping spaces and how much they charged. He came back in about five minutes giving me the thumbs up, and I knew we had a home for the night. The only thing I could think of was to take a shower and get my blister breathing and on it's way to healing. When you walk everywhere, you always want to pay attention to directions. When the park ranger told us to go to the road and turn left, we thought he meant to the end of the road. We did, saw where the campers and RV's were pitching up, I had a shower with my clothes on (hey, it was a HOT day) and then had to turn around and walk back to where our space actually was.

A fellow camper told us to take the first path on the right for a short cut. This sounded great to us, especially after making such a big walking mistake. The path was hard packed sand and gravel. After a little test, Morton decided to go for it. He did suggest that I take the short cut and he'd walk the long way.

Since we are a team though, we stuck together. Already we are relying on each other so much that it's hard to be away from the other one...plus, there was the sign. Coming in to this place a wooden sign announced, "Beware, poisonous snakes". Morton and I were definitely sticking together.

Pushing the wheelchair through the first part of the path was a breeze. We were commenting on how great it was, easy, be there in no time...then we came to the lose sandy sand...bogged down and cussing, Morton went in to off road mode. Turning the wheelchair backwards, using brute force, he pulled it out of the dry sand and up on to the edge of a rough grass. I was thinking, "Sort of the grass that a poisonous snake might like to wait in", so I kept to the squishy sand.

Finally, after some incredible scenery we would have never seen (wrong turns can sometimes produce the best scenery) we came to the boardwalk. This structure wound it's way over the growth of the key, and there were wonderful tent platforms that had roofs over them. Tonight we would sleep without the fly sheet, hence...less sweat. Our tenting pavilion was about 20 feet from the Atlantic and from where the sun was setting, we placed our tent to face what would be the sunrise. A cool breeze was already bringing the promise of a great night sleep. The boards would also keep out the snakes. The park ranger told us they were in another area anyway. As Morton set about tying the tent down, I was organizing our dinner of peanuts, trail mix and whatever else still hung out in our food bag. We are in need of a real grocery store. So as I'm about to get us something to eat, something starts eating us. My arm was covered in tiny black specks and a fleck of blood here and there. The bitey things are called "No See Ums" because you really can't see them. But boy can you feel them.

Morton started slapping and dancing as well and we both decided it was time to throw everything in the tent and organize it in there. Rushing, we kept the screen open no longer than it took to shove the backpacks and water through. Morton had to run to the toilet block and I took a moment to wipe my bloody arms off with my old wet t-shirt. Getting our bedrolls out and spreading the sleeping bags over them, I stretched out for a minute. My legs were aching and my blister on my right heel was stinging. My eyes started to read the book about where we were staying. I was trying to forget the sign about the snakes, I just have this old childhood fear. The word "Rattlesnake Key" jumped out at me and I imagined the critters under the boards where I was right now. Just then, I heard a noise outside the tent. It wasn't Morton. It had to be a gator or a snake. The sounds on the board were right outside a very thin piece of material called our tent. The footsteps of the approaching Morton made me feel a bit better. I called out to him that something was outside of our tent. Not sure what exactly, but he should be careful.

Stepping around the edge I prepared myself for the worst thing to happen to Morton's shadow. He bent down to pick whatever it was up. How crazy is he??? "Don't you dare bring it in here!" I shouted, as he unzipped the tent. He was already shoving the shape through the small hole in the tent. "Take it, it's yours!" Morton said. He pushed my empty bottle in that had been left out of the tent. The wind had been blowing it up against the side, making animal type noises. It was going to be a long night.

Morton and I actually spent a really nice evening watching the guys beside us come and go (they must have had rhino hide for skin or great bug spray) from their kayaks. They were talking about the fishing, the word "shark" was mentioned, and their lanterns on their heads and the stretch of the tent material actually made them look a little like aliens. Rather entertaining, but we were too sleepy to stay awake any longer.

When morning came, we were treated to a glowing sunrise. Packing our tent and gear, we headed north. In search of fitness, warm food and feet that are free from blisters.

Day 9 : January 9, 2007 - Tuesday MM67.5 Long Key State Park to MM75

Today was hot again. There were some big bridges coming up and anything could be in front of us. Our maps leave a lot to be desired, but we really just have to follow US1 north until we get out of the Keys. Things like cafes, stores and watering holes are noted on some, but sometimes the one you are counting on has closed or isn't open when you are walking past. I wonder what Lewis and Clark would have done with the internet? Just think of how far Marco Polo could have gone.

Morton and I have a few tourist maps, books with coupons, but we share one common thing with those early explorers. We have no car. Using just our feet, not even horses, we are trekking all over the places (sometimes in the wrong direction) and following a dream. What had been one of our biggest fears, the bridges of the Keys, have became one of our greatest pleasures. The walking area is always flatter and wide enough for us, the view is incredible, and on a hot day, you can't beat the breeze. Bring on the bridges, we love them now, not fear them.

After a cold shower with my clothes on, and Morton making a moonlight dash to the shower of the campground, we were both feeling a bit grubby. Still not lucking into any warm food, we drank lots of water and kept walking. We knew we were going to cross a big bridge, just wanted to have a fuller sort of stomach for it. When we first saw the bridge rising, we both sort of gasped at the same time. It was stunning. It had a curve and rise to it that was our highest to date. It was ready to have us walking on it, I could tell. The Atlantic was on the right, stretching out as far as our eyes could see. It was going to be fun.

We took a little rest before the bridge, but not long. With the energy from trail mix, water, a few strips of jerky and a handful of peanuts, we walked up on the bridge. It was high, seemed like we were just on it for a moment or two and then we were off it. I didn't look straight down at the highest point of it. Didn't want to get vertigo. Morton did hold the camera over the edge and take some pictures. It was odd being up on the bridge and looking at where we were about to walk. We could see clusters of houses, signs where we could hopefully get something hot to eat (even though neither of us are really hungry) and maybe a shop where we can get vitamins, more stuff for our food bag and band-aids that are specially made for our rain-caused blisters.

Getting use to walking on the flat road again after going up and down the bridge just takes a few minutes. Our bodies tilt at an angle to balance with the edge of the road. We see the trail from something (a plane, a rocket?) that seems to be going straight up in the air, fast. We wonder if it is the shuttle, but most likely just some very fast, very expensive, plane leaving a big carbon foot-print on the sky.

There are no stores, the place we stop to eat lunch/dinner is closed, maybe forever. You can't really make out from the signs on it. So we keep walking. My blister is hurting and we know we have another lengthy bridge in front of us, just not sure where. After all, who would have thought we needed an excellent map for the Florida Keys? Since we were caught out with night one of pitching the tent after dark, we have both vowed to NEVER do that again. As four o'clock approaches, we start thinking about getting a place. There are little villas, big houses with gates, timeshare looking places and not a lot on offer. We come to the path of a place that doesn't really say if it's a motel, campground, timeshare or apartments, but the sign that says "vacancy" is all that we need to go back the gravel trail. Poor Morton struggles with the chair, but we stick together. I have been elected to go and ask about a room for the night. There is a pool with lots of brown and red people at it and the office is on the top floor, up a grey wooden staircase. Trying to not look too grubby, I poke my head in the office, where a girl is speaking Spanish on the phone. She says something to the person on the phone (I have to learn Spanish) and tucks the phone under her neck.

Gesturing with her hand for me to speak, I give her the very short version of what we are after. "We are walking around the borders and coasts, do you have a room we could use for the night or a place we could pitch our tent please?" She tells me in a very rushed voice that they have a three night minimum stay, that each night is $200.00 and they don't give to charity. I never mentioned that we were a charity, again...just a 7x7 bit of grass without fire ants is all we are after. I said that we only needed one night and we would be very happy to just pitch our tent and be gone in the morning. She wagged a red fingernail at me and said, "No, no, no, sorry" and before I was even out of her office she was back chatting on the phone. Now I don't speak Spanish, yet, but I could tell it was a personal call. She wasn't out and out rude, but she was so short with me, it was a bit frustrating. Turning back I said, "Excuse me, can you tell me how far it is to the next motel heading north?" "Ten miles" she answered and then turned her chair around, so I couldn't even say "Thanks for the info". Back down the steps I did use their private bathrooms for the sun burnt swimmers and washed my face and arms in the sink quickly. Morton was waiting and I asked if he needed the bathroom. Camel man didn't. He could tell that I was disappointed.

Nothing but posh houses with big gate and "no trespassing" signs were everywhere. I told him about the ten miles and we both knew that we would be doing a bit of roadside camping near a bridge that night. No warm food again as well. We talked about the last time we ate something warm, it was at the campground at MM39 before the Seven Mile Bridge. The air was getting cooler and a wind was blowing. It might start raining again at any moment. The sky was getting dark and the was no way we were going to be able to do another ten miles. Impossible. We had just gone about half a mile, when there on the same side of the street was a resort with a sign that said "VACANCY". Ten miles? Was the woman on the phone really THAT bad with distances? Again, we shot back the path and to the office.

A little cage was in the front with a lizard in it and a little dog, BooBoo, with a blue bandanna sitting at the door. A smiling lady listened to what we were after and said that they were full there and she couldn't help us with a room, but there was a bit of grass we could camp on. Joy! Riding me to it in her golf cart (everyone in the Keys seems to have one) with Morton's pack on the back of it, Morton shoved the chair along to keep up with us. The spot was ideal, in the shelter of a tree and hedge, and we made about setting up camp as quick as possible. We didn't want to chance bugs at dusk.

Two guys with smirks on their faces listened as Morton told them about the walk. They looked in disbelief, but I don't think they understood what we were doing it for. The older one told me I'd be skinny after it. He also said that it doesn't sound like fun, sounds more like torture. I guess it's all down to what you think is fun. As we dove in our tent it was just 5:30 pm. There was no where around to get food, and we really never want to go asking someone for dinner. Not while I still have three years of fat reserves to live off of. Morton and I were both wanting to eat something other than trail mix, granola bars and jerky...but neither of us were really hungry. We talked for a few hours, read our horrible little maps, reflected on things, discussed using bikes for part of the walk and most importantly, our blisters were able to breathe for hours. As I was stretched out on my belly, my legs started to get cramps in them. Not little cramps, but horrible knots from top to bottom. I tried stretching them, rubbing them and even taking pain killers, but nothing worked. Our cell phones weren't getting great signals and I wanted to get through to my daughter-in-law to see if there was anything I could do.

When I reached her by phone, after walking around until I found a spot to get a signal from, she asked when the last time was we ate real food. I told her and she said I needed to get some food down my neck. Easy if you have a car, not easy if you are depending on your two feet. Learning that I wasn't going to die from these bad cramps, I tried to think about other things. Wishing my blister would start hurting worse than my legs so I could take my mind off them, I was remembering how my mom's legs use to hurt her at night. It was from her diabetes and poor diet and no exercise. She was in so much pain just a year ago that she was begging the doctor to cut them off. Thinking of family and how much things have changed in a year, my mind was distracted from the ripples of cramps and somehow, I managed to find sleep. The wind was whipping the tent a bit as we fell asleep somewhere around eight o'clock. During the night we'd wake up to hear noises that sounded like rain, or the flap blowing free, but in general it was a good nights sleep.

We knew just two and half miles up the road was a place that served breakfast, and for the first time since leaving my sister's house in Edgewater, Florida, we were going to have something warm for breakfast.

Day 10 : January 10, 2007 - Wednesday Lower Matecumbe Key MM75 to MM81.2 *Kon Tiki Resort*

Going to sleep so early has it's advantages. You wake up so very early, and we did. It sounded fierce outside. Wind, maybe rain and cold. While it was still dark, I unzipped the fly sheet and was surprised to see a million little stars twinkling at us. Morton told me the time, five thirty a.m., and we both had been in the tent long enough. Twelve or more hours in a seven by seven tent isn't something I recommend. Breaking camp quickly, we didn't have our usual breakfast of warm water, trail mix, power bars (we are out of them) or anything. We just walked up the bike path that wiggled beside US1. We were both thinking about the breakfast that was right up the road. Five minutes in your car, seventy minutes on foot.

The place was small, a counter inside with five or six stools, and just five or six tables. The waitress was nice and showed us a place where we could cram our wheelchair full of backpack and tent in the corner. It was a working corner though, and the whole time we were there she had to squeeze through. Good thing she was thin. Seeing the menu I realized how hungry I was. Starving really. I wanted milk, even at $2.50 a glass. I chose the plate with biscuits and gravy, eggs and hash browns. It was one of the least expensive things and looked like it would fill the gaping hole in my belly.

Drinking two glasses of ice water (big mistake) while we were waiting on our food, Morton enjoyed his first cup of coffee in ages. He had ordered a short stack of blueberry pancakes and we both passed the time waiting for our food by chatting to the people at the next table. They, like so many people we have talked to over the last few days, thought we were homeless. People really always will judge a book by it's cover. We don't mind people thinking we are homeless, but it would be nicer if they knew why we were walking. The couple were lovely and we had a nice chat, then their food arrived. We were almost drooling as we smelled it. Delicious. Soon enough, we were each getting our plates set down. Mine was a fair sized serving, but I was wishing there had been more. Then I started eating. After about 20 bites, I was full. Not just a little full, stuffed. It was all I could do to finish the milk. My stomach must really be shrinking from not jamming it full of junk each day. With well more than half still left on the plate, I offered it to Morton. Usually he will gladly finish my plate or anyone else's. There has even been more than one occasion where Morton and Graeme have come to an agreement to split the leftovers off my daughters plate. But not today. Morton was struggling to eat his own two pancakes. Trying a few bites of the sausage gravy, he loved it. It was fantastic, but we just couldn't eat it. This was a first for both of us. We agreed from now on, we don't get two meals, just one...splitting it and saving money. After he paid the bill we made a quick line north. There was another bridge coming up. A longish one. As we were walking I started to get sick to my stomach, then cramps. I didn't have to go to the bathroom. It was more like my belly couldn't handle the food. The last thing I wanted to do was to lose this breakfast. We had just spent more than our whole days food budget on it, and I needed it for real nourishment to my leg-cramping body. Sitting down on a bit of guard rail didn't work. It only made me sicker. Morton suggested laying the tarp out on the ground (we learned this after a bad experience with fire ants and my towel) and me laying flat on it. This sounded like a plan.

There was a perfect grassy bank, right before our bridge, and we spread the tarp that was still damp, out. This tarp is huge, way too big for us really, but Morton wanted to bring it. It is great for sitting in the middle of and being able to watch on the white if any creepy crawlies are coming to bite or sting us. Laying down on my side I pulled my knees up to try to get my stomach to stop hurting. Morton sat in watch while I rested. He learned the other day while we were taking a break for my blister, that fire ants get on you and bite you to bits in a second. A few had bitten me and I was still carrying around the blister marks to prove it. We had stopped for a moment and I was just going to spread my towel down to sit on. We searched the grass for their tell-tale signs of their homes by mounds of sand, but there were none.

Bending down, I put my hand on the ground to get my body down. Before my knee even hit the ground, my hand was covered in biting ants. Fire ants are aptly named because it feels like liquid fire wherever they bite you. Brushing and rubbing them off I jumped back up, screamed and Morton pushed the cart along to follow as I went up the road. It seems the wheel of the wheelchair was resting on their ant hill. Another lesson we've learned. Today with the tarp spread out and my belly doing back flips, there were no ants. I had my jacket on for the first time since the walk began. It was chilly, my blister was sore and I was wondering what on earth are we doing this for? Then I think about all the strangers out there who are grabbing a bit of inspiration, there are thousands of you now reading this. I also think about all the wonders and adventures that are waiting just up the road for us. Resting did the trick and in about thirty minutes, my stomach was doing fine. The food must have made it's way down. We walked and walked and started to come into real civilization. Stopping to read signs that you never normally read in a car, we learned how the one Key was settled ages ago with Indians. Interesting stuff that I took pictures of to really read later, when I wasn't walking. We sort of were walking to a place that I had been before. Years ago I was in the Keys with my nephew and we stayed at a place called the *Kon Tiki Resort*. It was beautiful, right on the water and has a special feel to it. It wasn't quite our ten miles that we wanted to walk, but with our lack of power and stomach cramps, I needed some extra time on the computer to catch everyone up to speed on the walk, make contact with some of the press we are going to be doing in Miami and check the email. The sign for it, on the Gulf side, was just ahead and it wasn't quite one o'-clock. We had walked a good distance today, just left as the sun was just coming up though.

Walking back the familiar path I had a real good feeling about this place. The big fluffy orange cat that was here the last time was no where to be seen, but there was another cat. The man in the office was fantastic, helpful and not only let us have a room for the night, but also let us use the washer and dryer that are in this very cool Tiki hut. After a shower, this one might have been a two-million dollar shower, and clean clothes, Morton and I went for a little walk around the resort. They have their own private lagoon with hammocks between palm trees and some of the prettiest views we have seen so far. Paradise is definitely here. Since I have so many pictures to do things with, I spent the afternoon on the computer. I'm not going to be able to upload them all until later when I'm in a WIFI spot because the connection that I get with my computer is seriously lacking. We didn't really have lunch and Morton was looking in the phone book and spotted a Chinese place that delivers. There were some places around, but remember our budget. There are not too many places that we can afford. Looking at their menu online we decided to split a meal. Half price and just the right amount of food. My intentions were to work on the computer and get updates online for the people following our journey on the web. But with General Tso's and rice in my belly, no cramps in my legs, a bed and the television on, I fell asleep about 8 pm utterly exhausted.

Day 11 : January 11, 2007 - Thursday MM81.2 *Kon Tiki Resort* to MM84.5 *Theater of the Sea & Pelican Cove*

The day started with a very short walk, just a little over three miles. We got a not too late start from the *Kon Tiki* where Morton had gone over the wheelchair from head to toe. He tightened loose screws, adjusted the breaks and cleaned everything he could clean on our pack horse on wheels. Weather was perfect for walking, not a hot sun, but a gentle sun. We talked about what was waiting for us on the stretch ahead and a sign showing construction reminded us of the dangerous part of road that is north of Key Largo, just a few days away. We have had police warn us against walking it. They said the cars really speed at that part and the construction has the edge of the road totally gone. We figured we would go into the tourist information place to see if we could get an update on the construction and a decent map. It proved to be a very helpful stop. First we passed where the old railroad caboose that use to house the Chamber of Commerce. It was lovely but lonely looking. The thought crossed my mind about how fun it would be to spend the night in it. We want to stay in some odd places along our journey and it would be a great one...maybe on the way back in three years. Waiting outside with our wheelchair, Morton went in to the tourist info place to get the maps. I gave a look at our books we have been using to guide us up through the Keys. The pages now meant things to me. We had seen most of the ads up close and personal as we walked by them.

The name, *"Theater of the Sea"* jumped out at me. I had wanted to email them earlier, but the last week and a half have been a whirlwind. Using the phone number provided, I called and spoke with Maureen. She was very helpful and invited us to come along and get some photos for the site. We also might get to interact with the dolphins, sea lions and sting rays. It looked like we were going to get a half a day off to see something along the way. After all, what is a journey if you don't stop to smell the dolphins?

Now a few years ago I drove straight past *Theater of the Sea*. I was on my way to somewhere in the smaller mile markers and didn't have the time. After today, I can truly say that was a mistake. This gem is not to be missed and has to go on all of your "To See" lists. Talk about a fantastic day.

When we first arrived, Maureen was gone. We had a bit of time to kill until she got back and Morton and I started thinking about where we were going to stay the night. After having a day off of sorts, we wouldn't want to get caught in the dark in the next bit of road that is north of mm 84.5. Looking again in our tour guide book (those things are really proving to be fantastic for us) we decided the place we were going to walk to was going to be out of reach. There was one hope. A place called *Pelican Cove* is situated right beside *Theater of the Sea*. Again, calling and explaining what we were doing, a lovely lady and her manager, agreed to let us stay in a room for the night. Pure luxury...two nights in a row in a bed. We could get use to this.

With our lodging sorted, we were able to relax and enjoy the day. The Theater of the Sea takes you on a journey from what feels more like habitats of the actual animals and birds rather then a show. It also doesn't feel plastic. It is a really unique place, ran by the same family since first opening. You really would love all the things to do there, yet all at such a relaxed and friendly atmosphere. The next time you are in the Keys, allow 2 to 3 hours to see this treasure chest.

Morton and I loved all the cats they have adopted, both inside and outside. Cats of every shape and size are waiting to be stroked and offer a huge range of purrs to say thanks. Once inside, you have a map that takes you from one show to the next, including dolphins, sea lions, parrots as well as boat ride in the lagoon, nature walks and even a special beach you can go snorkeling on. The first show we saw was the parrots. Not having our wheelchair with us felt good. It was stashed in what would be our room for the night. We held hands and laughed and were very entertained. Clever and informative, the show ended and we moved over to the dolphin show.

We sat in the very first row and when they asked for a volunteer, my hand shot up. Now in my 43 years, I have never been the one to volunteer for a show like this. First, you had to walk out on a dock, which I was afraid I might sink. Then we had to kneel down, again, this can be a task for me. The dock was a little slippery and I thought I might actually slide right in with the "kittens of the sea", as Mark Twain called dolphins. Kneeling I got to stroke the dolphin. It felt just like I had imagined. Waving at us as he went past, we got several passes with this slippery fellow. Then we were told to lean forward for a kiss. This was the part that I was afraid I would fall in. I kept well back from the edge, as I had fears of tipping us all into the lagoon. Talk about something that would be a shameful moment! All things went well though, he swam up, kissed me and I even turned from just a cheek kiss to a lips on nose kiss. The dolphin pushed against me and held it for the photographer to get a picture. Morton had our camera running on video and this brave and bold moment when I stepped outside my fat shell, is captured forever.

The rest of the day we spent enjoying the beauty of this place. The shows were all wonderful and I promise you, you will love it. Since we didn't have lunch really, we decided to eat early (about 3:30) at the cafe they have in Theater of the Sea. SMART MOVE! It was affordable, the freshest and best food I've had for ages and the lovely atmosphere of being there was delightful.

Walking back to our room, which is right across the parking lot, we took a stroll by the private beach. There were some Para gliders out in the ocean, music coming from their poolside bar and Morton and I rested on a swing for a few moments. It seems a million miles away from camping beside the road over the past few days. The walk has to be a balance of seeing things, doing things and always moving. There have been many beautiful things we have walked past already that we wish we would have had time for. Today, we will always remember, as our special "first" on the walk. In three years when we return, I'll get on the platform with the dolphins again, maybe this time in a bathing suit!

Day 12 : January 12, 2007 - Friday MM84.5 *Pelican Cove* to *Keys Wild Bird Center* MM93.6
Today started with a free breakfast, courtesy of the wonderful people at the Pelican Cove. We toasted our bagels, sat on their lovely deck overlooking the ocean, and for a moment, forgot that we had to walk 10 miles today. Breakfast and our stay were over too soon. We said our goodbyes and the lovely lady was kind enough to tell us to walk up OLD US1 to save some steps and stay shady. It was a brilliant suggestions. We met only one car, saw an iguana and the shade indeed was upon us.

Soon enough we were out on NEW US1, just in time for construction. There were a few seconds I thought Morton or I were going to get hit by a car or truck racing through (I pity the people that are working in there, SLOW DOWN!) and as we were crossing the draw bridge, Morton got the wheelchair wheel stuck. It wasn't his fault really, bad design. Perhaps the panic of it all made me so nervous I needed the bathroom NOW! It was a horrible feeling to be stuck between these concrete barriers, traffic and feeling Mother Nature calling. Considering using the porta-potty for the workers, I was given a slight reprieve and said I could make it to the next set of businesses. Surely there would be a shop with the cluster of signs that were still too far away to make out. Almost running, we spotted a real estate office. Leaving Morton standing on the side of the road I dashed for their door. Red in the face and sweaty, looking quite desperate, I asked the ladies if they had a bathroom I could pleeeeeeeeeease use. They did and I did. Then we all chatted for a few minutes about the site, the walk and how your bathroom is one of the things you miss the most when you are homeless. Earlier in the walk we had a similar situation and Morton went in a bank to ask for the use of the bathroom. He was just scouting it out for me and had kept his backpack on. He came back and told me I could use their bathroom and where to find it...again, I did the 100-yard dash. Later a lady told us they thought he might be trying to rob the place or blow it up...you know, with his WEIRD Scottish accent ;) but they saw me and our wheelchair full of STUFF and figured we couldn't make a fast getaway. Seeing how dangerous just 1/2 mile of construction with no side to the road was, we are going to be taking the bus from Key Largo to Florida City. After all, this isn't a contest, or a race with danger...this a life changing adventure that we need to stay alive.

Walking today felt great. The temperatures were good. There was a nice breeze, sometimes too nice and my hat got blown off several times. I keep my ponytail stuck through it though, so it never gets too far from me. Occasionally on big bridges I hold the hat in my hand. We don't fancy jumping over the edge to get it back. Talking about all our safety options today, we both agreed that as the journey continues, we will have to make little changes ourselves all along the way to fine tune things. As we learn and discover what works and what doesn't, we need to adjust. We also appreciate the TIPS people are leaving on the daily blog...we read and we like! Thank you all. We were passing the *Free PRESS* and went inside to do an interview with senior staff writer, Steve Gibbs. He was very helpful, took several photos of the pair of us and wished us well on our walk. Hopefully now some of the people who wonder who we are and what we are doing, will learn. One of our breaks today were in the side yard of a church. Benches, shade and people setting up for an art show happening the next day. Morton and I enjoyed the break and found it a bit hard to start walking again. My feet and ankles were swelling and the backs of my calves were so sore and tight. But we continued. Passing a real grocery store, we stopped to do a little shopping. Our beef jerky had run out and the only thing left in the bag was 4 trail mix bars and dried ginger (Morton likes it, I hate it!). You wouldn't think that we would bump in to someone we knew, but we did. It was the park ranger from a few nights ago on Long Key. He chatted with us for a while on everything from the dangers of traffic, the amount of traffic, Scottish kilts, wars - old and new and it was nice to see a familiar and friendly face. After about 15 minutes or so, I left Morton and him chatting to go inside and get our shopping done. Dry roasted peanuts, cereal bars, tuna salad in cans, crackers, trail mix that was on sale and 2 cans of ravioli with pop tops...we will eat it hot or cold. It felt pretty good to get the food bag fat again. Not that we have any real appetite after walking, we have to eat though. It's an odd feeling for me to tell myself to eat. A first in my life really.

While I was shopping I noticed a man following me around and obviously watching me. I would have put him down to a store detective if it wasn't for the fact that he looked so suspicious himself. Outside while Morton loaded our gear I saw the man, talking with another, watching every move Morton and I were making. I pointed them out to Morton who said that the other fellow had been watching him the whole time. These weren't fans of the website though. They were watching us with bad intent on their minds. This was confirmed as they followed us up the road, on foot, on the other side of the highway. We would stop, they would stop. It was really unnerving and I was ready to get on the phone and call the police when they both suddenly disappeared.

While we were heading up the road, studying our little maps, we learned that we needed to get bedded down in an area where there were still beds and people. We really feel so much better for walking when we have a bed to sleep in, I can work on the pictures, the site, charge the phone and so many other good reasons to have a room instead of the tent. The other reason that we really wanted to be inside tonight were the scary men who had been keeping such a scary eye on us. We tried everywhere but got nothing but "no" told to us. No room in the motel, one offering a special rate of only $119. for a night (that is our food budget for 12 days!) and we even asked to camp in a spot at a private club. The person we needed to talk to was out though, we had to keep walking. Finally, we decided to call the people at the *Keys Wild Bird Center*.

Little Changes   **28**   *Priscilla Houliston*

We wanted to see this sanctuary and rehab center for birds and hoped they might be able to help. The were able to help us with a spot to pitch out tent & get to enjoy the sights and sounds of the sanctuary. Magical and scary. We made our way back through injured birds in giant aviaries that were there mostly because of man. Legs of storks that had been caught in fishing line and had to be amputated reminded us of the turtle we saw at Theater of the Sea that will forever have to wear a life-preserver since two of his flippers have been lost due to careless fishermen. The birds that are here will mostly live out their days here, injured beyond repair and kindly cared for until they die.

There is a long board walk that winds around cages and feels like it goes on forever. We didn't stop to read about all these wounded creatures, but kept walking to our little beach for the night. Our little tent got a work out, camped on the beach between a strip of sand and the Gulf & a real wild mangrove! It barely fit and before dark we were inside, safe from the mosquitoes, listening to the wildest evening yet approaching. The center had closed for the day so we were left in total darkness, on our own with the wild things. The water was just feet away from the front flap of the tent, though I was assured it wouldn't come any higher by a professional photographer who was a regular here, taking pictures of wild and captured birds. Sometime during the night I woke up from a dream of everything being covered in water, floating in our tent. After patting the floor of the tent with my bare hand I was satisfied it was just a dream.

Laying back on my flat pillow I looked at the low light the moon cast against the side of the tent. Was it my imagination or was that an alligator standing on it's hind legs waiting to pounce on the tent? The image would move a bit and I shook Morton, to get his quiet input. He grunted it was a tree and to go to sleep. Still a bit spooked, remembering the fact that our tent is so very thin and would keep nothing but mosquitoes out, I fell back to sleep. Besides being woke up by two rain showers, we slept the rest of the night like babes in the woods.

Day 13 : January 13, 2007 - Saturday - *Keys Wild Bird Center* MM93.6 to MM100.3 & back to MM99.5 *Sunset Cove Beach Resort*

Popping our heads out of the tent we were greeted by pelicans, hundreds of them. Morton loves the pelicans and getting to be so close to them, he was like a little boy. They had all flown in for their breakfast, but Morton and I had nothing for them. Come to think of it, we could have eaten a fresh fish that would be thrown to them by kind keepers in just a few moments, but there was no time for sushi for breakfast. We knew we had to hurry because we wanted to get to MM100 early, contact different papers and television stations that are following our story and update them on the first 100 miles. Imagine that, I have almost walked a hundred miles under the blazing Florida sun. Even though we have clocked up more that 100 miles with all our criss-crossing, seeing the MM100 was a real rush. It felt like a true mile marker had been reached.

A year ago I would have never thought I would be able to walk a hundred miles. Really, not even one mile was within my reach. It was so depressing being encased in my big body that wouldn't even get up and down from a chair without a substantial amount of moaning and groaning. There is a internet coffee shop at MM100.3 and I've been jumping at the chance to upload all our videos for the public to see. It wasn't meant to happen today though. We had nine different email interviews and a few telephone interviews. We have decided to take the bus that runs from Key Largo to Florida City to avoid the construction on the 18 mile stretch the police have told us we shouldn't walk. We also have to rule out Card Sound Road because the website says you can't walk on the turnpike. I guess they wouldn't know what to charge us. So we made some phone calls which all turned in to "no" for the room for the night. We were keeping our eyes open for a safe looking piece of grass without fire ants to pitch the tent, when we passed the *Sunset Cove Beach Resort*. You first spot a big swan boat in the front, and the quirky look just spoke to me in a very appealing way. Entering the office, Sara (same name as my daughter) was very helpful. She would make the call needed to see if we could stay for the night. She took our phone number and sure enough, in about an hour, she called us with a yes! We were so thankful. By that time we were in the internet coffee shop and had to come south again, something we will do in the morning to catch the bus too. Morton was so impressed with our room (me too!) as it has a kitchen, bathroom and guess what...a PRIVATE BEACH! Morton insisted we suit up and swim. I just wanted to get a shower and get to the website. But the walk is a two person proposition, so I showered and we went down to the beach.

After all, my weight has kept me from doing things with Morton for years now that he wanted to do. The movies were out of the question because I didn't fit in the seats, but was embarrassed to tell him the truth. Instead I would lie and say that I wanted to watch it on DVD when it came out. As we walked the drive that led us between the rooms, we both noticed how much attention to detail is happening here. There are little coves set up everywhere with hanging comfy chairs, tables, even a giant Tiki bar with a waterfall inside it. Sofas and big chairs form seating spaces where people staying here can all take advantage of the "outdoor" rooms. There is a great dock, free use of canoes and kayaks and a lovely sand beach. Morton was worried he was going to leave the Keys without getting to swim. But fear not Morton, you finally got your toes wet. While I watched from one of the three Tiki huts on the beach, Morton waded out. He went slow at first, then jumped in and swam his little heart out. He tried to coax me in but I was clean from the shower. My hair was all untangled and I wanted to keep it that way. Besides, I'm more of a pool girl than a beach girl. The words *Portuguese Man of Wars* were still echoing in my ears from the park ranger just a few mile markers down the road. Coming out of the water Morton was very smiley. Odd for him...he always says that his relaxed expression is a frown. All he needed was a bucket and shovel and I think I could have talked him into building a sand castle. It is uncomfortable for me to be out amongst people in a bathing suit. I'm so hideous and fat I feel as if anyone that is within sight of me must be laughing or sick to their stomach. At this moment I try to cover as much as I can with my bulk. We went back to the room and I started working online trying to forget the looks that people give me. I can see the question in their eyes. How on earth did you get *THAT* fat? But of course no one ever really says this to me. Planning out what and where we were going tomorrow, locating maps and trying to put it all together consume the next few hours. We would have a much easier time of it if we had a crew with us, but it's just the two of us and Morton is about as much help on the computer as a chocolate fire guard.

Day 14 : January 14, 2007 - Sunday - MM99.5 *Sunset Cove Beach Resort* to Florida City, Florida

This might have been our scariest day so far. The scary part was a bus ride, not walking. We had made the decision to take the bus that runs from Key Largo to Florida City to avoid the construction. We made our way from *Sunset Cove*, south to the bus stop and waited. We were always going to do the SAFE thing out here, our number one goal is to stay alive as we are going on our journey around America. But actually catching a bus was really bothering me. It felt like I was cheating myself and cheating the people watching. After all, aren't we *WALKING* around America? The bus pulled in, 15 minutes early. We stashed our stuff in the undercarriage and boarded. It was clean, cool and really did feel like we were cheating. Morton and I watched the miles tick by, plenty of sidewalks and bike trails for us. We sort of gave each other the "big eyes" about maybe jumping off from this coach out of the Keys and using our legs. Instead we just sat back and watched. Before long, we saw it. The road narrowed, there was no edge on either side, and even being in the bus was a scary trip. It would have been a nightmare ending in tragedy if we would have walked these miles. We both gazed in horror as there became no edge to the road. I wondered how many hours we would have had traffic backed up, how many accidents would have happened. Taking the bus suddenly felt very right. Morton and I both smiled at each other now. We watched as miles rolled by at a speed that we were not use to after just two weeks of walking. There would have been no where to camp unless we were willing to wade across wet canal areas. It just wouldn't have been worth it. The forty minutes on the bus would have taken us about 3 days and might have cost us our lives. When the bus came to it's final destination, a massive super store in Florida City, we felt like we were fish out of water. Our lovely Florida Keys were far behind us and this was the city. Unfamiliar territory and changes in plans left us both a bit scared and confused. What were we going to do? Time plays a huge amount of our walk. Eight hours a day we have spent walking on average. Then searching for a place to stay. Then trying to get our web site taken care of. You have to remember, when we first started planning the trip, there were going to be eight of us on this adventure. My parents, my son & his wife and my daughter and her husband. We were going to have an RV that would act as headquarters. We were going to have bikes for back up support and we would have a car that would be a rescue type vehicle. Now it is just Morton and I. Things have changed. Lots and lots of little changes since we decided to trek America. It will work out, it just has to. To give you the short version of WHY the changes, my father passed away in September. My mom had another stroke in November, my son and his wife are now caring for her and my daughter, Sarah, became pregnant. All these things that would put a person off the idea of walking around America, only seemed to make us more determined to do it. Our family still supports us with phone contact, internet research for us and in every way they can, but they are about 1000 miles away right now. Not too good when you are a stranger in a strange place, with no real contacts.

So there we were, in the mega store, like lost little kids. Morton and I were more exhausted mentally than we had been since the journey began. To tell you the truth, I felt like crying and getting the first plane, train or automobile home, but we can't do that. As I said, we have learned so much more in our first two weeks of living on our own, on the road, then we did in any of our months of training. Nothing could prepare us for all the situations we have came across. Lack of water, limited budget, going days without eating warm food, going days without showers...all real life that although we might have thought about it, we didn't really think of mental anguish of this undertaking. Mentally and physically we were both utterly exhausted. So, as we walk we talk. Morton and I spend hours talking about various situations, conditions of the walk, what we are going to do, while never really able to plan further ahead than 24 to 48 hours. Heat, weather, blisters, food, water, sleeping arrangements...so many things to consider every single day - this is the topic of most of our conversations. As we walk we are passed by bikers. The kind on bicycles. Some pulling trailers. This looks like a great idea to us, well, me anyway. Our wheelchair isn't going to make another hundred miles. The wheels had the tread worn off in the first week and the wheels are now 1/4 to 1/2 inch smaller then when we began. Pushing it is also leaving Morton feeling twisted and sore in his shoulders and back. I know that even though I try to push it sometimes, it really wears me out. So on top of carrying his pack, he's forced to push mine. Again, when we were planning our trip, our "stuff" would be in the motor home...now, we have it all with us. Bicycles had been on our drawing board early in the planning stages, but we liked the thought of walking. Slower, easier and able for almost any-one to do. We both really like walking. We just didn't think about carrying all our stuff as we walked, and some-times, when you are walking, it's impossible to get a foot even on the road, let alone share it with the cars. Could we switch up and move to bicycles now? Would it work? What would the pros and cons be? This has been our conversation for the last week. Morton is very against the idea. The only thing he likes about it is the fact that we can keep moving, even with blisters. He also likes that we can get out of a dangerous situation easier on a bike then on foot. Though I always just talk about the positive things on here, walking can be very scary. When people stop, you are at their mercy. With the two men that had already trailed us on foot, we were both a bit scared. And lets face it...who am I going to be able to outrun? No one. But on a bike, we can cover between 40 to 50 miles in the same amount of time it takes us to walk 6 to 8 miles. We can still walk when we are at places that have trails and a safe place to store our gear. But would it be the right choice? The real things to consider are that A: Our wheelchair won't cut it   B: I can't carry my pack yet   C: Going home is NOT an option   D: Safety has to be our number one concern.

Morton and I walked around the store with our stuff, knowing that before we knew it we would have to think about where to stay for the night. The walking/biking discussion would have to be put on hold. We were in a big city that neither one of us felt comfortable or safe in. Calling the tourist info center, they gave us the number of a hostel in the area. Things worked out that we were even able to get a ride to it from the lady that ran it, she was stopping by the store to pick up some extra tents for their outside camping area. Setting up camp at our first stay in a youth hostel, Morton and I feel safe here. Our tent is nestled inside a wall with other friendly travelers. There are showers and even free pancakes if you make them yourself in the morning. We are going to take today to decide what is next. We are looking at bikes and trailers. I'm going to try out riding bikes, which should be interesting considering the last time I was on one I was fourteen years old. Though rid-ing a stationary bike is great for me, how is my big behind going to take 5 to 6 hours on a bicycle each day? This should be answered today as we experiment at several stores. While we are deciding what way the walk/ride is going to proceed, remember that life is all about change.

Day 16 & 17 : January 16 & 17, 2007 Tuesday & Wed Florida City, Florida to Coral Gables, FL

Spending a night in a hostel was a new experience for me. I almost worked at one in Napoli, Italy, but have never stayed in one in my 43 years. We didn't actually stay inside the building, we used our tent in the back. A private garden shaded with large trees and a stone wall that kept out the bad people, Morton set our tent up under a coconut tree.

After the experience on the bus and being dumped in the city, Florida City, we had to find lodging. Now what I'm about to tell you is a true story. It actually happened that the hostel wasn't my first choice on where to stay that night. We first called a local church and see if we could camp in their yard or perhaps sleep in their hall. I had my son look up on the internet (in Pennsylvania) the number for a church. After dialing, a woman answered. I briefly explained who we are, what we are doing and asked if they could help us with a place to stay for the night. Now I know the woman was still on the phone, because every few seconds she would say, "Uh-huh", not sounding too impressed. Not that I was trying to impress her with the walk, we just needed a safe place to bunk for the night. Pausing to hear her reply when I asked the question, "Do you think you would be able to help?" the line went dead. I didn't lose signal. She had hung up. Looking at Morton, who was looking at me, I said, "We must have been cut off" and I redialed the number. The same lady answered, I started to apologize for being disconnected and she said, and I quote, "NO!" and promptly hung up.

This was a bit shocking. I wasn't asking for money, food, clothing, even a bath, I was just asking for a place that was safe for my husband and I to put up our tent for the evening. Raising my eyebrows and dropping my mouth wide open, I looked at Morton and then started to laugh. "She said NO and hung up on me!" Morton didn't believe it. He thought I was winding him up. "I wonder what her boss would think of that?" I asked Morton. "You mean the pastor?" said Morton. "No, her BIG boss" and I pointed up to the sky. We both just sat a few minutes in disbelief.

Then I called my son again. He was off work, busy at his computer and sort of happy to help. He found a few more numbers for me and one was the hostel. One a stroke of luck, Nicole, from the hostel, was coming by the store and would be able to give us a lift back. Excellent. Smiling, she walked right up to us and said she just had a few things to pick up. We waited and then all rode back to the lovely old building together. Forget "youth" hostel, this place had all ages there. It was a really nice place, clean, cheap laundry and the staff were kind and organized. Morton made our camp and I jumped on the laptop and set at it. We found a place to get the bikes and trailers, but it was 19 to 20 miles away...time for public transportation. The next day we set off, on the bus, to our buy our bicycles. We lucked in to a sale and got two bicycles, two trailers designed for hauling children in and the bicycle pump for $440. Now we just had to ride them twenty miles back south to the hostel. It had been a long time since I rode a bike, what if I forgot? Morton and I figured that a "test ride" in the parking lot was in order. We positioned our bikes with the trailer hooked on and I leaned my bike over slightly and hoisted my leg over. It went over with no problems. A few months ago, this would have been impossible. I wiggled the pedal around to a good place to start from and went to get up and balance for my virgin ride. The trouble was, the trailer felt like training wheels of sorts. I lost my balance and tumbled over in slow motion. Trust me...it wasn't pretty.

Finding our way home to the hostel on the bikes was quite the journey. We forgot our water bottle at the store and I thought I was going to die from lack of liquid. Since we were racing the sun setting and didn't have lights on our bikes, we couldn't stop for much of a rest either. Maybe the bikes were a bad idea. Aaaahhhh, if only we had a set of instructions to follow. But then life wouldn't be as interesting, would it? Morton made a pit stop at a used car lot to ask if they had a water fountain or a soda machine. The salesman and a customer were in a heated argument (I guess used car salesmen will understand this!) and Morton was pointed to a machine. He decided to just buy a soda and get the heck out of there before bullets started flying. We downed the icy cold peach drink in record time and got back on our bikes. The sun was going to set and this was Homestead, Florida, time to ride faster. As we put the MBT's to the pedals (they work excellent on pedals, the cushion saves the pedal from digging in to the center of your foot) we knew we were fighting a losing battle. Stopping and calling our son James at HQ in Pennsylvania, he broke the horrible news to us, still six miles to go. That was it, we had to take the bus. But remember, we are on the tightest of tight budgets and Morton bought a soda! We had to count the change and we were 10 cents short of the fare we would need. Ten little cents! We couldn't really go on with night coming and no lights. Not only is it dangerous for being hit with a car, we could run over something that would give us a puncture and we have no flat tire kit.

On the trip north on the city bus to get the bikes, we saw a man using a bike rack on the front. We had to get on the bus and hope we could find someone with a spare ten cents. Is this crazy or what? The first driver that stopped was a bit rude, said, "They won't fit" and pretty much kept rolling. Morton was giving up and said, "Let's just ride!" But I wanted a bus...Morton didn't pay attention to just how bad of an area we still had to ride through. I didn't want to get mugged, hit with a car or run over a broken beer bottle (there have been dozens of them on the road so far) along the way. Waving my hand for the next bus, Morton was muttering under his breath about not having the ten cents and he didn't want to be a beggar. But at the moment, it was really our only option. This driver was not only helpful, he said to forget about the ten cents. He took us right to our door, and patiently waited as we loaded and unloaded all our things. He even told us to have a great evening! Customer service is what it's all about but you have to love your job to give good customer service, that bus driver obviously did.

Back in the sanctuary of the hostel, Morton pulled our big tarp over the bikes. We ate the last of our little tins of tuna salad on crackers. It is amazing really. You think I'd be starving, but the opposite is happening. I have to really tell myself to eat now. We had plans for setting out EARLY the next morning. Tuesday was going to be a good day. We could feel it. My backside was just a bit sore from the seat, which is actually more like a torture device. Thinking about it, the seat feels like a brick turned sideways that is covered with a piece of plastic cloth. The free-spirits at the hostel played the bongos in to the wee hours and in the early morning, the rain came. By our wake up time, the tent was drenched. The tarp covering our bikes was drenched.

Condensation had the inside and outside of the tent and tarp wet. We took the time to hang these up on the sunny line, so we wouldn't pack a wet tent. Good for the tent, bad for the time. About eleven am on Tuesday the 15th of January, we left the comfort of the hostel and headed north on US 1. We had the trailers loaded, but we were carrying a bit of excess gear now. The wheelchair and our backpacks had become superfluous. We needed to get rid of them and now my sisters house that was still three hundred miles north of us seemed way too long to wait. We decided that the first pack and ship place we spotted, we were going to post them to my mom's house. The extra weight is killing us and not just my body. Mom can use the wheelchair to visit places that don't have wheelchairs to borrow. She does really good with her walker and cane, but she does get tired out fairly easy.

Somewhere in Homestead, beside US 1, we spotted a shipping place. The girl inside was helpful and very chatty. The front looked like they were shut, because their shutters were pulled over. They had been broken into the night before. The thieves had stolen the computer and made a mess for someone else to clean up. We had to get boxes from various shops to pack the chair and backpacks. Her largest box wasn't big enough. Sheer determination and dooberizing (a made up Scottish word that means to MAKE something work) on Morton's part paid off, and an hour later we had a box to set up on the scales. 47.8 pounds. Hmmm, almost the same amount of weight I have lost since we started training for the walk. The box took two of us to lift to the counter. As the scales weighed it, the thought crossed my mind that my body, my poor abused body, had been lugging this weight around. Even more shocking, I still have FOUR of these boxes attached to me! With two-hundred pounds still to lose, my mind was reeling at the thought of all this weight pulling down on me. Why did I wait so long to understand what my excess weight is doing to me?

Morton and I were glad to lighten our load and we headed north, pushing the bikes for a while and chatting. The one thing about the bikes that I don't like is that we can't really talk on them. Morton and I are hoping to pick up some sort of walkie-talkie things that are headsets, but they are a few months and a few hundred t-shirt sales, away. Budget, budget and more budget! Before we knew it we saw the brown sign that marked the upcoming, *Coral Castle*. Now anyone who hasn't been here and doesn't know about this place, please visit their website and learn. This remarkable place was built by one man. A little man at that! As we entered, the man at the gate pointed me in the direction of Sylvia. We had been emailing and had even thought of camping out in the castle, but that will have to wait for another time. Sylvia invited me in to her office and asked lots of questions about the walk. She was so warm and wonderful and not only let us look around the castle, she even gave us each a t-shirt and posed for a picture with me. Like kids on their field trips, Morton and I parked our bikes and headed inside. Thoughts had been on my mind about the trip. Is it the right thing to do? Will we make it the many miles? Can my body ever get use to that hideous seat? Lots of fears and doubts had been with me all morning. Plus, I was really missing home. Homesickness is something that I fear will grip me a lot during this journey. There is a life-sized cut out shape of the man, Ed, who built *Coral Castle* as soon as you come in the turnstiles. You push a button and listen to what he is saying to you about it. Now I'm just paraphrasing, and don't quote me (or Ed) on this, but he was talking about how people would look at his size, just five foot tall and 100 pounds, and they would almost tease him about how could anyone so little, cut and move rocks that weigh tons? My ears perked up and I listened closely. Ed was saying how you could do anything that you put your mind to and had the vision in your head. Seeing what you want to achieve in your mind's eye, then being willing to work for it, anything was possible. This is just what I needed to hear! Walking past the old stone where Ed use to collect ten cents (just the bus fare that I didn't have) from people wanting to see this curiosity, I entered this tropical wonder with my mind's eye focusing on everything that was going on all around me. While I snapped the pictures, listened to the remarkable tour guide and strolled around the grounds, it was all crystal clear. Everything would work out. The walk, now bicycle ride, is just my destiny, our quest and above all, our passion. It's our dream that we are willing to work for, walk for, cycle for and do whatever we need to do to see it through.

Leaving *Coral Castle* I found that all my doubts and questions had faded. Smiling, we mounted our bikes and headed north for the unknown. We were really hoping for a room for the night, but really just a safe place to pitch our tent would work. With no real idea where we were (somewhere on US 1 north) the loss of mile markers that we depended on in the Keys, we could only guess. Evening wasn't far away and the three motels we asked for rooms or a place to pitch our tent had all said "no". We knew there was nothing but city in front of us and we couldn't ride at night. My stomach started to do belly flips when we asked someone walking where the nearest motel or campground was. He told us at least 20 miles north. Morton and I had stopped on a crossroad to ask a man for information. Seeing off a side street a building that looked sort of like a church or a school, we figured we would ride back and ask about camping. Maybe seeing us in person they would take pity on us. After the first whole day on the bike I was soaked to the skin with sweat.

There was a school and a church. After speaking to different people, we were told we could camp at a house across the street, in the fenced back yard. Sanctuary! A lady and man came and unlocked the fence and we wheeled our bikes and trailers to our home for the evening.

About the third day of our trip in the Keys, we met Captain Steven and his wife Jennifer. They had us camping, using their shower, giving us ice water and making us the only homemade meal we have had since we started. I was thinking how nice it would be if we could at least have a drink of cold water, but we will never ask. Just like the ten cents that Morton didn't want me to beg for, we won't beg for food or drink either. As we set the tent up and got nestled down before dark, I was hoping, crazy hoping, that at least a cold drink might come out of the house. But it didn't. In fairness, the lady in the office had said we could camp there. The people in the house had nothing to do with it. They probably thought we were odd and different, I don't know. But what I do know is that now, learning what I have learned these last few wonderful weeks, I will never walk by a homeless person again without offering them food and water. You just don't know what their situation might be. I'm going to be a Captain Steven and Jennifer! *Let hospitality rule!* We fell asleep at 7 pm. Both exhausted, not really hungry, we had a few handfuls of trail mix, it was wet and horrible in the tent. We had to keep the fly sheet on in case of rain and the temperature in the tent was nearly unbearable. Morton grunted appreciation as I fanned him with the Florida state map I had picked up for free off a tourist rack.

Morning of January 17, 2007 One of the advantages to going to bed at 7 pm is that when you wake up at 5 am, you feel great! Most of the time. This morning we got up hot and sticky and sore. The seats and using all our new muscles on the bike had caught up to us. We needed to be out the locked gate at 6 am, so it meant an early tear down in the dark. Managing to get everything folded while it was soaking wet, only made us feel more uncomfortable. The heat of the day was starting and our clothes were wringing wet as we climbed on the bikes. Going to the bike path that runs beside US 1 and the buses only road, we soon discovered it was dangerous to go in the dark. We might hit a nail or the roadside broken glass that litters the lane. Pulling into a bus stop we sat on the cool concrete seats and ate our breakfast of warm water, cereal bar split between us and some trail mix. Oh for a shower or even a big mud puddle to splash around in.

There was a store in front of us, though how far we didn't know. We had seen it the previous day on the bus and then passed it again riding home with the bicycles. We needed to stop to get a tire patch kit to have onboard for our journey. As the sun came up we started out again, to discover that getting to the store at 7:10 am wasn't a great idea when they didn't open until 8 am. We sat on the sidewalk (again, be aware of who you walk past...we looked like we were down and outs but we aren't, well...not all the time!) and waited. Inside would be food for our food bag, a much needed bathroom and the tire patch kit. As the clock ticked by, we talked about how wild the drivers are to bikes. They pull out in front of you (knowing full well you will stop) they block the bike path while they are inching forward to cross the road and worst of all, they come so close to you they almost knock you off the bike. We looked at all our bruises, cuts, bites and tan lines and tried to get the time to go as quick as it could. We both wanted the bathroom, bad. Morton offered me some more warm water, was he CRAZY!? Finally the magic moment arrived and we were in, one at a time, to take care of business. They had everything except the tire repair kit. More cereal bars, more packs of crackers with peanut butter and 3 cans of chicken salad. I couldn't face anymore trail mix for the moment, next time we shop perhaps. Heading north we made really good time. We knew we wanted to get to Coral Gables if at all possible. Remember, we are riding the bikes with traffic and have to stop at red lights, stop signs, to keep from hitting the sides of cars that go in front of us and other thrills of the road. We won't reach top speed on these roads. As we ride we pick up the patch with Morton's last $3.00 in his pocket from a car re. The food bag is stocked for a few days and we will get water somewhere. We pass lots of nice looking places to eat. Smells float to our noses and for the first time in ages, I wish we could go in and have a hot meal. But not today. Stopping by a park for our noon rest, Morton and I enjoy the shade. The picnic table we make as our home for the next hour (the sunny part of the day) is new and the wood smells nice. Butterflies float around us and the large tree that is giving us shade is also the home of lizards. Lots of lizards. The old me would scream and run, the new me just watched the show. My socks are drying in the sun and life is good. We share a warm bottle of water and my MBT's become my pillow for a few moments, tucked under my head as I lay on my back on the picnic table.

Each day our biggest concern has got to be shelter for the night. After last night, we are both hoping for a room. Any room. Any size. The shower could really just be someone's hose in their back yard. Just a safe place to sleep and some water to splash away some of the sweat in. Our needs are very simple.

We rode up and down the sidewalks, me in the front and Morton following behind. I turn to look at him and discover how hard it is for me to look backwards and not kill myself. I am still too fat to try to look under my arm like the pro's do, but give me a few months. My eyes spot a sign for a hotel and I yell "STOPPING" and head in with Morton on my tail. They are all full, the man says. Sorry. So we ride. Maybe we will reach the beach and will find a lovely spot to camp. Maybe. As I'm thinking about the traffic, the smells of food of every description cooking and thinking of where we are going to sleep, Morton lets out a scream. I stop the bike to look back. His trailer has tipped off the sidewalk and is out in the road. He's trying to get it sat back up and traffic is buzzing so close to him. I kick down the kickstand and run as fast as my fat legs will carry me to him. The important thing is that he is safe. We get him off the road and check for damage. Morton is looking at what made it tip, the broken curb of lawsuit fame. This was a close call. Lecturing Morton, who is telling me that bikes have as much right on the road as a car, I try to get it through his head that not all drivers really care. It is hard work trying to find courteous drivers, but we all think we are. Morton needs to know that never, ever, ever, can you step out on the road. Ever. This was me being scared and protective. I was just so thankful that he wasn't hurt.

In a few miles we spot something that might work for a room for the night. A hospital. Perhaps if we talk to someone we could sit/sleep in a waiting room. Maybe get a shower in a room that wasn't being used. The trouble was, it was on the other side of the very busy highway. Time to call our connection in Pennsylvania for a phone number. Don't worry, we are all with the same phone company and we get unlimited calls to each other....budget remember! The number I was given by Graeme just rang and rang. Even though this hospital was just a few hundred yards away, we didn't want to take the bikes over. Traffic was getting a bit crazier as people were heading home. Neither one of us wanted to cross the street and leave the other behind. So we got on our bikes and kept going. Whoever said "Good things come to those who wait" is a genius! Spotting the sign for the *Holiday Inn at the University of Miami*, we headed in, parking the bikes side by side in the check-in area. Morton waited outside and I went in to ask about a room for the evening. Stepping in the cool lobby, I looked back at Morton. He was hot and in the sun. What have I gotten my husband in to? He is from Scotland for goodness sake, they never have weather this warm there. Walking up to the counter, a young lady, Lizbeth, smiled and listened to what I had to say. She would have to ask someone and see about this. This is a very busy time of the year for them and they didn't have a lot of vacancies. She asked if I would mind waiting. It was a delight to wait on a chair in the cool. Morton sat a bench in the shade outside, ever vigilant over the bikes. While I was waiting a man and his wife arrived to check in. The man was older and the first thing that struck me were his pale blue "soft" jeans. My dad always wore these. I could hear my father's voice saying that he was having a hard time finding these jean anymore. For a moment, the memory of my dad and the realization that he's gone forever hit me like a truck. My heart hurt and felt empty. My eyes stung with tears. Taking the American Diabetes bandanna that says "Every 21 seconds someone is diagnosed with diabetes" on it, I wipe the tears in my eyes. I don't want anyone thinking that I'm crying at the thought of having to spend another night in a tent with no shower. Just then I look up and Lizbeth is smiling and nodding at me. She is waving me over. My heart soars higher then the planes my dad flew once upon a time. Almost running I thank her over and over for her kindness. We are getting a room. A real room. Now I'm sitting here, showered, using their free wireless to upload pictures and videos and catch our visitors up on our last couple of days. Sometimes life is perfect. This is one of those times.

The bikes are getting us further, the seat is cushioned with a little pillow that I put on it with a bungee cord we found beside the road and we won't stop. Like Ed back at Coral Castle, our dreams are going to be our reality...just give us a few years.

Day 18: January 18, 2007 - Thursday - *Holiday Inn, University of Miami*, Coral Gables, Florida to Miami Beach, Florida

Setting off in good time, the first part of our morning was glorious. We rode over pink sidewalks that zig-zagged through palm trees and flowers. It felt almost like we were at an amusement park. Shades of *Mr. Toad's Wild Ride* were stamped all on the feeling of the ride. My mind was thinking back to when I was a kid and my family would come to Florida in the winters. We had a little house in a little development that we would rent out for a week at a time when we weren't using it. My dad would always come in, usually on a cold Pennsylvania Friday, and announce to my family that we were going to head south. The station wagon would be packed in record time, we would gather our own clothes and things we would need for the thousand mile car ride, and we'd be off. Usually we would leave in the evening and be in Florida the next afternoon. My dad didn't believe in hanging about on I-95. He liked to get there, fast.

Once we arrived it felt strange for a few moments. You could be outside with no coat on. The orange blossoms were sometimes in bloom to make the air sweet and exotic. There would be just enough time for my brother and I to throw our things in on our bunk beds, then we would have to make the hard choice between going fishing with dad or staying at the house with mom and riding our bikes. Depending on what the weather was like, we would usually go fishing. But when we would be at the house, the bikes were never still. They were a couple of old bangers that had rust on them, loose seats and you had to make your first stop the 7-11 to get air in the tires. We would get just enough money in our pockets to get a treat as we filled the tires. A Slurpee (something we never got out in the country in Pennsylvania) and a bag of something crunchy and salty...maybe Taco Chips, and we were the happiest kids on the planet. Dodging cars and keeping on the sidewalks, we would ride for hours exploring the roads in the little community. This same feeling came back to me this morning. I was 10 again.

For anyone who isn't in Miami, let me tell you...the city is "Under Construction" everywhere you look. Cranes dot the skyline and the street in front of you. Machines roar, dust is made, sidewalks are sprinkled with orange cones and riding a bike is a bit of a nightmare. Since we are wider than a regular bicycle, we are hesitant to use the busy street. Instead we keep to the paths, walking our bikes through the parts that you can't ride through, dropping down over curbs that would stop a wheelchair in their tracks and the clock for the daylight hours is ever ticking. Still the black clouds are far away and the day is perfect weather for riding and walking. At one point, the sidewalk turned to leaves and grass and then just stopped at a pink wall. We looked at each other, looked at the 4 lanes of traffic whizzing north and south and knew what we had to do. Lifting our rigs down on the fraction of the road's edge, we literally stepped out in front of non-stop traffic and set off. We went as fast as we could, me in the front (since I'm the slow one) and Morton getting the brunt of the danger. Cars would come so close they felt like they were brushing us, horns blew at us, people screamed things out the window, but we had no choice. **SHARE THE ROAD**, for pity's sake!

At the end of this one mile stretch I saw the alien. A real alien, not like Morton, my alien husband from Scotland. This guy was about twenty feet tall, green, many eyes and was wrapped around a giant monkey. I had to stop and get a picture because no one was going to believe this image without a photo to back it up. It was the sign for the exhibition on at the Science Museum. We toyed with the idea of going in and having a look around. The time was still good and we had came further than what we hoped for. Looking in, we spied picnic tables in the shade. We were going in. Shady seats when you are living on a bicycle are too tempting to pass up. The next pedal around on my bike and my chain snapped. I said some words that I won't type here and so did Morton. He looked at it, turning his hands black with grease. "I think I can fix it." he said. Pushing the bikes to the shade and picnic tables Morton started dooberizing the chain. Fast and furious Morton became a bicycle ninja. At one point, I even saw a piece of string he had found beside the road being used. I helped him locate his tools and set off to see if I could borrow a yellow pages to look for a bike shop in the area. Leaving Morton to try his best, I entered the cool museum. The people inside were helpful and before long I was calling bike shops, explaining where we were, what we needed, could someone drop a chain off...etc. My first question to each shop I called was, "Are you near the Science Museum?" since I didn't know the area. The one man asked why I wanted to know that, then became very unhelpful and told me not to waste his time...he thought I was SELLING something! Whatever happened to customer service? After 30 minutes I decided that there needs to be a AAA for BIKES! Someone do this, you can make a lot of money. If you think about it, what DO you do when your bike breaks down? If you do this idea and make big bucks, remember dear old Priscilla shared it with you and maybe spot me a free membership. Morton was now in the full sun, the shade having slid across the lush green lawn he was working in, and he was covered with sweat. Laying down, not caring about ants, he was attacking the chain with *brute force and ignorance*, as he likes to say. He said he was having no luck. I thought we might have to ask for a place to pitch our tent or spend the night in a museum...might be fun. Going back inside to find a bathroom, I struck up a conversation with a really nice guy at the ticket counter. We talked about the site, the journey and the possibility of spending the night in the museum. After 15 minutes, I went back out to see Morton packing away his tools and wiping his hands. There was also a big grin on his face. "Fixed, but I don't know how long it will last." Morton said. We decided to give the aliens a miss and rode on, towards the beach. Not shifting gears on the bike with the bad chain, we headed north and then east. Through the city under massive construction, dodging cars, road work and a whole hot dog, laying in our path. Actually, the hot dog looked pretty good, but we just kept riding.

There is a big bridge that you have to cross to get to Miami Beach and A1A. It's tall and long and loads of people must throw bottles out of their car windows as they are coming or going from the beach.

We were walking the bikes up since we didn't want to strain the chain, and we were treated to a nice breeze and a playful dolphin that was swimming below us. Glass crunched below our shoes and bike tires. At the top we decided to ride down, slowly. I was trying to work out weight and mass and movement in my head and knew that if I just let my bike fly I would be hitting 70 m.p.h. at the bottom of the bridge, and who knows how or when the sidewalk is going to end here. It was nice not having to use the pedals. Gently pulling back on the brakes to keep from hitting warp speed, I nervously enjoyed the ride, stopping at the bottom to catch our breath. When we started off again, I stopped right away. My front tire was flat. Pancake flat. Morton pumped it up and we tried to laugh about our second bit of bad luck today. The tire seemed to hold and we rode. Crossing a long stretch of fast cars and semi-sharing the road with them, we were almost at the beach when we stopped for a breather. The tire had been holding but it did look like it could use a little more air. Morton pumped it up and then looked around the wheel. As he brushed away a little rock, a loud hissing sound started. We both watched in horror as the tire went flat. The rock he had just brushed away was really a piece of glass that had been sealing the puncture. Morton said he could patch the tire but it might be a real pain in the neck getting the wheel off the rim. What else could we do except push the bikes on the flat? I sat with my butt on this 2" bit of pipe that was guard rail. Looking at Morton I spotted a Coast Guard sign behind him. I had a plan! I would call the station and see if they had a 7 x 7 foot of grass for us to camp on.

Graeme, my son-in-law, didn't answer, so I phoned my sister. She found me several numbers and I started trying to reach this station. Finally, after speaking with a helpful woman at another station, she told me the right number and who to ask for. Crossing my fingers I dialed and explained my heart out. The man asked if I was in the service. No, but we are part of the *President's Fitness Council,* I explained. My son was in the Army, my dad was in the Army Air Corps and then the Air Force...even stationed in Miami beach in WWII. This didn't cut it, there was nothing he could do, good luck and happy trails. After all, we just might be terrorists. Sigh...what has happened to us America? Have the terrorists actually won?

Morton used his dooberizing skills nicely and proved to be the perfect man to have on this crazy adventure. The flat was fixed and he was wiping his hands off on a rag he had found roadside. Just then we heard a loud boom and a car stopped four feet away from us. Two young girls had just gotten a flat and landed on our doorstep of the moment. Winding the window down and disregarding any formal greeting, the passenger asked, "Do you guys know how to change a tire?" I thought of my own daughter and her best friend out in the car and this happening. I promptly volunteered Morton and his services. Their trunk was full of stuff, their spare seemed to be welded in place, their jack was the world's worst, but after 15 minutes or so, Morton had their tiny tire on and they were off. The operation had taken place in the right lane at a red light and there were so many people who were screaming at us for having the nerve to get a flat in this location. Calm down people...the next time it might be you!

We continued in to the Art Deco area of South Beach, high dollar area, and started doing the horrible task of trying to find a free place to stay. Condos, businesses and hotels were all that was around. After hearing, "My manager is gone for the day and I can't say yes" about ten times, it was dark. Morton and I started pushing the bikes because we didn't want to get in trouble or hit, riding at night. Spotting a chain motel, we went in and new that we would have to just pay for a night. The man at the desk gave us the best rate he was able to and said we could talk the the manager in the morning about comping it for us.

Day 19: January 19, 2007 - Friday - Miami Beach, Florida to Hollywood Florida

Exactly 4:30 this morning, we woke to a screaming man in the hall. He was drunk, banging on the door and his wife or girlfriend was refusing to let him in. His argument was that he had paid for the room and all his belongings were inside. She wasn't buying any of it. Morton, still not use to the fact that people carry GUNS in America, shouted at him to bloody well shut up. I pushed Morton and asked if he wanted to get us killed. Of course I said it in a whisper. The voice in the hall stopped for a brief moment and then right across the hall, the man began pounding on a strangers room. See, I told Morton, he's going to kick the wrong persons butt for telling him to bloody well shut up. Morton whispered "Sorry" and the drunk kept pounding. It seems he wanted the man inside to call someone and get him a new place to sleep for the remainder of his night. He had been out partying and the lady waiting wasn't going to take the bolt off the door. He kept yelling and pounding, but I didn't want to make a peep. Finally he started screaming, "FIRE!" and banging on all the doors. By this time he was being so loud, I couldn't take it anymore and called the front desk. After all, we didn't get a free room here, we had to actually pay for this and at a rate that is killing our monthly budget. Security consisted of two guys who told him to get out. He argued at first about his clothes being in the room and he had paid for it, but then went along fairly quiet. After that fifteen minutes of weirdness, sleep couldn't be found again. I just laid there for a while hoping I could sleep for another hour or two, but gave up and started working. We are disappointed that the press in Miami didn't even return our emails about interviews. I don't know about you, but I think a 390 pound woman on a journey like this is something that you really don't hear about every-day. There must be loads of breaking news that local that takes priority...maybe before we are out of this area I'll get the chance to watch and see what's going on. Maybe Miami doesn't want to see a fat lady walking or on a bicycle. Maybe there is no one in Miami that is overweight. Maybe the only news they show is bad news.

As we ride today we are taking our share of the road. It makes the ride go faster, but there are still red lights that we seem to catch. Construction is as plentiful beachside as it is on the mainland. And I'm sorry to say, broken beer bottles are big hazards all along the edge of the streets. Green glass seems to be the broken bottles of choice, but maybe they just stand out more. Right across from a mega condo they are working on, Morton shouts my name from behind. He has a flat on a rear tire. By the time we are done with the journey, it will be interesting to see just how many punctures he repairs. This is number two officially.

Strolling down to the beach for some pictures as Morton flips the bike over and sets to work, I see back over the miles from where we have came. Buildings that were giants when we were riding in front of them are now the size of blueberries. People are stretched out on the beach enjoying their day. A lifeguard tower sits still. I wonder who we'd have to ask to sleep in one of those for the night.

The manager at the place we stayed was of no help with comping the room. We had to pay the rate of $89. (a special rate mind you, normal was $159.) for the night, but with taxes, the room was $101. That is going to kill our budget. We didn't want to rent a room, trust me. This is the first we have rented since the start. We had no choice. There are signs posted everywhere prohibiting camping or even sleeping in your car. Beaches and parks everywhere, but not a place to camp.

Morton has the tire fixed and we go about 1/2 mile up the road. The road seems to have been going uphill slightly ever since we have left Miami Beach. Maybe it's just an illusion. So here we are 1/2 mile north of Morton's flat and we spot a fire station. I yell "STOPPING" and pull over. Just then a car gets a flat tire right beside us again. Is this going to be a regular thing on the journey? This time it is an older lady and man. They have a handicap sticker on their car. Morton knows he is going to be changing another tire. He walks to the car to volunteer and they only speak Spanish. They probably wonder where Morton is from. They look at me to translate and I try speaking slower in English. It doesn't work. A few hand gestures of a jack and a tire has Morton bewildered. The man is shaking his head no and waving his hands. Morton returns to our bikes and I talk him into going into the fire station and asking for a spot on their lawn to pitch our tent. I tell him they might take pity on him being from Scotland, stranger in a strange land and all. He returns in less than five minutes shaking his head no. The tire is being changed by two construction workers who do speak Spanish. We pedal on and leave them to it.

At this point we are really torn between our stomachs and our desire to get a room for the night. You have to speak with the manager to get a free room, but this is Friday and they all will be going home early. We stop at some big chains, get lots of run arounds and people saying to leave a number and we'll get called back on Monday. We will be 50 miles north of here by then. It just sort of shows me that they really aren't listening to what I was saying. The one lobby I walk in, the man actually laughed at me when I told him we were on a 16,000 mile journey. He eyed me up and down and laughed and said, "You?" Now it never ceases to amaze me how fast we are to see other peoples problems crystal clear. Hoping that he was going to give us a room, I couldn't say to him that I can lose weight, and *AM* losing weight. He'd have to pay money to get his hair back. He also looked like he never said no to dessert. But I kept quiet. No room from the rude man, we kept going.

The only good thing about going in so many hotels and motels begging for rooms is, we get to talk to the people there about what we are doing. Some are nice enough to even write down our site and promise to visit. The bad thing is it takes up so much precious time while it's daylight. The drawback of not having any pace car or camper with us. At the mercy of the road and can only go as far as daylight allows.

We continue north, finally coming to Hollywood. We've passed so many houses, hotels, condos and places that we could have slept. Once while we were stopped eating our cereal bars for lunch in front of a club marked "members only" we had a security man stop to ask if we were going to be sitting there long. You could tell by his face and manner that us sitting there was bothering him. We both said "no" at the same time and he grunted and drove off. Oh the life. It was a public bench and we weren't even thinking about crashing into his "members only" club, even though they did have acres of lawn we could have camped on. It was going on 5 pm and we knew that we had to get serious on the room. Camping isn't an option since it is illegal and we don't want to start knocking on doors or buzzing big gates to ask for lawn space. So we turned down a side street when we spotted a little place by the ocean. Old style rooms, mini cottages, the sign said cheap rates, and a little handwritten "vacancy" sign gave us hope. If the big chains were all saying NO, (Except *Holiday Inn at University of Miami* ... we LOVE THEM!) maybe a mom and pop would have a bit of pity. The young man listened and went to a back room to speak to someone about our plight. The rate was $79 a night and the best they could do was $59 a night. It was a take it or leave it sort of deal, it was their last room for the night.

Now I know I can live for about six months to a year on my stored fat, but Morton, he's having to wear his belt tighter now. We haven't been eating a lot and with spending so much on rooms, we will have to trim our food budget down. He and I both agreed we better take it.

Getting the key, we took to the task to getting everything inside the small room that was stuffed with a table and chairs, fridge, kitchen cupboards, tv with rabbit ears, microwave and two beds. The only way everything was going to fit was with Morton turning a bed on it's end to get the bikes in. The nearest place to get something to eat was in the distance. I remembered my daughter ordering pizza online. I searched and found and within 20 minutes we each had two slices of pizza, with two slices leftover for our breakfast.

Near sunset we took a little walk down to the beach. The wind had picked up and neither one of us had enough energy to even try to go swimming. Maybe further up the road we'll jump in the Atlantic. After all, it's going to be on our right side the whole way to Maine. The room left a lot to be desired. Old and shabby I can take, but moldy and dirty with giant bugs running around isn't nice. I felt like I should leave my clothes on in the shower and in the bed. We ended up rolling our sleeping bags out.

Day 20: January 20, 2007 - Saturday - Hollywood, Florida to Ft. Lauderdale, Florida

What a lovely ride we had today. Leaving our room early we decided we were going to start looking a lot earlier for a room today. The trouble is that there is a lot of tourists and locals that come to the beach for the weekend. There is also a big flower show in town as well as dozens of cruise ships that are in at the dock. We wish there were places that we could go and pitch a tent at. Seeing the whole big long beach makes you wish that the laws weren't so strict and we could camp there. My daughter suggested since you're not allowed to sleep there at night that we switch our days and nights around....sleep during the day and ride or walk at night. If it wouldn't be so dangerous, we'd consider it. But for the mean time, we just ride. I told Morton there wasn't hills in Florida, and there really isn't. What there is are bridges that go up and down. The going up we usually always push the bikes. We are still using the repaired chain and don't want to strain it. The coming down the bridge is equally tiring, we can't just let the bikes roll. We don't know when or how the path will end.

Of course there is always the danger of the broken glass, nails, bolts, pieces of cars, etc., to be on the look out for. It isn't just a case of a carefree bike ride. Today we stopped in a grocery store and I bought grapes and tangerines. We have to be careful with the fresh things we get. We never want to throw food away. Morton waits outside with our bikes and gear as I shop. There is no scale to weigh myself on. I'm a bit disappointed. Surely I must have lost at least 100 pounds in these last few weeks in sheer sweat alone.

Discovering there is a laundromat at the next shopping area, Morton wants to stop and do a wash. We both agree though that we have to keep going. We really have to try to get a free room tonight. Staying in places that we have to pay for is killing the budget. Laundry can wait. We stop not long after our shop to take a break on a bench and eat our lunch of grapes. As we are there we are approached by a man who asks if he can have one of the bikes. We say "no" of course, laughing I stand up and straddle the bike that he's closest to. If he's going to steal it, he's going to have to push my bulking body out of the way. The man goes over to Morton, still seated on the bench and says, "How about giving me a dollar for the bus then?" in a very angry tone. Morton didn't understand what he said and asked him to repeat it. The man seemed frustrated (I don't think he could understand Morton) and he waved his arm at us and walked on. Suddenly our shady bench on a side street felt less like a sanctuary and more like a good place to be mugged. What is happening to our country? Why can't you pitch a tent on the beach and not have to worry about being mugged when you are sitting on a bench eating some grapes in broad daylight? We vow to each other to send out emails to groups asking for their help as we go through their towns. We know there aren't enough hours in our day to do this, but it makes us feel a bit better. Cycling clubs, flower clubs, social clubs, churches, temples, organizations of every description...we just want a safe place to sleep at night that doesn't mean we have to go hungry for a week to pay for it.

We had to leave A1A to go over the US1 to bypass Port Everglades. This is a huge port that is filled with cruise ships of people who are now taking all the hotel and motel rooms. We want to get back to A1A and get a room, but maybe we should try on US1. It might not be as busy. But there was not a room to be had. Paying or otherwise. We really could get so much further if we weren't having to spend so many hours a day seeking shelter. I wish our original team of eight were out here, it wouldn't be as scary.

Calling my daughter for some computer work on upcoming rooms, I discover she's out with my son, his wife and her husband. The four of them are spending some quality time together and their voices and laughter make me feel like I'm on the moon. So very far away from them. Homesickness brings the tears to my eyes and I wonder what the point of this journey is. I didn't plan on it being this tough, resorting to begging for shelter on a daily basis and the real feeling of being homeless. Setting off over the high bridge that will bring us back to the beach and to A1A, we stop several times going up for Morton to take pictures. He's been using the camera a lot and likes it. There are huge cruise ships and one flying a British flag. It has the name "Hamilton" on the back in giant letters. This is from a place in Scotland, near Glasgow.
We both talk about how many lifeboats are on the ship. I think not enough to handle all the people that the big ship must carry. Didn't the shipping companies learn anything from the Titanic?

We finally find a room, beachside, but we have to pay again. We are really worried about this. I use the remainder of what I have on a gift card but it still isn't enough to cover the charges. But we have to have somewhere to sleep. Morton does the laundry in the hotel and I try to work on the site, send all the emails I need to send and upload pictures. We want to spend Sunday getting up the road as far as we can, so we don't stay up late. Morton is sleeping before me and I fall asleep thinking about tomorrow, what it holds, where we will be and all that waits in front of us. In the morning we do get a free (included in the cost of the room) hot breakfast. The trouble is, we really don't eat like we have done in the past. Exercise is taking away my appetite. Who would have figured?

Day 21: January 21, 2007 - Sunday - Ft. Lauderdale, Florida to *Holiday Inn,* Highland Beach, Florida

When I woke up this morning I never thought I'd get to see a family member today. We just had breakfast, set off and before long, this feeling just hit me to call my sister Cindy. It seems she was on her way south and was going to give me a call to see how far along we were. She had a book signing not far from where we were going to be heading for. When she was done, she'd call us and we'd go out to dinner. It was all happening so fast I couldn't believe it.

Covering the miles and using our maps, we guessed that we would have to do another 18 miles to meet with Cindy. Even a flat tire for the day didn't delay us long.
We flew by traffic jams, took very short breaks and drank our water fast. The day was hot and the sun kept shining out from behind the clouds. This was a day for smiles and celebrations. We were going to see family! The only real down side to the day was a group of people we passed heading for the beach in Lauderdale-by-the-sea. They sort of shoved and nudged each other to look at me and then they laughed. It didn't really bother me, not like it use to. Hey, I'm out here changing my life, not sitting on a sofa eating chocolate. Winding past houses that cost crazy money and boats that could feed small countries, we kept riding. We still get odd looks and I think some people still think we are homeless, which we are. Once we stopped by a park to ask about tenting for the night and encountered some very helpful people. A police officer who took the time to show us several places on a map but down the road a bit further than we were going today, a park ranger who brought us a glass of ice cold water and a few other people who were very helpful and kind. Perfect strangers. Cindy called when she finished with her business and I told her where we were. She was just going to drive south and meet us. We kept going north and for the first time I actually paid attention to the faces in the cars heading south, hoping to spot my sister.
I need to mount the camera on the front of the bike because you won't believe the ODD looks that I get. People point, stare, looked shocked, look surprised but everyone, and I mean *EVERYONE*...looks. I guess I do look like quite a site out there. Red in the face, brown arms and my body looks like someone who couldn't even lift her leg over the bike. I think, "If they only knew how far we were going, they'd really be shocked!" Let them look, it might shock them or shame them into changing their own lives.

Soon I spot my sister. She turns around as we find a spot to pull over. It all happens quick, we hug, I apologize for being sweaty. Her and I head north in the car, leaving Morton with the bikes. We are going to find a room and then go to dinner...sounds EASY! About a mile up the road is a place with a room. Fingers crossed, we might even get it comped in the morning. It feels weird leaving Morton beside the road, but there isn't any room in the car for all the gear, bikes and people. I'm glad when we get back to him and he's safe and sound. He tells me later he wondered just what he would do if I didn't come back. I guess I'm not the only one who is scared out here. Morton and I ride on to the room where my sister was waiting for us with her car. We store the bikes and gear and head off to find a place to eat. REAL food and seeing my sister in the same day...it feels like a holiday. Now my sister is on her way home, Morton and I are settled in for the night in a lovely *Holiday Inn*. All the ingredients for a peaceful nights sleep.

Day 22: January 22, 2007 - Monday - *Holiday Inn, Highland Beach* to *Queen's Lodge Motel,* West Palm Beach, Florida

This morning we got up early. Looking out our window at our fantastic view of the ocean, it was really tempting to go swimming. That's been a hard part of our trip so far, all the water and not getting in it a lot. This isn't a vacation and there are a lot of miles to cover on land. Maybe the next time we will swim around America. We had a few calls to make and some never ending computer work to get done before we started off. One of the calls was to the general manager of the Holiday Inn at Highland Beach who was wonderful and gave us the room for the night. It was a terrific way to start the day, saving our budget. With the WiFi at the hotel, it was tempting to keep working, but we knew that we wanted to make it to West Palm Beach.

As we rode our bicycles the storm clouds were gathering behind us. The sky was getting black as we pulled in to a landscaped park beside the ocean. We were going to just hold on until it passed over us, then continue with riding. Huddled under a pavilion, we hoped that we wouldn't hear thunder or see any lightning. When the rain started, it felt really nice and didn't last as long as we thought it might. Morton did a little adjusting to my brakes that were seeming to be stuck on, then we set off again.

We had two people shout out things today. The first was a lady who looked right at me and screamed, "CRAZY!" She was going the other way and I wasn't holding her up at all. The second was a man who again was going the other way. He screamed a dirty word that I won't trash up the page with. Let's just say he insulted me and a pig. When we stopped for our next break I asked Morton if he had heard the rude comments. He said he had and couldn't understand why they yelled. I told him the lady who screamed "CRAZY" must have either been well informed or she was the best judge of character I'd ever seen. The guy was just an unoriginal idiot. We had a little laugh about all the other things they could have yelled, inventing some seriously funny and original lines and then got back on the bikes refreshed by our own humour.

Anyone that has ever been on A1A might just think of the parts that are full of stores, shops and all the retail side of the beach. This wasn't the area we were riding in. There were huge pines with soft needles that made the road shady and welcoming. It looked like we were on a road in the middle of a forest for parts of the ride. Living in Scotland for several years, I have seen my share of castles. From the castles that people live in to the ruins of the castle on the edge of the famous Loch Ness, I really did enjoy them all. They are all so different. Testimony to a person's vision from a very long time ago, these fortresses are one of the things I miss the most about the United Kingdom, right after the people. Today it felt like I was looking at the castles of the future. Homes that were on the palace level with the stone palaces we've visited in Scotland. Maybe the sizes aren't as grand, but I imagine what they lack in square footage, they make up in levels of luxury. The royalty of olden times couldn't believe their eyes when they would look at the level of luxury that so many people live in today. The only draw back about riding through this incredible neighborhood is the lack of benches. You know I need my rests and the benches are a little slice of perfect when we find them. But there were none in site. No sidewalks either. Just miles and miles of homes you could spend hours looking at and wonder just how the people inside had made so much money.

We rode and rode until we got to the town of Palm Beach. Huge fountains, parks with artistic carved benches and me all sweaty and hot. Morton pointed and suggested sitting down for a moment in this surreal setting, but I declined. I just felt too smelly and fat to stick around. It was all so picture perfect I didn't want to get chased off for not being pretty enough. There was a point where we had to turn left to cross over to US 1. Of course this meant another bridge to climb up one side and then try to not let the bikes go to fast down the other side. As we were walking the bikes up, a very nice lady walking the tallest Yorkshire terrier I had ever seen, asked a question about what we were up to. Time slipped away as we told her what we were doing and she told us what she was doing. Just about twenty minutes we chatted, long enough to really feel like we had all really connected. She promised to write as Morton passed her a handwritten slip of paper that just said "www.LittleChanges.com". We get a real rush as we meet and talk to people about what we are doing. The excitement that they share with us about our adventure really does great things for us. As our new friend walked off, we rode off. I hoped I would hear from her online. *Ain't technology grand?*

Coming back to the mainland we negotiated the city streets and traffic. We had to take to the sidewalk as we headed up US 1 because there was no edge to the road and traffic was thick. Spotting a gas station we pulled in for the bathrooms and a cold drink. The public bathrooms are also where we fill our water bottles. There Morton started talking to a guy on a great motorcycle about the trip. He was really interested and Morton passed another little handwritten slip on with our website on it.

Passing great places to eat we knew that our priority had to be a room. Always seeking rooms or places to pop the tent up. The smells were so tempting and with our lack of real food during the day we were going to split a meal somewhere cheap, but nice tonight! Visions of delicious food danced in my head as the smells floated by on the warm breeze. It had been ages since we saw a motel and we were just thinking of try-ing to ask at the fire department. Morton said I would have to go in and ask, so I chose to keep riding. The fire departments all seem to say no, regardless of how hard you beg. There were a few motels on the other side of the road but I didn't feel like crossing traffic, which had gotten a lot heavier. Just then we saw the *Queen's Lodge Motel* ahead on the right and I shouted the key word, *"STOPPING"* to let Morton know not to run up the back of my trailer, which he does on occasion and blames me for not telling him. Parking the bikes in a space, I went inside to speak with the manager. She listened to why we were doing what we were doing and was kind enough to put us up for the night. She even put us in a ground floor room with a big sliding glass door that made it easy to get our bikes and trailers in to. Bliss! Getting shelter at the end of a day is such a wonderful blessing and thrill. The manager had lost her mother to diabetes. She has a sister that was just diagnosed. I told her about the statistic of every 21 seconds someone is diagnosed and we both agreed that a big part of the problem was people being unaware.

Coming inside the room I rushed into the shower. How I appreciate each and every drop of the water, set to as cold as I can stand it to cool my body temperature down a bit. It really is the thing that I miss the most out here. My legs were really sore from the days riding and I did some stretches to try to make them not knot up. Something that I want to share with you is the fact that I'm feeling so much better. Exhausted, yes. Tired, yes. Beat up by my bike, oh yeah. But I feel like I'm undoing all the years of damage I've done to my body. I've discovered the CURE for obesity! Eat smarter, exercise more.

Day 23: January 23, 2007 - Tuesday - *Queens Lodge Motel*, West Palm Beach to Hobe Sound, Florida

Great days happen! Today was one of them. This might have been the happiest day of our trip so far, even taking into account our bit of bicycle woes. We left our room in good time, the trailers still being packed from the night before. Hooking the bikes up to the trailers, I was away to turn the key in leaving Morton on his own. Even though Morton is a grown man, he's a bit naive when it comes to people around him. He doesn't understand that there are a lot of people who carry and use guns or knives in this country and might rob you for your broken Timex wrist watch. He is like the child who knows no strangers, he speaks to everyone. The night before a person told us to be careful in the area, which seemed odd since just a few miles ago we were driving past multi-million dollar mansions. But I guess you don't have to go far in this world to see social and economic differences as plain as the house on your block. Morton promised he would "be aware" as I took the key back, then hurried back to him. After all, we have to look out for each other and I'm very protective of my husband. He's the best in the world, so supportive and kind. The only downside is that he always looks grumpy (his natural expression) but I have to say, he's smiling much more now.

We got on the bikes and I cringed. My torture seat, even with my makeshift pillow I have bungee-corded around it for added fluffiness, isn't cutting it. It feels like it's made of concrete. Lumpy concrete with a few stones in it. I move around in the seat trying to find a spot that doesn't hurt to sit on. The bike wobbles as I try to make the adjustments. In a few miles my backside will be numb, so I just grin and bear it and peddle. We cross a drawbridge, a semi-scary thing. We like to push our bikes up because I'm too out of shape (though not for long) to ride. Looking through the metal grate you see down very far to the beautiful blue water below. Boats come and go and I hope that I don't trip up on the grate or get a shoestring caught in it. I also hope that the person sitting in the booth can see us and won't start raising the bridge while we are on it if a tall ship should sail along. Once we past the crest and take some pictures, we climb back on our bikes. Getting braver with each bridge we cross, I use the brakes less on the downhill and just let it roll. After all, we are out on the road so we shouldn't have to stop on a dime. The wind blows and flaps my sweaty wet t-shirt almost dry. The one bridge we come to has a power station below it. I think about all the times that we came to Florida as a child and my dad would love to fish right below the station. Something about the water being warmer or the fish being familiar with the noise of it, so it was easier to catch fish there. I wondered if dad had ever fished by this station.

We decided we were going to actually eat something today and I had my heart set on finding a taco salad. We passed a place about 9 am and I was still full from my cereal bar and the morning exercise. Oh well, we did get in to a grocery store and Morton did the shopping for a switch. I waited outside on a bench that really was concrete, but still 100% better than the thin torture-shaped bike seat. Coming out of the store with a bag and a box of food, I remembered that I forgot to warn Morton about buying too much. We are limited to what we can hold. He managed to get it all crammed in including a bag of oranges from California (he didn't know this was a no-no in Florida!), a bunch of green bananas, some new looking foods and several cup of noodles that he got at the bargain price of 29 cents each. Tonight, if we find hot water (or at least warm) we would eat them. Funny, but it sounded like a great meal.

Right after we had been to the little grocery store chain, I spied a big grocery store that has the giant scales in it. On impulse I pulled in. "Why are we stopping?" Morton asked. "I want to weigh myself and use their bathroom" I explained. Never before would I have even gotten on the scales in private, let alone in the front of a store. There wouldn't have been any amount of money to make me do it. Now I was jumping on them, anxious to see what was happening with my weight. The scale only goes to 300, but then there is a ten pound gap and it continues on. I know this from Key West. I got on and watched, almost as if the scale was in slow motion. It stopped at what would be 304 pounds, but you have to add 10. This couldn't be right, almost 30 pounds in 23 days? I stepped off, let it go back to zero and tried again. The same thing happened. I had lost 29 and a half pounds. Smiling and floating outside to Morton I told him my weight. Again, this is something I would have NEVER done before. He had no clue that I weighed 440 pounds in May of 2006. Morton ran in and discovered he weighed 188. He was 199 back in Key West. No wonder he is now needing his belt to keep his shorts up. I know I said I wanted to wait until February 1st to weigh in, but I'm so glad I got on them. I needed the scale to tell me what my body was saying. I never thought it would be a good thing to be happy about weighing 314 pounds, but I know I'm just going down from here. Soon I'll crack the 200's - somewhere I haven't been in many moons.

As I was peddling up an incline it felt even harder then normal. I missed a stroke and the bike almost came to a stop. It felt as though my brakes were on. I looked for a safe place to pull in and saw a little fresh fruit and veg market. Added bonus, a bench! We took a space in the parking lot that really wasn't a space big enough for a car and Morton set about trying to fix my bike and get the brakes unstuck. "It feels like the brakes are sticking." I explained. Morton lifted the back tire off the ground and tried to spin it. No joy. "Hmmmm" he thought out loud and began to mumble about tools and not having the right ones. I took the camera and phone and went to park my backside on the bench and try to contact a lady with the Florida State Parks in Tallahassee. We have learned to make the most of our down time on the bikes to keep the day moving along. Voicemail was all I was able to get, so I just sat there watching Morton work on the bikes. He gets lost in his own little world as he works magic on them. Morton wasn't needing my help and I've learned to really just step in when I'm needed. He has a specific process that he does when he's fixing something and I didn't want to be in the way, plus the lure of a bench is something oh so tempting to me now. As he was making his final adjustments, he needed me to steady the bike. I held the handlebars as he experimented with how quick the brakes would grab. Just as he was putting the finishing touches on his handiwork, a couple came over to us. They asked if we needed help and we all fell right into a conversation. They felt like friends in an instant and before we knew it, twenty minutes had passed. Donna and Gary wished us a safe journey and we said goodbye and headed on our way. They had offered us use of a washer and dryer, showers and had even given us money towards food. They had also told us some nice things to see along the way to the state park.

Morton and I rode and talked, the best we could, about how kind and generous they were. We had talked about everything from diabetes to life in Scotland and how they should visit. It was great, but short. It is the kind of conversation that makes you think of what a world it would be if everyone were like this couple. Talk about the easy solution for world peace! These people were really treating others, perfect strangers, as if we were close friends. Riding was less sore, I hadn't taken any pain pills today. Morton offered the suggestion that maybe with less fat on my backside, I was riding on bone. I assured him I had at least another 100 pounds plus to go before this could be the case. The fact is that two of my eighteen bruises and black-and-blue marks on my body, are located on my backside, courtesy of the seat. Truth is, it's my weight on the seat that is the problem. The only thing I can do about that is to lose it.

At a lovely bit of housing and shopping area, we spotted *Wendy's*. Pulling on to lush, thick dark green grass, Morton crossed the street to get our order. We spread our tarp out and had a roadside picnic. A late lunch of one of my favorite things, but I couldn't eat it all. Morton had to finish it for me. It feels so good to feel full! Packing up we rode on for the park. Up some steep hills, down the other sides, passing the turtle station we wanted to visit, but there were very dark clouds gathering on the horizon and we wanted to set up camp before the rains came. Finally we spotted the brown side ahead that announced the state park and we rode even faster. It was a left hand turn so we moved through traffic to cross US1. Going downhill in to the park after the long time in the saddle felt excellent. We parked the bikes and headed in to the ranger station to get our space assigned.

As I was getting ready to head out a lady who worked there said, "Someone was here looking for you and they said they'll be back." Now the only people who knew where we were was my daughter and her husband and the couple we had met earlier. I smiled and knew that it must be Gary and Donna going to drop in to say "hello!" Telling Morton about it (he had waited with our bikes) he agreed it must be them. We rode on to our site and set about setting up. Morton is becoming the tent expert too, though he says it goes up differently each time. I had the laptop out and began working on the website, when a pickup truck pulled in. Sure enough, it was Donna and Gary. Not only were they coming by for a visit, they brought their grill, a cooler full of food and drink and chairs. We had the most amazing evening with new found friends that a person could ever hope for. Gary did the grilling and Donna had made green tea with mango (my favorite drink). Donna also gave me wonderful tips for my pregnant daughter, Sarah. Being a baby nurse, she has this kind and caring nature that is so incredible. Donna also makes jewelry using gemstones and presented Morton and I each with a necklace that contains a circle gemstone. The circle is a symbol of our journey and the gemstones she chose were things she thought would help us. Mine is calming. Just what I need while riding in heavy traffic! As the evening went on, it really did feel like we were visiting friends we hadn't seen in a long time. We traded information and stories and I hope that we keep in touch. They are responsible for giving us something that money can't buy and is seldom duplicated...a perfect evening. The storm clouds had disappeared and the stars and moon were out. Donna pointed out the lovely moon. It's the kind I call a "Cheshire Cat" moon. Just a slice of a smiling moon looked down at us as we ate and drank and enjoyed the beautiful Florida evening almost as much as the company. Saying goodbye was almost like saying goodbye to my sister the other night. It was a bit sad, but you hope that your paths will cross again in this life. We can't say thank you enough to people like this we are meeting. Words haven't been invented to sum up how we feel when we come across these human angels. Now it's off to bed, with leftovers of our feast for breakfast, and a day of stopping and resting in front of us. No matter where you are, we wish you a friendship encounter like this with people that were just strangers a few hours ago.

Message from Morton:

Hi there...hmmm where to start? I have to say I'm not the best at writing. The last few weeks have been amazing. We have met a huge amount of wonderful helpful people. We have been having a few teething problems with the bikes, problems that under normal conditions and access to a tool box and a vehicle wouldn't be as bad. Having a chain come apart with only pliers a spanner and nuts and bolts to use as clamps was a perplexing problem but as usual a modicum of brute force and ignorance helped me through. The chain is now back together and will hopefully stay that way because without a link joiner I'm stuck.

The bottom bracket slackening off without a C-key wasn't as big a problem more of an irritation to fix. Spanner (*wrench* in American-English) as a hammer and pliers in the turn notch always works wonders (I at least paid some attention to my Dad's *You haud it and I'll Daud it* School of engineering- haud meaning hold and daud meaning hit- and Scott from the print factory....*if you don't have the correct tool try a hammer!!!*). The pedal coming slack was a more major annoyance though...you need a socket to tighten it properly and the thread hasn't been made eccentric on that side, so any slight movement makes it naturally work its way loose. A gentleman called Rudi kindly turned his car round and stopped to loan me his tools to fix it but even after tightening it really hard it still came slack again. Fortunately Gary who came to visit us with his wife Donna had tools in his truck....we have adjusted the fit with a hammer and tightened it with the socket now....hopefully that will have done the trick, if not I'm at a loss what to do to keep it from slackening off again. One repair I'm mightily sick of is punctures. I wouldn't mind if they were from stones thorns or bits and pieces fallen from cars or from accidents on the road but they all so far are from broken beer bottles thrown into the road or left along with other rubbish by irresponsible fishermen or day-trippers. *PLEASE TAKE YOUR RUBBISH HOME WITH YOU OR PUT IT IN A RUBBISH BIN!!* Cheerio the now Morton

Day 24: January 24, 2007 - Wednesday - Hobe Sound, Florida

Trying to not get too excited about a real day off to do nothing, we polished off last nights leftovers for our breakfast. There would be no breaking camp...let the tent stand. It needed a good airing out after being packed away damp from our stay in Florida City. Morton and I studied the maps of the state park we are in and saw miles of trails for bikes and people, but nae cars! Nae is Scottish for no. It looked like paradise. We were also impressed with the variety of wildlife that is around here. We had woken up to a squirrel sitting perched on a palm tree outside our tent, nibbling away at something. Our first wildlife spotting for the day! Heading off on just our bikes and leaving the trailers tarped in case the rain came on, Morton and I explored. We both said our son-in-law Graeme should be here for this part. There was a sign about no pets beyond this point because of the alligators. The bikes ride so wonderful without the hundred pound trailers holding them back. I felt like I might actually hit warp speed going down a little hill. It was like being a kid again and the adventure led us to a pavilion that is perched on a natural ridge. It doesn't look out of place in this natural setting. Large timbers make up the roof and strong wooden posts look like it will be here in a hundred years. The floor is smooth concrete and there are seventeen very sturdy wooden picnic tables inviting you to bring your family and friends and enjoy it. Bathrooms in the corner and electricity everywhere, make it the perfect place for me to set up an outside office for the day.

There is the email to get through, the site updates, the press interviews, there are a few newspapers and television stations following us on a regular basis now and the never ending task of taking care of my pictures. Morton takes the camera and goes down a trail looking for some of the critters he has read about. I warn him about poisonous things that bite and he gives me as wave and keeps going. On the island that is Great Britain, at the top where Scotland sits, there aren't any dangerous critters. You can poke around in the heather, the fields, the forests and you don't have to worry about getting stung, bit and killed. Just maybe attacked by the midges. Sort of a tiny biting flying insect. But Morton is a long way from Scotland here in south Florida. The ranger told him about a family of alligators living under a bridge by the river and I'm worried Morton's natural curiosity will get the better of him. But he's out of site now and my mother hen warnings are out of his head already I'm sure.

Working on the computer outside is so wonderful. The breeze, the sky which is getting a little cloudy is always changing. It's a great space to work in. You could do great things in this pavilion looking over the natural landscape. I wish I had my paints and easel with me. But there is only so much you can carry in a bike trailer or backpack. Morton has been gone for about 45 minutes and I start to think of the family of alligators. Like coming between a mother bear and her cubs, I imagine a mother alligator would be pretty protective too. Looking out over the trail he went down, I can't see any trace of him. Keeping busy with my postings and the PR side of the walk (help me out by contacting your newspapers, Oprah, tv stations, etc) I forget about Morton and the gators and get lost in my work. Jumping almost out of my skin when Morton shouts, "Look at this!" I have a fast flashback of my little brother years ago scaring me with a snake. Surely Morton isn't daft enough to pick a snake up. Leaping up from the picnic table with a considerable amount of speed, Morton is on top me. He's only holding the camera, not a snake. Talk about relief. He flips through the pictures on the camera and explains what he has captured in pictures. My heart is still pounding a little from the fright that he didn't mean to cause. He had no luck with seeing alligators.

Trying to hurry up with what I am working on, Morton sets out our lunch. The weather is just right as we munch our way with "new" food from our red food bag. Half working and half eating, we half chat. Morton stretches out on the sitting part of a table and closes his eyes. I feel a little guilty about working right now and not enjoying all that is around us. We should be off cycling 20 miles on a trail, but I just need a day for my bruised backside to take it easy. I've even been alternating sitting on it, right cheek and then left cheek and laying on my stomach to work. After his wee nap, Morton wakes up feeling bored and anxious. Maybe we should have just ridden today he thinks out loud. We talk about the journey being a journey and not a race. We also talk about the weather. We are going to be getting in to a lot sooner now that bikes are in the journey and we aren't just on foot walking the whole way. Our coldest weather gear is still at my daughter's house in Pennsylvania. Everyone has been telling us to take the time to smell the roses, so a day of just sitting a bit and working isn't a bad thing. We need days like this. Morton calms down a bit about the journey and looks off over the burnt trees and various colors of green that sweep down to a small lake. I continue writing on lappy. Breaking the silence, Morton scares me for the second time as he grabs the camera and jumps up. "Look at that!" sends chills down my spine as I turn to look behind me. It's a huge gopher tortoise. Morton is over and quietly walking through this growth about two feet tall. I shout at him about spiders and snakes, but it's too late. He's in it and not caring. "Look at the size of him!" Morton shouts in a whisper. "Uh-oh...that's not good!" Morton is whispering very loudly. He's switches off the camera and shoves it in his pocket. With both hands he's reaching down into a region I can't see. What on earth is he doing? Didn't I warn him about snakes and spiders here? He straightens up holding the giant tortoise. "Come on, leave that alone." Morton is talking to the shelled creature as he sets him down a few feet away.

It seems there was a plastic fork the turtle was going to try to munch. He must have smelled food on it. The sad thing is, there is a trash can just 200 feet away from where someone threw this fork down. Morton set his new friend down and went back and picked up the fork, a bit of glass and the remainder of a plastic bag. The tortoise watched him. I think he was mad at Morton for taking his lovely smelling fork away. The big creature stayed in one spot. He was nibbling on flowers and grass that surround the pavilion. Morton couldn't resist the temptation and picked him up again for a picture or two. I told you he's like a school boy sometimes. I told him you are not suppose to touch any creature and I think he might be breaking several state and federal laws. He sat his friend down, almost where he had first picked him up. "I only moved him so he wouldn't eat the fork!" Morton said in a quiet tone. "That was the first time, what about the second time?" I asked. "I was just putting him back." Morton explained. His friend came back over towards us. We later learned these creatures are endangered. If they are this friendly to everyone, it is easy to see how man could take advantage of them. I told Morton about a time when I was 15 and accidentally ate gopher.

It was at a boy's house I had this huge crush on. They were friends of my parents and I just thought their son was the cutest thing going. He had dark eyes, dark curly hair and this devilish grin. He was a real Florida native, as were his parents. He wasn't scared of anything that came from the swamps or the groves and I was thrilled to be asked to dinner. As his mom dished up what looked like chicken and dumplings on my plate, we all made table chit chat. About halfway through with the meal his mom asked me how I liked the gopher. It was all I could do to keep from spitting it out. "Gopher, like the furry brown animals, gopher?" I asked in shock. "No, no, no" the mother said and the table started laughing. "The gopher turtle, Danny caught this one himself!" Oh my gosh! These people were monsters! My stomach or brain wouldn't let me take another bite. My crush was over. I just wanted to wash my mouth out and never think about this gopher stew supper again. Morton laughed and asked how it tasted. "Like chicken of course!" I told him. I could never understand all the exotic foods that people claim taste like chicken. Why not cut out the middle man and *JUST EAT CHICKEN*!?

As I worked and we rested, Morton and I got treated to a variety of wild birds, but no alligators. We got a special treat when the park rangers came along to change this creative trash can. They warned us that it would smell and we might want to move, but we held fast on our front row seat. The ranger explained there would be 8 or 10 feet of bag coming out of this can. They used a tractor bucket with ropes attached to hoist up the long bag with a wooden disk on the bottom. It was indeed long. It was also covered with huge red fire ants. If you have never heard of them get informed. The ants that bite you and their poison is stronger than that of a cobra. They have been known to kill grown men. Taking care, the ranger put some poison of his own in the bottom of this garbage can pit and said that should take care of them. Morton snapped some pictures and I kept working on the computer, while keeping a watchful eye to make sure a line of giant red ants didn't sneak up on me.

After ages we decided we better go back to our tent. I closed up shop and we mounted our bikes and rode down the lovely trail. Once back at our camp I dug out my jacket, it was getting a bit cooler. This is something that I haven't had to do up until now really. The weather is changing and it isn't for the better. Morton was going to put dinner together but was too shy to ask the people next door for some hot water for our pot of noodles. We would be eating cold stuff tonight. Flipping my laptop open for the last time for today, I was happily working when a nice couple stopped for a chat. They are down here from their sheep farm in Ohio. I can't remember her names but his name, or at least his nickname, is Turtle! After Morton's little adventure with the turtle earlier, I thought it was quite cute.

We talked about laptops, connections, Scotland, sheep, taking movies of wildlife and the journey we are on. They were really nice and later Morton kicked himself for not asking them for hot water. We have to learn how to really talk to strangers but years of our mothers telling us not to have taken their toll. When they had walked on their way, we, well Morton, popped the lid off a can of cold ravioli. This is something that I was dreading, but it actually tasted alright. It was food and it WASN'T trail mix!

Darkness started falling and by 6:30 pm when I would look away from the screen it all seemed quite black out. It might be fun to work away in the dark, as long as the bugs would leave me alone. Just as I was thinking it, a huge bug flew right to the screen, hit it and then flew right in my face. Just as this was happening a huge raindrop hit my arm. We both leapt in to action and I was unplugged and in the tent in a matter of seconds. I used my body to shield the camera and laptop. Morton just made it inside when it started raining hard.

With all my time on the computer today I had looked at the forecast. Rain, and lots of it, with the temperature falling for tomorrow. Rain on a roof is a nice thing. I remember listening to it on my sister's metal roof in her old farm house in Pennsylvania and liking it. I can also remember the way it would sound on my pony barn while my little brother and I would be sitting out a thundershower above my ponies stall. Rain on a tent roof in Florida can be a scary thing. You don't know how hard it's going to rain, how strong the wind is going to blow and how long it's going to last. The other thing that worried me was lightning. It kills so many people each year and our tent would offer us no protection. Peeking out the little window I saw the lights glowing inside the motorhomes of happy and dry campers. "We need a motorhome." I told Morton. "Sponsors" replied Morton. We lay there on top the sleeping bags talking about the pro's and con's of a motorhome. It is all pretty pointless though, unless we would have another person or persons along. It would take away the real sense of adventure the journey has, but it would make a lot of sense too. A place to sleep safely each night, time saved every day from packing and unpacking and I wouldn't have to beg for shelter each and every day of my life. After twenty minutes or so we changed the subject. The rain had slackened off a bit and we even thought about going outside again to see if we could see any stars. But Morton was falling asleep. His big adventure walk must have taken it out of him.

About 10:30 pm a loud noise woke me out of dreamland. It was our neighbors who were either coming or going. It felt like we had slept the entire night and it should be dawn soon, but we were far from that. The lights flashing on the side of the tent wasn't lightning, but just headlights. Dozing again my phone rang. I had just found it and answered it when it stopped. Listening to my voice mail it was my daughter-in-law saying she was sorry for calling so late, didn't realize what time it was...they all know that 10:30 is late for us! She said we'd talk tomorrow so I tucked the phone away in a baggie and fluffed my pillow up that I had unstrapped from my bicycle seat. Morton was already snoring and I wasn't far behind. It had been a long and enjoyable day off, but we were both worn out.

Day 25: January 25, 2007 - Thursday - Hobe Sound, Florida

It rained last night, hard and pretty much the entire evening. At least every time I woke up during the night, it would be raining. I would feel around in the dull light for any leaks on the floor and try to find a comfortable position to get my body in. Spreading my towel out on our hideous sleeping bags was a great idea. For the first time since using them, they don't feel like sleeping on a plastic trash bag. In the morning the sky looked like the rain had washed all the color out of it. The word *gray* wouldn't even cover it. There were some black clouds on the north east horizon and I knew we had to move fast. The wind had whipped the fly cover for the tent almost dry and we raced the weather to get tore down and packed up. Morton had set out our food for breakfast, along with a leftover bottle of Donna's home-brewed green tea with mango. We both agreed to eat after everything was stuffed in the pouches and pockets, safe from the weather.

Just as we finished folding our huge white tarp the big drops started falling. Making a quick judgment call, as quick as you can at 8 am anyway, we unfolded the huge white tarp and covered our bikes, our trailers and ourselves at the wooden picnic table. It was almost cozy under the tarp. The rain was playing a very fast melody while tapping away and we munched away at our breakfast. "It will blow over", I told Morton, being ever the optimist that I am. Watching his watch, we waited. The rain kept coming then it's companion, the wind, showed up for good measure. We were now wrestling the big white tarp against the cold and rain. It was going to be a beautiful day! Hard to believe just a few days ago we were dying from the heat. Putting our heads together, it helped to keep us warm and let us hear each other, we discussed what we should do. Take our chances with road spray and ride? We still have no lights and people come so close to us in the sunshine I have even got a white shirt with a permanent mark on it from a van who thought he owned the road and brushed against me while passing me at forty miles an hour. What would happen if we pushed to get up the road today and the rain got worse? This part of the highway doesn't even have guardrails to sit on and cover up from the weather. We both agreed that the wise thing to do is to stop for the day. Again. It was the only logical thing really. After all, it's not a race or contest. Our only real rule is to be safe and stay alive!

Deciding that the pavilion we had spent the wonderful day in yesterday would give us sanctuary, we made a run for it as the rain slowed. Covered in wet sand and sticky from the rain, we set up our outdoor office once again. This time closer to the wall that would hopefully break the wind for us. The same ranger came by that we met yesterday. We talked about the fire ants and he gave our bikes a good once over. Leaving in his pickup, we kept working. Morton was working on trying to find us warm clothes as the temperature was really falling fast. In about a half an hour a female ranger appeared. She asked if we had camped there during the night. They had reports that someone camped in the pavilion. Nope, not us. We were on space 44! As she left, Morton and I agreed that ranger number one must have thought we had just worked on the laptop through the evening. It's a good thing they are diligent in watching, makes you feel a lot safer when it's just you and your tent. Morton and I remembered that they had cabins, or so said the sign by the road. They are actually ran by a concession, *Jonathan Dickinson State Park River Tours*. Maybe if we called them they would be kind enough to let us use a cabin for the night, which has a forecast of showers. Tomorrow the sun will come out and we can ride. But tonight we couldn't face the thought of the wet tent and another night of worrying about the water leaking in. Calling the number, I spoke with Tina. She listened to my story and sounded very sympathetic. She could probably hear my teeth chattering from my outdoor office, still with a great view, only slightly damp now. Tina said she would speak with the appropriate person and took down all our details and phone number. There was nothing to do now but wait and shiver.

The bathroom was quite warm and Morton took sanctuary there. He was doing double duty and letting the phone charge too. After all, you have to make every second count, right? I kept working, watching the birds fly about and hoping to see the friendly tortoise again. Coming out of the bathroom and talking to himself, or so I thought, Morton handed me the phone. It was Tina. She was telling me the excellent news that we would have a warm and dry cabin for the night! Now we just had to get to where she was, by bike, in the rain. While we were discussing waiting it out or riding, the weather seemed to break for a moment. Now or never was our cry as we jumped on the bikes and pedaled like fiends. We had no idea how far we had to go, just that we had to go back from whence we came and head for the river. The lovely Loxahatchee River. The break ended as the skies opened up again and washed every grain of sand off our bikes, our trailers and even the soles of our shoes. It poured.

Adding discomfort to this uncomfortable situation, my pillow on my torture seat had been stashed in the trailer to save it from being soaked. I had to scoot sideways in the seat to keep from screaming. Side-saddle I suppose you could call it. It wasn't pretty or nice, but it did make riding semi-bearable. There were no clues as to how far we needed to go. There were signs here and there assuring us we were headed to the river and the precious cabins. Oh for a friendly person in a pick up truck! But we kept on under our own steam. Crossing a little bridge we saw a sign about alligators and not molesting them. This must be where the ranger meant when he told us there was a family of alligators living under a bridge. Wishing the camera wasn't packed away and was waterproof, I hoped we wouldn't see any. I wouldn't want to miss the picture. Surely alligators are clever enough to not come out in weather like this but then they have the gear for it.

I could see roofs through the trees. Hopes soared as we kept up with the rain. We steered towards the buildings and my flushed face broke into a smile as we spotted the cabins. The cold was gone and I was burning up with the energy of the wild ride we were just on. Stopping right at the first cabin I offered to wait with the bike and two trailers if Morton would unhitch and go find the spot we check in at. He went for it after a bit of begging and pleading on my part. I told him that my butt could only take so much more of that seat. Did I mention I have the best husband in the world? Just as our furious ride stopped, so did the rain. Morton unhitched his trailer and set off to get us checked in for the night.

Waiting in this wild spot on my own, it was so quiet. The noise of US1 was too far away to hear. We had ridden over the railroad tracks ages ago and it too was silent. The Orange Blossom Special train wasn't running at the moment. Just me and nature. My cell phone started ringing deep inside the trailer, safe from the weather. Letting it ring I looked at where we had landed for the night. Breathtaking. Stunning. Seeing the trees and the low brush dripping wet from the storms, I heard the song the drops were making. It was a rhythm of an odd beat. Wishing I had something that would record it, you'll just have to take my word that it really was music to your ears. I was completely enchanted and smiling. Two birds, both with red heads and dove gray bellies, came from out of nowhere and landed on the tree in front of me. They pecked at insects that must have been driven out by the rain. Feeding like they hadn't eaten in ages, they worked their way up and down the tree. I thought of our big giant woodpecker in Pennsylvania and how you could watch him for hours. That is top quality entertainment. My ears perked up when I heard another noise. It was Morton coming from around the corner and a woodpecker with the soft gray chest and red head swooped right in front of him. My hero had the key to our home for the night. He was so intent on his riding and returning, he didn't even see the bird.

Stepping inside I got the phone, camera and laptop out. Setting up office on the table, the phone rang as Morton was heading to the camp store to get something to make for dinner. It was from the same number I had missed as it was buried from the rain. It was a reporter from a newspaper in Stuart, Florida.

Filled with the energy from the ride and the rain, I rambled on and on to the reporter. I kept apologizing for talking so much, but said I couldn't help it. I feel so passionate about what we are doing and the feeling gets stronger with every passing day and mile of our journey.

After ages of me not shutting up, Morton returned. He had found one of his lucky pennies right outside our door. Finishing the interview, Morton set about making our dinner and getting our Zen hooked up. We haven't had music for days and we both miss it in our lives. The first song on was *"A Rainy Night in Soho"* by one of my favorite Irish bands, *The Pogues*. As the music played on, I recounted this day for you. I started thinking that I was glad no one was here with us to get wet and cold, but all things considered and now a warm dinner in my belly, I wish you were here. It's been an amazing day.

Day 26: January 26, 2007 - Friday - Hobe Sound to Stuart, Florida

The cabin we stayed in was brilliant. It had a living room, a real kitchen, an actual bedroom and a great table and chairs for working at. It also had a squeaky clean bathroom...if you want to get up close and personal with nature, make sure you visit Jonathan Dickinson State Park. When we woke up the pale green curtains were pulled. We couldn't really tell what the weather was at 6:30 am. Peeking out a curtain the sun was saying it was going to be a perfect day for riding, and it was right! The night before after I did the phone interview with the Stuart newspaper, their photographer called us and made arrangements to meet us in the morning as we were packing. He was going to get some photos of pre-trip and then as we ride. We met him outside our lovely cabin and he went right to work. Chatting with him, we just needed to get on our bikes and ride. He was going to go in front of us to get some action shots.

It was chilly and for the first time I had long pants on and a long sleeve shirt. Morton found his hat, but opted for just shorts and a t-shirt. Riding was great, no chain slips or flats. We had several miles to backtrack to get back to the road at the entrance of the state park. There were lots of times that the photographer stopped in front of us, but we just kept riding as his camera clicked away, capturing our unposed smiles from the joy of a sunny day. On our way in we passed a boardwalk and viewing platform where the family of alligators live. Morton and I stopped at this and the photographer stopped with us. He was nice enough to take some pictures of us together on our camera too.

Not long after we left the photographer from the Stuart newspaper, we got a call from NBC Channel 5 wanting to do a story. We were thrilled and made arrangements to meet up the road. Morton did his daily battle with the chain and the gears as we headed up US 1. Still making good time, we met up with Tania Rogers of Channel 5 and her cameraman. The interview was really good and as we rode off and they were getting their last shot of us, Tania even passed me a bottle of water out the window of their news van. Talk about a great time! Before long we came across a nice park, public restrooms and were enjoying the new bottle of water. A kind groundskeeper asked if we wanted some ice, but we don't have any facility to hold it yet. He did give us great directions to find the big and cheap store where I might find a bicycle seat and we said our goodbyes and kept riding north. Just the thought of a nice seat that didn't feel like I was sitting on a broken brick was enough to keep me going. Morton trailed behind, letting me set my own pace. Poor Morton, he has to get sick of looking at the backside of my backside.

Reaching the store, Morton waited outside and gave the bikes a once over. Inside I avoided a shopping cart and decided to only carry things in my arms. It would stop me from getting more than we had room for. I felt the bicycle seats they had for sale and looked for the biggest one to fit my butt. The bike seat felt good but I was wondering if it would really deliver all that the label on it promised. Outside Morton put the seat on and we ate our dinner. Loading the food up in our trailer, we kept going to who knew where. The seat felt so much better and looked nicer than my make-shift comfy seat of my bed pillow wrapped around it. We had stopped earlier in the day to do our laundry and had to go fast to make up for lost time.

Riding to Stuart, I started asking in hotels and motels for a room for the night. It could be an empty room with no furniture, one that they were refurbing, we really didn't care. Anything would suit us. It wasn't looking good and sunset was coming. We sort of feel like vampires in reverse...we need a place to get in before darkness falls. Safety is our only priority when night falls. After getting loads of "no's" we did find a room for half price. It is still a big chunk of our budget, $75.00, but we really don't have a choice when we have no where to camp and sleeping at the side of the road is not an option. There also weren't any houses in our path to ask for a piece of yard. Now we are tucked up, watching the news and waiting for our piece to come on. We've seen the teasers for it and Morton looks GREAT on camera. Me, the camera **does** add 10 pounds, so I have to ride harder. And the bike seat report is good, it is actually wonderful. It doesn't hurt anything (yet) and I'm going to go to sleep and have happy dreams about a nice long ride north tomorrow.

Day 27: January 27, 2007 - Friday - Stuart to Ft. Pierce, Florida

Coming up to a red light there was a man yelling out his window at me. He was also smiling and waving. Odd combination really. The most wonderful thing though, is what he was yelling. "Hey Skinny, keep up the good work....keep going!" Woohoo, he had seen the news! The power of the press was among us. Our day was filled with toots, waves, shouts and lots of well wishes from people. It was nice to have people know why we are sharing the road with them. Morton even had a guy shake his hand and thank him for doing what he's doing for diabetes. The man explained he has Type 1 and doesn't do enough to help people get educated.

Spying a bike shop as we rode, we went in to see if Morton could pick the person's brain who repairs bikes. The man, Jeff at *Pro Cycles* in Stuart, put the bike up on his bench and determined the wheel axle was bent. There was nothing really that could be done for it. He told us that there was a store (the chain that we bought it from) in front of us about four miles. The trick was to be able to get the bike there.

With a little luck and a little walking, we finally made it. The store was on the opposite side of the road and Morton nearly gave me a heart attack as he just gave a hand signal and started moving. There were horns and swerves and the two of us dodging cars to get over. Hand signals really didn't work. Once we pulled in, I dug out the receipt and Morton took the bike inside. There was a guy on a bike who had pulled in to talk to us. He had seen the news. Disappearing inside, Morton went to return the bike with the bent wheel axle. I was glad it was his bike and not mine. It would have been very embarrassing to think my weight had bent an axle. The truth was though, it had been bent since the time we bought it. You really do get what you pay for. Outside the store, I chatted with the man from New York. He was telling me about bicycles and the area. It was good to have company as I waited, and waited. Morton came out after the man had cycled away, he was looking a bit disgruntled. Explaining that they couldn't repair the bike, they did have others just like it in stock. They didn't want to exchange it though. Even though it was just twelve days old and even though we had the receipt. Morton didn't understand why, so I asked him to wait outside with our two trailers and non-broken bike and went in. I'm a big believer in being nice to people. Treating people just as we want to be treated. But I also am a believer in not letting people bully you. What I encountered was a bully, first class. This manager told me we had abused the bike and he wouldn't replace it. Period, end of discussion. He made suggestions that my weight had broke the bike. I asked him to read the blog and see that Morton had to do things to it almost daily to keep it going. It was Morton's bike that was the trouble, not mine. After about five or ten minutes, I knew that we were getting no where. He wanted us to leave the bike and when it got fixed, it would be fixed. Maybe a day, two or three. There were parts that his guy would have to order, perhaps. All very vague. Why can't we just exchange it for a bike they had in stock? The identical bike! They had two of them in stock. But no, this man wasn't budging. I had to remind him, we had the receipt, we didn't abuse the bike, and while I was waiting on him, I watched the girl at the counter exchange items for two different customers, with no receipt. One had even said her child broke the lid on the toy box by bending it backwards. When I mentioned this, the man grunted and said to the person behind the counter, "Just exchange the bike" then turned to me and said, "Don't try this again. We won't replace any more bikes for you." He turned and walked away before I could tell him to have a wonderful day. I wasn't trying to pull one over on the man, or the giraffe, for that matter. This was a bike. We had it for 12 days. We did not abuse it. My fat backside did not bend it. I wondered why the bike company didn't put some warning on their bike, "Don't ride daily" "Don't ride on sidewalks" "Don't ride on the road" and above all, "Don't abuse or use the bike". The bikes were something we got because we were really worried about walking through Miami. Safety and speed were what we were thinking. We aren't naive enough to think they will last forever, but we did think they would last longer than 12 days.

After losing at least an hour in negotiations at the store, we were back on the road again. It's easy to let a bad experience ruin your day and put you in a bad mood. This didn't happen today. It was sunny and I had a nice seat on my bike. I was wondering though, just for a second, about what would happen if my bike died. Up ahead we could see the road narrowing and the bike lane disappearing. The traffic was heavy and we had to keep a fast pace and hug the shoulder that had a concrete barricade running beside us. Cars were blowing their horns again, but not because they were spotting us from the news. They were honking because we were taking up thirty inches of the road, their road.

Morton shouted that we had to stop. Slowing down, I stopped and he was right behind me. He jumped off the bike and started running his hand over his new back wheel. "I cannae believe this!" he exclaimed. Looking close, I didn't spot what he was seeing. The tire, the brand new tire, was coming off the wheel. Was it the road construction? Was it Morton abusing it? Was it a defect in the tire? Who knows. Before you could say "Snap" Morton had his kit out and was back on the fixing wagon. There was a bench in the shade and I pushed my bike and trailer over to it. The bench had my name all over it. Morton was lost in the bike repair and I figured I would look at a map and figure out how far we could get before we called it a day. There was a woman walking near me and I asked her some information about the road in front of us. Important things like campgrounds, motels and construction. Being so very helpful, we started chatting about the journey we were on. She told me she had some friends that needed to hear this. She walked to the nail salon where her friends were just getting finished. Their nails all looked great when they came over and we had a great talk about all the little changes they could make in their lives. One was going to start riding her bike again. One was going to start taking walks. They all promised to keep in touch on the site.

Once the tire was sorted, we tried it again. As we rode I thought about all the things that we really want to do on the walk. I love talking to people and we need to get more connections going to talk to more people each day. The press is a great way to do that, and so is the website. The trouble is the time that it takes to make all these things happen cuts in to our riding time. I wish I were real twins instead of just the size of two people. Looking for a room now jumped in to my mind. I asked Morton for a time check and knew we had to start being on the look out. As I said before, this can be a real time consuming part of the day. I don't want to bore you with the details, but we heard five flat out "no's" in a row. One man, after listening to what we were doing, said he read about us in the paper. Why weren't we going to camp, why did we want a room? The thing we really do want to do is to camp in people's yard. Explaining this and asking for a bit of space behind his motel, I heard my sixth "no" for the day.

We did have an offer from a man who was six sheets to the wind (a wee bit drunk) to come home to his house and put the tent in his back yard. He was a little intense and said his wife might not like it, but he didn't care what she said, he told us if his wife gave him any lip, he'd "take care" of her. I didn't want to see how he intended to do that, so I said we wanted to keep riding. Morton asked me up the road why we didn't go pitch our tent in his back yard and I told him that he didn't want to find out what a drunk man meant when he said he would take care of his wife.

The best we got was a reduced room. We could try to go further, but there might not be anything. This is what really is the crunch time of our day. We think that we will soon have state parks to camp in, I will soon have family to camp with, and we keep hoping that the message gets out about who we are and what we are doing and we soon get offers from people who are at least semi-sober to sleep in their back yard, with their wives' permission of course.

Morton goes over and tightens all the lose bits on my bike. Screws that are going rusty after 12 days are getting tightened and wiped with a clean dry rag. He knows he has to take good care of our bikes, because as the man said, we won't be getting any more from the store. Tomorrow is Sunday and we want to have a nice ride up beside the Indian River. I'll be coming into territory that feels a bit familiar. Who knows, maybe we'll even find a place we can actually pitch the tent for free.

Day 28: January 28, 2007 - Sunday - Ft. Pierce to Vero Beach, Florida

As we left the shelter of our room, the sky was dark and cloudy. Rain started spitting on us as soon as we stepped out the door. It's really hard to feel motivated and good at a time like this, but there really isn't any other choice then heading north. We have a very long way to go and the forecast was saying that it would clear up. Before long we were back on the bikes and in the zone of riding. Within a mile Morton lost his pedal. Seems there is a flaw with the design and instead of being an eccentric bolt, which would never come loose when you pedal, it is the opposite. It comes loose as you pedal. You have to wonder how this one got past the designers and inspectors. He must have a Monday morning bicycle.

Since it was Sunday, the places we past were closed that might have a new bolt we could get to re-place the dud. As we left US1 and headed east to get A1A north, we knew that our odds of finding a place beachside just got a lot slimmer. Signs kept pointing out a Navy Seals Museum, located on A1A between Ft. Pierce and Vero Beach. Each time we would pass one, Morton would read it out loud and ask me if I fancied that. This is code for..."I fancy that, let's stop!" After a few pedal repairs and a small triumph for me, we were at the entrance to the impressive museum. My small triumph is that I was able to ride the whole way up and over a bridge. I didn't have to walk the bike. I know this sounds like no biggie, but I was grinning like the Cheshire cat coming down the bridge. Weeeeeeeee, I'm a child again in my forties! There was a bench in front of the museum and Morton and I decided to have our lunch on there. The sun was out, though a bit more on the chilly side, it felt nice to sit and eat our canned tuna. Benches are like our sofas now, even the hard ones with bird crap on them are a welcomed sight to us.

Morton went inside the chain-linked fence to take some pictures, but when I offered to sit with the bikes when he went through the museum, he declined. He really does love places like that and I think he knew he just couldn't go in and out. He would have to read every sign at every display and hours would be lost. I did suggest asking them if we could sleep in one of their wild vehicles outside, then it wouldn't matter how long he took. He still declined. While he was inside the fence snapping pictures, I was holding down the bench. A lovely couple from Michigan stopped to say hello. They were driving to the airport and had seen the news. They offered us a place to sleep when we get there (hopefully this summer) so stay tuned for that. Their little twins sat in the back of their car patiently as we shared stories with each other about fine tuning our lives and the journey we were on. Morton returned to the bench beside the road and a man named Bob stopped to talk too. He had read the story in the paper about us. He was out for his own walk, using two canes to help him along his way. He was really inspiring to us. It was so much harder for him to get out and around, and he was still doing it. His walking will add years to his life and let him see and enjoy the lovely Florida seaside.

There was a fantastic path beside most of A1A and save a few pedal repairs, it was great riding. Ahead I spied the brown sign for Avalon Beach State Park, gave the hand signal and pulled in. Morton wanted to see if he could borrow a proper tool to try to get the pedal tighter than he could with just pliers, from one of the motorists pulled in the parking lot. Nothing like having the wrong tool, wrong bolt and dodgy pedal to make your Sunday sour. The park was a little piece of paradise. Nice surf, clean beach, not too many people on it and these lovely pavilions with picnic tables that provided a place for me to stretch out flat on as Morton set about bike duty.

For the last two days my right hand has been numb on the pinky, ring finger and middle finger. I had twisted my back and I think (I hope anyway) I pinched a nerve. I just need my back flat and to click back in to place and the numbness and tingling should go away. At first I was afraid I was having a heart attack, but there are no other symptoms. Is there a doctor in the house?

After about an hour break with no relief for my back and tingly fingers, we were just about to head out when Morton said, "Oh bugger!" His trailer tire was flat. There was a giant thorn sticking in it. At least it wasn't broken glass. I kept my white feet in the sun for a little while longer as he repaired the flat. My MBT shoes sat to the side as my toes wiggled in freedom. The last few hours of our ride were a nightmare. The weather was brilliant. The path was wonderful. The nightmare part was having to stop every half a mile or less to put this pedal back on. We got it down to a science where I would keep riding slowly as Morton would pull in and attach it again. He would then catch up with me just in time for it to go slack again. The whole horrible scenario would then repeat itself in this never-ending journey of delays.

There was a *Holiday Inn* on our horizon and they have been the only real big chain who have helped us on our journey thus far on a regular basis. We crossed our fingers and hoped for some more help as we limped along on the bikes. I might mention that the bike with the horrid pedal is less than 3 days old. Morton hasn't abused it, but he is tempted to throw it off a bridge!

Pulling in to the *Holiday Inn at Vero Beach* just off the A1A and right on the beach, I felt so happy I could have cried. It really was near sunset and I had hit my wall ages ago. My legs were aching, my hand was tingling and the fear of being trapped by the road with no pedal had been getting to me for the last two hours. I just wanted a place to sleep, a place to work on the site and a place to be safe.

The girl on the desk, Chistiana, was so very helpful. She couldn't authorize a complimentary room, but she did help us with a special rate and let us know who we would need to speak with in the morning. She also suggested their restaurant, *Mulligans*, as a good place to eat. Getting our gear in the room we decided we were both starving. It hadn't been the hardest physical day, but talk about a stressful one with all the repairs. I called home and talked to my kids, Sarah, 25 and James, 24, and both of their spouses, Graeme and Mari. It was what I needed to feel very good. Their voices are all excellent medicine for me after a long day and helped heal a bit of the ever-present homesickness I feel on the road. Have I mentioned I have this problem with homesickness? The real pain in the neck is that I know that going home is the only thing that cures it. Heading to *Mulligans*, we were lucky enough to get Jen for a waitress. If you eat here, and we both highly recommend it, ask for Jen. She was so very wonderful. Her mom had seen us on the news and just earlier in the day, had told Jen about what we were doing. They had spotted us on the road to the south of here. It was a wonderful conversation with this very clever and caring person. Jen gave us a coaster that she had put a lovely message on the back. She suggested collecting them from our journey, which we are going to do if we get the chance. I have to mail home to my daughter, DVD's from all our photos and videos, so they will pack quite nicely in with them. It will be great to look back at them when we finish in a couple years. Thank you Jen!

This waitress, who is really an angel in disguise, also bought our meal for us. We were so shocked and grateful to her. This was one of the kindest gestures I have ever witnessed in my life. My only hope is that Jen emails and we keep in touch. When we get back to Key West, and have a HUGE party we need all these wonderful people that we encounter along the way to come!

Heading back to our room as the breeze was blowing off the ocean, the stars were all shining on us. We held hands and walked, enjoying the evening. Our bellies were full with the most delicious food. They do the best house salad I've ever tasted, and the company of our new friend Jen, as she took care of her customers, was just wonderful. The perfect way to end a less than perfect day.

Thank you so much to everyone who TOOTS, WAVES, CLAPS OUT THEIR WINDOWS and says HELLO along the way. We love it when that happens. It tells us what we are doing is a good thing, not a crazy thing. Your support is just the most lovely thing I think I've ever seen.

Day 29: January 29, 2007 - Monday - Vero Beach to Sebastian Inlet, Florida

Morton really scared me this morning. We were setting off from the Holiday Inn and needed to go away from the beach and pick up A1A north. I was in front, as usual, and Morton was following behind. Riding about 3 blocks, something made me stop and look back. No Morton. I felt like I had lost my child. Looking there and not knowing what really to do I thought maybe he had turned right out of the parking lot and just headed north on the beachside street. Just then his bright orange flag on the trailer came into view. He was sitting at the hotel getting ready to follow. Breathing a sigh of relief, I almost pushed off to start riding again. Something made me stop and turn around just in time to see Morton heading north on the beachside street. He didn't see me! Have I lost that much weight?

Getting separated out here is something we both fear. We have to depend on each other and be in visual contact at all times. It's not always a nice world, and two is far safer than one. Turning my bike on a dime while straddling it wasn't a pretty picture. I started going as quick I could. My mind was racing as fast as my feet as I feared Morton would be going as fast as he could to catch me. He also had BOTH our phones with him. Not clever and very poor planning. Thank goodness he had lost his pedal. He was not too far ahead trying to get it to tighten as best he could. When I caught up, breathing heavy from my frantic pace, I scolded him for not seeing which way I went. I was so scared and angry and he didn't understand why. Obviously Morton has never been a mother.

From there on we stayed thisclose, not sure if Morton was worried about scaring me again or wanted to catch my backdraft. The wind was blowing hard from the north and it felt like we were going uphill in a gale force wind the entire day. There were stops with the bike, the usual pedal problems. At a park with a nice sunny bench I called the company and asked for someone in management. The girl on the phone said she'd try to help, so I explained our woes. She was absolutely brilliant. She took all the details and is having the new parts sent out to my sister's address here in Florida. We would only have to limp along a day or two more with the pedal problems. We figured the trouble arose when the person putting the pedals on the bike at the toy store got a little off track or cockeyed with it and put it on at sort of an angle. Enough to make the threads on the bolt pretty useless. Morton, who was doing a great McGyver impression, took some copper wire from a church maintenance man and made a make-shift bolt that held up for the rest of the days ride. The scenery was excellent, though I wished the cold wind would change direction. For the first time we rode in the sun hoping to get warm. My fingers were tingling on both hands, just the ring finger and pinky fingers. Morton offered his nasty leather gloves, but it would have meant stopping and digging for them. They are his old work gloves he insisted on bringing and never really uses.

At last we were seeing our signs for Sebastian Inlet. My heart leapt. It had been a long day. Then my heart sank. It was another brown sign that said, "Camping 2 miles" The bathroom was calling and all my body was aching from the cold wind. It was going to drop to 39 degrees tonight and I could just think of a warm tent and cozy sleeping bag. Finally the horrible sleeping bags would come in handy.

When we saw a warden locking the gates at the treasure museum, we stopped to ask how late the campground was open. The person we talked to was so kind and helpful. She told us all about the treasure museum that we hope to explore on Tuesday, and said she'd see us at the campground. Just a bit longer, I could make it. Staying on the nice sidewalk that we didn't have to share with cars, my mind was on my dad. Sebastian Inlet is a name from my childhood and fishing trips from the past. It was one of my dad's favorite places to put his little boat in the water and go out and try to catch the big ones.

It has only been since September that I lost my dad and I don't know if the sadness will ever leave.

Why didn't I video his tales of all the old stories that I use to dread hearing again and again? He would have gotten a real kick out of telling them on film and my children's children could have seen old Pap in action. I suppose I was always thinking that dad was always going to be here. He was such a fixture in my life that thinking he'd be gone was something that never crossed my mind. Enough about thinking of what I should have done. You can't change the past but they say you can learn from it. Missing moments is something that I'm going to strive not to let happen in my life any more. Knowing who and what is important is something that I want to remind myself of every single day of my life. Time is short, no matter who you are or where you are.

Before long we were spotting the big bridge. We knew the campground sat at the foot of this tall bridge, on the south side, thank goodness. My dad was fading away from my thoughts as we pulled into the campground area. Then he was there again, in full force, as if his ghost had stepped right out in front of me.

It was a board with the tides and the times on it. Dad lived for these things. They are what old school fishermen set their clocks by. Dad should be here now. My mother and father should have been in front of us to set up their motorhome. Dad could have gone fishing for our supper as Morton and I struggled with the wind and the pedal. But life isn't always what it should be.

Walking in to the ranger station we got ourselves sorted and the lovely ranger from the treasure museum even showed us right to our spot. The area was grassy with a nice block of shrubs and small trees to help shelter us from the wicked wind of the north. Pitching our tent fast (we are pro's now) and climbing inside to set up our home for the next two nights, I heard all the campground sounds. Cars returning with boats after their days fishing. Kids laughing and playing. Women chatting as they were going for a walk around the park. Home sounds. Morton worked the outside and I was finally out of the wind and warm for the first time today. Spreading out our sleeping mats, then making sure I zipped the two bags together to form a fleecy cocoon, I wished we had a way to get hot water. One of the few things left in our food bag is hot chocolate mix. *Oh to dream of such luxury!*

There is no power at our tent site but we think if we walk over to the spot where you can wash your clothes, we could hook up for our 9 pm chat on the website. Morton gets inside the tent and I'm thankful that his body is always throwing off heat. I swear it gets 10 degrees warmer as soon as he enters. Tucked inside the sleeping bag, but still sitting up, we have our canned tuna dinner. The cold weather has us both still hungry, but we know that we have to save our last two cereal bars and single pack of crackers for breakfast. A few raisins are still left in the bag for the morning. Slim pickins.

Just a few moments to snuggle and close my eyes, then we'll get up and head over to the power for the chat. It's just 7 pm as we pull the bag around us. Morton comments that we seem to have more room in them now. Between us, we have lost over 50 pounds since the last time we had them zipped together in Pennsylvania. Each night we use them in Florida, until now, has been too roasting to even think about being under to cover. Before I know it I'm grabbing around in the dark to answer the tune of the Smurfs. My phone is ringing and I get to it just in time to see it was a missed call. It was my son's number. Calling back, it was his wife, Mari, who had called. We were talking about a home they are looking at. Oh the joys of being newlywed! Morton said that we had slept past the chat time and I had been snoring. We both thought about getting out and going to find the power, but we just didn't have the energy. The wind was blowing and our little tent was sheltered by the trees and bushes. This was the first time of the entire day I had felt warm. Snuggling on to my Scottish heater, I decided the day was over and adjusting my pillow, I fell back asleep.

Day 30: January 30, 2007 - Tuesday - Sebastian Inlet, Florida
My feelings on today are so very mixed, I really don't know where to start. I woke up thinking about what was in front of us here while we were in this place that holds a lot of memories of my dad. We had an interview and several follow up via emails, interviews. I also wanted to try to write a story about a day that my dad, my little brother and I had shared some thirty years ago. The birds were singing outside our tent, they like us, had survived the cold night. The sun was doing it's job of heating our tent up as Morton and I began stirring. Wanting to catch up with a reporter that hadn't phoned me back yesterday, I dialed his number. That is when my day really started taking an ugly turn.

Hearing a phone conversation that I shouldn't have heard, where this reporter called me "f**king fat" actually reduced me to tears. I'm not a crybaby, but I do have feelings. This man wasn't a professional and his language could have made a sailor blush. Sitting at a pavilion that is surrounded on three sides by water, and trying to get my mind to focus on all the things I wanted to get done today, I have to admit, those hateful words kept creeping into my head the entire day. Still, there were so many things to be done, I tried not to think about it and managed to get a little writing done, a little picture taking and even an interview with said station, minus the reporter who can't operate a cell phone. People kept saying hello and talking about what we were doing and I was unusually quiet. Morton carried most of the conversations while I was unnaturally quiet. I was in sort of a state of hurt and anger. There were so many things that the reporter didn't realize about being this heavy. I wanted to phone him just once again to explain myself. Explain how I got this fat. Explain why I'm giving up two years of my life to be away from my family. Explain why we are sleeping in a tent and begging for shelter, homeless and sometimes hungry.

Then a light went on over my head. Someone left a message on the blog about the situation that put it all in to perspective for me. This person was the one that needed to do explaining and soul searching. Not me. I'm on a mission. Fat, but with purpose. I'm a "fitness witness" putting myself out here to be poked fun at, cursed at, talked about being the butt of joke (yes, yes, the BIG butt of jokes) and there is a reason why I'm doing this. My mother almost died from taking her health for granted. I have a friend who just lost her second leg to diabetes and still needs to get the wake up call to make her own little changes. There are MILLIONS of us around the world who feel like we are not worth taking the time to "fix" our own health situation. I'm here to tell you otherwise. No matter what size or shape you are, from Twiggy to the person who holds the current record for being the heaviest on this earth, YOU can do something about it. No one, no pill, no magic cure will work. Only YOU can fix this. Just like I'm the only person that can fix my body.

Let the Todd's of the world (sorry to all named Todd, no disrespect meant) say that I'm STILL F****** FAT! I, sir, can lose this weight. I AM losing this weight. You and your cruel comments will be what you are. They are not what I am. If we look around us there are beautiful people in every corner. This has nothing to do with being a size 5, this has to do with what is inside your heart and soul. Some people will say hurtful things to us, but never let it get you down. Keep doing the right thing, be proud of who you are and where you are in life. Todd, the offensive reporter, has his reasons for saying what he said, whatever they might be. An apology would be nice, but only if he even knew why he was saying he was sorry. Me, I'm going to keep moving, keep on our incredible adventure and welcome people into our lives with open arms and eternal gratitude. We have met hundreds, if not thousands of people now, who can relate to what I'm going through and why I'm doing this. Morton and I were going back to our tent to try to warm up after a day of sitting exposed to the wind. We were talking about the sparse food bag when the lady camping across from us came over. She asked if we had anything ready for dinner and would we like some homemade vegetable & beef soup. This dear friends, was an angel on earth! Alice is down from Missouri, has an lovely smile and makes the best soup we ever tasted! Well, at least as good as Jean's, our next door neighbor in Scotland, who makes incredible soup! Sharing and connecting, promising to visit our website when she gets home, we said goodbye to Alice with our bellies full. I was finally warm inside my heart again too. Now the trick was going to be to stay awake until our 9 pm chat! We hadn't really thought the time thing through, it's a bit past our bedtime. We took a walk around the campground and headed down to the water. There is a place you can clean and gut your fish and he was sure he spotted an electric socket. I said it couldn't be, as electricity and water really don't mix, but we went closer. The wind had died down and the moon was just coming in to view. As the sun set we discovered a lot of birds but no electricity. Heading back to the camping area we were going to go with plan B. There was a washer and dryer area that had a nice big sink with a counter that would be perfect. I'd be standing the whole time, but it would keep me awake! My daily routine of loads of exercise has me wanting to be in bed at 8 o'clock now. We got sidetracked by the very first ranger we met when we came here. She's an amazing person who has been through so very much and still have the most positive attitude. We talked a little about how other people can try to drag you down, but you really have to decide what is or isn't going to affect you. A line that I can't get out of my head comes from the song, *Caledonia, "Lost the friends that needed losing, found others on the way."* It really has a lot of truth to it. Dougie is a clever man and a great singer. Along our journey we are going to find the pure treasure of friendships that will last for the rest of our lives, no matter where we are. That is just a bonus for all the other things we are learning out here.

Setting up the laptop, Morton started chatting in person with a man who is a firefighter from Massachusetts. He was so helpful, gave us some great advice and I got the laptop open and set for the first live chat of our adventure. I hoped that someone, just one of you would come along for it...you didn't disappoint me! There were about 12, then 8, then more, plus I was getting lots of instant messages from people who didn't have Java and weren't able to use the chat room. The hour sailed by and Morton even managed to type a bit. Thank you to everyone who helped turn a very sad day into an amazing day that ended on a wonderful high note. We both know we are very lucky to be doing what we are doing and to just be alive!

Day 31: January 31, 2007 - Wednesday - Sebastian Inlet to *Beach House Motel* , Indialantic, Florida

This morning was just lovely. We had nice clear weather, the little songbirds that woke us up and a special treat as we were leaving the campground. Two fishermen were cleaning their catch and the pelicans and storks were on call to get handouts. There was an intense moment when a pelican thought my camera was on the menu too, all while my camera was rolling. He almost ate it.

Riding off from the special inlet was tough, but that is the thing with what we are doing. You might get lucky enough to be in the same place two days, but we always have to move on. This incredible journey only works when we are moving. As Morton reminds me each day, we have a long way to go.

As we got to the top of the bridge that spans the water, you could see for miles behind us where we had ridden. The beach was almost deserted and I was sorry we hadn't taken a walk along it. Fishermen were spread out on the bridge that was below us and I regretted not doing any fishing either. No time for regrets now, Morton is right, we do have a long way to go.

We ride to the first store where Morton had cycled to the day before. Time for a bathroom break and a cold 99 cent drink. There was a picnic bench that we took a nice little break on and chatted to a nice couple. We wrote down the website, as we do for lots of people, and hopefully they will keep in touch.

 Riding on we were approaching a Publix grocery store on the left and had to do a pit stop for my weigh in and to replenish our food bag. Just before we got there a woman in a Corvette started tooting and waving at us. She was motioning to pull in, and we were soon stopped in two spaces and talking. Her name is Sandie and she had actually been praying about which way to go to find us. She chose north and if it would have been just one or two minutes different, we would have missed each other. This lovely lady asked if we had a place to stay (her friend lived near by) but we were still ready to ride a few more hours. Sandie also gave us a donation for our walk, which we put to good use in the grocery store. After about 20 minutes of chatting, we parted ways. Our paths were destined to cross and timing was indeed everything.

As I shopped, Morton waited with the bikes. He met an 89 year young man who rides his bike daily. They were chatting away when I came out of the store the three of us chatted on about it's never to late to get healthy. He was really an inspiration. He looked great, still played tennis and really has found the fountain of youth. Get moving and keep moving. As we were riding our bikes north we heard a little "ding ding" of a bicycle bell as our new 89-year-old friend passed us. He left us eating his dust and Morton and I both said we can only hope to be that healthy and fit at 89. Amazing!

Miles later we started thinking of a room. There is no way to really describe how scary it is not knowing where you are going to sleep each night. We are happy with a bit of yard, but we were in condo city and gated community-ville. A few campgrounds were a no, they only took motorhomes, not tents, as were a few motels and even a lovely B&B. There were lots of people that wanted to help but didn't have the authority to say yes to a free room. After several hours riding I start getting really tired. My face was gritted with sand, salt and sunscreen. The weather had changed from freezing cold to sunny hot and my body was crying out for a rest. I knew though that I couldn't stop to rest until we had a place for the night. Morton suggested we try a fire station ahead, but my heart just wasn't in asking. There really was no use in asking there and we both knew it. Holding my bike handles like some sort of divining rod, I hoped it would point us into a room or tent space. The knees and legs were aching and my backside was ready to walk the bike. Time would run out soon though, so we had to keep looking. We had lost track of the number of *NO's* we heard before pulling our bikes into the *Beach House Motel* in Indialantic. Speaking to Rocky, the great guy here, he was willing to help us. Not only did he get us settled in a room, he came to the room and asked if we needed something for dinner. He offered to get us a sub or a pizza. Is that too kind or what! We have full food bags though and had a lovely dinner (using the microwave in our room) that included FRESH strawberries. Oh what a night.

MONTHLY TOTALS... And did I mention that I got on the scale in the grocery store? Morton did as well and weighs and amazing 182 pounds. This is 17 pounds lighter than when we started on January 1! And me, I hear you ask...what did the scales say for me? I'm so pleased to tell you that they said 304. It's not a typo, 304 pounds! In just 31 days I have lost 39.5 pounds in 31 days. To say that I'm thrilled is the understatement of the century. Now I know my weight won't always come off like this. Loads of it is water weight I'm sure. But I am seeing things on my body that I haven't seen in ages. My knuckles, my ankle, the lump of fat just below my knee is leaving and I feel like I can do anything. Absolutely anything. Our computer says we have gone 355.75 miles, but it's actually been a bit further. That is an average of over 10 miles a day. I know it's not fantastic, but it's FANTASTIC for me. Nothing short of a miracle!

Tonight we sleep in a warm bed. We have a shower. We bought a jar of the powder Gatorade, so now we can have a few bottles each day (Don't worry Sarah, I'm going to keep up our electrolytes) and our food bag is full again. Actually, it runneth over. In a few days I'll be enjoying the company of my sister Cindy and my niece Katie for a day or two. Cindy is kind enough to work on new slips for us so we don't have to hand out hand written slips that say "LittleChanges.com" and people we meet along the way will be able to find and track us online. We have a date to have pancakes for breakfast. But that's still a few days away. Tonight I'm going to get a great nights sleep, enjoy everything I have to be thankful for and count all of my blessings. Tomorrow we ride.

Day 32: February 01, 2007 - Thursday - *Beach House Motel* , Indialantic to *Luna Sea Motel*, Cocoa Beach, Florida

It has warmed back up, so we were both in t-shirts. My jacket hangs like a banner behind me now, fading in the sun, on the back of my trailer. The words, LittleChanges.com will hopefully be seen by a few hundred people each day. Perhaps their curiosity will get the better of them and they will find us online. As we rode I started noticing all the different mailboxes. You might see a rusted box that is barely clinging to a bent pole in front of a house that costs several million. Perhaps after paying the mortgage they can't afford a new one. You go a bit up the road and see a hand-carved tiki totem pole that is holding a mailbox in it's mouth. From dolphins, sea turtles coming out of their shells, giant iguanas, post trucks and even a surfboard with a hole cut in it and a mailbox shoved in, we really see a wide variety. If it wouldn't bother the people in the homes, we might start taking pictures of them.

Moving north the big difference today was that the wind was coming out of the south. It really helped us make excellent time and saved my sore knees. I had taken a pain killer this morning to be safe, but on this magnificent day, I didn't really need it. The names on some of the streets seemed familiar. During my childhood we would sometimes come to this area for a day trip, on the way to fishing or just to have a drive. There were some signs at some stores that seemed like I might have seen them before, but it was 30 years ago when I was here. There was one store sign we recognized and headed for, a massive chain leader but not one of my favorite places. We were bargain shopping though.

Morton needed a tool for the pedal, some other bits and pieces for his ever growing tool box, and was only too happy to run in while I stayed with our bikes. Since starting he has found a pair of pliers, a wrench, a screwdriver, a tape measure, a hammer, a mass assortment of bolts, nuts and bits of wire. Like a little pack rat, he stores them all away in a green box that he found early on in the Keys. Quite often when I see him stopping and bending over to pick something up, I give him "the look" that makes him explain why he needs to save this paperclip. Hey, if he's willing to carry it all around and might be able to use it, let him pick it up. It had just been litter before Morton got a hold of it.

As we got close to *Patrick Air Force Base* there was a big old plane that was making circles over our heads. We stopped to take some pictures and a video, then moved right along. Morton asked me what kind of plane it was, but I have no clue. Maybe someone out there could tell Morton. I was remembering a time that my family had came down to watch the planes that fly here. Dad had our family Super8 camera out and was filming when someone from the Air Force came over and asked him to stop. I guess you really don't have to worry about that now. With technology you can see almost anything on this earth you want to.

There is a little park, right across from the base that has the most wonderful shady picnic tables. We decided to have our lunch there and didn't sit too long before heading north again. Looking through our free book about motels, which is how we are navigating as well, I made a few telephone calls hoping for a room tonight. We actually got lucky twice. First there was a helpful man that was going to take my number, make the calls to the owner and call me back. He actually did this, got us the room and called me back, the trouble was, my phone put him right to my voice mail. We must have been in an out of signal spot. So I had called what I *thought* was the *Holiday Inn* on the beach, but it was actually the Holiday Inn that was over 10 miles west. The general manager said yes. The next *Holiday Inn* we came to, we went inside and they didn't have a clue or a room. The lady suggested that I called the other Holiday Inn, ten miles west of us, which I had. Yikes! Talk about a mix up. As I left the Holiday Inn beachside, thinking there was no way to get to the other one, Morton handed me the phone with the missed call. It was the *Luna Sea Motel*. They were just 1 mile in front of us. I breathed a big sigh of relief as I headed the bike north.

Calling the man who had said yes at the *Holiday Inn at Cocoa*, I felt like a real idiot. He was very understanding and I said I would put his link on our sponsors page anyway since he had been prepared to give us a room for the night. Everything worked out perfect in the end. We are in a lovely room with a fantastic bathroom, refrigerator with freezer (ice cold water for tomorrow), microwave and all the comforts of home. Did I mention FREE wireless internet?

Morton went to *Wendy's* to get us dinner. I ate as I worked on the computer, unable to stop. When I spend days without being able to upload, it takes ages. I might even be burning the midnight oil to catch up on all the videos. With a little luck, tomorrow we will be on the mainland and heading towards Titusville. If I get close enough, I have some cousins that I might get to camp out with. Just cross your fingers the thunderstorms miss us tomorrow and the film crew catches us.

I almost forgot something really odd that happened to us today. Earlier in the evening I posted just where we were staying at on our website, something I do on a regular basis. Before tonight I hadn't really thought anything of it. About 11 pm while I was sitting on one bed with my laptop covering the tops of my legs, a knock came on our door. Morton was fast asleep in the other bed and something made me pull back the curtain just a bit and look out. It was a man carrying a bunch of flowers.

It seems that the website has attracted a potential boyfriend or two for me, even though every day I talk about my husband, show pictures of my husband and in no way am I looking to replace my husband.

This man thought we were made for each other. I was a bit flattered, but really just freaked out. It never dawned on me that by saying where we were staying would bring the locals out looking for us. It was just a bit of confusion I guess. He thought I was looking for Mr. Right and didn't realize I had already found him in Scotland ages ago. I will learn from this though and perhaps not post on the internet where we are. It was very odd and a bit alarming, but at least he didn't take it badly. He just went off into the rainy night with his flowers and will hopefully find his Miss Right.

Day 33: February 02, 2007 - Friday - Luna Sea Motel, Cocoa Beach, Florida

There are times that you want to just kick your feet up and take a day off. Right now, it doesn't feel like that time. Watching the weather outside out window from 7 am on, we kept switching channels hoping to find the one that would tell us it was going to be sunny with a south wind. We couldn't find that forecast. We were watching the local news and all the reporters in Florida were covering the destruction of the weather. The change in temperatures were wrecking havoc all around us as we were caught in the middle of deadly weather. I'm not quite sure how many people were killed yesterday, 14 was the last total we heard. It was more than enough to teach us a valuable lesson about respecting the weather. There are cases where you just have to take the day off, even though your body tells you to ride.

With my laptop at the ready, I gave it a big workout. Finishing all my videos to date (huge job) and moving my pictures to DVD's, my computer now has a bit of room on it again. It was warm on my lap as I kept trying to get just one more thing done. From 7 am until 11 pm the computer was doing something. It was the longest day I have put in online since the days of old when I would work at the computer all day, skipping breakfast and lunch and then eat like a hungry wolf when I came home.

There is a big connection between my lack of exercise and my hunger. Without spending any time doing real exercise, I was actually hungrier than when we would be out walking or bicycling 7 or 8 hours each day. It might have something to do with the difference in the amount of water I drank as well.

It was the first time in a long time that we had late night snacks. Morton kept saying all day that he was "peckish" and would poke in the food bag looking for something nutritious yet that would taste great. The best he could do was some amazing Indian River oranges that he would peel and split between us.

There are so many things to do each day, besides walk and ride. It's up to us to do all the photographs, videos, make the new page(s) and update the site. We also need to email the local press, go over things like weather forecasts, road closings, maps that we are going to be using and get all out our gear and do the daily things on it. It really is a task that many should be doing that is left to just the two of us.

Morton does the tear up, tear down, keeping us going with the tasks like cooking, packing, organizing, laundry and my baby is the computer. My baby is very demanding and does take a lot of time.

We got over the feeling of staying or going yesterday, then I was able to dig in and get serious without looking at the clock. There just isn't enough hours in our day to do all I need to do. Sometime today I would get through this mountain of videos. I worked and worked, finally finishing all of them. Now I get to upload them all to *YouTube*. Perhaps along the way we will have a proper day off here and there, but I have to warn you, I always make the mistake of turning on the computer to check just one thing. Before I know it, the hour or the day is gone and there are still things to be done on the computer.

Day 34: February 03, 2007 - Saturday - Cocoa Beach to Titusville, Florida

When we left the room this morning, we collected a free slip for breakfast at a place that was about a mile north of us. Just as we crossed the road that we should have turned left on, my front tire went flat. It was also just starting to rain. Great start to the day.

Morton fixed the flat in record time and we debated about forgetting the free breakfast and just heading north on A1A. Since we never really know when we are going to get a warm meal, we decided to go for the free breakfast, then just head west to the mainland and follow US 1 north. Pulling in to the place, the food smelled great. We parked the bikes and Morton waited on a bench outside while I went in to see if we could get our breakfast to go. The lady who was working the cash register said they didn't normally do take out on the free breakfast, but they made an exception for us. Moments later we were eating the delicious sandwiches when a couple came outside and asked where we were going. This was one of those chance meetings that we seem to be having so many of. Bob and Janech, who have made about 60 trips cross-country on bicycles, were standing in front of us letting us pick their brains. We were the luckiest people in the world to meet them. You can see just what it is that they do at *www.WanderingWheels.org*. Janech, who is a brilliant mechanic, went over the bikes with Morton and gave him so many tips that only years of experience can bring. They are also experts at crossing the desert, so we asked lots of questions and they were generous enough to answer. They were also generous enough to give us a bright yellow jacket for Morton and a cash donation. After asking their advice on helmets (I wanted them, Morton said no, not enough money) they said that we should really have them. Morton also listened as Janech explained about tightening things TOO tight. We could have spent days absorbing the knowledge these two have. They said to call them if we need help. They have friends all over America. How incredible is that? Parting ways as the rain was starting, they rode off on their lovely 15 pound bicycles and we headed west. Smiling at our luck of meeting these professional experts, I didn't even mind the rain.

Before long I was seeing sights I have seen before. The hospital that my dad took my brother to when he cut his finger with a filet knife. Paul was putting together a little balsa wood plane and got a very sharp knife out. He sliced his finger and came out to my mom holding a cupped hand under the bleeding finger. "I didn't bleed on the new carpet" he announced. Riding along to the hospital I helped get Paul checked in. Dad was in a bit of a panic and said that he was 17 (he was really 7) and it was one of the rare times that I saw my dad flustered. He must have been worried about getting the whole thing behind him as quick as possible, since my dad had given my little brother the knife. He did tell him to never play with it.

We also came across a department store and I went in and bought Morton and I each a helmet, finally. We took some pictures in them and headed off. I felt so much safer and they are really comfortable. It is something we should have had all along the way, but better it happened this way. It was destiny really.

Scenery was changing, but filled my head with so many memories. There was the mall that we would go to sometimes, the familiar bridges and then US1 in Cocoa. It is a lovely little town filled with antique stores, art stores and wee cafes. Morton took a nice picture outside one of the antique shops and while we were stopped a man came out to ask where we were going. Chatting to him for a few minutes, he pointed us in the right direction and wished us a safe journey. He told us he was making little changes in his life that didn't have to do with eating and exercise, but with his problem with alcohol.

US 1 is a busy road. I was hoping there would be a nice sidewalk or path, there is, but it's a bit random. Here and there and on the south side of the road. So we stayed in the north lane riding out bikes on the edge of the road. There were some horns that were tooting, but in general the only problem we had was the north wind pushing us the wrong way.

Port St. John was where my parents had their home that we would come to in the winter. They bought it on one of our visits to my aunt who lived north of Titusville. I think they paid $14,000. for the 3 bedroom, 2 bathroom cement block house with two stunning palm trees in the front yard. It was rented out to people from Pennsylvania who would come down for a week or two at a time. My aunt would make sure it was clean when they left. It held a lot of fun family memories and made my heart ache with that too familiar pang of homesickness. As we approached this village, I felt like I wasn't in Kansas anymore. There were loads of stores, a strip mall and even some red lights going in to it. The only thing that I could recognize was the red roof of what use to be the 7-11 that Paul and I would ride our bikes to for treats. We would always buy Archie comics, a Slurpee and odds and ends that we never got in Pennsylvania. It was pure dead brilliant, as they say in Glasgow. Thinking that I might drive down the streets and find our old house, I considered asking the people if we could camp in the backyard for old time sake. I would want to look inside too, to see if the big brick bar was still in the rec room with a giant letter M on the front of it. A real accent point from the swinging Sixties. But we really wanted to make Titusville by tonight, so we kept going.

I hit my pain and exhaustion wall several times today. I think my legs were so sore because of my day "off" yesterday. I would let out a scream or a big *"UGHHHHHHH"* and keep pedaling. Morton was getting worried that I was going to just get off the bike and pitch camp by the road. It was tough against the wind too. At one point on the road, in front of us, a car stopped. It was a bit worrying, but we hoped it was someone kind. It was actually Lori, the fantastic ranger we had met at Sebastian Inlet. We hugged and it felt so good to see this special lady. She was taking her father to a relatives for a visit and couldn't believe she saw us. I told you it's really wild how we keep meeting and re-meeting some people. The good feeling that you get from the people who are connecting with what we are doing is just the thing that I needed. It kept me going and thinking about all the paths, roads and trails there are to be crossed. The adventure is just really beginning and already we have seen and done so much

.   Morton has been complaining a little that the only armadillo he's seen has been squashed ones beside the road. Today on the ride we saw two. Both living. We pulled over for the first and Morton snapped pictures of the little critter who was busy eating grass or ants, we couldn't tell which. He was so busy eating, he really didn't notice Morton following him, close, with the camera. When he did see him, he turned and ran to a ditch. There was water running in it and the shelled creature jumped over it, bounding once in the water but springing up like a kangaroo. Safely out of Morton's reach on the other side, he started eating again like a hungry little wolf. Morton wanted to follow him and keep taking pictures. I doubted if Morton could have bounded over the water. There also might be an odd gator or two lurking in the dark water, so he was easily talked out of chasing Mr. Armadillo for more photos.

Soon, as we rode on, the rain came back and I squeezed into my orange poncho. My hands were cold since it was only about 56 degrees today. The feeling in my legs was a little like Jello. My knees were really going up and down as the wind blew harder. The bad thing about being a little familiar with where you are, you know how long you still have to go.

Finally we saw the sign for Titusville. Sweet. Soon we were playing the "room for the night" game. Morton even asked, a first for him, but we were just getting a lot of "no's" - after all, it is another Saturday night. Trying to stay as tight to the side as all the cars started switching their lights on, I was getting scared about getting caught out after dark. Please, please, please, I thought as I stepped into the *Riverside Inn*.

The lady at the counter asked where we had came from and listened as I told her what we were up to. She had seen us on television and was very helpful and supportive. She arranged for us to have a room for the night and not just any room. It is brilliant. A king sized bed, so much room we can get around and have our choice of working at a desk or table (I chose the table...Morton can join me once he fine tunes our bikes) and a shower that looks fantastic.

There is a *Taco Bell* across the street that we already know what value meal we are going to get and split. We have been doing that with a lot of our meals and find that it is just right. Plus all the miles that we did today seem to have the most amazing effect on my hunger...I really don't have any, so sharing a meal is fine by me. A few months ago I would have bitten Morton's head off if he would have suggested sharing food. Meeting new friends and seeing a friend from a few days ago, today has really been a good one. Even with the rain and sore muscles, it feels so right doing what we are doing. I highly recommend following your dreams, no matter how wild, strange or odd they might seem to the rest of the world. You will surprise yourself if you try.

Day 35: February 04, 2007 - Sunday - *Riverside Inn,* Titusville to Edgewater, Florida

When will I learn to NOT check my email in the morning. I can't help it though. There might be a person inviting us to camp in their yard or a reporter wanting an interview. It is an important thing to do. It sucks me in though, getting lost in the mass emails, answering questions and all the other things that come with it. This morning we were up early, ready to go on our big 30 plus mile ride today. My sister's house was waiting. We were riding to Edgewater and best of all, my niece Katie was there! Talk about your motivation to keep going. When we left our lovely room at the *Riverside Inn*, we met the Randall family from Minnesota outside. They were heading out for a day of beachcombing with the crew. We had talked the night before, so it was nice seeing them all again. The mom told us that the four youngest were quadruplets! Imagine that! Morton and I had never met quads before. They were all so very friendly people. Hopefully we will get to see them again when we get up to Minnesota.

It dawned on me too late to say, but the older sister of the quads, who is 16, is a very special young lady. Can you imagine having not one, but four new babies come into your world when you are just three years old? Talk about a wonderful family, it was so nice speaking with them we could have stayed for hours. But we just snapped a few pictures and promised to keep in touch, and we all rode away.

Going through Titusville is like stepping in to a time machine. As we were coming through the night before we passed an A-frame building that has held up against countless winds and hurricanes, from my childhood. It was called Jungle World or Jungle something and had been owned by the man who played the original Tarzan on television. Once and only once, my dad took my little brother and I there. Dad was not partial to what he called "tourist traps", a forerunner to theme parks. He felt that for the cost of a fishing license you could get all the entertainment and dinner that a person could stand. But today, he took Paul and I to the depths of this JUNGLE place. I don't remember a lot about it other than it had a little train that you rode. It jumped the track and my dad and several other men helped get it back online. These were the days before crazy lawsuits and rules and regulations that would prohibit people from pitching in and setting things right. We all climbed back on the little train and it took us the rest of the way without incident. There was also an arcade room with pinball machines and snacks. Dad did enjoy both of these things. I can remember the thing I absolutely hated about the place. Cages of snakes. It was sheer panic and gripping fear when I saw them and I have no clue as to how I got out of the building they were in. Paul was fascinated and had his face pressed to the glass. Yesterday Morton and I rode past this building, the backyard "jungle" looking a lot like a real jungle now. I wondered what ever became of the man who played Tarzan.

But this morning I was seeing things that reminded my of my Aunt Gladys. Aunt G had a house a bit north of Titusville, but Titusville was most definetly her stomping grounds. She new every shop, where to buy what and everyone that ever met her can never forget her smile and her generous heart. There were many of times we camped in her backyard and there were several occasions I got to go all on my own to her house for a few weeks or even a couple months in the summer. Riding past streets that we have shopped on in her metallic green car, I can still see her dark tanned arms waving at people she knew. She would fill me in on who they were, where they were from and how she knew them as we drove to our next destination. The thing I remember most about my Aunt Gladys was the way she could tell a story. She was a treasure that all the world missed out on. Talk about missing her calling, Aunt G would leave you spellbound as she took you back to a house she lived in, in a big northern city somewhere, and tell the tales of when my uncle (her little brother) had came to stay with her. My aunt had made the transition of going from a farm in Pennsylvania to this big scary city, but my uncle (her little brother) never got the feel for it. He would have to walk home, through the dangerous and dark streets, after working his late shift and rattle his metal lunch box to make lots of noise to scare the baddies away. My aunt would tell us how he would talk in different voices, pretending he was an entire crowd. After all, there is safety in numbers! Maybe Morton and I should try that. One night my aunt had planned a horrible joke for her brother. While he was busy at work, she was busy setting the stage. Climbing out a window on the top floor, laying on her stomach on the porch roof, she waited with her surprise. She listened for the familiar "voices" of my uncle returning and shoved the object closer to the edge. As my aunt told us this story, we would wait for it. I knew what was going to happen, but my aunt had a way of building it up that we almost jumped out of our own skin waiting. Poor Uncle Gene, I thought. He didn't stand a chance against my Aunt G. At the crucial moment when my uncle was just going to step on to the safety of the porch, Aunt G let her plan fly. She shoved the dummy she had made out of a stuffed pair of trousers, sewn to a stuffed shirt, with a head made from a pillow case and a felt hat shoved on it, out through the darkness at my uncle below. As I said, he didn't stand a chance. Aunt Gladys filled the night with a scream that she could still create all those years later to delight and fright us. We would always jump, but I imagine nothing compared to how my Uncle Gene must have jumped. Aunt G would punch and thrash to show us just how her younger brother fought to the death from his attacker. He threw it to the ground, jumped on top of it and didn't stop until he had knocked it's block off, or pillow case. In all the commotion, he looked up to see his sister sitting with her legs dangling off the porch edge laughing so hard she nearly fell off the roof. He was not amused and went back to the safety of the farm the next day. It all worked out in the end. Uncle Gene now lives happily up the valley he has spent his entire life in. He's a wonderful man who recounted this same story to me just a few years ago. I had always wondered if Aunt G had perhaps embellished a bit, but after hearing his version of it, she had been spot on.

Smiling, we passed a park that I have had more than one picnic in with my lovely aunt. I'll never forget this special lady and it doesn't feel the same knowing that she's not with us anymore. Sadly she passed from cancer a few years ago. I wanted to tell Morton about her, about all these special things we were seeing, but we can't really talk on the bikes. Instead I just kept going and was chuckling and crying thinking about my uncle killing the dummy.

There was a bridge that I wasn't able to ride over at the north end of the town, so we pushed. Staying clear of all the broken glass, nails, screws and other things that can bite tires, we climbed back on the bikes at the top and for the first time today we actually made good time. The wind was that strong though, at the bottom we really had to pedal hard to keep going.

Going past the little town of Mims where my aunt stayed for all the years that I knew her, I wanted to stop in and visit my uncle Robert. It was church time and I knew he wouldn't be home and we also had a full day of riding still waiting. I promised myself that tomorrow I will call him and have a chat. It's not the same though as being able to give someone a proper hug around the neck. It's been a good 15 years since I've seen him, so maybe I'll find a ride to head back down to collect that hug.

We stopped to get a picture of Morton under a sign that read the towns name "Scotsmoor" thinking it would be cute having a Scot in Scotsmoor. I had just called my niece to tell her we were on our way, but had no way of knowing how long it would take us. We had things like flat tires, jumped chains and the weather to think about. I assured her that we would be there today, however long it took. Morton posed for the pictures and came back to his bike and left out a yelp. He had a puncture on his trailer tire. Jumping into action, he pulled it off the trailer as I snapped some pictures. Looking south behind us, a white pick up pulled off the road. The man in it pulled on the grass and right up beside us. He had passed us earlier in a big tow truck, thought we had a broken axle, went to his business which was just ahead of us on the right, got in the pickup and came back to lend a hand. Talk about a *GREAT SAMARITAN!* His name is CJ and he and his finance have a towing business, *C&L Towing* in Scotsmoor Florida. We chatted a bit about where we came from and where we were going. It seems they had just been in Key West at Christmas, where he proposed to her. We just missed each other by days down there, but here he was at the side of the road, ready to lend a hand. Talk about your good guys!

With the flat fixed, we kept our bikes pointed north, right into the wind. It was chilly out, only reaching 60 for the day and the wind chill factor had to make it even lower. The rain kept away, with only dark clouds blocking out the sun, our faces still got hot from the work out the wind was giving us. Uphill all the way. After I tell you about the sights we see and post the pictures and videos, it dawns on me that the one thing I can't really share with you is the smells that we encounter. Some you can be glad of. The road kill that the buzzards are feasting on, the water that has gone stagnant beside the road to breed mosquitoes and the smell of seaweed that has came in and piled on the shore in a rotting state, are things you would rather not smell. Then there are the smells that we would love to share. The breeze that carries the salt air off the ocean that can only be described as "beach", the smell after a rain, when we have a walk in the woods and you can almost smell the plants growing and making the air that we breath, then my favorite smell so far, the orange blossoms.

When I first asked Morton if he could smell the orange blossoms, he said no and argued a bit that I must be mad. There were oranges still on the tree, both green and orange. How could there be blossoms? This, I can't explain. But as I type this to you, I'm setting my eyes on a tree in my sisters backyard that has oranges and blossoms. The scent takes me back again to childhood. Florida is filled with memories of escaping the frozen winter of Pennsylvania, loading up in a big station wagon, and waking up in the land of Dixie. There is a shop that we are cycling past that has a tale from my childhood dripping all over it, pushing me back in time and I smile then remember.

When I was about eight years old we stopped in to Manny's on US 1, just south of Edgewater. It is an old concrete block building, now not used for anything. But going back thirty some odd years ago, it was prime Florida nostalgia. The shelves were stocked with exotic gifts for every taste and budget. Lamps made of shells with plastic pink flamingos and the word "Florida" hand painted on a big shell that would hide the little bulb. Little wooden crates that would fit in your hand that were filled with tiny oranges that were actually chewing gum. Rubber alligators that looked like miniature versions of the big gator out back that you could look at for *FREE*. These were the sights, sounds and smells that old Florida was to me. My parents never sprang for the shell lamps, which were a bit pricey. But I did get the odd shell or sand dollar on occasion. There was also the time that I got my most exotic and tropical gift that an eight-year-old girl could ever hope for. A bottle of genuine Orange Blossom Perfume. This was pure class from head to toe. The clear bottle was a smart shape, exactly like an orange, with little dimples all over the glass. The bottle was only about 3 inches tall. A little dab would definetly do you of this scent. When you removed the lid, which was a tiny hard plastic orange with wee green plastic leaves, you were transported to the center of a thousand acre grove in full bloom. You could almost get drunk from smelling this intoxicating fragrance. The sample bottle would be tilted and dabbed all over my arms, neck and behind my ears making me feel like a real Hollywood starlet. My dad must have had a cold or at least a blocked nose when I took the packaged bottle to him and begged for this rare treat. He wasn't a big fan of perfume or makeup and I didn't get my hopes too high. If he would have caught a whiff of me, reeking with the concentrated stuff, he would have said no. Looking back I can almost picture oranges smell-waves rising up from my neck as I asked for the perfume. Taking the box that held the special bottle, Dad flipped it over and saw the price. $1.00. Not too much at all. He was pushing a cart that held enough oranges to feed an army and a few gallons of fresh squeezed juice. *"Put it in the cart, it'll get paid for!"* Dad said.

Now my attention could focus on the woman who had the best job in the world. This is the very first job that I can remember wanting. When I laid eyes upon her, I knew what I wanted to be when I grew up. This lady was sitting almost up on a little stage. She had crates of oranges surrounding her and a big machine in front of her. Someone else, an underling I imagine, had already sliced the oranges in half. It was this special ladies job to take the oranges, and in one swift motion, grind them down onto the spinning machine and that fast juice, fresh squeezed, would shot out and into this tank. Brilliant! For ages I stood mesmerized by this magical process. The words, *Fresh Squeezed Orange Juice*, always conjure up the image of this lady with her hair net, surrounded by mountains of sliced oranges. Talk about a glamour job! I dreamed about this until the day I saw the people shucking oysters beside the raw bar at the seafood place we were having lunch at. That would be my new dream job. Just think, instead of bonuses, you got to keep all the pearls you found, or so the man who was shucking told me. My dad bought a bushel of the oysters and although I never ate any of them, I used the short steel blade on the thick round wooden handle to open the entire bushel. No pearls, maybe the next time.

If only I could find a way to ride my bicycle and write. There are so many small seconds of things we see each day it is quite impossible to remember them all. The thoughts that filled my head were all sweet-nostalgic and knowing that real family was waiting just up the rode, my heart really pulled me along through the wind. Before I knew it we were making the turn left into the large development that my sister lives in. The last five miles is usually the toughest of the day but today they were the sweetest and easiest.

My niece met us at the door with her lovely smile and we got lost in hours of conversation, the best meal I've ever tasted and fell asleep way after midnight in the feeling of family. Leaving here is going to be our toughest thing we have done to date and knowing it might be years before I see Katie again, I won't think about that now. If this journey is teaching me anything, it is to enjoy every single moment we are given. Live in the now, think about your future and your past, just don't make the mistake of living in either of those places.

Day 36: February 05, 2007 - Monday - Edgewater, Florida

Waking up in familiar, homelike surroundings was very pleasant. Earlier I had heard Katie leaving for work and thought about getting up, but I was really worn out from the day before. Not just the physical side of the day, it was very emotional as well passing my aunt's hometown, my parents old house and remembering all the people I loved that were no longer on this planet. Once I got up, Morton wasn't far behind. He set about working on various functions that keep us going. I had a lot of work in front of me for planning out our first Must See Cities stop. St. Augustine was a natural choice for our first stop. It's the oldest city in America and one of the most charming. Morton has never seen it before, but I've been lucky enough to. Walled, ancient (for America anyway) and not far away, all my thoughts focused on this town by the water.

Planning just what we are going to do is hard. There are so many things. St. Augustine is made for walking of bicycling around. Money plays the big factor in what we are going to do. Since our budget is so small, we have to rely on the generosity of businesses to help us. We are pleased to announce that in St. Augustine, southern hospitality is alive and well. We have had the most wonderful luck with getting lodging, food (incredible food) and the most delightful things to see. Spending the entire day on the computer (very bad for me, very good for the website and journey) I was pleased with what all I got accomplished. There were a lot of email interviews to catch up on, the videos and making contact with places that we are going to be going through. Morton did some odd jobs around the house to keep busy. He really does love doing that. Katie's dog, Nola and her kitty cats kept us company as she was at work, then out to a friends for dinner. As the evening came on, we talked about walking to get Chinese food, but our budget couldn't really handle it. Plus, the computer still needed several hours of work. Raiding my sister's cupboards, with permission of course, Morton whipped up a really good meal. He just boiled the pasta, added a can of clam chowder and drained green beans. Warm and delicious, the fact we are able to do laundry and have a shower, I'm quite overwhelmed.

I think living on the road is leaving me a bit shell-shocked and it is tempting to just stay in this warm glow of family for the rest of my life.

It was a quiet evening and as we headed for bed, we knew we needed to wake up early. Very early. We were meeting a reporter and photographer, had to pack and load and go 30 miles north. As I fell asleep my thoughts were on my family and how hard it was going to be to leave in the morning. This isn't as easy as it reads. It is heartbreaking to ride away from this Florida oasis of the comforts of home and a roof over our heads.

Day 37: February 06, 2007 - Tuesday - Edgewater to Flagler Beach, Florida

When I woke up this morning, I would have never guessed that we would travel 43.3 miles today. The sun was out, it was very cold and it was way too early to be waking up. Last night I was too wound up to sleep. Twisting and turning, I couldn't seem to find a place to fall asleep. So when the alarm on the phone went off this morning while I was in a really good sleep, I just wished for another hour. But not today.

We met with the reporter and photographer and then had to wait for a bit before we left. Hoping to catch up with a different reporter, we waited for another 30 minutes or so, then headed out. We learned the lesson to keep riding and let them catch up with us. We are HAPPY news and take a backseat to any bad news that might come along. First though before we left, we hugged Katie so tight and got some great pictures. Hopefully at some point on this adventure she will be able to come out and move with us for a little while. Fingers crossed.

Staying as close to the river as we could, we stopped at a lovely park where we had been almost exactly a year ago. My mom and dad, son and future daughter-in-law were all with us. We had spent the day out looking around New Smyrna Beach and finished the day with my son grilling fish on my sister's grill. We didn't stay there very long, but I did make a call to my mom. I needed to just talk to her for a moment. It was reassuring to hear her voice, even though she is 1000 miles away. She is north, just the direction we are heading. In New Smyrna Beach, right beside US 1, Morton and I stopped and our jaws fell open. We were looking at the path that the tornado had cut through this area. It was the most shocking thing I have ever seen. Trees were snapped like toothpicks, pieces of houses were stuck in tall branches, the wind having swept them like they were paper napkins on a table. This is the weather that we had missed by sheer luck. The power this thing carried was something that could still be felt. We took some pictures and we spoke some quiet words, but it just felt wrong. This storm had taken lives, forget the dollar value of damage it has done, that means nothing.

Reaching Port Orange we turned right to head out to A1A. There were still the images of the tornado damage in my mind. I thought of it as we looked at a group of mobile homes that were beside the water. It would have been very frightening to be in one of them during a storm like what just happened here.

Just a day or two different in on timing and we might have been camped here in the path of the tornados that kept us pinned down in a motel in Cocoa Beach an extra day. Timing is everything in this life.

Soon we were at the edge of the Atlantic Ocean. After a thrilling ride down a tall bridge with just my front brakes, we both wanted to make some time. We wanted at least 30 miles today and the only way to get it done was to keep our feet on the pedals. And that we did. Minus a few flat tires, a brake adjustment or two, little stops for breaks and food, we flat out rode today. Like a couple of kids getting ready for summer vacation, Morton and I talked about what all we were going to see and do in Saint Augustine. It was a brilliant idea to stop for a few days in incredible places along the way and we weren't sure why we had felt the need to make this journey a race. The sun was going down and we were in an area where there really weren't any rooms, campgrounds or even houses. It was condos and wilderness. Sort of wilderness. So we kept on the lovely wide bike path and hoped to see some neon lights soon. There was a park that we were going to camp in, but we both left out a groan of despair as the gates were locked and shut when we rode by at 6 pm. We had no other choice then to keep going. The growth beside the road was thick, but there were paths here and there. Maybe we should sneak in and pitch the tent. Who would know?

Just a bit further and we saw a motel that had rooms still available. We had to spend $35. on the room, employee discount, but we really didn't have a choice. It is going to be really wonderful not having to worry about where we are sleeping for a few nights once we get to St. Augustine.

You know, if someone would have told me a year ago that I would have rode and walked 43 miles in one day and not died, I would have never believed them. My body is surprising me every day with how much more it can do. It makes me really feel that our goal of 50 miles a day on the bicycles will soon be met. Unless we have a major problem with the bikes, we will be in St. Augustine Beach tomorrow.

Day 38: February 07, 2007 - Wednesday - Flagler Beach to *Holiday Inn, St. Augustine Beach*, Florida

Waking up beside the ocean was a fantastic way to start the day. We were also happy to see the sun with not much wind. This was a day made for two people on a massive fitness quest. The sights we saw today were spectacular. There are no words in our human language that can sum up the mixture of what I was seeing and how I was feeling. I will give it a go, but I warn you, it was a million times better then what I'm about to tell you.

First, picture the waves coming in on the never ending beach. They are sapphire blue with snow white tops that curl under to meet the sand. The sound they are making is always the same, yet never the same. You can see sandbars and seagulls sitting on them, all on a canvas of brilliant blue sky. Pelicans are flying in formation, low, over the breaking waves. The second in line mimics the first one more efficiently than any pilot. They dip together, each give one flap of their mighty wings and climb on the invisible breeze just a few feet higher. Now try to put yourself in my place for how I'm feeling. Just a year ago I was in a horrible state of depression over my body. I had felt like when I turned 40, almost 4 years ago, my body was falling apart on me. It was hard to admit that it was my own fault. Food and more specifically, massive amounts of food with no exercise, left me heavier than ever with my spirits lower than ever.

Yesterday we rode 43.3 miles. I know we have already told you this, but please try to understand what an accomplishment this is for someone like me. Someone who had considered going to the refrigerator too much work is now riding a bicycle and walking for several hours daily. On the road with all these elements coming together and the thought of St. Augustine waiting on us, the grin never came off my face. It's a good thing the bugs aren't out during the day or I would have had a mouth full of mosquitoes. Able to cycle small bridges in a single bound, I rarely have to get off and push it now to crest a bridge. Unless of course we are taking a break to do some purpose walking. We are also taking fewer and shorter breaks now. It only happens once or twice a day that I really feel like I'm hitting a wall and today I was able to sail through all my walls like they were made out of wet tissue paper.

There was a shaded path that twisted and wondered through huge trees that were draped with Spanish moss. This part of our ride was really stunning. It felt like we were getting to peek at the real Florida, prior to all the condos crowded on the beaches and the plastic influx of signs of man. The only hint that you were near civilization was the paved path you were on and the picnic tables that were sprinkled along the trail. Morton took a lot of pictures, we did some videos and wished that we had time to just ride this same route daily for the next couple of weeks, or at least until the snow stops where we are heading.

We did a little shopping and got lunch at a grocery store. Taking advantage of their shady picnic tables, we shared a little bite and chatted with a group of people on vacation. People really make our day. Meeting so many nice people and talking about a variety of things (today's topic was green tea) makes our world go round. As we got further north I realized another reason that I was feeling so happy today. Sure we had some flat tires. Sure we got pushed around by the wind a bit. But one thing that was missing from today was that we don't have to go searching for a place to stay. We know right where we are sleeping, not just for tonight, but we actually have a place sorted until Sunday, giving me a few begging-free days. Without the worry, my mind is free to just enjoy the ride. Without the feeling of my health going downhill fast, I feel my body listening to what I'm doing. The journey is really one of mind and body, one won't ever work right without the other. Making just a few pit stops for bathrooms, a drink here and there and of course pictures, we were at our room in St. Augustine Beach at another *Holiday Inn* by 3:30 pm. Superb!

We even had time for a stroll on the beach to look at the sky turning into evening. Morton touched a jellyfish. I thought about swimming, for a brief second. The perfect end on a day of such. Even though swimming is one of my favorite activities, there are still too many things that need done to let my hair down and put the bathing suit on. With a day like today to think about when we are riding and walking out there, I really do know that anything, and I do mean anything, is possible!

Day 39: February 08, 2007 - Thursday - *Holiday Inn, St. Augustine Beach* to *Agustin Inn Bed & Breakfast*, St. Augustine, Florida

Magic happens when you start chasing dreams. Today was proof of that. Morton believes in prevention. He likes to tinker at night and make sure everything is just right with the bikes, and last night was no exception. He "rotated" my tires on the bike to provide equal wear. It took him the time that it took me to tinker with the website. As we were leaving the *Holiday Inn* he discovered however, the brakes weren't quite right. They were actually sticking on. So we sat for about an hour after our start, until he got them just right. After all, there would be a bridge to come over and the last thing I want to do is go down a bridge again with no brakes. The last time I did this I had to cross my fingers that the light at the bottom would stay green long enough for me to sail through it. I have no idea what I would have done with no brakes if the light would have changed. I suppose I would have gotten hit by my first car. We rode and thought we could maybe pick up something to eat along the way. Our stomachs were growling so we drank lots of water and gatorade mix. Every once in a while we would catch a smell of something lovely, but food eluded us all morning.

The view today was again dazzling. Soon the lighthouse was coming in to view and we knew we couldn't be far away from the amazing Bridge of Lions that would take us in to the ancient city. As we near the famous bridge we discover that there is a new bridge beside it. A temporary bridge. We learn while crossing the new bridge that the old bridge is being restored. The new bridge will move again once the Bridge of Lions is safely back in place. Today we push the bikes over, as the sign instructs, taking lots of pictures and chatting to a few people on the way.

Once we are on the other side if feels like we have stepped back in time. Forget prefab construction here, this is the ancient city of Saint Augustine. We are in the old country, surrounded by pure history. Certain streets are made of bricks, the oldest stone fort in America stands guard and the tiny lanes in the historic district are perfect for walking. Morton and I ride our bikes along the water and head for *Ripley's Believe It Or Not*, before checking in to the *Agustin Inn B&B,* which will be our home for the next few nights. The great people at Ripley's have been kind enough to provide us with tickets to some of the best things in town. While everything is getting sorted out, I look around the entrance to this castle. Memories of a previous trip flood my mind and for a moment I'm ten again.

We would always see the sign for *Ripley's* on the interstate as we would drive past St. Augustine to head south to my aunt's or Cocoa area. No matter how much my little brother and I pleaded, we couldn't convince dad to make the car stop. That was until a certain trip down in the winter I was 10. For whatever reason, dad relented and pulled us in to St. Augustine. Mom waited in the car with a book, dad sat outside probably thinking about all the fish he was missing and Paul and I got to go through the museum. The only condition dad had was that we were out in an hour. We promised, just one hour, then headed in to see the wonders of Mr. Ripley's world. Paul and I were greatly impressed, read every sign, tried every puzzle and we were nearly finished exploring when my dad caught up with us. We had stayed over the hour. We had to get shuffled out and back on the road. It was still great seeing what we did, but there were so many things to see inside, an hour just didn't cut it.

Oddities, comedy, tragedy...Mr. Ripley really was the first great investigative reporter/artist in our history. His artwork always fascinated me in our local paper and I just loved the way he went everywhere. Morton and I got a tiny taste of what was in store for us by going through the amazing redwood four bedroom house. It's our dream to get to sleep in it some day. I would even love to live in something like it. Imagine a tree so big you can lay it on it's side and make a home inside it! *Believe it or NOT!*

We headed off on our bikes for our last ride in a couple of days. Finding the *Agustin Inn* was a snap and like finding treasure right in the heart of the historic district. Standing outside this beautiful inn, we just sort of both looked at each other as we saw it. "Brilliant" said Morton. He was right. It's better than brilliant. We were shown to our room by the lovely staff and got all of our gear stowed. We were like anxious kids waiting for the school bell to ring. There was so much to see. But the charm of the Agustin Inn made us slow down a moment, sit in the shade and just catch our breath. Imagine getting to sleep here for three whole nights, breakfast in the morning and explore the city. It feels so fantastic, we are both walking on air.

There is a *Red Train* that takes you all around the city so we figured this was a good place to start. When you come here go to Ripley's FIRST, they sell excellent packages and if you choose the train option, you get free parking for three days and free train riding for three days...talk about a deal. The RED train is a great way to see the entire city. You can hop on and hop off at any one of it's many stops. Don't worry, you can still get loads of exercise if you wish.Morton and I decided to go full circle, see the sights while sitting and deciding what all we MUST see. This is not an easy task. At each turn there is something else that we really want to see. About 10 minutes in to the train ride we decided that once our big journey is over we are going to come back to Saint Augustine for at least two weeks. It really is the best kept secret in Florida. Our friends and family in the UK that have been to the states have all MISSED St. Augustine. If you ask them where they went in Florida (and a LOT of you are probably like this!) you will just hear "Orlando" and maybe the Keys. I can't understand why everyone doesn't discover this place. There are so many incredible things to see and do here, the beach is one of the nicest, if not THE nicest and add in all the history and there really is something here for everyone. If you want to understand the history of America, get yourself to this special place. The feeling of time is really here. Morton was so impressed with everything he was seeing, but I kept surprising him with the video. He calls it, putting him on the spot, I call it getting his gut reaction. I want to know what he thinks of it all! After all, this is my country we are in now. Up until now, Morton had really only seen Florida in the movies, television or for a week in 2002.

The evening came quick with the two of us sitting by the water. We were watching the sky and all it's colors, melting like the Northern Lights, swirling with pinks, golds and purples over the skyline of the city. Horses pulling carriages got their lanterns lit, the street lights came on and the lovely city started to glow like the special jewel that it is. Morton and I were still in for an amazing treat. A magnificent treat. We walked the short but beautiful walk over brick streets to *La Pentola* for dinner. There we stepped inside a candle lit courtyard, with linen table clothes and felt the Med calling us. This place was beyond compare. We can both safely say this was the best meal we have ever eaten. It is the meal we will dream about when we are far from food. The meal that we will compare all others to. The menu is perfection and everything is made from fresh, natural and the best. This is what people should be eating when they dine out. Nothing processed or added. Just the most incredible meal. I have to stop talking about it now or I'm going to make myself hungry again. The soft music playing and impeccable service added to the entire experience. This is an evening we will never forget and smile whenever we think of it. Thank you so much Chef Jorge for your kindness and culinary skills.

Walking the short stroll home to the lovely *Agustin Inn*, Morton and I talked about all the nights we had cold tuna from the can for dinner. We are going to have many more nights like that in front of us, but now we will pretend we are back at the *La Pentola*. But I don't think anyone's imagination could be that good though. When we came back we tried out the corner spa for two in our room. Bliss! Again, this is something that is going to spoil us rotten for the road ahead. The days when we were so aching and sore at the end of the day seem a million miles behind us, not just a few short days ago. Our muscles relax as the warm water massages our bodies and I wonder how on earth I could carry one of these along on my bicycle trailer. The bath was sleep therapy for Morton. As I downloaded the pictures from today, he was sleeping before the camera had even empties. I wanted to upload, tried to upload and timed out from the upload. Too many pictures! Recording the moments on this journey through photos and film seem like an easy task, but it requires so much work each day. It must be done though.

Day 40: February 09, 2007 - Friday - *Agustin Inn*, St. Augustine, Florida

Sleeping in a bed so comfortable has to be a good thing, right? We both wake up and still have to try to get our head around the fact that we aren't riding 30, 40 or 50 miles today. Today we are *EXPLORING!* But only after we have breakfast. The *Agustin Inn* does everything right. Actually, better than right, whatever that is! The breakfast was delicious, fresh, homemade and presented in a room where you are all seated together. This is really a nice way to get to mingle in the mornings. If you have never stayed in a bed and breakfast, you are missing out. There were several couples at the table and we all enjoyed a wee blether (little talk) before starting our day. People from very near and far come here to enjoy this special spot. I know we will be back again for at least a week when we finish the journey.

Morton and I set off walking. We wanted to visit *Ripley's Believe It Or Not* first. It was a wonderful weather day out and we were holding hands and walking. It did seem odd not to be pushing a bike, pulling a trailer and the fact that we could go in a building together was really something special. Funny how you forget the little things. The experience was incredible. I can just say, if you visit *ANY* Ripley's in the whole wide world, make it this one. It's the only one that Mr. Ripley ever stayed in and the collection is mind boggling. We even got to make a wax cast hand...talk about fun! We could have stayed the entire day, but we have so much to see here.

We keep moving. Yesterday we had the chance to visit the Catholic church in town, but there are several others we want to see. There are also other buildings and experiences we want to explore.

Lunch today was at the *LaPentola* for our second visit. Talk about getting spoiled rotten. Morton and I really hoped to get to meet Chef Jorge today. After a lunch that melted in our mouths, we got the pleasure. This wonderful chef came out and spoke with us about cooking, health and we hope to meet him again. He is so talented and creative in the kitchen you just have to visit to believe it. It wasn't just Morton and I that were singing his praises. There were several other diners that were as amazed by the food as we were and were in the process of telling Chef Jorge this as we were leaving.

Walking down the old streets Morton and I made our way, with really no where in mind really to go.

Little Changes   **67**   *Priscilla Houliston*

We took pictures, talked to several people and found our way back on a RED TRAIN! We were going to try to get in to see something that was just closing when we got there. It will go on the list for tomorrow!

We walked back to the *Agustin Inn* and started downloading pictures. Trying to get an early start for tomorrow will mean an early night tonight. We decided we were not going to actually eat a whole dinner tonight, just have a little plate of the treats they have here on the weekends. It was really nice meeting some more of the people that are staying here as well. Tomorrow we will go on the Ghost Train, visit Flagler Church, visit the Old Town and try to see as much as we can. We might even get a visit from my sister Cindy and her student from France, Samir!

Food for our day Breakfast: Agustin Inn : fruit cup that was very fresh, quiche, lean bacon, muffin, toast, orange juice *Lunch:* Morton had grilled tuna sandwich with flan with orange sauce, Priscilla had lobster ravioli with the most incredible sauce, asparagus and cannoli with pistachio that was just beautiful. Again, this was a meal prepared by Chef Jorge at *LaPentola Dinner:* We just had the light tidbits (that were delicious) that the *Agustin Inn* has in the evenings. Fresh fruit, cheese, veggies, 3 meatballs, some crackers

Day 41: February 10, 2007 - Saturday - *Agustin Inn,* St. Augustine, Florida

Saturday, our last full day in St. Augustine, came way too fast. It feels like we have just gotten here and the first thought that crosses my mind is, "Just one more night." Staying in a place like this has been just wonderful. It really does feel like our batteries have been fully recharged and today we have a real surprise in store. My sister Cindy is coming up from DeLand, Florida for a visit. It does sort of take the sting out of the thought of leaving this beautiful place. Morton and I went down to the lovely table for breakfast. I really like how they do the three choices of breakfast times, we like early, since our day will be quite full. It is a really nice time to get to speak with people and again we make some new friends who will hopefully keep in touch. The food is fresh cooked and perfect. Even Morton can't make waffles as good as these were. The fresh strawberries were huge and sweet and served in a separate silver cup. This was really nice because the waffles stayed hot and I would just cut off a portion of the chilly berry to eat with the waffle.

With our bellies full, we headed out. We had a free ticket thanks to the wonderful people at *Ripley's Believe It Or Not!,* to see a recreated old Florida living museum. The museum is very hands on and we both enjoyed playing, trying, reading, talking and getting to really feel how the three different types of people lived in this area so long ago. Morton even had me wash a shirt on a washboard.

From there we headed for the Flagler Church, built for the memory of Henry Flagler's daughter who had died shortly after giving birth. The church is not only her final resting place, but Henry himself is there too. This church is something that you must visit when you come here. The stained glass is remarkable and the interior is as stunning as the exterior. Morton said it reminded him of a church he was in once in Scotland. We could have spent ages there looking around, but we had a lot to do and we were also going to have a lunch, courtesy of *95 Cordova.* There had been a person talking about how wonderful it was earlier at the *Agustin Inn.* We were both really looking forward to a treat, and we were not disappointed. The interior was wonderful, the food was brilliant but the very best thing about lunch was our waiter. He really made the meal special and we even got a picture together. A transplant from New York, NY, our lovely waiter loves to travel and is going on his own tour of Europe this summer. Hopefully we can keep in touch with all the brilliant people we are meeting. I just have to give him a warning that Morton told him about...watch out for the flying baby trick! For those of you who have never heard of this trick, it goes like this. Someone, a thief, has a fake baby wrapped up. You, the unsuspecting tourist who are busy guarding your valuables will let your guard down to catch this fake baby the thief tosses in your direction. Morton explained this as the waiter and I had a good laugh. Neither of us had ever heard of this scam but we will both think twice if someone tosses a baby in our direction.

After lunch and an explore around the Lightner Museum compound where we walked inside the largest swimming pool of it's time, drained now and turned into shops and cafe, we went to meet Cindy and her friend from France, Samir, at the *Oldest School in America.* Spotting my sister through the very crowded street, we started waving like mad. People were looking around to see who and what we were waving at. Speeding up, we gave each other giant bear hugs and went in to explore the old school and grounds. Massive trees draped in Spanish moss filled the backyard that was alive with squirrels and fellow tourists. It was interesting and Morton and I both learned things we didn't know. Like even though we might have been a wee bit naughty in school, we never had to sit with a rat under the stairs. That would have been punishment enough to make anyone study a bit harder. Leaving there we walked and talked. The city was at our feet and we just got lost in all her charms. We varied our walking partners and our topics and kept moving until everyone wanted dinner. The first choice was booked full, it was Saturday night after all. The second choice was an English pub. The conversation kept us all going until we realized that Morton and I were going to be late for our Ghost Train and Cindy and her friend from France had to head back down the road. We all walked to the traffic lights in front of *Ripley's Believe It Or Not*, hugged tight again, then went our different ways. The last few hours had seemed like just a few seconds. Time really does fly when you are having that much fun.

The *Ghost Train* was so much fun and guess what, I think I even got a picture of a *real* ghost. There were loads of people on the train and at a point in the tour where the guide was telling us about what had happened on this spot so many years ago, I was snapping pictures and only half listening. Digital cameras are amazing and I was doing a quick review of the picture I just took and was shocked to see three orbs hanging below the long stretched branch on what the guide was saying was the hanging tree. If you look at the picture, you can see the orbs are right about where the heads of the unlucky would have been.

The tour on the train was brilliant but the best part was coming back to the museum that houses Ripley's famous collection, when it was closed, the lights dimmed, and getting a tour around the place. It looks quite different in the dark and the cases glowing with shrunken heads and oddities of every description send a chill down your spine. It was on a certain staircase as we were coming down and I was snapping away that I really got a shot of a ghostly image. I showed it at once to the stranger who was behind me snapping away with his own camera and he held his camera out and snapped another, pointing in the same directions, just a few seconds after I captured my wee ghost. The picture on his camera was a green orb in the same spot. Not as detailed as mine but there was no explanation for why it was there at all. We showed our guide who was impressed and asked us to email copies to the office. They might even use them in a slide show of odd images people have taken in this place that is said to be haunted.

We walked home from the museum under the stars and past the cemetery that sits right outside the gates that lead you into the old part of St. Augustine. Again, I snapped a picture and sure enough, above the grave that is suppose to be so haunted the guides won't even take you there now, there was an orb floating just a foot or so above the tombstone. Do you believe in ghosts?

Back inside the lovely glow of Agustin Inn, Morton and I chattered on about this amazing day filled with the spirit of family, new friends and maybe a sideline of capturing the most haunted places in America as we are on this adventure. The evening flew by in a lovely ending of a sleep that was much needed in a real bed.

Day 42: February 11, 2007 - Sunday - St. Augustine to Jacksonville Beach, Florida

Going down to our delicious breakfast for one last time at the *Agustin Inn*, I was feeling very sad about leaving. The weather was lovely, we were still all excited about our adventure on the *Ghost Train* the night before and it just felt like the best vacation in the world coming to an end. But we do have places to go and people to meet, so we said our thanks and goodbyes to Lori and the ladies at *Agustin Inn* and headed down the brick street one last time. Lori had given me a card to open later. If there is one place we really want to go back to, it's there!

We made one final tourist stop at the oldest drugstore in America. Even though we had lots of riding to do, we just both had really wanted to peek inside. It was from a time when things in the world of medicine were really different. Bottles filled with potions and elixirs sure to cure almost anything still line the shelves as well as a few coffins for those who are too far gone to be fixed. When we were getting ready to set off again, I remembered the card Lori had given us. We opened it to find the nicest note of well wishes I have ever seen, along with a tiny silver angel. Lori had said to keep the angel as long as we needed and then pass it on to someone we met who needed it more. What a very wonderful person and a lovely thought and gesture.

Today we rode right out the old gates, with sand instead of sidewalk. It was hard not to stop for one final look at the 4 room log house in the giant redwood that sits in *Ripley's Believe It Or Not!* parking lot. I'm quite smitten with it and really hope we can spend a night in it some day. We want to start staying in really *unusual* places, like that giant redwood. We rode over a big bridge and were back on A1A, north of course. The ocean looked so pretty today. It's brilliant when you can actually see the ocean and not just condos. St, Augustine has a rule that no building can be above a certain height and I think it is a great one. Share the view. The ride was straight into the wind, but we only had one flat tire for the day. It was also great to stop and talk with a real cyclist that is familiar with the area. He gave us some great tips on where to go and where not to go. Construction, bridge work and traffic is one of the the things that the locals can tell us that no computer program will ever come close to. Even though I don't feel like a real bicyclists, I love speaking to them for information.

Before we knew it, it was getting time to start hunting a place to sleep. We were in Jacksonville Beach and needed to call it a day. I started doing my nightly begging for a room or a bit of lawn. After lots of no's, I did get a great guy named Tim, who helped us with a special rate at a motel. Every little bit does help but I can't stress enough how much we need the help of the public. We really want to camp in backyards but people just look at us like we are mad when we ask this. This room, even at a special rate, cost us about 7 days of our food budget, so we are going to be eating a fair amount of pot noodles and tuna to help make it up. I managed to get a decent amount of work done, but there are never enough hours in the day for the computer side of the walk. The images, the videos, the pages...it is VERY time consuming. If only I could do certain things while I was riding the bicycle, but alas, that would be far too dangerous. It's an early night tonight and up to meet with a television reporter in the morning.

Day 43: February 12, 2007 - Monday - Jacksonville Beach to Little Talbot State Park, Florida

I had this very odd feeling when I woke up this morning, with the light just peeking in behind the curtain. Almost as if I had no clue as to where I was or what I was doing there. Days mix together this early. I guess that is what is to be expected living the kind of life we are. The oddity of sleeping in the same bed for three nights in a row must have had me unadjusted to waking up in strange places. Back to the ever-moving adventure. Sometimes it just strikes me what we are undertaking. It is a huge quest. It is something that isn't for the fainthearted. The things we see can be very scary and there are times where you sort of wonder what it is that is calling us on. Are we answering the call of the wild? Perhaps it is more of the call of nature. Or maybe it's just the call on my cell phone. This morning as we were getting ready to leave our room, the phone rang. We were going to meet with a television reporter outside and had to kick it in to high gear to make it on time. Morton was fast and furious at packing the gear and getting everything down and outside. He also swung by the breakfast room, ate his breakfast on the fly, got some for later (breakfast for lunch) and I pleaded at the front desk to be helped with the room for the night. I was told that the general manager didn't have to power to do this. I should have spoken to the corporate office months ago to get the okay. In the end, we have a tax deduction for eighty dollars and about 7 days of our food budget is shot.

Why oh why don't these big chains (except YOU, my lovely *Holiday Inns*!) get with the program and HELP US! They could talk about what we are doing in their newsletters, encourage their staff to get involved with the website and making their own little changes. Come on corporate America. Get BEHIND what we are doing and PLEASE help us with the free rooms that we need. They can be rooms you are remodeling, rooms without a bed (we have sleeping bags) even conference rooms...we are not choosy and we really do need your help. The reporter, Mike Bunker, was just fantastic. He was very generous with his time and listened to our tale of travel. Hopefully he will keep in touch throughout our journey and hopefully just ONE person (more would be better) will see the news story and start making their own little changes. We filmed the piece in front of the motel we had just stayed in, but I'm learning enough about advertising to ask if he could NOT get the motel in the background that hadn't helped us with a free room. Why put them on the news when they didn't want to help?

Riding north on A1A, we head into Mayport. It is historic and has a lighthouse, but all we really see in the Navy base and the ferry that is going to take us across the St. John's River. It's a short ride for only $1.00 each and we just have enough time to chat with a group of people who were on their way to a real plantation. One of the women invited us to look her up when we come through her part in Maryland, and again, we hope she gets in touch when we get closer. We love backyards and don't get to stay in enough of them. The ferry was something that the local bicyclist told us to take. It would avoid all the congestion and traffic of Jacksonville and keep us so close to the coast that we enjoy hugging. It was a smart ride and a great choice. When we ride our bikes off of the ferry (we were first on, last off) we turn right and go up A1A instead of turning west to go back to the busy highway, 17. The thought of seeing the historic plantation is too tempting for me. Morton follows along behind, leaving me to decide the routes. Soon we spot the brown state sign directing us to turn left. Passing under massive live oaks full of Spanish moss, we ride for miles before seeing a sign telling us the plantation was in one and a half miles. By this point our road has turned to hard packed sand and we are out of the sun, in the shelter of the shade of the giant trees. Morton shouts something about it being far and out of our way. I give a shrug and keep pedaling. The journey is the adventure. If we add a few miles on to our ride, what will it matter. You don't get to bicycle past something like this every day. Plus the fact that it was all a wild chance that we were here, seemed like something we just had to see. The first thing that comes in to view are the slave quarters. These are so striking, set in a semi-circle under massive trees. Some have been restored a bit and some are no longer with us. We park the bikes and each walk our own separate ways in silence. This is a place where humans were owned. It is a place that we can never forget. Morton is reading the signs and I'm snapping pictures when I come upon an armadillo that is having his lunch beside the slave houses. He munches without one little pang of sadness in his head about what happened here. I take some pictures to try to take my mind off the seriousness of the long ago situation. Morton comes over to see him and we decide to head up to the big house.

With very mixed feelings, I was feeling so moved by just the mere sight of the slave quarters, that I really thought about turning around and not even looking at the house. This plantation however, was different. The house wasn't any larger than a regular house. There was a barn, a kitchen house, a garden that was already growing various plants, including cotton. But what made me feel a lot better is when I started reading the story about this plantation. It seems the owner of Kingsley Plantation was married to a black woman. He was also, or so the information said, a person who argued that blacks be treated equal. He wanted people to not be judged by the color of their skin. He was so worried at what would happen to his wife and children when he died, that he moved to Haiti, where he knew his wife and children would never be slaves. I had never heard a story like this before. Incredible people really. I'm going to do a bit of research about it on the internet and pass any other information on. Why hasn't Hollywood made a movie about this place?

Making a new friend of a volunteer there, we spent way too much time looking around. We also had our picnic by the garden before jumping back on the bikes and heading back towards A1A on a different side of the island. The sky to the west was looking a bit cloudy and Morton told me the shocking news that it was twenty past four. Yikes! We had to move it into high gear. We were going to be pitching a tent tonight and I didn't want to do it in the dark. Way too hard. There are only so many things that our little wind-up flashlights will show us in the dark and I don't want to land on a nest of snakes. There were so many beautiful vistas and the ocean was teasing us to take pictures, but we had to press on. Sunset was coming and maybe the rain. Headlights were coming on in cars as we turned into Little Talbot. The ranger on duty was a wonderful man who took care of us and got us on our way to the campground. Hopefully he will email, I love when I get email from people we've met on the road. Actually, I really love getting any email that isn't trying to sell me penny stocks, a diet wonder drug or to make my hair grow back. Our space here is the most beautiful view, breathtaking and pure Florida. We enjoyed a sunset, without any rain, then ate our dinner at the picnic table as the stars all came in to view. Afterwards, we had a little stroll to the river and then to the bathrooms before tucking in to the tent for the night.

Day 44: February 13, 2007 - Tuesday - Little Talbot State Park to Gross, Florida

My dad would have been 83 years old today. He should have been along with us on this journey, with my mom watching out the window of their motorhome, providing us a moving "headquarters" with our group of eight. But his heart didn't hold out. Age, stress, diet and being 82 had a lot to do with it. He went very quick. Someone told me the other day that was a good thing. It was good for him. He didn't suffer, but we didn't get to say goodbye. This past summer as my dad worked long and hard in the garden, his therapy from everything, we had this little joke between us. I would tell him to come in from the heat, drink water and remember, I could only take care of one parent at a time. I didn't want him getting sick on me as I took care of my mom recovering from her stroke. If I would have had any idea it would be my dad's last summer on this earth, things would have been so very different. I would have hugged and kissed him every chance I got. I would have asked to hear all the stories that he liked to tell so much, just one more time. But know one knows when our call will come. The only real thing you can be sure of in this life is the certainty of death. My dad got his call on September the third. It was a Sunday morning that will never fade from my mind, even if I'm lucky enough to make it until I'm 82. Dad was going to climb a ladder and clean the chimney. I wanted him to wait for my son or Morton to return from cutting up a tree that had came down at my sister-in-laws in a storm a few days prior, but dad didn't want to wait. He was spry and fit. Coming on to the porch, the phone rang. Dad answered it and that quick, in a twinkling of an eye, was no longer here. Morton and the police officer that arrived gave dad CPR for a good twenty minutes before the ambulance arrived. I sat on the porch with my mom. Deep inside we both knew what had just happened. The night before my dad left us we spent the first and only time together on the computer that we ever shared. He and I were looking at my laptop at Glacier National Park, one of the places we were both excited about visiting. Dad didn't really like or understand computers. As we looked up things like fishing reports, 360 degree views from the campground we were going to stay in, dad looked across the table to my mom who was sitting quiet at the end. "Did you know all this stuff was on the computer?" he asked with the wide eyed innocence of a child. Mom who is very computer savvy smiled and said of course she knew.

My dad was a lot of things. I could write thousands of pages about him. One thing that I will never forget is that dad told me I could do this journey if I really put my mind to it. When I hit my wall each day and feel so tired, I think about his exact words. "It will work as long as you don't give up." And I won't.

Today as we broke camp and were on our bicycles by 8 am, I was thinking of the date. The first time in my 43 years that I don't get to wish dad a happy birthday. It's hard not to let my mind wonder and ask myself all the "what if's" but they do no good at all now. We pass little pieces of water and I see people out in their boats. That is just where my dad would have spent most of his time out here. He would have loved what I was seeing today and I'm sure we would have had a day off to go fishing.

Looking for the right road on a map I remembered how dad would put the map in my hands from the time I was old enough to read and say, "You're the navigator, what road should we take?" and I would get to figure out the best way to get to a fishing hole in Florida or Canada. We lived in Pennsylvania, but dad didn't fish there. He said it was "all fished out" and I would wonder why people still went out in boats.

The map we are using leaves a lot to be desired. We picked it up for free at a tourist stand some-where. Someone had told me that certain roads weren't on it, so when we came to a cross road that I thought we should go left at, we were lucky enough to ask a man on a golf cart who was collecting cans. He helped us with directions that were spot on and and we followed them with no trouble. I wondered how old he was. Does he remember to take his medicine? Does he have someone to look after him? He was smoking and I wanted to beg him to stop, save his life and then be on my way.

Riding and thinking a million miles away, I kept one eye open for 17 north. I kept the other eye on the sky. The forecast said it was going to rain, thunder and even some lightning bolts were going to dance in the sky. We needed to be in a place early today. While we were still on A1A Morton spotted a dollar store, where everything inside is really just one dollar. He loves them. He has also been bugging for a pair of hair clippers. Why pay someone to cut your hair when I can run the trimmers over it, he asks me. I sit outside with the bikes as he goes in to search. I'm thankful he just has $5.00 in his pocket. I have learned to not let Morton do the grocery shopping without me. He doesn't remember we have a small area for food and tends to buy more than we can carry. Sitting on the curb in the shade I think about how easy it was getting in and out of the tent this morning. The first time I practiced in a tent in Pennsylvania, I couldn't get in or out on my own. I can sit on curbs now too without having to think about getting a forklift to stand back up. The exercise is really working and I don't need a scale to tell me how good being healthy feels. Morton returns grinning with his treasure in his hands. At this moment I'm on the phone with my daughter Sarah, learning that my son, James, has had his finger crushed at work. He has a hairline fracture and he has lost his nail, gotten stitches and the doctor tells him his nail most likely won't ever come back. Nail bed damage. I'm cringing as Morton is showing me a pair of hair clippers he has just bought for $1.50. He can't believe it, the buy of the century. Sarah is saying that James is fine and they are getting a snow storm right now. My lovely daughter also warns me about a storm in our area. I look to the black sky and have to agree with her. We will be careful, I promise and say goodbye to my daughter. I would give anything to be able to hug her and my son at this moment. We could all go collect my mom and take her to dinner. I only hope mom doesn't know what day it is. If she looks at the calender though, she will see my father's birthday looking back at her.

Knowing that we are so close to Georgia feels incredible. One big state is almost done, well, at least one side of it. This will be a real milestone for us. We soon come across 17 and head north. Trying to just re-member all the very happy times with my dad isn't working. There were hundreds, if not thousands of them, but they are making me cry as I cycle. Not a safe combination. Dad wouldn't want me crying, or anyone. He would want us happy. He really didn't do sad, but I couldn't help it. Saying just a few words now and then to Morton about glass or nails, I kept quiet in my thoughts. Poor James. His finger sounds so sore. It was his ring finger. Then I start to think. My dad had a finger that had been crushed. It had a weird and ugly nail on it that never grew right. I try to remember what finger it was on him, but I can't.

I give up torturing myself with sadness and try to focus on the state border coming up. We could see 95 in front of us and it is just a little past that. It's been a great riding day, I think to myself. No punctures, lots of friendly little toots from people who saw us on the Jacksonville news last night. If only it wasn't February 13th, I could have really enjoyed it all. We stop on a bridge over a swamp. *McQueen's Swamp* to be exact. Morton gets me to take a picture of him in it for his friend in Scotland who has the last name McQueen. I didn't tell Morton that today is dad's birthday. Tomorrow is our anniversary, four years, and then in just five days after that, Morton turns 40. Thank goodness there are so many great dates mixed around this sad one. A very kind lady turns around, comes back to us as we are eating a lunch of boiled peanuts (dad preferred peanuts salted in the shell) and she wants to make sure we are alright. She warns us about the approaching storm. Morton talks and for the first time on our journey, I don't speak to the person. I was just afraid that I would burst out in tears for no real reason. A car passed us with a little dog sticking it's head out the window that looked just like Max, our family wiener dog.

The kind lady told Morton about some upcoming campgrounds and we started going towards them. Just as we saw a billboard, the heaven's opened and we were drenched. We pulled in to a closed business and took advantage of their roof overhang. Sarah supplied me with the campgrounds phone number, I called and they don't do tents. Sorry. They didn't even have a bit of grass for us to pitch the tent on. I'm not sure why people think everyone has a camper, but they don't.

The sky is black. Even though it's only 3 o'clock, it looks like it is night falling on us. We have to just try to get a room at the 95 intersection. It's our only hope. We pedal and the sand that we had gathered on our bicycles from earlier in the day is washed off. It will save Morton time and energy later. Thanks nature.

It looks like there are two motels, great, one of them might have a kind bone or two in their body. But alas, the first one we go to is closed. The second one can give us a discount price of $59, but no free room. I walk out to ask Morton and the sound of thunder is heard as the rain gets a little harder. Who needs to eat for 6 days anyway? I want to lose weight don't I? We have to get the room. We are a million miles from friends and family who could help.

As we head for the room I tell Morton to look at the parking lot. There is not one car in the whole place. But this is a 95 motel. It fills when people are too tired to drive any further. I know this kind of motel well from trips to Florida from Pennsylvania. Later as the storm gets worse and night really does fall, it will fill up. I wish we could have slept in the closed motel, I have a feeling it would have been just as clean.

When we come in the room I have my shower since they always make me feel better. Today however, it only feels good and gets me clean. I still feel so sad I could just burst into tears. Morton, for the first time today, asks me what's wrong. When I tell him, he understands and quickly changes the subject. Morton is British after all, they really aren't known for their deep emotions, but he's coming around.

Morton asks if I'm going to call my mom. I have to but I hate to. If she doesn't know what day it is, she won't be feeling sad like I am. But even though my mom's stroke has left her having trouble knowing the day, after nearly 56 years with dad, I know she will know just what day it is.

Tomorrow the day will be different, our ride will be different, the weather will be different and it will be our wedding anniversary. If I can just make the phone call, have a good cry and then get busy with all the work I have to do. Heck, we are in a motel room with a television. Maybe we'll try for some mindless entertainment.

Our Zen player is filling the room with music and Morton has cut his hair and had a shave. He feels much better knowing that he only had to spend $1.50 on his hair for the next two years, or as long as the clippers last. *Matchbox 20* is singing the song, *Mad Season*, and I hope that I can get through mine. I'm going to call my mother.

Day 45: February 14, 2007 - Wednesday - Gross, Florida to Woodbine, Georgia

The day started a bit later then we would have liked, but hey, it is Valentine's Day and our anniversary. We slept until the late hour of 7 am, shocking! My computer kept losing connection and there were so many emails to get through. We are also trying to get good weather reports, find some places to stay in the next week and make sure we have a good map to use.

The winds were so strong today so the ride was going to be tough. We had also been told that the roads were going to be very unfriendly towards the bicycles. Check! We didn't expect the bike to lose it's chain, have several flat tires (so many that I lost count) and in general, have our toughest day yet. Any day you wake up is the best day of your life and I now know this.

Crossing out of Florida felt great and happened before all the bike woes. Morton took some pictures, I took some pictures and we felt like we had been in Florida for at least 100 years. Morton cut his hair and little beard way too short for his liking. The good thing about hair, well most of it anyway, is that it will grow back.

The terrain in Florida is really different from Georgia. In Georgia the pine tress are a big source of business. You see trucks running up and down the road all the time loaded with them. They smell great, but boy do they go fast. Combine that with the edge of the road just being about 12 to 18 inches wide and you have the combination for some real thrills.

When we were stopping for all the flat tires we discovered some lovely woods with little blooms starting to come out on vines. It also really reminded both of us a bit of a fall day. It was chilly and even with the sun out, still cold. Some of the trees still had colored leaves clinging to them from last autumn. It was hard to tell what season we are really in.

Morton missed the armadillo that was eating beside a swamp. We both kept stealing peeks at the woods that would turn into a swamp, then back into woods. We were both hoping to see an alligator, but I have a feeling that today they would have been hiding somewhere warm. The houses and the landscape were all so different now. You can really see what happened to US 17, the coastal highway, when the interstate 95 came to town.

You could make out signs that had once welcomed tourists, buildings that had once been used now were empty here and there. The homes were of every style and description, most of them were very well taken care of though the tourist trade would never past by their front doors like it once had done.

Soon we were passing through a little town that had a tourist information center. Morton went in for a Georgia map and then I went in to use the bathroom. Someone must have been having a lovely lunch because the whole place smelled delicious. The smell of food only seems to really get to me when I've been living on a lot of tuna and crackers.

There were little shops that looked inviting, but we didn't have time to visit. We needed to get up the road and the wind was really killing our time. Our wheels seemed to barely be turning as we struggled to pull along our trailers behind us that felt like 1000 pound anchors. We considered that walking might be a bit faster, but stayed on the bikes as long as the tires weren't getting punctures. The little towns would have to wait for another time.

As we kept going the sky got darker, but no rain came. There were long stretches of nothing and the feeling of where we were going to stay was setting in. There were a few houses here and there, but we were still miles from the town we had hoped to get to. The sheer terror of having to face a cold night in a tent beside a swamp really was motivating me into riding, regardless of the wind. If we have learned anything since starting, it is to roll with the punches. If your bikes need work, you have to stop. If we don't get as far as we hoped, there is no sense worrying over it. Just get on with the journey and tomorrow really is another day.

Speaking to Sarah in Pennsylvania, I learn the update on the snow they got. It has a layer of ice on it now, with more coming. Ahhhh, winter. Maybe being stuck with flats by the road in chilly Georgia isn't that bad at all. At least we don't have any ice or need a snow plow.

We pass a fruit stand but Morton only has a few coins in his pocket. I'm pretty sure they wouldn't take credit card, so the fresh fruit and veg need to wait. There should be a little town coming up on the horizon. I strain my eyes and hope something good happens as the mile markers go up. We never really know what is right in front of us until we ride there.

Morton is elated to see mile markers again. He got use to them in Key West, missed them the whole way through Florida, now it looks like he'll be happy once more watching the miles slide by us.

Soon we spot the signs of civilization. More cars, more houses, a church here and there and sidewalks. All good things. Then we spot a billboard for the motel in town. It wasn't very far and with any luck we would still have some skin on our faces from the wind when we get there.

The man at the motel said he couldn't help with a room. He also said there were no other motels or campgrounds. As we were talking about the room, the rate and the journey, the weather station was saying that there is another storm passing through. He was able to give us a rate under $40. and that was the best he can do. The room is really big, but to tell you the truth, I'm really getting tired of rooms. We would be so much better off if we were in the tent, free, and only had our food to worry about. There are nights though, like last night and tonight, that we really don't have a choice. Darkness was going to come, there was no edge to the road and the bikes really needed going over. All things that require shelter and we can't be picky about where we are staying.

Getting set up, I decided since there was no wireless internet, I would take advantage and do a t-shirt design. I combined all the best flower shots from Florida and made a great design out of it. Morton and I talked about some other designs we wanted to do for each state, flowers, critters, beaches & people. If we can get a couple of great shirts, our sales can go up and we won't have to wrestle with the idea of sleeping under a bridge in the cold. The t-shirt sales on the website are helping to fund the journey.

If our budget was unlimited we would be in the safe shelter of a motorhome each night, surrounded by friends or family and the weather wouldn't bother us. But that isn't our case. The budget is so tight it squeaks and we know the brutal truth that when we spend on a room we have to cut somewhere else, which is food.

Day 46: February 15, 2007 - Thursday - Woodbine to *Guesthouse Inn and Suite,* Brunswick, Georgia

This morning was our chilliest yet. We could see our breath as we suited up with our warmest jackets and left Woodbine. When we stopped here yesterday I was really wanting to make it to Waverly. I have learned though that trusting your gut is the most important thing you can do out here.

Intuition. It is a weird thing how it seems to be working with us, but it struck me as we left the one motel that there wasn't anywhere else we could have gone. As we rode along the rode there wasn't a nook or cranny we could had tucked the tent in. Maybe if we were willing to drag the bikes back in the woods, but we won't do that just yet. They are too heavy to go off-roading and the trailers would never make it.

The road was a lot quieter and there was an extra lane here and there that made it feel a lot safer. There was a steady smell of pine in the air and combined with the chill I wondered if it would be Christmas soon. The beauty of the countryside was really something that you should see. Get off the main road and see how things look on a road less traveled.

We had to stop to make a slight adjustment and there was a picnic table that doubled as a work bench for Morton. He pulled out all his tools, some that he found, a few that he bought and one that he had just picked up about three miles back. There was a tiny post office and a wooden house up on blocks. Such a quiet little place. I wonder what it would be like to live here? There were houses dotted here and there. It was easy to just pay a little attention to the road and still stay safe.

We were startled by a big black dog that wasn't on a chain. It came charging at us and Morton yelled, *"Oi! Stay"* and it did. I hope that trick works with bears too.

As we rode the phone rang with a person in Savannah inviting us to come and have dinner with them. I had spent last night sending emails to different places looking for things to do while we are in the beautiful town. The trouble was that I got so carried away with my planning for our visit, it was 2 am and Morton was snoring when I really looked at the clock. It would be fantastic if we had someone to plan the details of this trip, but then it wouldn't be so surprising. It would be easier, but it would take a lot of the fun out of it too. This is like a reality television show without the tv or budget.

As we reached the turn in the road that was Waverly it was a good thing we had stopped where we did. There really was just a gas station and a turn. There was also an intersection. Perhaps if we would have turned that way there would have been something, but it was another time that my gut feeling was spot on. Never missing the chance to use a bathroom, we stopped at the gas station that was also a little store. Morton waited outside with our bicycles. As I headed in removing my glasses so I could see, I had to stand still for a moment for the shades to catch up with me. They should be reactor lights and go lighter as soon as I come out of the sun, but it takes about five minutes. More than enough time for me to trip and fall in the dark. I always leave my bike helmet on because it tends to pull out some of my hair every time I take it off. That wouldn't be so bad if it just pulled out just the gray hairs, but it tends to pull out a little of both.

The bathroom was always my first order of business and with that out of the way, I had a little look around the shop. There was this delicious smell of chicken. Fried chicken. Looking at their price sign I went to consult with Morton. After all, we hadn't had anything warm to eat since Sunday night and that was just pot noodles. He agreed, as long as they would take the credit card. I think we have about 47 cents on us in cash. Going back in and having a little chat with the nice guy behind the counter, we got a 4 piece dinner to split. The man serving at the counter told me about a couple he had seen that were moving from Wisconsin to Florida and were on bikes with one suitcase. He said the bikes looked they were from a yard sale.

Taking our warm meal outside, we used the picnic table to have our feast. Eating everything except the rolls (we would reserve them for dinner later) we washed it down with our horrible tasting water. Since we fill the bottles up in bathrooms along the way, we are always taking a chance as to the taste of the water. Really all we care about is that it is wet. It felt good to have food in our bellies as we rode off and turning right, we headed east towards Brunswick.

Morton had picked up a free magazine with special saving coupons for motels in it. I took the time to look through it while we had to stop at a church for more bike adjustments. You know, if our bikes really were horses we might have to think about shooting them. The book and the map gave me an idea about where we wanted to end up tonight.

I had looked on the web for a campground and there was nothing. Asking people for their backyard is really tough. We have never had anyone say "yes" that we approached. It also is a bit like begging and we don't want to get in trouble with the police. Morton is telling me that there is no way we can afford to pay for a room tonight. If we don't get a comp room, we have to just put the tent up somewhere...anywhere.

Since the ride and walk for the day was almost over, the book with the coupons needed to be consulted. Pulling over we just sat on a fresh poured curb. There are some motels that have discount coupons for $39 a night, but our budget is already running over this month. Morton says no, absolutely no. It makes me a bit angry. What if we can't get a room? Does he really want us to put a tent up in a city corner?

This is one of those moments where I want to cry and then run home as fast as I can, but I can't do either. Going on is my only option.

There are a little cluster of motels near 95. Three that we can see. I need to start doing the tough part of the day now. They are all chain motels which are really hard to get a room at. Our luck hasn't been that great with them, except with the Holiday Inn properties. It's easy to feel like what is the point to all of this. It is very hard work. Today was very cold and my nose was sniffling all day. The tops of my thighs were frozen as I went to go try my luck with motel number one. There were two lucky pennies we came across earlier at one of the breakdown spots. I wished I would have had it in my hand, but I trusted my gut only and walked into the lobby at *Guesthouse Inn and Suites*.

The general manager was in, Kailash, and willing to listen to my story of what we were doing and why we needed a room. She was very understanding and said that she would be happy to help. I wanted to squeal with pleasure and rub my lucky gut for the feeling that led me to this motel first. Kailash was even kind enough to put us in a room that was so close to the door for getting all the gear inside.

When I checked my email I was thrilled to see that we were getting some emails from Savannah. So far we have one ghost walk (this should be great) a pampering session at the *Savannah Day Spa* for Morton and I (this should be sheer perfection, can you say "massages"?) and best of all, we have a great contact with the visitors center who is going to really help us get to the best of the best in Savannah.

The fact that things won't always fall into place is all part of this crazy journey, but sometimes they will. That is something I have to remind myself of.

Day 47: February 16, 2007 - Friday - Brunswick to Fort King George, Darien, GA

Today started of fantastic and just kept getting better. As we left our room stuffed with a nice hot waffle made by Morton, the chill didn't even bother us. The sun was out and even though there was wind, it wasn't a gale force wind. A day for riding and smiling, taking on the glow of good health. Looking around at the beauty we were riding through, Morton and I seemed to miss the bulk of the city altogether on our route. Little bits of civilization here and there would pop in, but basically it was a ride in the park.

There were a few dodgy bits around some construction and I would cringe whenever I'd catch sight of I-95 with all the heavy traffic on it, all in all it was a terrific day for riding. Morton took a few pictures of a paper mill that my little brother and I had called "the pollution factory" when we were kids and would ride by it. It still looked the same but there was no horrible smell today.

I was able to ride up all the bridges today, such a big deal for me. Sometimes though, I still like to push the bike. Your legs need a nice stretching after all.

There were a few wild dogs today that would bark and chase us for a bit. As long as we keep going I think we'll be alright. Morton does talk to them and that seems to confuse them. They most likely can't make out what he's saying with his accent though. We joke that he doesn't need to outpedal the dogs to avoid their bite, he just has to be able to outpedal me.

Each day we have a goal of where we want to get. This is always flexible and depends greatly on how the bikes behave and how tired I get. It gives me untold pleasure to report that I'm not taking as many "huff and puff" breaks now. It is usually a break that is less than five minutes and I try not to sit down. My body is really getting so much stronger. A miracle really considering how hard I abused it with food for decades and virtually no movement.

We ride through a wild bird refuge and see spectacular sights of flocks of ducks taking off from the marshy water. Huge wading birds will flap their wings and take lift off. The impossibly large birds move fast to move easily in front of us. There size is something you don't expect to see flying. Sort of like me on a bicycle. When the cars are gone there is a peacefulness in this place that can not be matched.

Morton sees something worthy of a photo and says, "Go dead slow!" I know this means he will snap a picture of my back as I coast and wait for him. Sometimes it's a piece of trash he is picking up. He can not pass a 6-pack ring without grabbing it to put in our trash bag. Seeing what these things can do up close and personal to birds while we were in the Keys really made a lasting impression on us both.

There is an amazing plantation that we get to have a picnic at and met a group of four people just finishing with the table sitting in the sun. It is a group of four people who all belong to a hiking club that turn the table over to us. They all looked so great and guess what!? Exercise is *their* secret! They are Elouise, Cedric, Suzanne and Tim and they are an inspiration to exercise with what you *love doing*. We didn't get a chance to see the house, there are way too many things to see. We keep going and I try to hold in my mind the important thought that if you do an exercise you love, it will never be hard to keep at it and keep your health.

Before long we spy a tourist information center coming up in a little town called Darien. We love to stop at them to see what is waiting before us. We like to ask them about campgrounds in front of us. When we pull in there is a metal sign telling us about *Fort King George*. We see that it was actually manned by Scottish Highlanders. Our interest is raised but it's getting a bit late in the day to play tourists. We have to think about camping. In the visitor center I find a flyer and a number for a campground up the road several miles. I call and talk to a nice lady who passes me over to a man who says they have donated before and don't do that sort of thing anymore. It seems there isn't anything in it for them. I guess a bit of grass holds more value than I thought.

We took this as a sign to just go with out gut feeling of seeing this fort that was just a mile away. We were looking at a brochure and I decided to give them a call to see if they do camping. The nicest lady ever, Trisha, was wonderful. She said they have a spot that the Boy Scouts use and we could pitch our tent there. Free. Hopping on our bikes we ride down the prettiest street we have seen yet. Every developer in the whole world should see this street. They make the road split to accommodate the huge live oak trees that not only line it, but reside right in the middle of it! There is a spectacular church we want to stop and look at, but we race by to get to the fort. If we hurry we might have time to see it before pitching the tent.

We meet the marvelous Trisha who is kind enough to call the local reporter for the newspaper. Our story really does seem to touch a nerve with everyone who hears it. People are sometimes so kind to us that it just proves that the whole world IS a wonderful place, if we would only let it happen. Sandy, the associate editor for the *Darien News*, asked us lots of questions, took our pictures with this fort that had called to us from the sign in the background and then we were like kids and off to see it. Trisha told us that we could camp across the street after we had a peek through the fort. There were some historic reinactors down in the primitive area, but Morton and I wanted to head right for the fort. This is a very special place and something that you must see to believe. We felt like kids that got separated from their school group as we roamed this amazing place after hours and all by ourselves.

When we had our quick look through, we followed the trail and the voices to meet the people who bring history to life here. Trisha had talked to them about us popping our tent up for the night, but they actually invited us to spend the night in the fort with them. Talk about a bonus that we weren't expecting. This night was going to be one of the best.

Patty, George, John, Rachel, Katrina and Phil are our group of new friends that have shown us one of the most wonderful nights yet on our journey. Picture this, these people, who are all experts and take time out of their lives to present history in the flesh, put us up in the building that would have been used by the fort as a hospital. The night was going to be in the 20's with frost in the forecast and our private room has a roaring fire in it, built by George. His wife, Patty, gave me this lovely homemade lip balm and healing lotion as if she was a mind reader. I really did need to get something for my windswept lips. Maybe they had stood out as lips in need of a bit of therapy.

As the night wore on, we talked, ate, drank warmed lemon drops (so very good and warmed by the fire) and boy were we entertained, one and all. It was as if these were long lost friends that we just happened to run into again. All because the sign that was pointing from Highway 17 sounded like somewhere we should see. Following your heart and trusting your instincts is the only way to live our lives.

After sitting around the fire until midnight, yes, you heard right...we stayed up until midnight, Morton and I headed out of the warm big building into a sea of stars. It was moonless, but there were at least a million stars that were twinkling at us. The smoke from the fires smelled so good and when we opened to door to our cabin, the fire was soon stoked up to a nice warming roar.

Using a mattress stuffed with straw that was laid out on the wooden floor, this was as authentic as you could get. Money could not buy us an experience like this and we will never forget it. Soon we fell asleep in the warm building with this feeling that we were in the set of a movie. A five star experience that we were lucky enough to be invited to take part in.

Going back in history tonight has made us both want to explore this world and what has happened in the past so much more. Travel inspires a real desire to learn.

Day 48: February 17, 2007 - Saturday - *Fort King George*, Darien to Richmond Hill, Georgia

Waking up early this morning, Morton and I got our gear stored and headed out fast. It is like taking a band-aid off fast. These new friends that we made are tough to say goodbye to. They are all so lovely and interesting it would be easy to spend the day with them, helping them tidy their camp, cut wood and forget that we were on this great adventure. But we have to ride. Morton and I set off with a great speed and the name *Midway* on our mind. It would take us within 30 miles of Savannah, which is where we need to wind up on Sunday for a free room.

There were so many peaceful moments as we were riding today we might have been the only two people on the planet. The birds sang and played beside swamps of standing trees. The sun melted all the frost that was out this morning glistening back at the fort. Feeling supercharged from our wonderful night, we rode and smiled heading ever north. We had a place lined up to stay our very first night in Savannah, but after that, we still have to find lodging. We are trying to learn not to worry too much about things. They really do all seem to work out on this magical journey.

We passed the smallest church in the USA and went inside. We wished we were closer to where we would stop for the night. It would have been perfect to camp behind. Though inside, with very limited floor space, there wouldn't have been enough room to sleep. Even though we went over 40 miles today, it seemed so short. Before we knew it, we were coming into Midway. We didn't know much about it, but we knew enough to know there is a museum there. Maybe, just maybe, we could camp there. But there was no joy waiting for us. They didn't allow things like that and the girl told us there was a campground 4 miles ahead. We could do four more miles no problem.

We needed to get a move on, get camping and get cozy before the temperature fell. It was going to be another chilly night, or so we were told today by everyone.

Riding and riding, we clocked off four miles and both started wondering if we missed it. Sometimes things aren't signed great, but we had no choice other then to keep riding. Oh how we rode. The four miles turned out to be a lot more. After ages I saw a busy road on the horizon crossing the path of US 17. Could we be back at I-95? I didn't think we met it again until we got to Richmond Hill. Could we have really gone that far? Stopping to consult our map, we decided to run down the list of motels that would be bunched up where the highways meet. It was going to be very cold and the elusive campground was still no where to be seen. We gave the phone a work out to call ahead rather than going in to the counters to beg for a room. The Daytona 500 is on. Everyone was booked up. Even though we were several hours north of it, people were not too far to drive to it from here. All the signs on the motels welcomed the race fans.

The sun was starting to look like it wouldn't be long until it disappeared. I kept dialing. There were a few that had one or two rooms left, all out of our budget range. When a special event comes to town, or in this case, just passes through, the rates go up accordingly. There was one motel who had a room, just for one night, at a reduced rate of $30. We thought about going off the road and into the woods, but with the bikes and trailers, this is impossible. The room it is. Maybe they have WiFi, I thought! Always a selling point to someone who is battling her super slow connection through AT&T on the laptop.

We came to the room and found that the last room was on the second floor with no elevator. Morton, poor Morton, had to climb the stairs carrying the bikes and trailers, with just a little assistance from me. He is brilliant and is really the glue that holds this trip together. Now we are tucked up in the room, a million miles away from our dream night last evening. Morton is sleeping and I'm going try to untangle myself from the computer and join him.

Day 49: February 18, 2007 - Sunday - Richmond Hill to *Olde Harbor Inn*, Savannah, Georgia

Escaping from the second floor with two bikes and two trailers loaded with all the gear is a tough trick. I nearly came crashing down with my bike and then volunteered to wait at the bottom with the bikes like I had done on the way up the stairs last evening. Morton is a real gentleman anyway and would have it no other way. Finally after all these years I found a KEEPER!

It was cold, nothing new there. Since Morton picked up two pair of gloves at a store the other morning after camping at the fort (they are both bright green) our hands were at least warm as we rode under Interstate 95 and headed to Savannah. Riding without peace and quiet, it was impossible to try to have a conversation, so we both just kept quiet. I was dodging glass, screws, nails, bits of wood and would occasionally shout a warning out to my hubby. By the time he heard me he was usually running over the thing I was warning him about, so I gave it up as a bad job.

The odd dog barked at us and the children that were brave enough to be outside playing, pointed at us. The sky was brilliant blue and the trees all looked like they were cold and sleeping, waiting on a spring that might never arrive.

There was a rather steep bridge coming up and we had to get off and push. One of the bikes have a bad habit of losing it's chain whenever we climb any sort of incline, hill or bridge. We were able to speak at this point, but instead we both kept quiet. Morton was searching the ground for lucky pennies and bits of treasure. Me, I spotted a spark plug that sparked a childhood memory.

My parents, actually my father, had a friend called Harry. Harry lived alone with no family in a lovely stone farmhouse in Pennsylvania, not too far from us. I'm not sure of how they knew each other, but Harry was a lonesome old guy who would come and visit.

He had a sister ages ago who lived with him, but she had died, leaving him on his own. Harry always wore bib overalls that were blue and white striped and a straw hat. He always smelled like raspberries that had gotten moldy and horse manure. He was famous for telling "Har-Har" jokes. Really BAD jokes, not dirty, but BAD. For example, Have you heard about the thing that killing all sorts of animals by the road? It's called CARS. When he would say this punchline that made no comic sense he would throw his round head back and laugh really loud until his cheeks would become a bright pink color. That laughter would make everyone who had heard the terrible joke laugh too. Everyone was happy. Harry thought his joke cracked us up. No harm, no foul. One day Harry drove to our house just to ask my dad to stop over at his farm. He was excited and in a very secret mood, he pulled away in his old rusty red pickup with the round big fenders on it. Dad wondered what it was about, maybe he had a bumper crop of something he was growing. I was curious as to what Harry wanted to show my dad and bugged to go along. It was back in the days when I was still cute enough to bug and not be annoying. Dad relented and let me tag along.

We set off, just the two of us, in our family station wagon. This was the same station wagon that had teeth marks in the dashboard where I would bite it when I was younger. Now at the age of 12, I was embarrassed by the marks and had the tendency to put my hands over them to cover my shame. Sort of like wearing big and baggy clothes now to cover the body I have created out of sheer greed for food.

Pulling in to the stone farm house, Harry came rushing out to the car. He was telling my dad that he wasn't going to believe what he was going to show him. Harry was saying that he was going to be a millionaire. Dad raised an eyebrow of disbelief or wonder, I'm not sure which. We followed his musty raspberry scented form into the house.

Now I had never been inside before. I had heard about it from my dad. He said Harry needed help getting it in order, a good spring cleaning. What dad should have said is that Harry needed to borrow my dad's bulldozer. The house was a tip inside. Things were stacked to the ceiling and there was only enough room for a person to walk on the little paths that created mazes around the room we were in. I wasn't even sure what room it was. I loved it!

Boxes stacked on boxes, tied with twine and things dangling about the place. Herbs and flowers hanging in clumps on beams that were thickly covered with cobwebs. Sacks over lumpy shapes. There could be ANYTHING in this room. Harry went right to a pile that was only as tall as he was. He opened a box that looked brand spanking new next to the other ones in the room. I now realized that the ROOM was what smelled like rotten raspberries. Harry just smelled like that from living here.

Opening the box, Harry pulled out little metallic pink spark plugs, only 1/2" long. "Just look at them!" he squealed. Now my dad's eyebrows went all the way to his hat. I thought that they must be for a very tiny car that one of the other boxes must be hiding. Harry proved me wrong though by grabbing another box and yanking out a woman's head. Not a real woman, but the head of a dummy. She had rubber sort of ears and he stuck the wire that held the little pink spark plug through the lobe of one. I was mesmerized.

We weren't allowed to get our ears pierced and this was as close as I'd come to seeing it done for many years. The little plug dangled and the lady looked fantastic. If only I had my ears pierced I would have put a pair of spark plugs right in. "What on earth is it?" my dad questioned. "Fashion!" Harry snapped in a rather insulted tone. My dad was ignorant to fashion. He didn't believe in primping or putting on any show for any person. Dad couldn't recognize this trendy thing, but I did. At that moment I would have traded my two front teeth for a pair of these pink spark plugs. True, I didn't have holes in my ears, but a friend in school said all you needed was some ice cubes, a potato and a pin to fix that.

It seems, Harry explained to my dad, an inventor had approached Harry to let him in on this ground-floor, earth-rocking chance to invest in these pink plugs. Dad wanted to know how much Harry had sunk into the new trend. Harry got shy at this point, he ground his shoe into the floor with his hands buried deep in his pockets. Dad had to coax it out of him as I stood watching the earrings shimmer in the plastic ears of the dummy, backlit by the sunbeams coming through the dusty window. Any amount Harry said would have been a bargain. They were sheer genius. Finally Harry came out with the number, his whole life savings, twenty thousand dollars, was the amount he told my father. My dad was floored. He told Harry to call the police, cancel the check, this guy was a cheat and a phony. Harry had nothing in writing. Just a box of 100 pink spark plugs. It seems that was all Harry ever got for his money. Just a box of pink spark plug earrings and the head of a dummy to display them on. At that rate they cost him $200 a pair.

The inventor has strung poor Harry along for a couple months. Harry held faith in the hope that any day all the stores would be selling the pink wonders. Dad urged him to go to the police, but I think Harry was too ashamed to do this. He told dad, "It's only money and I can always make more."

The spark plug I saw today wasn't pink. Who knows, now it might be a big thing. Put the name of a NASCAR racer on it and even the guys would buy them!
It's funny how our journey is reminding me of all of my life. It feels good and keeps the homesick blues away or calls them close to me, depending on the mood of the day.

Approaching Savannah on bicycle was a first for me. It was lovely riding down the streets of old houses, huge trees and smiling faces. We nodded and said hello to so many people as we rode past. Before we knew it we were at the Savannah River.

It seems that Factors Walk, where our room for the night is, is right beside the river. The location of the *Olde Harbor Inn* is perhaps the best in Savannah. Morton and I pinch ourselves to make sure we aren't dreaming. We are still a bit early to check in, so we find a bench, there are hundreds of them in this lovely city that feels more like a hometown. Sitting in the sun, we eat our lunch and look at the river. It is a great time to silently count my blessings.

Even though it means we will have to push them back up again, we decide to ride the bikes along the water. It was worth it. Just so very nice out, even though the digital thermometer at the bank we passed said it was only 54 degrees. We talk to lots of people who are out walking. One young man is riding his bike down to Key West. It felt good to be able to share some information about the road that might help him.

Before we knew it, time slid by and we were checking in to the lovely *Olde Harbor Inn*. From outside you know it's special, from inside you know it's spectacular. Places like this never look as good in the photos, you have to see them in person to believe it. The lovely man gave us our room key, invited us to come for wine and cheese at 5:30 and we were off to put the bikes away. I thought this was going to be a room, but I was wrong. It is a suite. A living room three times the size of our living room in Scotland, a kitchen with everything in it, very tall ceilings, stunning bathroom and a bedroom with a four poster bed. The window in the bedroom looks out on the river and the windows in the living room look out to the moss covered trees. How is it that we keep getting SO lucky? Maybe it is all the lucky pennies that Morton keeps finding. He says that he heard a saying in Scotland ages ago. When we say, "Find a penny pick it up, then all day you'll have good luck" he says, "Find a penny and pass it on and it will bring luck and friendship to both." I like his saying better. Passing on good things and lucky pennies is better than keeping them all for yourself.

The bedroom in our suite has the most comfortable pillows I have ever felt and lovely bedspread and curtains with a pattern that I want to have some day. The print is very nostalgic, with lovely soft colors and monkeys all over it, doing all sorts of things. Playing musical instruments, eating grapes and more. Even if you live in Savannah, you need to stay here. You will be impressed.

After doing some quick updates on the site, we had a little walk, then went for the wine and cheese. I don't really drink, but red wine is really good for you. This wine actually tasted wonderful. The cheese was great too and there were even little sandwiches out. The best part though was meeting the other guests. A couple from St. Augustine. A couple from New York. Friendly chat and the looks of disbelief when we say where we are from, or more to the point, where we are going. Flabbergasted is a good descriptive word for the reaction we get. After a little chat, we head back to the room. What I love best about it is that Morton can watch his Sci-Fi shows in the living room and I can sit on the bed and use the laptop. And guess what? I actually am getting my LAP back to work on. For years I wouldn't have been able to work like this, now I can even cross my legs again. It is all of these little changes in my body that make me smile and realize that my dream is finally coming true. With my music playing in my headphones from my little Zen, I work on getting pictures up, edited, writing, email and all the other upkeep on the site. It is a big amount of work, but it flies by. Looking at the clock just now, for the first time, I see that it is nearly midnight!

Little Changes　　　　**80**　　　　*Priscilla Houliston*

I haven't told you the very best news. My daughter and her husband are coming for a visit with us this week. There is a television crew that filmed us last summer when we were training to do this together. They wanted to film us in Savannah. Sarah is being the best daughter in the world and giving up a few days pay to come do some filming to support her crazy mother on our wild journey around America. I get to see how big her tummy is getting with the baby, hug Graeme and best of all, we will all be together to celebrate Morton's fortieth birthday. Maybe I better pinch myself again. This all feels a bit too much like a dream. Hopefully I won't wake up freezing in the tent camped behind a billboard somewhere.

Day 50: February 19, 2007 - Monday - *Olde Harbor Inn*, Savannah, Georgia

Happy Birthday to Morton. Make that Happy FORTIETH Birthday to Morton.

We woke up to a lovely cooked breakfast at the *Olde Harbor Inn*. When we looked out our windows we could see the tug boats coming and going, see the people of Savannah waking up and most of all, see the sun shining. Today we have an interview with Melanie from Channel WTOC/CBS in Savannah. It is going to take place right outside the inn, handy and lovely. Melanie and her camera person, Tania, arrive right on time and are lovely. We do lots of questions, show them the things we have packed in our little trailers and they set off in the car to do some filming of us heading out to Tybee Island. We are happy, smiling and trying to avoid the traffic. There are about 14 miles in front of us to ride but the ladies from Channel WTOC stay with us for only about a 1/2 mile or so.

Yesterday when we arrived at *Olde Harbor Inn* I discovered this massive logging chain Morton had picked up from beside the road and draped over one of our trailers. We already look like we are homeless and with him adding this to our load, I got a bit cross with him. Since today is his birthday I let him get away with keeping this chain that he claims we will use to secure our bicycles on the condition that he carries it in *HIS* trailer, since it weighs a good twenty pounds. It made a funny story to show the television people, but I have to tell you, if the cameras wouldn't have been rolling, I would have made Morton leave this found treasure behind.

Morton and I stop to tighten the trailers after going over a railroad crossing that was rough enough to rattle them lose. Something compels me to telephone the place that said we could stay until Friday. My heart sinks and I almost burst into tears as the man tells me that his wife had said they couldn't do it actually.

We would normally not stop for the several nights, but since we were going to do some press, see the lovely city and catch up with newspapers that we are keeping up to date on our journey, we really had to stick around. We had someone from Washington DC coming down to do some filming and my daughter and her husband were in route to meet us for Thursday in Savannah. It would be the first time I saw Sarah and Graeme since December. Now all our plans seemed to fly right out the window. Typically we are so use to not knowing where we are going to sleep. It's an everyday thing to us and we take each day, each moment really, as it comes. But now was different. We had to stay in Savannah for the press commitments but we couldn't afford to stay on our budget.

Explaining what was happening to Morton, he was stunned. He didn't understand when they decided to not help us with a place to stay, why they didn't call us to tell us. There was nothing to do but to get on the phone. We had so much work to do on the computer that I needed 4 or 5 hours minimum today to be work time. I telephoned Glenn at the *Olde Harbor Inn* to ask for his help, again. They are very busy, with good reason, it is the prettiest place in Savannah and talk about location, location, location. He was kind enough to be able to help us for one more night. This was a lifesaver. It would get us the time to take care of the computer, search for new location (plan B) and go knocking on doors asking to pitch our tent if we couldn't find somewhere to sleep.

As we waited on a bench like two lost children, my cell phone got a work out. The weekend before we had sent emails out to lots of different places asking for their help. Savannah is really pretty at this time of year though, actually it's pretty in every season, so there were not a lot of vacancies.

Turning towards Tybee Island again, because we really did want to ride to the beach at Savannah too, the very first person I called, Deb, at *South Beach Ocean Rentals*, was just looking at our website. She had gotten the email, was looking to see that we were doing and thought the journey was a really good idea. She might be able to help, but it would be up to Michelle to decide. Deb promised to call me back and it sounds odd, but I quit panicking and started focusing on all the other calls I had to make.

It is our goal and desire to let as many people know as we can about our journey. Really we want people to know that there is always HOPE. As long as you are breathing, there is HOPE. We all have the power in us to change our lives, we just have to not be afraid to do it.

Morton thought I should keep calling for a place to stay, but I told him that it was all going to work out. I had to take care of work for the next couple hours or it would cut in to our touring time in Savannah. Since we really do have a lot of work to do along the way, I did need to keep on my present task.

As I was talking to newspapers up and down the east coast, I got a beep on my phone. I finished my 10 minute interview in about 2 seconds and took the call. It was Deb. She had talked to Michelle and they said they could help us out with a condo for our stay in Savannah. Best of all, it's right on the beach.

We had seen Erica at the *Savannah Area Convention & Visitors Bureau* earlier in the day and she had helped us with tickets to see the most incredible things in Savannah. Their building is this beautiful old bank that has a huge safe in the back and ceilings that seem to be 50 feet high. Things were really falling in to place and Sarah and Graeme were heading south. It was a good thing too. The one bike had been over a rather rough patch and the one spoke that was broken turned in to five spent spokes. We couldn't ride it around town anymore, let alone around the country. We would need the car that Sarah and Graeme would be arriving in to rescue us.

The rest of the day we did all the press we could do on the phone and by email while sitting outside on benches overlooking the Savannah River. We sent images and updates to a growing list of people in the media that are following our journey. How I wish we had a media person with us to take over this task that I'm having to learn as I go along. I lost hours on the computer uploading pictures, sending big 300dpi images to newspapers and trying to keep up with all that we do. Morton watched television and slept a little. After all, it was his birthday.

We both came to life at 5 pm when the news was coming on and we were watching from our room in the *Olde Harbor Inn*. It is always good to be able to see the reports. Tonight was one of the best. Melanie really did an excellent job at telling our story as we feel it. It was great to hear the lead in and lead out on it too. The news team all were very supportive of what we are doing.

Snapping a lot of pictures of the television, Morton and I were really impressed with how much footage they used and how much time they spent on the story. I know this is our baby and we are very passionate about what we are doing, but this IS something that needs told. They aren't just words when I tell you, "If I can do it, anyone can!" The other thing we want to happen too is to have hundreds, thousands and even MILLIONS of people doing this "journey" right along with us. The very first journey you need to take is the one that leads to better health.

Smiling and finally finishing on the computer, Morton and I set off on a walk. It felt good to stretch our legs. After all the stress of the morning with the bike wheel breaking and the "no room" incident, we had really been up and down the rollercoaster. Walking always helps de-stress you. Walking beside the Savannah River is an instant cure for all that ails you.

My phone started to ring and it was Sarah saying they were approaching the city. Could this day get any better? Even with all the bad things that happened, there were far more positive things going on. When life whips a roadblock in our faces we are learning to just find a way around it, not stress over the roadblock itself. Savannah has many charming things to offer, but one of the nicest is a stroll. Sarah and Graeme were kind enough to take us for a proper meal for Morton's birthday. This was really feeling like a dream now. Seeing my little girl, with her belly really showing now with her first child, it was just so perfect.

Morton and I order a meal to split. We get a chicken dinner that the restaurant is famous for. The waiter brings it, sets it in front of me, then says he has to go get the other plate. Morton and I start dividing the plate as he sets another plate down in front of Morton. The kitchen had already split the meal for us and it was huge. It goes to show you that you can SHARE a meal while you are out and still be very full. Most places that you eat out at give you way too much food and sharing it is a nice way to save calories and money.

Today while in the charming Savannah, we learn some really important lessons that we will hopefully be able to remember the rest of our lives. The first is that things always work out if you just let them. Panic and stress need to leave our lives.

Second, there are very kind people out there who care about strangers (we meet them every day) and it is the best way to live your life. The golden rule is the best rule and call it what you will, it is how we now are living our lives.

Day 51: February 20, 2007 - Tuesday - *Olde Harbor Inn*, Savannah to *South Beach Ocean Rentals*, Tybee Island, Georgia

Packing and moving from Savannah to Tybee Island *SHOULD* have been by bike. The only trouble is, one of the bikes had broken beyond repair and couldn't be rode. So we had to go to the car, thanks to Sarah & Graeme, to get everything shuttled out to the lovely condo by the sea. We couldn't have continued our Savannah and Tybee Island tour without the help of Deb & Michelle. Their generosity in the use of the condo was perfect timing. Things were just working out, as they seem to always do on our incredible journey.

Morton and I arrived to the condo by the sea with our first load. This was the items out of our trailers and the trailers themselves, folded up to take up less space and fit into the trunk and backseat of a Volkswagen. We were met by both Deb and Michelle and after a few hugs and our eternal gratitude, we made up way to the condo. This is somewhere very special that you could have a fantastic vacation in with friends and family. The condo has a view to the ocean that is out of this world. Inside it's light, spacious and puts your in such a tropical state of mind you can almost hear the steel drums playing. From the porch that overlooks the ocean that has a big porch swing and various furniture, to the well appointed kitchen, two bathrooms and two bedrooms...this is paradise that we really needed! Morton was thrilled to see the *full sized* washer and dryer! This means we will have clean clothes without the cost of a laundromat. There is also various WiFi connections that we can pick up. Perfection.

We get our things out to the island in two trips, then head back into Savannah. We have an appointment for the *Savannah Day Spa* for 3pm and we need to get a bite to eat. Sarah, being pregnant, needs to eat on a schedule. After all, she is eating for two.

Sarah was also in for a treat from Morton. He had said that he would be happy to give up his pampering at the spa for Sarah. That way we could spend some rare mother/daughter time together. She was thrilled and I think he was a bit relieved that he wasn't going to get a massage! Even though he says he doesn't want one, I know his body would love it. But he has never done this before and is kind enough to give his shot at it to Sarah. It was decided that Morton and Graeme would use the car and visit a museum, explore the Colonial Park Cemetery and see a bit of Savannah while Sarah and I were being spoiled rotten. As they dropped us off in front of the prettiest house in Savannah, we trotted up the stairs and in to paradise.

Let me tell you, I have been lucky enough to see the inside of houses, mansions, castles and even palaces from all around the world. This house that has been converted in such a wonderful way to become the *Savannah Day Spa* is one of the most incredible places I have ever seen. The owner of the *Savannah Day Spa*, Celeste, is this amazing woman who had this incredible vision that is just a real oasis in the city of Savannah. Their team of fantastic professionals pamper you and spoil you in ways that you thought weren't possible. Customer service, well-being and total relaxation are the order of business here. Best of all, it's set in a house that you will not believe. Elevators take you up and down the five stories of spa pleasure. Your tensions melt away as the time ticks on in this truly stunning setting. Everything inside and beyond the grand entrance felt like we were in the most beautiful dream you can imagine. We were given drinks of refreshing ice water with cucumber as we came in. We met several of the staff, answered a few questions on a sheet. It was also a bit of a wake up for me about how horrible I am to my skin. I don't use any moisturize and should! Since I use nothing but sunscreen on my face, exfoliated by stuff flying up off the road and a big daily dose of sweat, my skin isn't really looked after. We sat on the most wonderful chairs surrounded by lovely furniture from the period, yet very up to date. There were so many goodies to look at everywhere, I would have been tempted to treat myself if I wasn't living on a bicycle. My skin really needs some help, the daily routine of sunscreen and sweat with a little sandblasting from passing traffic isn't going to help me win any beauty contests. Celeste showed us to the amazing bottom floor at street level. This part of the house is just breath-taking. We entered a room, a huge room, with candles lit everywhere, superb lighting, waterfall showers, private sauna, a tub for two that I'll never forget that had it's own waterfall and every detail you could possibly think of.

We had an hour in this palace of luxury. Sarah said, "Morton should have been here with you." But I don't think she *really* meant it. There were rose petals on the floor, a chilled pewter platter that was filled was arranged with fresh sliced pineapple, grapes, oranges and huge strawberries. Cashmere robes were there for our use and Sarah and I squealed like two high school girls as the door closed behind us and all of this was ours to enjoy for the next hour. Since Sarah is pregnant, she couldn't do the hot tub. Shame for her, but more room for me. After a waterfall shower, I came out to find Sarah munching the fruit and saying that I can only have one strawberry. She is in love with them. But this wouldn't be the first time Sarah falls in love today with something at the spa. Climbing in the tub that was filled with the most lovely scents you can imagine, I pushed the button to the quiet almost silent hum of the jets. This also started the waterfall. Laying back in the water was pure sheer bliss. Sarah gave me my one strawberry and I burned this feeling in my brain. This is what I'm going to think about whenever I hit a hard spot on our journey. What a moment.

After lots of talking, giggling, enjoying, and ooohhhing and aahhing about all the perfect little touches, we put on our lovely cashmere robes and headed to the waiting room. It really is a relaxation room filled with loungers, chairs, chilled water and of course, decorated with superb taste. If you look pampering up in the dictionary you will see *Savannah Day Spa*.

It wasn't long until someone came to take us to our first treatment. Facials. We each rode up in the elevator to another level of pampering, so relaxed from where we just were. Sarah headed to one room and I went to another. The facial was so very relaxing that I think I might have went in and out of sleeping. My face was in spa paradise as I was given a head massage, face massage and all in expert hands.

The spa is set up to really do whatever you want. From just a little pampering to several hours of pure luxury pampering. This is something that everyone should treat themselves to, often. They also cater for couples, which is a wonderful experience. Not just the ladies get pampered here.

Next on our journey was the massage. Oh yes, the massage. Again, Sarah and I rode together to another floor that was stunning, into rooms that were so peaceful and serene. Again the treatment was perfect. I had forgotten how wonderful massage feels. I really do need to have more massages. My muscles ache after what we do day in and day out. If I could find a massage therapist who likes bicycle rides, I might be set.

The person doing the massage was a real expert. She knew just what part was sore before I could even say. She kneaded and pushed all the stress and soreness out of my back and shoulders. I really wanted to ask her what she was doing for the next two years and if she fancied seeing the coastlines and borders of America. The time slid by and when it was finished, I was taken to the top floor for the last treatment, a pedicure. You can imagine how my feet feel after bicycling and walking for about seven or eight hours daily, seven days a week. As I got on the most comfortable chair and my feet went in to the whirling pool of warm water, I wanted to purr. This was the real icing on the cake. Sigh.

Sarah wasn't in the room yet, but they were getting a chair ready for her so I knew she wouldn't be long. Little did I know she was on a waterbed getting a massage from Ken. Ken had popped in to say hello to me, we had spoke on the phone last week. He was very kind and according to Sarah, has the most wonderful massage technique. Sarah is quite the little expert on massages as well. She is a person who enjoys them and gets them whenever she can.

She was glowing when she came into the pedicure room. Smiling and saying "*that was amazing, did you have a waterbed?*" and all the other chatter that kept us buzzing through this social part of our visit. We were so thrilled with everything that we decided Savannah makes the list. Our list of places that would be a great city to live in, just to be near this incredible spa. The most spectacular house filled with the most incredible people...who could ask for anything more? As we finished our pedicures, got out of the cashmere robes and back into our clothes, we really were new women. We both said our goodbyes and thanks to these wonderful people and slid down the stairs back to the streets of Savannah. Words were gushed about how incredible, perfect, delightful and amazing our afternoon had been. I'm not sure if the guys understood this, but we did. The other thing that only I understood was that it was going to be something that will never happen again, as so many things in our life are. I appreciated every second of it as the treasure that the experience was. We walked and talked the rest of the evening. Shared a six inch sub on the old streets and kept walking a bit more. The spa had both relaxed us and energized us.

When we got back to Tybee Island there was a lovely moon over the water. A Georgia moon. It looked into my bedroom window as I fell asleep so happy knowing that my daughter was sleeping in the room next door and my grandchild was sleeping in her tummy. Perfection.

Day 52: February 21, 2007 - Wednesday - South Beach Ocean Rentals, Tybee Island and Savannah, Georgia

Today was a tough one. My mom is in the hospital with heart failure and there is nothing that I can do. We are set to explore the Savannah and I'm torn about just catching the first plane back to my mother. I am assured there is nothing I can do and my sister is with her. Such stress on an already stressful adventure is tough to deal with, but there is no other choice.

Sarah and Graeme are here with us and it feels like we aren't even on our journey now. This feels so odd. Why aren't we moving north? Why am I looking at my little baby? I try to get my emotions under control and get on with it.

We head to the Visitor's Center in Savannah, park the car and take a trolley tour. There are many companies to choose from, pick the one that suits what you want to see. There is a lot on offer.

Hollywood tours, spooky tours, pirate tours, history tours and so many other choices. We all climbed aboard a trolley and headed off for a narrated tour of the largest historic district in America. It is a fact that I never knew before, even though I have actually lived in Savannah for a brief period. A million years ago of course. I should mention that Savannah has a lot of remarkable things in it to bring you here. The charm of the people, the food, the location, the history, the weather and a million others. And, the beach is just a 20 minute drive to the lovely Tybee Island. Our trolley guide was really from Savannah. She knew her stuff, told her jokes and was lovely. Now I don't know if it was the fresh air or the fact that we had food in our bellies, but Morton ended up very sleepy on this tour. We were all sitting across the back seat and looking over, I saw Morton nodding off. My camera was up and I was going to snap a picture, but just then we were passing something lovely. That's easy in Savannah. The squares that are dripping with Spanish moss in huge live oaks, the azaleas that are in bloom and the interesting statues in the centers, make these wonderful subjects for your camera.

As I was clicking, the trolley was stopping and Morton, who was ready to start snoring, fell forward. He actually fell right to the floor, waking up on the way down. The lady driving asked if he was alright. He was more surprised then hurt. If only I would have had the camera set to video and captured it. The four of us started laughing under our breath and for the rest of the day we would put our hands and arms in front of Morton as if we were stopping. Graeme was the only one who wasn't really laughing about it. He actually joined in a little when Morton told him if it had been *him* that had fallen asleep, Morton would be laughing. It was a "you had to be there" moment that will make us all crack up for years to come.

We left our trolley tour at the Savannah River. There we all hopped on board a paddle boat and went up and down the river, hearing about the rich history. Savannah is still one of the busiest ports in the USA and we saw so many huge ships. The air was a bit smelly from the fumes of the papermill, but when we got to the other end it was pine scented.

There we saw giant stacks of logs being scooped off an enormous pile and put into a giant chopper. It was really fascinating to see all the trucks, like the ones that had passed us so close on the roads, lined up with their trees. It also makes you think about things like *recycling*! It would have been better to see old papers getting scooped up. If you don't have recycling where you live, do something about it. Get it there and *USE IT!* When the river tour was over we headed down River Street. A must do for all.

Sarah had spotted a gelati shop and wanted to compare it to Italy. It was really great but it wasn't like our little favorite shop in Volterra, Italy. We were all ready to move there for the ice cream. Of course the ice cream would be mixed with healthy doses of walking so I wouldn't end up weighing over 400 pounds again.

Walking to our next trolley stop we decided that since we had a car at our use (Sarah & Graeme's) we should take care of trying to get our bike sorted. It makes a huge difference having a car and other people as support out here. We knew it wouldn't last long so we had to spend some of our precious time together doing "journey" things as well as filming with the crew that is making a documentary about our adventure.

The bike place was really fantastic. They said it couldn't be fixed, gave us our money back and we were off to locate another bike. We had looked in the same store but there was nothing in our price range, less than $90., that would suit. There was the 24-hour super store from a world-wide chain we would visit after our ghost trolley tonight. Hopefully they will have a bicycle that we can use.

But for now we went to have dinner. It was an all you can eat place, or as Morton likes to call them, *"Eat 'til you burst"* feeding hole. I just had a sensible salad, very small portions of the pizza and pasta and was going to skip anything sweet at the end. Morton came back with three desserts on his plate. I scolded him for doing that, so he cut them in half and I helped him with his calorie intake. We still did have some walking to do, but I don't want any of my old "pig out" habits raising their ugly head.

We went back to the ghost trolley just in time to board and depart. It was really brilliant and we had the best host. Tonight nestled with my daughter I had the pleasure of being with my family. The stars were all out and dancing when we got back to Tybee Island. You could hear the ocean on the sand and we considered going for a walk, but I am falling so far behind on my pages and photos I opt to work on the computer. We talked for a while, then worked on what we will be doing tomorrow. There is going to be the press, pictures, filming and all things that make it feel like it isn't a vacation after all. Just a very brief stop in paradise. Though the ride is taking us places we have never imagined, it is still tough.

Day 53: February 22, 2007 - Thursday - South Beach Ocean Rentals, Tybee Island and Savannah, GA

My mother is heavy on my mind. I had this dream about her and I wake with this sense that I have to go back to take care of her. Remember that from May to November of 2006, we were staying with my mom and it was as if our roles were reversed. I was the mother, she was the child. I was and will always be, very protective of her. It's hard when you realize that sometimes there is nothing that you can do about someone else's health. I had to focus on my own now. The morning was spent crying and telling Sarah, Graeme and Morton that I had to go back. My sister is there on her own and I know first-hand what a huge job it is. We all talk, I cry some more and then the clock jumps up in front of my face. There are so many things that we have to do today. It is also our last full day together with my daughter and son-in-law. My heart is already breaking at the thought of them driving away.

We go through the interview, filming and photo shoot. It was a lot shorter than I expected. It really makes a difference when you are working with the pros. There is even time for us to grab a mini walk on the beach. Then, we split up, Sarah and Graeme drop us in town and head off to get up to their own things to do. Morton and I wanted to see a few more things in Savannah and have lunch at the famous *Clary's,* where the locals eat. The food was delicious and it reminded me of the brilliant movie, *Midnight in the Garden of Good and Evil*, with Kevin Spacey. It was set and filmed in Savannah and if you can't get to the city, watch that movie. Great flick and Kevin is brilliant as usual.

The day went faster then any day of my life. Before I knew it our tours were all over, the filming was finished and Sarah and Graeme were picking us up from in town and we were heading back to the beach. My mind was thinking that this had been the fastest few days in ages and the next time I saw my daughter, her belly would be bigger with the baby and mine should be a bit smaller. Hugging my daughter and holding her hand is something that I've always done. I will never stop. In my mind she will always be that little curly headed girl in a pale blue dress giving me big hugs around the neck.

We go and eat dinner at a place filled with alligators, for Graeme, he does love his gators. The night is wonderful and the hour slips away. I try to take a few pictures, but everyone really does get annoyed at all the pictures I take. Instead I try capturing the moment in my minds' eye, to think about while I'm out on the road and she is home feathering their nest. There are brief the moments back at the beach while we are watching television for distraction. We all know saying goodbye in the morning is going to be a tough job to do. We also all know how important it is what we are doing out here.

Everyday I get so much email from people I have never met and most likely will never meet. They encourage us, tell us we have inspired them and after all, this journey is something that is so long overdue. Without it I would have gone to an early grave from my own fat. With it, we might just be able to help a person or two along the way.

As hard as it is to say goodbye, we must. There is still so far for us to go on our adventure. No one really knows what is in front of us, but we can look back on where we have been with the satisfaction of knowing that we aren't just talking, we are walking.

Day 54: February 23, 2007 - Friday - South Beach Ocean Rentals, Tybee Island to Savannah, Georgia

Outside their car was pulling away. We are left all on our own again. Sarah stopped to wave goodbye through the windshield before heading off on their long drive back to Pennsylvania. It is a feeling that is just horrible. This is what I knew we were in for though, homesick feelings, missing out on everything that is happening at home and many times feeling like, "What on earth are we doing?"

Morton is making the the motions of moving our gear back in to our trailers and hooking up the bikes. As we were getting ready to set off we got a chance to talk to the lovely Michelle, who had made our stay on Tybee Island possible. She wished us well and asked us to come back to see them when we were done.

We took a few pictures and then were off. I was trying not to think about Sarah and Graeme leaving. They had to go back to help my son James, who is moving on Saturday. It was really lucky that we had even got to see her, but it was so hard now. Why can't we just appreciate the good things and not feel or find the sadness in situations? It is a tough request.

Riding off of Tybee Island we have to make our first photo stop for the day. They have a lighthouse that is not to be missed. It's the tallest in Georgia and it is stunning. We rode off our route and north to it. There was a moment that I was really scared when Morton said we really needed to climb to the top. Time and knowing my legs had to hold out for the biking today. I reminded him that it costs money and we had just $20. in cash to last us for as long as we could make it. The week in Savannah had been fantastic for our budget. I think we spent $13.00.

With the help of the *Visitors Center* and our help with the rooms and meals, and other things Sarah & Graeme were paying for. It is an odd feeling, having your grown-up child pay for your lunch or supper, but they said they wanted to, plus they really believe and support what we are doing. Our rooms had been sponsored by *Olde Harbor Inn* and the lovely condo from *South Beach Ocean Rentals* on Tybee Island, we had been given passes for all the things we had seen and done, so spending the money to see the lighthouse wasn't in our budget for this time.

As we approached Fort Pulaski, Morton asked from the next bike back, "Isn't this on the pass?" He had made a comment every time we passed this massive fort that he fancied a look inside. Since it was on our pass and we were doing good with time, we decided to head in, have a look and our lunch. We got lost for several hours inside. There were lots of people who were chatting with us, so many things to see and Morton even got to see an Enfield being fired. We had our little picnic and then started back on the bikes.

I wish I could say that I was over Sarah leaving by now. I wasn't. It was so sad thinking of things like, when is the next time we will see each other, will we ever see each other, all I can say is, it was so very lonely. I missed her, my mom, Graeme, my son, my daughter-in-law Mari and my entire family on both sides of the pond, so very much. Sorry to go on about it, it is the hardest part of what we are doing though. My husband won't see his family for almost two years, so I guess I should stop whining about not getting to see enough of mine. Sarah had called me as we were bicycling with tears in her voice. It was a call to please not go over the big bridge. It had barrels all over the side, we would have to push our bikes, then when we got off the bridge, she told me that the road had no edge, traffic was flying on it and she was worried about us. I told her that we have to ride on the roads that bikes are allowed on, whether they are safe or not. We have no choice. Since I don't really talk about it that much, you have to hear it now.

Morton and I have a massive fight after I hang up the phone with Sarah. Her tears and fears on top of my own ball of emotions churning in my stomach was more that I can take. I beg Morton to let me call her to come back and get us. He tells me that he is putting his foot down, end of story. We ride in silence, my anger at my stubborn husband pushing out my homesickness. The really bad part is, I know he is right.

Heading back towards Savannah we make a pit stop at a store that we had just been in two nights ago with Sarah and Graeme. Not only did they buy us the cereal for breakfast, they bought us a surprise gift of bicycle patches. Today we needed to fill our food bag back up. We did, but as we did I kept thinking, "Just two nights ago I had my little Missy here." My heart wasn't in it and I didn't really care if I ever ate again. I'm too busy hating Morton.

While they were here we had passed the sign for *Bonaventure Cemetery* several times. We had wanted to stop in to this historic burial ground to look at the stones, the moss and take some pictures. Today was the last time we would be passing the sign, so Morton and I decided to have a look. Stop three on our last bit of Savannah. I turn in and Morton follows, quiet as the grave.

It was lovely, the azaleas were blooming, the moss was swaying and it was so very peaceful. We knew we had to keep riding though and didn't have time to ride through the whole massive place. The next time we are in Savannah we will climb the lighthouse steps and explore the graveyards as they should be. This final resting place helps me check my anger. Why am I mad at Morton, he is only doing what I asked him to do. Keep me on track. Life is short, ride faster.

Leaving Savannah was proving to be tougher than I thought though. The day was wearing on and we still had to cross the massive bridge to get over in to South Carolina. As we made our way past the familiar streets, we were sad to be leaving this beautiful place. Fate stepped in though and Morton lost his chain. It was going to be a big project. A several hour project. The pedal assembly had worked it's way loose and he was worried about even pushing the bike. We needed a room for one last night in Savannah. And it was Friday. Not a good night of the week to find a vacant room.

We started making phone calls. The first eight places were all full. We were at the edge of a street that a lower priced place was on. I knew the city is busy all the time, so you have to book early. We went inside and they did have a room. One room left. They couldn't do it for free, the could give a ten dollar discount, but it would still make it $130. We asked them what was over the bridge, hoping it would be campgrounds or cheaper motels. We were told it was lots of nothing. With the misbehaving bike, it meant we needed to get inside for the evening. There is nothing you can do sometimes but bite the bullet and fix the bike. The weekend, late booking equals you have to take what you can.

I called Sarah and told her about the massive blown budget. They were still on the road. Her ankles were swollen and they still had several hours to ride. They will cover the same distance in just several hours though as Morton and I have came since Key West. What a difference it makes in a car. I guess the old bicycle couldn't stand the thought of staying together while it rode beside our new one. Pulling the bikes and gear inside the room we have a safe place to fix the bicycles. Morton sets to it on his bike and before the hour is up, he has it surprisingly back on track. We still have lots of things on our pass to see, including a different ghost tour. We decide to go for it.

Eating our pot noodles for dinner, we wait outside for one last tourist trip. The trolley picks us up in the dark and we set off. Morton doesn't fall asleep, I forget that my girl is hundreds of miles away from me and for a moment, one last moment, we just enjoy Savannah.

Day 55: February 24, 2007 - Saturday - Savannah, Georgia to Beaufort, SC

Do you believe in miracles? I do. We see them so much every day that I think sometimes I might just take things for granted. But we won't let that happen. Tonight, I count my blessings. There are so many it would take ages to tell you all of them, the biggest is just being alive.

Today when we left Savannah, we had a tough time doing it. It seemed as the city, bathed in sunshine and very mild temperatures, didn't want us to leave. First, the big bridge we were going over had a sign at the bottom proclaiming bikes and people on foot were prohibited. We had to find another way to get over the Savannah River. The option of riding west and north didn't seem like a good one, it would take us about 60 miles out of our way. We decided to try to cross the water by ferry.

We discovered that there is this free ferry that would take us to the convention center. We went for one last time down to Savannah and waited for the ferry. There were a few others there and we chatted as we waited for this free service. Docking, the crew sort of looked us up and down. I could tell what they were thinking when they looked at our bikes and trailers, will it fit? The other people went on first and we were helped on board by the friendly crew. There were no major probs, just a short slide across the river and we were nearly in South Carolina. The road and I had been warned by Sarah, got really narrow. There was the white line, then just a few inches, then the grass. It was so very close. The cars and trucks felt like they were brushing us as they passed.

We had a long way to ride and the weather was just right for it. Never mind the wind that pushed on us from the north and east, it felt great to be back on the bicycles. Riding was great therapy and cure for missing my daughter who had just left Savannah.

We did get shouted at, cursed at, honked at and even had something tossed out a window at us today. It had to do with how narrow the road was and the non-existent bicycle path. It wasn't our fault, we had no choice but to stay as close to the edge as we could. There were times though that the road had about a 8 to 12 inch drop off. If our trailer wheel fell off of this, I know without a doubt, that we would wreck the bike.

It was a thrilling ride. Up US 17 until we came to a cut off that we *thought* was the right direction. The signs were a tad confusing, but it worked out fine in the end with only a few extra added miles. We had our lunch on a bridge that sat over the prettiest swampy marsh. Trees were just pushing their new leaves, the air was warm and we couldn't have asked for anything more. We were sad though with all the litter that laid at the banks of this otherwise pristine place. There was a refrigerator sticking out of the pea green plants that floated on the surface. This didn't just fall out of a window, someone brought it here to lay it to rest. Littering fines, of huge amounts of money, need to be handed out along with the minimum of six months of picking up trash from beside the road. Not to be too hard on the culprits, I'd be all for making them collect the rubbish that is chucked out of windows for just eight hours a day, every day, for the entire six months.

If this didn't cure them of littering, nothing would. At first we had started picking up trash while we walked in the Keys. This only happened a day or two. We were finding that we would need a trailer to do this.

The things like bottles, cans, plastic bags and cigarette butts will *not* go away. Your children's children's children will still see them. Please put it where it needs to be, recycle it and reuse it. While we were in Scotland, I had written a guide for turning trash into arts and crafts. After thinking about how to reuse and recycle, I was amazed. There were over 400 different things I came up with in the name of arts and crafts that you could make out of rubbish. Think about things that you can *do* with your garbage and for pity's sake, when you are out in a car, the window is not a trash receptacle. Enough of the litter lecture, we just see so very much of it.

The broken glass produces so many flat tires for us. It isn't that I want to turn my bicycle into a soapbox to shout about the wrongs of the world, I just have a lot of time to think as I'm sitting there with my knees going up and down. We knew where our 30 mile mark was and were really shooting for that. There is so much to see out here in the lower coasts of South Carolina, but not a lot of building. There are lots of tidal marshes around us and we need to just keep riding. The views are great and though we are feeling sore, we feel so good today, the miles just melt by and my homesickness is leaving with them. Birds sing us along, even the people honking don't bother us. We just keep moving, ever north and east. Life is very good and we have so much to be thankful for.

As the 4:30 pm hour approaches we start thinking our daily thought, safe place to sleep. We know the sun will light our way until about 6:45 pm, but don't want to push it. There is a landscaper on the right and Morton pops in to ask how far until a campground or motel. I wait with the bicycles and watch two robins flying and singing. They are darting in and out of the moss covered live oak canopy. I wonder where they will go in the spring to build their nests and lay their bright blue eggs. Maybe they will be the first robin of spring that you see this year if you are in the north. Morton trots back to the bikes. The answer is 5 to 6 miles ahead. We both sort of just shrug at that. Not far, but we know how people think about mileage in their car. It could be a lot further and we both voice this concern, but since there is nothing we can do about it, we simply ride.

There is a familiar name coming up, Lemon Island. I remember seeing it on my detailed internet map. I wish I could remember how much further it was beyond our 30 mile point. I did remember thinking, it's too far for us to reach today. Here we were riding on to it. It was a long strip of an island hanging right off the coast. It should be on a postcard for the pure beauty of it. The sun was sinking down fairly fast. I kept pedaling as fast as I could manage and our eyes searched the sides of the road for a safe haven to pop the tent up.

Ahead of us we could see a bridge curving to the left. It was a big bridge, fairly high, but not impossible to ride over. Beyond it might be our motels. We had gone about 10 miles since the man had told Morton 5 or 6. Like I said, we had no choice but to just ride. I felt in my heart we would be fine. Just as we were crossing this spectacular bridge, the sun was setting. The sky was filled with so many brilliant colors and bright light shafts as the last bit of sun shone out to our bridge. It lit the area, but halfway across, it seemed to just slip below the horizon. My vision suddenly became murky and it was hard to pick out the safe parts of the bridge to ride on. My bike went over something metal and sounding like wire. It clanged in the tires and I heard Morton hit it too. Please, no punctures in the darkening evening.

As we came off the bridge we could see a gas station about a half a mile in front of us with its lights glowing in the dusk. All the cars headlights were on, when they passed us we would catch a glimpse of the dangers in front of our bike tires. Thank goodness this bridge was pretty free from litter. Ahead of us, just before the gas station, there was a van pulled beside the road. It's headlights were on and a man was getting out and walking towards the road and us. We just knew he was there to talk to us. It was darker now and even though we should have been scared and in the past we would have been, we stopped.

The man, Mike, told us about a place to camp. He also warned us there was a storm coming through. The campsite, where he has gone with his kids, is a two mile ride, in the dark and off the main road. He told us directions, said he would go home and double check the forecast. Then he would meet us back by the camping site to shine his headlights for us. Did I mention that Mike was a complete stranger to us?

He set off and we turned off the main road to follow his directions. It was dark now. Not dusk. Dark. Morton and I were both terrified of being hit by a car on this narrow road with no edge to it, but there was really nothing else we could do right now. We turned right, looked for a street name and then we found the dirt road we were going to camp down. Morton and I both voiced a bit of nerves about what we were doing and I told Morton I had a good feeling about Mike. As we stopped at the sandy path, we met a man who was out walking his beagle. We talked for a bit about what we were up to and he told us that there were some people that would drive down the path and get a bit rowdy on the weekends. He told us to be careful there and also told us about the thunderstorms. Another man joined us and soon Mike was pulling up, in a pick up. Mike knew and went to church with one of the men.

Our group talked about what we should do. Mike offered to go offload his work ladders and come back, haul us and our gear to the motel that was about 5 miles in front of us. The man with his beagle had us come into his driveway to be safe from passing cars and be out of the dark path of traffic. He also went inside and brought out another dog for us to pet. When Mike came back, the guys loaded up our gear and we were off. Mike invited us to go to church with him in the morning when we were at the motel. He also went inside and paid for our room. Miracle in action. Our needs were not just met for the day, they were exceeded. Mike was so friendly, so positive and such a wonderful person. He had actually seen us earlier and was worrying about our safety. In our experience out here, living day to day not knowing what or who is around the corner, we have seen miracles happen daily. Mike was our miracle today and not getting hit by a car or truck was another.

Day 56: February 25, 2007 - Sunday - Weatherbound in Beaufort, SC

Daylight came and Morton and I turned on the television to double check the weather report. Still severe thunderstorms for today, with Monday due to be nice and sunny. It was a bit of reassurance that we were doing the right thing by staying put now.

After a hot breakfast, Morton called Mike and he gave us the time he was going to pick us up to go with his family to church. It will be the first time on the journey that we actually go to a church while they are having a service. Mike is a man who goes out of his way to help others. His wife Amanda and their three children met up with us all after the service. It was really wonderful to get to interact with this caring family. Being so far from home and family, it's just a really nice feeling to be part of a family for a bit. They are really amazing people with such big hearts and great attitudes. After church we went to have lunch at a local restaurant. The meal was really nice, but the best part of it, without a doubt, was the company. It turned in to a lot of people and the place actually opened up their banquet room for us all. The time slipped away as it always does and we were saying goodbye to the people we had lunch with. Mike and his family invited us over for supper and he was kind enough to give us a ride back to our room.

The skies were cloudy, but it seemed the weather man had missed the storm, or the storm had missed us. I decided to work online for a while and had my headphones on listening to music when I heard the first crash and saw the flash. It was as if the heavens had just opened up and was now pouring. Clever weatherman! There was almost a need to turn a light on it had gotten so dark. I quickly unplugged my laptop and mp3 player from the socket and kept working on battery power as Morton took the camera. He was going to take pictures, one anyway. He was afraid to stand outside under the overhang. It was loud and crashing, but only lasted about 30 minutes. It would have been horrible to have been riding in it, even if it was short.

Since we had decided to wait out the storm and the storm was really scattered, there is no telling where we would have been when it all happened. It might have rained even harder up ahead, or it might have missed us completely. You just never know with weather and can only go on what you think is the right thing to do. Before long we were with Mike heading over to his house. He stopped at a grocery store on the way and Morton and I got our cans of tuna. Sounds like boring food I know, but it keeps well. Check back with me in two years to see if I can even eat tuna again. Amanda, Mike's wife, had made us a lovely pot of homemade chicken noodle soup with veggies and really nice noodles. She had also made a loaf of bread. It was hard to just have one slice of this treat. I could have eaten more, but didn't.

Their dog, Daisy, eventually got use to Morton. Everyone does in the end. I think it might have been his voice that made her a bit worried. The kids played and for a few hours, it felt like home. It was really good for being homesick as well. A nice treat for a mom who is a million miles away from her kids.

We had found out earlier that Morton's brother George and his wife Elaine, have had a baby girl in Scotland. We are so very happy for them, but it makes me sad that we won't be able to see the baby until she's almost two. Family is the biggest thing we miss being on the road, so it feels good when we are around people that make us feel like we are part of their family. At least for a few hours. Saying our goodbyes, Morton and I came back to get all our gear together. We had to get things organized, uploaded, stowed, ship shape and ready to roll when the sun comes out tomorrow.

Life for us will keep moving, as long as we are breathing. Our journey is turning in to so much more than just exercise, fitness, seeing the sights and feeling homesick. This is really a quest where we are learning more about ourselves and others than we ever thought possible. I'll leave you with a quote from G.K. Chesterton, "The Traveler sees what he sees. The Tourist sees what he has come to see." We want to be travelers who remember to appreciate the moment.

Day 57 & 58: February 26 & 27, 2007 - Monday & Tuesday - Beaufort to Broad Street Kosher Guest House, Charleston, SC

As Morton & I left Beaufort after our time there, we realized that we hadn't really seen it. There was a historical part to it that we should have rode through, but didn't. We had 80-something miles to cover in two days, depending on which sign you believe. The road signs all have a way of saying one mileage on one, say 73 miles, then you see the next sign after riding a few miles closer to the destination, and it will say 75. This worries us, but what can we do except keep pushing the pedals up and down on the bikes. Little by little, we go far. South Carolina is stunning. I keep hearing the words to Jimmy Buffett's song, *"Prince of Tides"* in my mind. I remember the book and film and wonder why I haven't really explored this state before now. I have driven through it countless times and never, sadly, stopped. As we ride through the countryside, sharing the road with the cars and trucks that pass us, Morton and I comment back and forth about how pretty this or that is. Let me tell you what it looks like right now. The marshes that go on forever, dotted with trees that are tall and of course, lots of them covered in the Spanish moss. The grass is still brown a bit from winter, but you see tinges of green everywhere. Buds pushing on trees, green in the swamps and birds are everywhere.

The signs that people actually live here are far and few between. We get lots of long stretches of road today. All good for seeing things, but it makes you wonder just where you are going to be able to stay. I don't fancy sleeping outside in the low country. The bicycles, both of them, got more then their fare share of punctures today. We also had to do lots of pit stops for Morton's chain. All in a day's ride though. We have learned to take each stop with the attitude of "it's meant to be" and not rush the day along. We make the most of each stop, drinking, checking the phone for any missed calls and other incidentals. There is also the bathroom situation. Sometimes out here there isn't always one when we need it. For Morton, as is all men, it's easier. For me I have to be brave enough to walk back into the bushes or trees and hope I don't encounter a sleeping beastie while nature is calling.

As the sun gets lower, we ask someone at one of the rare places of business we come across if there is anywhere to camp. He tells us about a place a mile ahead. After about 2 miles, we see the sign for it. It was the oddest experience camping we have ever had. The campground was like a ghost town. There were about forty campers in it, not a car or person in sight. There was a little sign when we came in that said if no one was there, choose a place and pay the person in the morning. The sunset was in high gear and we had to rush to find a location. Since there was no one or lights around, we chose to stay close to the bathrooms. They were clean, had showers (which we didn't use) and they did have an outside light. It felt so odd being the only people there. It was quiet and very still as the night fell. I jumped in the tent once it was up and Morton started tossing stuff in to me. It's funny how much better I'm fitting in the sleeping bag and tent in general. Getting up and down from the ground is so much easier too. The lighter me is loving it. We decided to call it an early night and I called my kids with instructions to call the police if they didn't hear from me in the morning. They both gave me some words of comfort and said maybe someone would show up during the night. Actually, that wasn't a very comforting thought.

While we had been riding, we were against the wind and with a frustration after frustration with repairs, we had to just lay our heads down and we were sleeping by 8 pm. Soundly sleeping. But not soundly enough to sleep through the noises we started hearing about 10 pm. There was something outside of the tent moving around. I think it might have even bumped *into* the tent. Shaking Morton I asked him if he heard it. Right on cue, the little critter started running around the outside of the tent. It thumped to the ground after tripping on a guide line. What is it, I wondered to Morton. He felt certain it was an armadillo. I was going to say that I wasn't sure if they were up this far, but we were both back to sleep again. Come 2 am we woke up again. This time it was a car and I was really scared. The car circled us on our little island of grass by the bath house. I was hoping it was the police or the people coming around that ran the place. We will never know who it was, it drove off and I couldn't get back to sleep. Morton was snoring before the tail lights were out of view. It seems I'm the only one that was worried.

Come morning on Tuesday, our tent was freezing inside. Anything that wasn't under the sleeping bag was cold. My arm and face felt like they were made of ice since they had been dangling out of the thin sleeping bag that wasn't built for this kind of weather. Outside we could see our breath as we packed up our tent. There was still no one around. I looked online to get the address of the person we were going to stay with while we were in Charleston. The bad news was, the address was 55 miles north of the city. This wouldn't work. Panic didn't just set it, it jumped up and smacked us around the face a little.

Quickly I set to work on looking for a place to stay. Everything else was secondary. We have been working with a great man who had arranged some press that we were going to do in Charleston and we can't let something like no where to stay, stop us from seeing the city that I have only ever gotten to drive through before. While I was still sending out emails, I got a telephone call from a lady who was going to help us. She would be able to help us with a place to stay for our entire visit.

With big smiles finally on our freezing faces, we could both breathe a bit easier. You know that sleeping quarters are the big worry when we stop in a city. After our mix up in Savannah, we didn't want to take any chance. Now the fear was erased and we could focus on the ride. As we got closer to Charleston and civilization started coming in to view, we stopped at a place that had a sign out for clean restrooms. Always a good thing. We popped in and met the nicest lady who was from Ohio originally, then ran a B&B in Michigan. She had moved to South Carolina and told us the most enchanting thing I want to share with you. Do you know where mistletoe comes from? Do you think it grows in bushes? I did. Do you think it grows on vines? Actually, it grows in balls that are high in the trees beside the road. They are green and lush right now and here is the really odd part. People actually shoot them down, or so said this kind lady who shared the tale with us. A few miles down the road and sure enough, there were several balls of mistletoe high above our heads.

Our map from Georgia had just enough showing in South Carolina to direct us to Charleston. There we will pick up a new map that will guide us on the rest of our ride through South Carolina. Today we sort of have to guess for mileage. We also have the usual tire repairs to add to our time.

When we were pulling out of a red light, something was coming really close to me. Really close. I leaned to the right, but I couldn't go off the edge of the road. The pickup truck that was pulling the boat must not have realized that the boat had about a two foot overhang on it. He was going slow and that is what saved me from getting whacked on the head. If the curve of the boat would have been any different, I would have gotten it. And by "it" I mean a concussion. Instead my bicycle or trailer just got bumped. It happened so fast, even at his slow speed, it was hard to tell.

There was also a rather hairy time when we were driving through construction, only had the edge of the road and a truck pulling a trailer had to really lock his brakes up. Tires were squealing behind us and it sounded like the noise that happens before a loud crash. I yelled to Morton to follow me and I drove off the road into a grass area and bumped into a barrel. My handlebars also bumped into my stomach on the already black and blue area. Morton nearly wrecked into me and the cars and trucks all floored it, one of them even squealing their tires. The truck pulled off the road in front of us at the end of the construction zone and I was really afraid. You never know what someone is going to say or do. He was on the phone as we passed him yelling into it and we just kept riding. When we were well out of the danger of construction we pulled over for Morton to check over the trailer and bike. Everything was fine but my stomach was really sore. People have to realize that *"Share the Road"* signs are more than just decoration. We will always choose a cycle path or side-walk if we can, but when we can't we *have* to share the road with you.

Morton and I were more than just a little relieved to see the bridge that would take us into downtown Charleston. It had been another really long day and we were anxious to get to meet Hadassah, the kind woman and owner of *Broad Street Kosher Guest House,* who has given us accommodation. Riding down Broad Street has to be experienced on foot or a bicycle. The homes are all unique, palatial and have such style to them. This is one of the prettiest, if not the very prettiest streets, we have been on yet.

We entered the guest house that had once been the detached kitchen to this grand home and Hadassah showed us what will be our home for the next few days. The antiques and interior is just stunning. The bed has carved thistles on the end posts of it, a touch of home for Morton. After all, the thistle is the flower of Scotland. The shower tonight was worth at least two million dollars. It was a sunny days riding and we hadn't showered at the deserted campground. All this with WiFi too, if I am dreaming I hope no one has the nerve to wake me up! Tomorrow we are off to explore, doing some television with a very special Charleston man, Louis, on Thursday and want to see all that Charleston has to offer...or at least as much as we can cram in the next couple of days.

Day 59: February 28, 2007 - Wednesday - Broad Street Kosher Guest House, Charleston, SC

Morton and I woke up early in our lovely room. It was actually as I said, once the kitchen for this great house in Charleston. It was common practice to have the kitchen in another house altogether. Things like heat and fire made it practical. Today it is the most special place to call your holiday home. Decorated to a standard that could grace any cover page of your beautiful homes type magazine, it is just so lovely. From the soft rich brown hardwood floors, with the gorgeous rugs that cover just enough of them for comfort, no detail is left undone. The wallpaper in the bedroom is a series of perfect tones and shades to bring the whole room together, found repeated in a subtle pattern here and there. The color of muted green on the kitchen walls is my new favorite shade, broken with creamy white wooden trim, real wooden shutters that work on the insides of the large windows. The kitchen, without a doubt is another thing of practical beauty. You can't imagine and I know the pictures won't show you, just how lovely this is. It is a very long way from our tent pitched in the abandoned campground the night before.

The woman who owns and runs this spectacular home, and yes, it does feel like a home, is also an incredible cook. We discover this at breakfast which is a real feast. She has baked healthy pumpkin bread, cured the lox herself, just the evening before and the whole lovely breakfast is served on lovely Spode china that comes all the way from Stoke-On-Trent in England.

At breakfast we meet a couple who flew from their home in New Hampshire a few years ago, to Jacksonville, Florida. They then proceeded to ride up the east coast all the way to Maine. They followed a different route then us, but they were still able to give us the kind of advice and stories that you just can't get from a book, not even this one. Hopefully when we are in New Hampshire we will get the chance to see them again.

After a wonderful breakfast with such a fun and varied conversation, we set off, on foot, to discover Charleston. There are a few similarities to Savannah, but the two can never be compared. The closest thing I can find is they both are old, historic cities in the South, near the water, with a fort in close proximity. That is where it ends. As we walked towards the visitor center we headed up Meeting Street. What a vision. Houses, buildings with huge earthquake bolts through them, cobblestone streets and everyone saying, "Good Morning" to us was a wonderful start to our day, showing us the Southern hospitality is alive and well.

Once inside the visitors center, we picked up our passes to some incredible attractions from Katie with the media department. The visitors center has a movie, *Forever Charleston*, about this lovely city, which was just starting, so we popped in to get a very entertaining history lesson. So many firsts happened here, but the one that stuck out in my mind from school a million years ago, was the first shot in the Civil War, which was anything but civil, rang out here. Fort Sumter sits out on an island off the edge of Charleston and it's said that while the first day of fighting went on, not one person died (just one unlucky mule) and the people watched from their windows as if it were just a bit of entertainment.

After the film, which I would recommend seeing, we headed outside to check out a bus tour. There were many of them, but none were leaving within the next five minutes and I needed to see Charleston *now*! This city is made for walking, begs to be walked and walk we did. Within just a few short steps we were inside the *Charleston Museum*. This was a big mistake to bring Morton here, but after putting him through such grief when we were leaving Savannah, I figured I needed to do something nice for him. The *Charleston Museum* offers a unique look through objects and presentations, of the low country. There are so many things to see and Morton was not understanding that we just have so much time. You need to allow two to three good hours to spend in this place. Your children will love it too. There is an entire area just for them, with a mini scale grand house they can even go "inside" and play games or have a tea party, which Morton and I did.

Right beside the museum is the *Joseph Manigault House*. You need to go insides this house just to see the staircase, chandeliers, furniture and paintings. The house itself is very impressive too. We were told how there had once been a gas station tight up against it and they were kind enough to give back the land to be turned back into the garden and had left the garden structure standing for us to enjoy now. Sometimes progress does do the right thing.

After all this walking we were ready for lunch. The first stop on our taste of Charleston was the *Wild Wing Cafe*, located on Market Street. This is the place to come if you like wings and specialty sauces, not to mention excellent service. Our waitress was really helpful and recommended some of her favorite things to see in Charleston. That is a good thing to ask your waitress, if you had only ONE thing to see in this town, what would it be? We even got to meet the manager who promised that he would peek in on the site. Their coleslaw was some of the very best I have tasted and the chicken was so tender. Morton had pulled pork with Old Smoky sauce. It was a first time for him and he was in hog heaven.

Heading through the market is a must when you visit Charleston. It is in a lovely part of the city, filled with everything you can imagine, including places to book tours...HAUNTED tours! We did this with *Bulldog Tours*, to see the old city jail, said to be VERY haunted indeed. We would find out for ourselves later. The market is also the place that you find the lovely horse and carriage tours that is the second best way to get around the city, the first way of course, being the things at the end of your legs with toes on them.
We went to *Palmetto Carriage Works* and right into their stables. We followed the yellow horseshoes to the bathroom before boarding the carriage. It was a bit surprising to see that our carriage, which seated 14, was pulled by two enormous mules with rather long ears. Aren't they suppose to be as stubborn as my husband?

Our guide started us off slow. He actually did very little talking, which startled me. I had things I wanted to *LEARN* about Charleston. After stopping by some sort of ticket or license plate bureau for carriages and he knew what route we were taking, he opened up a bit. His words were worth the wait. Lots of guides do a "push and play" tour. They almost sound like they are reading from a script and a rather dull script at that. Not this young man. He not only drove the mules well, but spoke to us from his very heart about what we were looking at. He told us tales in a quiet way about the houses and buildings around us. It was a journey that everyone should take. We had the very back seat to ourselves and Morton had asked for a blanket when we were back at the stable. The sun was out and it was quite warm, but our mule driving guide had warned us it would be windy down by the water. Even though Morton is a hearty Scotsman, he was wearing shorts and didn't want to take any chances with the weather. As a true Scotsman, he is all too familiar with how the weather can change. As we clip clopped past *Rainbow Row*, an extremely old row of house, maybe from the revolution times, we could feel the breeze picking up. By the time we hit Bay Street it was blowing down a gale.

The river beside us was capped with frosty white looking waves. It felt nice and snug under the blanket which Morton was kind enough to share even though I had scoffed at him for wanting one. The carriage ride lasted a good long while, showed us houses that we knew we had to go in and the easy way the guide had of speaking made us loose track of where we were. It seemed too soon to be back, but an hour or so had actually passed. He had told us it would take us nine hours to see the whole bit by carriage and by gosh, if we could have, I would have. Since Morton had his shorts on, we had to walk back to our lovely place of lodging on Broad Street so he could get changed. The night was coming with a ghost tour of the haunted old jail and before that, we were having dinner at *Bubba Gumps* on Market Street. We went on other streets and were delighted. Every street in Charleston will show you something different and delightful. Wear good shoes when you visit and expect to say "OOOHHH" and "AAAHHH" a lot.

Consulting our map, we returned to Market Street, once Morton had put the long trousers on. We wanted to make sure we were taking still another route. That again is the beauty of the city. Always many different roads to get you around. When we got to *Bubba Gump's* we were seated outside at our request, in a really snug corner. Anyone who has ever seen *Forrest Gump* has to come and eat here. Even if you never saw this movie, you will enjoy this very friendly and fantastic place with great eats. The waiter explained the signs on the table, license plates, that said, "Run Forrest Run" and "Stop Forrest Stop". It was showing the RUN sign and if you needed anything, refills on drink, to ask a silly question, anything...you just flipped the sign to STOP. Makes perfect sense! My eyes caught hold of the Coconut Shrimp on the menu and that is what I had. It was delightful and they really do know how to do shrimp. Morton and I even split a lovely piece of Key Lime Pie, sorry Graeme. The service and food were both excellent and we would love to try another *Bubba Gump's* (they have them all over!) and see if it had the same fun flair as this one.

Don't worry about me putting on weight here in Charleston. I think I might have mentioned this town begs to be walked in and since our bikes are getting to rest their wheels for a few days, our feet are hitting the pavement. And cobblestones and bricks.

Following the map that was our ticket to get in, we went to the old jail house to meet our tour guide. There was a whole group outside of folks waiting to have a peek inside. I hadn't seen the building in the daylight, but under the moon, let me tell you, it was *CREEPY*! This was going to be fun.

Earlier, when Morton was changing from shorts to trousers, I downloaded the pictures but hadn't been able to take the time to recharge my battery. This meant I wasn't going to be able to take unlimited photos. I had to stretch it out. Before the tour even started though, I think I took about fifty. What did I do before digital?

Our guide showed up bang on time. Another delightful guide. She didn't read from any script, just let the things we were seeing speak for themselves and gave us a real education on this horrible prison. I made a mental note to read more about it. The guide said they could never find any records for the prison, very unusual, unless there were things to be hidden. I imagine there were quite a few. We entered the gated yard and got the full view of this building. Usually I love all big old buildings, but this one really felt spooky. Creepy and yet calling to us. There were windows in the front part where the guards would have stayed, some even lived in it back in the day. But when you went around the prison, just bars and the windows open to the elements, bugs and the such. Just as it would have been for the prisoners.

Climbing the steps and going in the prison was quite the scary thing. People were laughing and joking, but I think everyone would have told you they were a bit scared if they would have told you the truth. I know I was. I held on to Morton's arm and learned about the horrible days of old. Walking from cell to cell, and they were huge, holding many people, you could really feel how bad these poor prisoners had it. We were even locked in one, the whole group, while our guide was outside. She flipped the light off and you got the feeling of just what it felt like to be in the dark with a group of strangers. Only difference was, we weren't with prisoners, just other visitors. Everyone opened their cell phones and tried to make it lighter. There was a lot of nervous giggling here. After about 45 minutes we left the building. The guide told us how to make sure the ghosts didn't follow us home. I did as I was told and wiped my hands down my arms and asked the ghosts to stay where they were. Hey, you can't take any chances, right?

Coming back, still another way, we were charmed back into our lovely Charleston by the flicker of gas lights on houses. We peeked in windows as we were strolling, into lit rooms of grand designs and I held Morton's hand quite tightly. It wasn't scary though. Charleston is one of the safest feeling cities I have ever been in. Back in our beautiful room I downloaded pictures, got things charged for tomorrow and now I'm going to sleep on the lovely bed, in the lovely home of one lovely lady who was kind enough to let us stay here. Charleston feels like home to us and we will never forget this wonderful lady.

Day 60: March 1, 2007 - Thursday - Broad Street Kosher Guest House, Charleston, South Carolina

Where to begin. We could really write a book about just what we did today, but I will try to behave myself and give you the short version. But believe me, nothing about today was short. We visited the most lovely houses in Charleston, after having one of the best breakfasts we have had at the lovely B&B on Broad Street. Just a very short stroll and you are right on the doorstep of three fantastic homes, all from different time periods and all breath-taking. Location, location, location. The houses we saw were the *Nathaniel Russell House, The Heyward-Washington House* and the *Edmonston-Alston Home*. There are so many more, but alas, we only have so much time here. We took pictures of what we could and as always, I kid myself into thinking I can remember all of this wonder we are taking in.

There were countless flowers that held all the scent of spring, people that we spoke to in these incredible homes and the morning just slipped away. We walked by the water up East Bay Street. This is one of our favorite streets, with good reason. If you have been, you'll know why. If you haven't been, consider this your quest. We could walk this street several thousand times and always see something new.

There was a building that we both wanted to see, the *Old Exchange & Provost Dungeon*. It did not disappoint. This was the last building that the British built for us, right before 1776 and very important historically. Inside it is like a brilliant blue piece of sky, tall windows with excellent views, resident pirate and Brit to guide you through it and of course a dungeon. In the old dungeon you can actually see part of the ancient city wall and hear the tales of the pirates that were held there, later to be hung in public.

Heading north towards the area of the IMAX theater, Morton and I were watching the sky. The weatherman was calling for storms and it did look like they were brewing as we headed further north from our room. We split a 6" sub and popped indoors while one downpour happened. Then we caught a patch of rain-free sky and made a break for it to the IMAX. Morton had never been before and I was so very happy that on our pass we had been given, there was something on it for a rainy day. The film we were going to see was *Sharks in 3-D*. Very impressive indeed.

Morton looked a bit like Elton John in his glasses, sorry Elton, and me, I like to think I looked a bit like Sophia Loren (on a very bad day after she had gained 200 pounds) as we sank in to the seats and waited for the show. The sights and sounds were amazing. It was just 45 minutes, but really good. When we left we were at the very top of this tall building by the water. What the weather was doing outside was shocking. Our little drizzle and cloudburst had turned into buckets of rain. We decided to just have a seat on a comfy couch and I turned on the laptop. Low and behold, I even got the internet there.

As we were sitting to wait out the storm, a very nice lady named Dee who worked here, and I do mean VERY nice, started talking to us. When people ask us where we are from, it's hard to just say. There is no standard answer we can give. When we tell them what we are doing, they sort of go into a bit of shock. Dee was no exception. We chatted and we explained we were waiting out the storm, with very limited funds and really couldn't even afford to take a bus back to where we were staying.

The next film, *A Night in the Museum*, was getting ready to start and she told us that we could go ahead and watch it. As we sat in the back and it was just coming on, this kind woman handed us a bag of popcorn. *"There's no butter on it"* she whispered. Morton and I both said thank you and she was gone. What a great lady. We sat there in the dark eating our popcorn, watching the film and waiting out the storm.

When it was finished, so was the storm. We walked to our temporary home on Broad Street, the prettiest street in Charleston and had our homemade red velvet cake for dinner. It was given to us at breakfast by the lady who owns the B&B and is an excellent cook. The cake reminded me of something my gramma use to bake when I was a child. After a day so perfect, there couldn't be one fault found with it, we fall asleep to the sound of the rain that was kind enough to wait until we were indoors to start again.

Day 61: March 2, 2007 - Friday - Broad Street Kosher Guest House, Charleston, SC

This morning at breakfast we made the sad discovery that we should only be three to four more days in South Carolina. It's good that we are moving right along, but I tell you, we could really just stay in Charleston. After what was without a doubt, the tastiest and healthiest breakfast we have had, we head out to meet our new friend Louis at the Charleston Food and Wine festival.

Louis runs an organization called *Louie's Kids*. They work to help tackle childhood obesity, one child at a time. The support camp scholarships and other programs for obese children from low-income families designed to help them lose weight and keep it off. If you would like to learn more about this fantastic organization, please visit Louie's Kids online and help them.

After getting a link to our website from a friend, Louis contacted us in Savannah and invited us to meet with him when we came through Charleston. He was even kind enough to arrange an interview on television with us on *Low Country Live*, with the local ABC station. We met at the beautiful Marion Square, a park that had been filled with large tents to house this very popular event. Louis is such a kind and giving person. He is a real inspiration and the passion for what he is doing is easily seen in his eyes. Dedication like this is rare and special. *Louie's Kids* has a tent at this event to show families how to enjoy healthy snacks. The interview is fantastic, it is our first live broadcast. Louis makes it feels so very easy, just like a chat with friends. He is friends with the man from the station that is doing the interview and my "live" nerves flew right out the window. Hopefully in the morning we will be able to stop by the festival and say goodbye to Louis, but we will keep in touch throughout our journey. We want to help raise awareness to the very important work that *Louie's Kids* is doing.

Heading off to the visitor center, Morton and I pick up a map of South Carolina. We will be needing it for the rest of our trip. We also decide to take a tour of the city to see it just one more time. We use our pass for Grey Line Tours and have an excellent adventure with a really good guide. Charleston is batting 1000 for terrific guides. After the tour, we have a fantastic lunch at *Joe Pasta*, thanks to Harrison. It was really good, fresh and it's easy to walk to from the Visitor's Center. The atmosphere was really nice and all the other dishes that were coming out for the other patrons looked incredible too. Morton and I were both so stuffed, but knew that we weren't going to be having dinner and doing lots of walking.

The sun was out with no trace from the rain last night. Heading to the water we were hoping to make the last tour of *Fort Sumter*, but we missed the boat. Oh well, our pass got us in to the *South Carolina Aquarium* and we really both enjoyed that. I loved the jellyfish, so lovely to watch. There were also otters that we could have watched play for hours. We got to see a diver feeding the fish while in the tank and have a good look around. There was just enough time to step inside the *Military Museum*, located in the same building as the IMAX theater. They walk you backwards through our military history with uniforms, memorabilia and unique presentations. Morton could have stayed there all day, but I wanted to get back. Sadly it is our last night, for this trip anyway, in Charleston. There is lots to do on the computer and Morton is going to make sure the bikes are ready for us tomorrow. A flat to fix and the packing of our dirty laundry. We need to find a washer soon or Morton and I will be knocking rocks on our clothes at a creek.

With March upon us, we want to make sure that as we go north, winter is leaving or we will have to put snow tires on the bicycles. We would both gladly stay in Charleston for many seasons, not just one, but the road is calling.

Day 62: March 3, 2007 - Saturday - *Broad Street Kosher Guest House*, Charleston to *KOA Kampground*, Mt. Pleasant (north), SC

The saddest part about leaving Charleston or anywhere for that matter, isn't the place that you are leaving behind. It is the people that we have met. For a brief moment we feel like we know the streets, know some friendly faces and it feels like home. That is really how we felt in Charleston and it just dawned on me as we were leaving that we are going to feel this sad feeling every time we leave somewhere that we have met people like the people we met in this special city. We rode past the Food & Wine festival in full swing at Marion Square we stopped to take pictures. I really wanted one of the banner for *Louie's Kids*. Sadly we didn't get to say goodbye in person to Louis, but we both know we'll meet again. Hopefully on Oprah.

The bridge was crowded with people walking, bicycling, jogging and then there was us. We were going to try to ride up it, but I couldn't. I'd like to blame the bike, but it's my lack of being FIT! Next time I'm in Charleston I will bike the whole way over that brilliant bridge. It was so very well thought out. We have to say it is the *BEST BRIDGE* we have been over thus far. A whole lane was dedicated to the walker, runner, biker and their safety was in mind.

Taking a survey as we crossed it, I counted 76 people using it along with us. I might have missed a few here and there, but that is excellent. Talk about a great way to see the city. Morton, with his eagle-eye, even spotted two raccoons far below us hunting in the marshy island for who knows what.

When we came off the bridge we spotted a television station. NBC affiliate, channel 2, so in we went. We were helped by a lovely lady, Sara, who did an interview with us and called for someone to film us bicycling around their parking lot. It was nice to be filmed in a safe location for a change rather than on the side of the road. The interview, like all of them, is fun and I try to imagine my words and the journey actually getting through to people. I want the light to come on for the world.

South Carolina is a wonderful state. Beautiful things to see, beautiful and hospitable people, so I can only assume that the people that were passing us today on Hwy 17, once we crossed the bridge were from out of state. We got so many mean honks, close brushes with cars and trucks and we even had a FIRST!

We got stopped by a police officer in Mt. Pleasant. She thought that bicycles weren't allowed on Highway 17. After a phone call, she said that we were indeed allowed on the road, just please be careful. Trust me, safety is our credo. We hug the side of the road as tight as we can, but there is such a thing as sharing the road. It sounds good in theory, but doesn't always happen. Since the interview, traffic and a late start were all sort of stacked against us, we didn't get as far as we would have liked to today. We have learned to be patient on this journey though. We can get just as far as we *should* every day.

In Mt. Pleasant we had our lunch on a bench outside of the visitors center. A helpful man told us about a campground up ahead and we called them. It should be perfect timing for us to arrive about 4 pm. On this road we couldn't chance being out after dark. The manager was kind enough to let us use a space for the evening. As Morton was putting up the tent, I was checking the email and doing the computer thing. Imagine my delight when I discovered that at the *KOA in Mt. Pleasant* you get wireless internet access! Joy!

We moved from our picnic table beside the lake as the sun was setting, to the clubhouse where Morton can happily watch television after a nice hot shower. My shower was really a million dollar shower. After it though, I discovered that my feet are in horrible shape. Layers of skin are peeling, the toes all look deformed and from not pushing the pedals but walking so much each day, there isn't much I can do with them. The bicycle riding will sort them out. It was fantastic after the first day back in the saddle. Life is better than good tonight, it's BRILLIANT. Just like the stars that are shining over our wee tent!

Day 63: March 4, 2007 - Sun - *KOA Kampground, Mt. Pleasant* (north) to Francis Marion State Park, SC

Make no mistake, it was cold last night. We had to wait a bit to get the top sheet on the tent dry and then we set out. A melted bit of frost was the hold up. To say the road today was a bit rough is an understatement. There is a little sliver of road between the right line and a drop off. That is it. Sometimes the drop off puts you on grass scattered with sharp things, sometimes it drops you several inches onto stone and rubble. Either way, it's a tough act on a bicycle. We struggle to ride that thin line between the certain death that awaits us if a car gets us and the slow and painful slow motion falling off our bicycle at the edge of the road. Weather is perfect today and I'm lost in my thoughts when we hear a bang. There was a car going past and we both sort of ducked thinking that people might have got tired of swearing at us and screaming at us. Maybe they were going to start shooting at us. But we couldn't be that lucky...it was a blowout.

I never heard a bike tire blow out, but boy, this one did. It had a nice two inch plus slice in it. An aftereffect from being rode over a hole in the road that had actually pulled the tire right off the wheel. Anyone that thinks for one second that we are just having a picnic out here needed to be with us today. We pushed the bikes about a half a mile to a store where Morton could safely tackle this foul flat without getting hit. He wasn't too happy when he saw it but Morton soon went after it, while I rocked away on a chair on the front of this store. I like to keep out of his way. The tube might not be able to be fixed. We have no spares. We are so far from anywhere without a car or way to get a tube.

We're almost broke. I dial my Sarah on the phone. She can tell at once that something is wrong. All it takes is her asking what it is and I burst into tears. Everything I'm trying to do out here I am doubting. Our finances are jammed up with money that is overdue us and I can't keep asking my pregnant daughter and her husband to help us. The financial part of this trip is the ugly side. We don't require a lot, but we rely on t-shirt sales and the kindness of strangers and advertisers to make it happen.

Sarah talks me though the reasons that I'm out here. These things I know, but I can't help it. Our immediate future looks very bleak and we are still not sure if this tube can be fixed. After about 10 minutes of Sarah, I feel much better. She is so wise beyond her 25 years. How did I get so lucky to have this little angel for my very own daughter? Morton says he has the tire fixed and for a moment, all is well. He has used the blown tube he found beside the road a while ago to make the patch.

We have very limited funds but decide to splurge on two, $1.50 hot dogs. They come with free chili so we load the dogs up so high with the chili we need a fork to eat them. Our water is still cold from the morning and after my cry on Sarah's shoulder (through the phone, next best thing to being there) I do feel better. There is a campground we are going to head to in a big National Forest. We still have a good bit of riding, but hey, the tire seems to be staying up. Besides the many close calls with the cars and trucks, the ride goes nice and smooth.

When we get to the campground they let us stay in overflow camping. We also hear some tales about how dangerous our ride is going to be on the Canadian border by a mother whose son rode it. We always listen to things people tell us and take them on board. You never know when the information will come in handy. Setting up far from the showers and bathrooms, Morton and I made our way through various sizes of fire ant mounds. We chose a semi-sheltered spot and set up camp.

Sleeping outside is something I love to do. But we were not expecting what happened tonight. We had a heavy frost and woke up to the tent being covered in a thick coating of frost. I felt like we were in the North Pole and a reindeer should walk past the tent at any moment.

Day 64: March 5, 2007 - Monday - Francis Marion State Park to Hopsewee Plantation, South Carolina

After letting the tent thaw enough to be packed away, we had to stay bundled up as we rode. The sun was out but the temperature was still really cold. We were both hoping the big blow out from the day before would hold until we could get a bike tube. It dawned on me that riding around without spare tubes for our three different sized tires, we were doing a massive journey with no spare. We wouldn't do this on a car, we really can't do it on the bikes. The spares HAVE to become a priority for us. There is a state park that we want to get to for budget sake, but we stop about 2 o'clock and something tells me to have a look through one of the little books that we've picked up along the way. There is an ad for *Hopsewee Plantation* and I think back to sleeping in Fort King George in Georgia. After all, we want to spend the night in unusual places. Calling the plantation, the owner himself actually answers the phone. I explain what we are doing and he says that we can actually pitch our tent on the plantation. Best news of all, it's just over the next bridge. We ride our bicycles down the shady lane towards the large white house by the river. This house is full of history and I don't want to spoil it for you, you need to visit their website and learn all about it. The really unusual thing is that there have only been five owners over the last 300 years and the fifth has been kind enough to let us stay the night. I asked if we could sleep in the houses that were once used to house the slaves, but they were being restored. To the tent! First there is a lovely tour of the house that takes you from basement to attic. It also has some of the most stunning views I have ever seen out a window. Morton and I sat on the back porch and you could almost picture the Southern Belle's in their big skirts sipping mint juleps on the lawn. Today we felt like we were on top of the world. The fifth owner of Hopsewee talked to us for a bit about how dangerous riding our bicycles on Route 17 is, he had also called a reporter from the newspaper in Georgetown that was coming by the plantation to do an interview. Morton and I had put our tent up and kept our bicycles untarped until the reporter had been. He might want a picture with them, but it turns out he took advantage of the incredible setting and sunset and we had our pictures taken down on the beautiful dock on the river while small boats played in the setting sun dancing on the water. We talked until it was almost dark and then said our goodbyes. The day had been really long and the cold night before had us tossing and turning all night. We went into our tent and we were sleeping by 8 pm. Not quite the late night we had with our reinactors in Fort King George, but still an excellent way to end the day.

BIG Milestone today...we clocked up our 1000th mile on the journey. It feels so FANTASTIC and time, along the the miles, have flown by. We were somewhere near Georgetown when we passed the 1000th mile.

Day 65: March 6, 2007 - Tuesday - Hopsewee Plantation to Pawleys Plantation, Pawleys Island, SC

The plantation looked so lovely bathed in the rising sun. There was no frost to be found on our tent so Morton and I were able to really just pack up and be on the road by 8 am. We were a little worried about the early morning traffic, but to be honest with you, the road in general is very hard on bicyclist.

We did our usual of keeping to the side as tight as possible. My ears stay well tuned for the sound of approaching cars. After a bit I realize something. When I hear a car or truck, it only takes about three seconds for it to reach us. Only three little seconds. This is a troubling thought. I keep this thought to myself though and ponder on it as we ride. Passing a grocery store, Morton goes in to do some shopping. I wait with the phone and touch base with my mom. She's out of the hospital and home now. She has a friend staying with her for a visit while my sister is in Florida on business. Everything seems to be fine there and I wait a bit longer for Morton. The only good thing is that he only has $20.00 to spend on food. A lady stops and chats about where we are coming from, where we are going and I can tell by her questions that she can't quite understand why we are doing this. Some people get it and some don't. It's alright, I feel the same sometimes. Morton shows up and discovers as he puts his $12.00 worth of groceries in the little trailer, that the bad tire has gone flat again. He pumps it up and we set off after drinking his bargain buy on chocolate "drink", kinda sorta milk. It is horrible, but was cheap.

In just a few hundred yards, the tire goes down again. This time right outside a lovely garden center. While Morton set about fixing the flat, I went inside to take some photos. I discovered more than flowers though. There were three cats, a parrot and a wonderful lady working there. We had a chat while Morton worked away. George, one of her new cats, actually jumped up on my back when I bent down to take a photo. He sat there like a parrot of a pirate. We weren't fast enough to get a picture, but I did manage to get some of the lovely cat. The lady also told us where there was a discount store that would have bicycle tires. It meant us having to go out of our way and double back, but we really did need that inner tube and Morton did have $8.00 left. Traffic was so very bad. The sidewalk was not able to be rode on. We just had to keep going as we were and hope for the best. The "best" being not killed. Morton bought a $3.00 sub to split. It was 12" so we each had a whole 6" to eat. It was so good, piled with fresh veggies and some kind of meat. That and bike tube. Nice. Back on the bicycles, we headed towards another night of not really knowing where we were going to wind up. All the stops for the tire had taken it's toll on our time. My back muscles were so sore from being tense from the heavy traffic and close calls with the cars and trucks. My legs were aching but we have no choice. We can either sleep by the road or keep going.

Coming over a bridge, the last bridge, when we were leaving Georgetown, something terrible happened. We were almost over it, the very end really. It happened fast. Really fast. A truck, a small truck, came so close to me that our wheels touched for a second and my bicycle went to the right, the wheels rubbing against the concrete of the bridge.
A thick knot doubled my stomach over and I felt like I was going to be sick. It didn't knock me off the bike, but it put a fear in me so strong that my life indeed did pass before my eyes. We stopped right after the bridge. Morton hadn't even seen my close call. He didn't understand why I was so upset, but what happened has happened many times before. A truck or car swerves the to left to miss Morton, then they swerve back to the right, almost hitting me or worse still, bumping me.

I grabbed a piece of paper and the pen and started writing with shaking hands. Morton tried to read over my shoulder and I asked him to stop. I jotted down what I was feeling and then stuck it in the front pouch on the bicycle. The words really just came out. The words are a bit morbid. I had to resist the urge to call my children and tell them that they might lose me out here. But not today.

Three Seconds To Die
The sound in my ear,
Three seconds, you're here,
I know my great fear,
Can you see me?

You fumble inside,
A CD for your drive,
Oh where did it hide,
Can you see me?

Thoughts blend I've known,
I'm floating when thrown,
Falling hard on the road,
Can you see me?

You come to my side,
The tears you can't hide,
I'm bleeding inside,
Can you see me?

I'm wondering "why?"
My children will cry,
Three seconds to die,
Can you save me?
by Priscilla Houliston - after a near brush with death

Today we kept riding, then we think about a room. As boring as it might feel reading, on the bicycle when we were thinking about a room, it is never boring. There is a generic motel and I get told no, they can't help...it's alright. I've heard it before and I'll hear it again. I don't take it personally, I just keep going. Morton does not like to go in and ask. He actually never has. He says he feels odd about it, leaving it all on my shoulders. It does feel a bit frustrating, but I have a good feeling that if a truck doesn't get me, we just might get a room for the night. There was a lovely sign pointing to the right, advertising *Pawleys Plantation & Golf Club*. They had the word "Lodging" on the sign and a phone number. It might be an interesting place to stay, even though we wouldn't be golfing. We have a lot of people watching the website who are golfers and something felt right about calling.

Brenda answered the phone and I told her what we were doing. She was kind enough to listen and even kinder to pass me along to the person that could hopefully help. Jan listened as well, then asked me if I would mind holding for a minute. Crossing my fingers and toes, I hoped upon hope that they might have a spare space for us. When Jan came back on the line, she said they could help.

My day had been so up and down, my shoulders so sore after three cold nights on the ground, that you can imagine how it must have felt to step inside the most beautiful one bedroom palace that overlooked the golf course. I could have cried tears of joy.

Being terribly selfish, I told Morton that I just had to jump in the shower. Now do you remember when we were in the Keys and after walking in the hot sun for about 10 hours, I discovered how a million dollars feels as I got a shower? Today might have been two million. The shower was the best I've ever had. The heat and the pressure took all the knots out of my back. The truck that almost got me seemed from another place and time. Internet access, a list of services as long as your arm and best of all, the views and comfort are second to none. Morton gave the biggest grin I have seen in a long time when Brenda told us there was a washer and dryer. He replied his simple yet effective one word summary, *"Brilliant!"* One night in paradise.

The great feeling we have been given tonight has taken away all my bad feelings from today. The flat tires, the close call and my realization that we might meet our end out here doesn't matter now. I have a bed, a real bed, calling my name. I won't wake up with my arm or nose ice cold tonight. It is amazing what a bed can do for your head.

Day 66: March 7, 2007 - Wednesday - *Pawleys Plantation*, Pawleys Island to Murrell's Inlet, SC

Today was perhaps our VERY BEST yet. But you know, that seems to happen to us all the time. We think we can't get any better of a day, then we are surprised. We also live seriously in the moment now, helping us make each day the best of our lives.

Starting with breakfast in the beautiful clubhouse at *Pawleys Plantation*, I thought about the next time I get to go golfing. I want to start going again, without the golf cart and use it as entertainment and exercise. We walked back to our lovely villa and as Morton got our gear ready to go.

Our phone rang as I was turning the laptop off and it was Helen from *Brookgreen Gardens*. Helen was kind enough to let us explore the fabulous gardens. We just had to do the almost nine miles and we were there to the largest sculpture garden in America.

Morton and I headed out the lovely entrance, past the men and women out driving golf balls, with so many squirrels running and playing. It was one of those rare places where man and nature really do co-exist. We had even seen black squirrels there. They have also left so many huge trees that the houses and villas seem to disappear in their surroundings. Heading back on Hwy 17, we stick to the side. There is a bit of an edge, then a bike path, then back to the road. We knew we had about nine miles to ride and our bag of food for lunch that was riding in Morton's trailer, felt more like a picnic then just our normal stuff in a plastic bag.

There was a large shaded bike trail that was winding and twisting beside the north bound lane. It felt more like we were playing then doing part of our massive trip. We would even shout, "Woo hoo" as we were going up and down the little hills and around the bends. It was just like being a kid again. I kept looking to my left to spot the entrance to the magnificent *Brookgreen Gardens*. Soon I see it. A huge sculpture of men and horses. Such a grand entrance, but it still doesn't even give you a clue as to what you are going to find inside.

On our bikes, we headed down the daffodil lined lane that wound back into the welcome center. The smell from the flowers were intoxicating. Once there, we just had to tarp our bikes and trailers at the bike rack, then we were off to explore. It felt like we were kids on a field trip. We even had a packed lunch with us and our ever-present laptop that Morton carries everywhere when we stop. We can't afford to lose it.

There is a beautiful film that shows you an overview of the history of the gardens. It shows how the couple who established them over 75 years ago, used the same butterfly lay out and kept these giant, sweeping live oaks. It really does take your breath away. This is art and nature working as one here, turning in to one and the same thing. We enter this world of sculpture, and really do lose ourselves in art. We see really famous and beautiful sculpture, all from American artists. How is it that I have never heard of this place? As we stroll through a combination of art, landscape courtesy of nature and flowers blooming and screaming "spring!", it's easy to lose all track of time. They do something really great here. When you get a ticket, it's good for seven days in a row. That is the best idea that I've ever heard. When you come here you realize that you want to come back, again and again. We only had a few hours. We tiptoe through the tulips, watch the water fountains and scope the sculpture. It is such an incredible place. We see young and old, people from everywhere, out enjoying the day. Morton is reading each sign about the sculpture and I wish that we could come back in every single season. I know it has to change with every passing hour, imagine how different the seasons must look here. This is the secret to making your exercise fun. Find that lovely place in your area and take walks there. If I lived in this area, I would become a member and walk here at least once a week. This place feels so different with a different sculpture waiting around every corner. The azaleas are just budding up here and will be in full glory soon. Make sure if you are anywhere near here that you come and see this. Our words might tempt you, but you can't even begin to imagine the size and scale of this garden. The clock ticks on and I know we have to keep moving. Morton and I are now in a special children's area which is charming beyond belief. The thought that went in to displaying each piece is remarkable. Ivy covered arches frame the background. Tree branches frame the statues and the moss hanging from the trees makes a statement so quiet you have to be very still to hear it.

Making our way back through the paths and gardens, we sit on a bench for one last time. I wonder if we'll ever be back this way again. I wished I would have taken more pictures. If only I would have read each sign as Morton did. I'll have all of these pictures with no idea of what the sculpture is, but then with his memory, I'm sure he won't remember either. Hopefully we will be back here one lovely day. We leave the lovely gardens and wait for about 10 minutes to cross Hwy 17. Traffic is heavy and we think that we should just camp for the evening. There is a state park near and we head there. Down a long lane, we go to the desk and ask if there is any overflow area we could camp in. We don't need a proper space, just a bit of grass.

 The man we talk to can't make the decision. He heads off into the office to check with someone else and comes right back out. They appreciate what we are doing, but it is going to cost us almost $20.00 for the night. Since Morton's wallet only holds $5.00, we have to keep riding.

One good thing, we have a lovely bike path. Shaded, up and down, winding under the trees and far from the dangers of the road. We really enjoy this bike trail. It's such a drastic change from the other day. We stop at the end where Business 17 splits off to the right, where a local gives us some advice on which way to go. He tells us about road ahead and we continue. There is a bike lane right beside the road now. So very good and every road in America should have one. More people would bicycle or walk if they were safer doing it. We calculate in the quietness of the road, how far we can travel while the sun is still up. I catch glimpses of the main road to the left that seems to have lots more commercial things on it. I wonder if we shouldn't be on that. We might miss a campground or a motel.

Then ahead on the left, we see a sign that says *Brookwood Inn*. It's a lovely courtyard of rooms set under tall trees. It looks so inviting I cross the road to ask about a room. A kind man listens as I explain what we are doing. He says *yes!* They have only one room left and he gives it to us for the evening. It was so fast and I came back to Morton so quick, he didn't think that I got the room.

As I pulled my bike towards the room without telling him, he got on his and got ready to ride. "Where are you going?" I asked. "We got a room!" Morton jumped off and said that it was brilliant. As we pulled the bicycles in, without fear of the sun setting on us, I realized what a perfect day this has been. We even have a microwave which means *warm* canned ravioli! I look back over the photos from the day and remember the garden. Today will soon just be a memory, but I don't think I'll ever forget the smell of daffodils filling the air whenever I see these pictures.

Day 67: March 8, 2007 - Thursday - *Brookwood Inn*, Murrell's Inlet To *Court Capri*, Myrtle Beach, South Carolina

This morning the weather person said we were going to have sun and the temperature might crawl into the 60's. Packing up and leaving the *Brookwood Inn*, we felt like it was in the 30's...tops. The sun was no where to be seen and we made sure the tarp was well over our "waterproof" trailer. The wind, we had been told, was going to be light. *Wrong*. Strong and blowing right in our faces. Why can't we get a good wind from the south? It would add so many more miles to our day. We must have looked a sight. No wonder the dogs bark and the children point when we ride past. We look nothing at all like the real fit people that ride along the road. Morton and I were both bundled up in our layers of t-shirts, long sleeves, jackets and Morton was even topped with a bright yellow windbreaker. We had on our matching lime green gloves he had gotten at a dollar store, with black grip dots on them. We discovered we had to turn them around with the dots on the BACKS of our hands, making them a bit tougher against the wind. It also stops our fingers from tingling as we ride.

The road had a bicycle path. *"THANK YOU South Carolina!"*, traffic was light and despite the icicles that were forming at the corner of my eyes from the steady stream of ice tears that were coming out of my eyes, it was going to be a great ride. When the wind is this strong we make rubbish time though. I go slow as it is and with the wind pushing us back, I nearly stop. I could actually use a GIANT set of training wheels to keep me upright today. With the bike in medium gear my legs were warm anyway. Our map shows us that North Carolina is really close to Myrtle Beach. Not far at all. I'm thinking that maybe, if we have no luck with getting a room, we will just keep going and catch up with the press later.

We love press, let me make that *REALLY REALLY* clear. It never crossed our minds though how much time from our day would be spent updating, doing phone interviews, doing live interviews and the such. It is the vital part of our journey though. We want the whole wide world to wake up and say, "Hey, if she can get out there and do this, I can take a walk each day" and who knows how many people will have the light go on over their heads.

For years, decades even, I knew I had to do something about my body and health. It was more than I just didn't fit in my old clothes. Going up stairs was a real chore, walking was painful on my knees and even the largest size in the clothing stores designed for big women didn't fit me. At a size 32, there was no where to go but the internet and magazines to get larger clothing. For five years I went without buying anything new to wear. I would make the old clothes stretch, literally, even cutting some on the neck and sides to fit in. Living in Scotland where obesity is just really taking off (thanks to fast food, bad food and a few "buffets" popping up) I felt a lot of times like I was the heaviest person there.

Being in denial is a horrible thing. We can lie to the people around us, as well as ourselves, but when we get out of the shower and see the person in the mirror, WE know there is a problem. In my case, a deadly problem. I would get really bad chest pains and be short of breath several times a month, but I ignored it.

When we got the phone call in May 2006 that my mother was in the hospital with a stroke, I didn't really know what to expect when I was crammed in to the plane seat flying back to the USA from France. I had experienced with my dad a long-distance stroke. His happened while I was living in the United Kingdom and he was out of the hospital and home in a week. He was talking on the phone and even driving. The only leftover from his stroke seemed to be the way he would drag his left foot a bit. Mom was different. She couldn't talk, walk, sit up and she kept her right hand in a fist and pulled to her chest. This was going to take months, maybe years of rehabilitation.

When I saw my mom, in the hospital bed with four nurses having to roll her to move her, *THE LIGHT FINALLY WENT ON OVER MY HEAD*. This was going to be my fate. My chest got tight and I got worried. Really worried. Being fat, really fat, deadly fat, was something that I needed to change NOW.

But where do you start when you have almost three hundred pounds to lose? Be honest. Get on a scale and learn how much you weigh. Then, decide what your options are. I thought (very briefly) about surgery. The death rate on it is 1 out of 200 people. That is way too high and I wanted to AVOID being in the hospital. My answer was at the end of my legs. I would start walking. Just a little, building up what I could do. It was during these very first walks, some taken as I was waiting for my mom to finish her three-hour therapy sessions, that the thought of going around the entire coastline and borders of America, came into my head. From the second it was there, I knew I had to do it...to save myself and hopefully many others. So what is the sense of doing it if we don't get the press, to tell the people (YOU) about our fantastic and free website, www.LittleChanges.com that you can watch the two crazy people (Morton & I) doing this incredible journey? Things were planned, routes, important things were NOT planned (budget) but I knew that everything would fall into place. Somehow it would work. It had to. After all, our needs are simple, our cause is just, things will work out. In that I have 100% confidence. Most of the time. Just on cue, a dollar type store appears as we are riding. I head in to buy tuna, peanuts, cheap noodles and spend a whopping $12.00. When I come out Morton is pushing the phone at me with a missed call. I crossed my fingers mentally that this would be a room in Myrtle Beach. I felt bad that I had missed emailing and telephoning all the press that wanted to know when we crossed the 1000 mile mark. There were also calls that we had to do with our press that we will be doing when we get to NYC. You can't imagine all the work that is going into the PR side of the walk. Sarah helps with what she can, but 90% of it happens out here on the road, by little old me, trying to talk over the roar of trucks and cars going by.

Debbie, from the *Court Capri* in Myrtle Beach had called. They could help us with a room. Sweet and wonderful Debbie! Returning her call I got the address and got on my bike. Suddenly the wind, though still there, didn't feel so cold. My thoughts turned to all the work I would be able to get done, being in a place with POWER. Electricity was maybe the greatest invention and vital to us to keep our batteries charged and the world updated. We were still about 12 to 14 miles away and the sky was looking very threatening, but I didn't feel threatened. We had a room! My heart soared and I went back to making my mental list of what all needed done. When our bike lane left us, my thoughts had to turn back to traffic. You really do have to watch out for the other guy out here. Or the other girl. There was a red sporty car that was heading south, when the blonde driving got a hankering to head north. She was going to make an illegal U-turn right in front of me, nearly on top of me. She was smoking, cigarette dangling from her red lips, head tilted and crunching a phone into her neck. We could also hear the stereo blasting through the rolled up car windows.

Morton was shouting from behind me to look out. I was on the very edge of the road, but the option of falling off the edge and into the sand seemed better than becoming her hood ornament. I turned right as she didn't even have the courtesy to look at me. I'm way too big to say she didn't see me. Without missing a beat, or falling over, I steered my bike back on the edge of the pavement wobbling as I went. Morton called her some censored words as she drove off to the north. She had priorities, was multi-tasking, I told Morton. Don't be so hard on her. Obviously she was smoking, talking, rocking, had probably just put her lipstick away and driving was the *last* thing on her mind. At least that is how it looked from where I was sitting.

Morton's theory that he is the one that is going to get hit the hardest, because he is in the rear, is *BLOWN*! It is official now, after the events of this last week. All bets are on me being the first one actually hit by a car bad enough to go to the hospital, since I seem to be the bigger target.

Laughing this scary event off, we kept going. The clouds were getting darkish and I didn't want to get wet today. There would be a shower waiting inside the room for us so I won't need one from nature. Before we knew it we were turning right and heading for the ocean. We had been catching glimpses of it, peeking through the ends of streets. It felt good to get away from traffic and closer to the sand and shore.

We pulled in to the parking lot for the Court Capri and met the manager, Tim, who was just great. He pointed us in the right direction and I was soon in the lovely lobby checking in for three nights. My eyes went right to the indoor heated pool and bubbling spa. They were both calling me and I knew that I would be using these later. Hopefully.

Debbie was the person who helped us get the key, told us how to get our gear to the room and then we were off. Our room is on the ninth floor with the best view we have ever had of the ocean. There is a huge balcony and a table right inside the huge glass doors that open on to your very own viewing balcony. Morton kept saying over and over, "This is BRILLIANT!" as he explored the room. The room has so much space, a kitchen, a great bathroom and a living room/dining room area. I chose the table beside the glass doors to set up my mobile office on. Morton set about putting out our food that we would be eating for the next few days and I was stunned. The food, our tuna, noodles, peanuts and pasta, amounted to just a little a pile. This would have been just one day, or even one afternoon of eating for me, before the light went on over my head. Moderation is now a word I know and use.

As we looked out over the ocean, Morton with his eagle eyes, spotted dolphins playing. We stopped setting up the office while we watched the show. These sleek and playful creatures were running in with the surf, diving and twisting, turning around and doing it again. We could have watched for hours, but then they moved south and the show was over. I got right to the email, setting up the schedule for the next few days and spent a good few hours working, eating lunch with one hand as I was answering emails with the one-handed typing technique that slows my 90-words a minute down to a halt. After a few hours with Morton looking like he was going to go to sleep at 6 pm, I made a move to my bathing suit.

We still needed to get my monthly bathing suit pictures, then we would go to the pool. I want the bathing suit pictures, front, back and both sides, to show my weight loss over the two year trip. I know the bathing suit will have to change in the picture...it's already gotten very loose. We decide to brave the cold outside temperature and go on to the balcony to get the pictures.

There we see a new sight. This is a man who has written his confession of love for a girl in the sand.

He looks up at a balcony north of us and since our balconies are all very private, we really can't see her. After writing that he loves her, he wrote with a piece of driftwood in large letters, "Marry me?!" and had even gone down on bended knee. How very sweet. We don't know if she said yes, but I was still feeling warm and fuzzy about that as Morton snapped my bathing suit pictures. I looked at them and my warm and fuzzy feelings left, FAST! *I'M STILL FAT!!!* How is that possible??? I know I still have 150 pounds to lose, but in my mind I'm not really thinking about that. I know how I feel (so very much better) and that all my clothes are loose on me now. I run the risk of certain pants falling off me when I wear them, but I still *LOOK HORRIBLE* in the bathing suit. I keep these thoughts to myself as Morton and I head down to the pool and spa. My jacket covers my fat and flabby arms and my pants, baggy ones, cover my fat legs. True, they are getting toned under the fat and I can feel muscles now, but I'm still FAT. The people at the pool won't know that I'm losing weight. They will just see me as a fatty who should have the common sense to NOT come out in public like this. Did I mention that I have a BAD body image? Getting a look at those pictures of me in a bathing suit wasn't a smart thing to do before going swimming. Morton gets right in. He strips off his shirt and has just the slightest trace of a belly now. He looks fit and fine and swims like a sea otter. I tell him I'm cold and sit on a chair hoping everyone looks away or leaves. Then I could take off my coat and pants and jump in quick. But the pool is lovely and people are enjoying it. Not a huge crowd, but enough to make me feel very bad about exposing them to my horrible body. What have they ever done to me?

There is a lady who asks Morton where he is from. He starts talking to her and oh no...he's explaining to her what we are doing! What is Morton thinking. You can't tell people how much I weigh when I'm sitting here in a bathing suit UNDER my clothes!!! She is kind and smiling and tell me what a great job it is that I'm doing. I try to look smaller and smile. Oh Morton, how could you! Morton is getting wrinkled from being in the pool. "I would have just kept watching the movie if I would have known you didn't want to swim" he told me. I felt bad. Here I was lying to him. I wasn't cold, I'm FAT. I didn't want to get in and show the world my body that is still, after months and months of working on it, my body is STILL fat. This reminds me of the olden days in Scotland when I would lie to Morton about not wanting to go to the movies. I didn't have anything against the movies, I just didn't fit in the seats anymore.

The people that had been in the spa got out. I decided that I just had to do this. Flabby and fat, but the spa looked so very tempting. I went to a chair beside it and snuck out of my jacket and pants. Then at the speed of light I got into the spa. It was 104 degrees and bubbling at just the right speed. It was worth stripping off for. After the 15 minute cycle ended, we just sat in the quiet for a while. The other people that had been in the pool had left. We were all alone and there was no excuse for me to not go into the pool now, other than I was so tired from the cold, the ride, my knee had been sore from a combination of the cold and the hard riding and I was ready for bed. It was 7:30 pm after all.

Day 68: March 9, 2007 - Friday - *Court Capri*, Myrtle Beach, South Carolina

Today was a rare day. We got to watch the sun come up right on the water. The Atlantic Ocean at Myrtle Beach, to be a bit more specific. Usually when we wake up this early it means pulling down a tent and packing gear. Not today. The waves that were coming in made the sounds of the ocean speaking. It was soft and constant, floating right up to our room. Perfect time to write, reflect but most of all, listen.

Morton was going to click the television on to see what the weather was going to do. He knew that we were going to be on the beach building a sand castle and needed to know. Asking him in a very nice, quiet voice (which probably really scared him) to please turn the television off, "Listen" I almost whispered. He got a startled look on his face but did indeed flip the tv off.

He came close to the big glass doors that have nothing, absolutely nothing, blocking the view of the magnificent ocean. "What is it?" he asked, with a bit of worry in his voice. Now keep in mind we have had quite a few scary moments on our travels so far. We even heard gun shots while riding our bicycles in Florida City. Being from Scotland, Morton never knows what to expect when I ask him to listen.

My smiling face gave it away that there was nothing scary lurking on the horizon. Just the sound of the water, the occasional seagull and if you listened really close, you could hear the wind. Morton smiled as much as he could for that time in the morning. It was early. But then I have so much to do today, I needed to be up with the sun.

With television off limits, Morton crawled back under the covers, but he didn't sleep. He just listened. Now the click, click, click of my computer could be added to the morning melody.

There were so many things to do on the computer that I won't bore you with all the details. Basically, cleaning up room by putting photos on to DVD, sending out almost 5,000 email updates, sending out dozens of press email updates, making videos ready for the Internet (the one thing I didn't get done today) and then reading our email and responding.

But now, with a bit of the computer side done, we donned our swimming gear, I opted for actual SHORTS over the swim suit, and we headed downstairs. We got to say hello to Tim and Debbie at the front desk and let them know we would be out back. There were two local news stations that we might be hooking up with today and in case they showed up, we wanted them to find us.

When we walked on to the beach, I did have my shoes on. It was chilly, breezy, but oh the sand was way too tempting. We stuck our orange trailer flags in the soft sand, I kicked off my shoes and set to work. I wanted to make a huge LittleChanges billboard in the sand, surrounded by sand castles. This wouldn't take a long time since it was just shaping letters, easy really. Not like the massive mermaid and octopus I made on a beach with my kids one day long ago in Florida. That was a little project that ended up taking about 6 hours. It was fun though, we just kept adding to it and going and going. People stopping that day thought we were professionals and we had the sand sculpture photographed by so many. I didn't even think of it until right now, I was in my bathing suit. Today, even though my legs were sticking out, I was too lost in the job to pay attention to who was looking. The people walking by were all taking rather brisk walks though. Morton was the one who was chatting and handing out slips for LittleChanges. We had divided the job and he had the task of making the large, outer, castle wall. Really just mounds of sand shaped inside a little plastic cup. The letters took ages, were a lot harder then I thought, but as I was approaching the "DOT", as in .com, Morton shouted a startling discovery. The tide was coming in he figured. The waves were getting closer. He said we had been at it for almost two hours and figured that we only had a few minutes before the tide would eat our sandy billboard.

Sending him up to our balcony to get the pictures, I went at super speed to do the "com", while a group of spring breakers walked up to me. They asked what LittleChanges is. They had spotted this sign from their room above and were lured down out of curiosity! Success...that is just what we wanted. You see, what we are doing is pointless if people don't know about it and use little changes in their own lives.

Morton managed to snap a few pictures of us together, at one point they were lined up and waving at him, in another few seconds, they were all pointing at the sandy sign, but alas, Morton was distracted by a seagull that was flying close to him so he didn't get any of the posed pictures. The spring break students all promised to have a look at the site and keep an eye on us. I also snapped a picture of their group for them. Very nice people out enjoying the morning and their lives. Morton made his way back down to help me gather up the gear and head back to the room. There were a few telephone interviews coming up. With the sound of the surf, the telephone interviews couldn't happen on the beach.

Brushing the sand from my legs, I put my shoes on and headed up for the room. After a quick shower I made a great discovery. My feet, which had been cracking and peeling on the bottom, were all smooth. Very smooth. The two hours in the sand did them the world of good. My mom always said that a walk on the beach was the best thing for your feet. Wow! I have to remember to do this more often.

The rest of the afternoon just sort of ran in together. There were phone interviews, one really funny one where the person could not understand Morton at all! He had to get me to repeat all his answers, but I was happy to translate. I forget how different he sounds and when he is on the phone he does tend to talk faster. The tide never did come in to wash away our little sand castles and sign. They remained all day and people even stepped around them, pausing to read what it said. Though I was working, I was seated at the table with my eyes facing forward to the ocean. I would glance up often to see and watch the changes in the sky. The water changed in color with the light that would be on it. A storm had moved in, but never rained. It did fantastic things to the sky and water though. This would have been pure entertainment to just have the luxury to stare at this wonder all day. They say no two fingerprints are alike, no two snowflakes are alike and now I know that no two waves are alike. They are mesmerizing, but you will be proud to know that I kept on task and worked while all this wonder was going on around me.

As for Morton, he did his dooberizing on the bikes, out on the balcony. He organized and read a book, keeping it nice and quiet for my telephone and concentration on the work I was doing. It was an easy day that went by way too fast. When the sun turned the outside light off, I thought about going down for a swim in the lovely pool. I would jump right in, I thought. Who cares if people are shocked at my body. I even went so far as to put my bathing suit on. But I didn't go. The computer really did need so many things done on it and I didn't feel right about leaving it. At the end of the day, about 11 pm, which is way past my bedtime, I turned it off. I had put in over 12 hours in total on it, with an easy 12 hours of work still to do. Just the sheer number of emails that we get are so time consuming, but all worth it. We want people to know WHY we are out here.

It is the question we get asked by everyone that meets us...why? It's the toughest question we get asked, but to sum it up in a simple statement, here goes. We are doing this to show there IS hope. If someone like me can change, anyone can. It is a journey that we both feel so strongly about, nothing short of getting splattered by a car or truck will stop us. We are doing this not just for ourselves, but for everyone who is watching this adventure unfold on their computer, day by day, finally reaching the goal that is *fitness*. The journey isn't about just names and places on a map. It's not just about getting healthy, losing weight, motivating ourselves and others. The real story is the people we are meeting. You, you are the story.

Day 69: March 10, 2007 - Saturday - *Court Capri*, Myrtle Beach, SC

This was a day for work and more work. The poor computer got quite the work-out, but I didn't. Since the biggest part of the day was just spent working, I only have one real highlight for you. Morton had gone down to the desk to return a disc with the graphic on it for Court Capri. He of course got talking, no surprise there, with Tim the manager. Morton came back to the room and said in a very coy tone, "Do you know there's a spa on the top of the building in the shape of a heart?" He was trying to lure me away from the work...and it worked.

He was soon off to the roof to scout it out. He returned to say there were three guys using it. I didn't know if I could take the trauma of the whole bathing suit in public, but my muscles were sore from sitting and working on the computer. Morton busied himself with the bikes and he tossed my bathing suit on the bed. It was another big hint. "How big is the spa, will it hold us too?" I asked. Morton tried to remember, but said he didn't want to stare at the guys in the spa. He thought it would hold more people. Turning the laptop off and giving it a rest, I put on the bathing suit and just my jacket on top. I was even leaving my shoes behind. Just a quick unzip of the *LittleChanges* hoodie and I'd be ready to get in the spa.

Morton was behind me by a few minutes. He had forgotten to take his watch off. I turned the timer on and climbed into the lovely, warm, HUGE heart-shaped spa. There was no one there and I had it all to myself! Morton soon appeared though, with the camera. He wanted to take some pictures of the incredible views, he said, but was clicking away at me. Good thing it was bubbling! From a person who never wanted her picture taken, I'm actually smiling for the camera now. After a while in the spa, we decided, wait...I decided, I would make a break for it while no one was around. There had been a few guys up and I was gulping hard at the thought of them getting in and me having to get out in front of them. I want a shirt that says, "I'm working on my weight" to let people know that this is me going down the weight ladder.

While I worked in the evening, we got to watch *"Breakfast at Tiffanys"* one of my favorite films. Morton of course, fell asleep. With my laptop ever on and sending images, film clips and more, it was almost relaxing. It was a splendid, productive and bubbly day.

Day 70: March 11, 2007 - Sunday - *Court Capri*, Myrtle Beach, South Carolina to *KOA Kampground*, Sunset Beach, North Carolina

We started the day off with an interview. An *excellent* interview by a lovely lady named Lee. She asked wonderful questions, got great shots and even went in front of us, taking more footage, with a bit of a warning about how the road was ahead. Before Lee arrived, Morton and I had moved all our gear downstairs and at the front of the hotel. It was a lovely sunny morning and yes, we saw the sunrise again. The view from the room was too good to not take advantage of it. We had also said goodbye to Debbie, who handed me a collection that they had taken for us at the front desk! I was really surprised and touched by this. It is the first time that this has happened and we were so grateful. It meant we could get the spare inner tube and some groceries on our way, without dipping into the credit card.

Morton and I headed north, stopping once and a while to chat with Lee, who was still leading the way and would film us going past. It felt really good to be back on the bicycles and I could feel my legs using all their muscles again. They really are changing. I can now see a hint of an ankle bone. There were stores, so we popped in and got $6.00 worth of food and a spare inner tube. It felt really good to have the spare again, because the other tire had blown and Morton was unable to fix it. The slice in it was about 4" long. Unpatchable, but Morton refused to throw it away claiming we might need it some day.

The state line was somewhere up ahead of it and boy was it calling me. I really wanted to cross into North Carolina. We had a bit of a late start and then the shopping, which always takes twice as long when Morton goes in the store. You know, I think he pokes around to give me a rest, but I'm always anxious to just ride. Especially today. The days in Myrtle Beach were fantastic, but there is this urgency to move on this journey. I never liked to move like I enjoy now, it's a fantastic feeling.

Traffic was really bad. We had a bike path for a while, then it just up and ended. There was still enough of an edge to the road that we only had to have one trailer wheel over the white line. It was still enough to get honked at, shouted at, even screamed at by a very angry young lady. There were several guys who were hanging out the side of a pickup and yelling abuse at us. They took the abuse a step further and threw empty fast food containers and bags at us, hitting me with a cup of ice.

Where, oh where, do they want us to go? If there is no sidewalk people, we are *SHARING* the road with you! Tooting at us or yelling won't make us disappear. We saw the signs first for the welcome station to South Carolina. Of course, it was on the other side of the road, but we knew this meant that North Carolina was just ahead. Did I mention the hills? We are starting to hit some upgrades, but on a good note, I've been able to cycle up them and coming down with my weight and the trailer pushing, I almost keep pace with the cars. Sweet Morton asked how I go so fast down the hills. He had to know it's as simple as weight = speed. Hasn't he ever ridden on a sled with a heavy person before? Same principal.

We took some pictures as we entered North Carolina, then started thinking about a place to stay for the night. Always a worry. Tonight it was really a worry because I know the balance in my account is just $5.00. Not enough for a room if we would have to pay for one. Our phone rang and we pulled over. It was my Sarah. She was asking Morton for my account number and he said, "Why?" without missing a beat she told him she wanted to steal our last $5.00. Morton called her *"Cheeky"* and passed the phone over to me. She was putting funds in our account. I felt a big sigh of relief coming on. I still wanted to camp tonight, hopefully in a back yard, but now at least we would have an option.

Someone had asked me in an email if we didn't have the money, would our journey end. NO! Even if we have to sell blood, get jobs until we have enough to keep going, whatever it takes, STOPPING is NOT an option. We do have funds coming in from t-shirt sales (we get $2.00 for each shirt that sells) and from banner advertising. We have been alright with our food buying, it really is the hotels and motels that we have had to pay for that kills our budget. Money doesn't make miracles happen, people do. Today Sarah and Graeme, with their beautiful generosity, was nothing short of a miracle.

There was a sign for a *KOA* turning to the right. We called them but there office was closed for the evening. The road ahead didn't look promising and it was almost 5:30, time to get in somewhere. We decided to go and see, hopefully we could talk them into being a sponsor for us and letting us have the space for the evening in the morning. Cross your fingers that they say YES! As we were bicycling down the road that leads into the *KOA*, I noticed the sun was still fairly high. I asked Morton what time it was and he answered that it was 6 pm. Ahhhh, *SPRING FORWARD*! I told Morton that we had an extra hour now at night. We could have kept going up the road to chance the next town, but setting the tent up on this mild evening would be fun.

In Scotland, in the summer, there are a few weeks that it stays daylight until 2 am, then just gets like twilight until 4 am. I miss that. It was so beautiful to go down to an old castle after being out and walking after midnight as if it were daylight. Just lovely. Much like tonight.

We were picking the space to put our tent up and I spotted something in the trees. It was the mistletoe balls I had told you about before. There were dozens of them. I took some pictures and blew them up and it *REALLY* is the real thing. Tonight we are under the stars in North Carolina. Please be gentle with us if you see us on the road. We don't mean to hold you up or cramp your driving style. *Hello North Carolina!*

Day 71: March 12, 2007 - Monday - KOA Kampground, South of Shallotte to Motel 6, Wilmington, NC

Today started great as we broke camp after our first night in North Carolina. Waking up in the tent, we seem to always have that feeling "Where are we?" It's familiar inside, but what is waiting outside? We woke up to a brilliant morning and the *KOA Kampground* were kind enough to donate the space to us for the night. Whew, we are so thankful when that happens. Especially right now, as our funds are so very tight. While Morton packed us up to head north, I kept working. We had a lot of emails to answer and send out press info to various papers and television in Wilmington.

As we started riding we saw these gorgeous blooms on trees. Various fruit trees that all seemed to smell delicious and look like Spring! We had to stop of course, where Morton captured some brilliant pictures. He is getting quite good with the camera. He always says he has no talent, but he is one of the most talented people I have ever met. The road became more like an interstate. It had a wide edge to it, plenty of room for us, but the speed of the cars and trucks going by was a little scary. Several times the wind from a truck would hit me so hard it would give the bicycle a good shake and whip my ponytail around to smack the right side of my face. The sky was a little cloudy at points but mostly the weather was perfect for riding. I only encountered one hill that I wasn't able to ride over and it always feels good to get off and walk the bicycle. When we were passing various restaurants during the day, we discovered just what happens to your stomach when you don't have the ability to go in and buy a meal. As we would smell things grilling, broiling, frying and smoking, Morton and I would drool. We would both start talking about food, not the smartest topic. I kept thinking about the lobster ravioli we had at *La Pentola* in Saint Augustine. I wished we had more in our bag then just pop tarts for lunch. We did drink loads of water and Morton's mixtures yesterday. He had gotten a bottle of lemon juice a while back and had picked up packs of artificial sweetener along the way. He would mix these into the water (though I prefer just plain water) and at the rate we were going through the water, the lemon stuff needed drank as well. I'm not sure if it was lack of food or the water and mixture we were drinking, but I started to get really bad stomach cramps. It was far between places and I was almost ready to go running for the woods when we finally saw a gas station in front of us. The sight of a clean public toilet will always bring a smile to my face. While I was waiting for Morton to come out, I called the first television station on our list. We were only about 12 miles south of Wilmington now and I wanted to make sure they had gotten our email. I was lucky enough to get through to Nicole, who was just heading out to cover a story in our direction. While we were heading north, they were heading south and we met along the road. It was a really great interview. It's amazing how that happens. You think that we would always just talk about the same things, but the interviews all seem to be like our days...no two are ever alike. They filmed us as we were riding and while we were having our last chat beside the road I started to feel very sick to my stomach. I leaned on the bicycle seat and hoped I wouldn't lose my pop tarts in front of them. Hopefully there would be a room in front of us and a store that we could pick up some actual food. I was really hungry for some fresh fruit and veggies. Something warm in my stomach would feel good too.

Nicole had told us how to go to find a hotel, the trouble was, I took the wrong road. I stayed on Business 17 and the feeling in my stomach got even sicker as we were crossing the lovely drawbridge into Wilmington. As we pushed the bicycles over the grating, you could feel the vibration of every car. Combined with that feeling, my stomach that was already really dodgy and the setting sun, my hands and legs started shaking. Traffic was really fierce too and we know this is a bad time to be on the bikes. Business 17 turned out to be a lovely way to go through Wilmington. We got on the sidewalk since it was really getting too dusk to be on the road. We rode past beautiful homes and even passed a Bed & Breakfast. I stopped and asked for a room for the evening, but was politely told no. The lady did tell us where to go to find the motels and thank goodness, it was right on Business 17. Morton took a picture or two but the light was really fading. When we got to 16th Street I remembered that Nicole had told us about a motel that was on there. Trouble was, we came into town backwards and didn't know which way to go.

There was a pizza delivery place on the corner and Morton went in to ask directions. A man was sitting in the window of the shop eating a whole pizza. He was probably wondering why I would want to stare and drool, but my stomach was now actually talking as it growled..."FEED ME!" A person looking at me would never guess that someone this fat was actually hungry, but I was. Morton came back and said the delivery man told him if we kept straight on we would come to a cluster of motels. He also commented that the smell of the pizza was killing him. He said that if we had one, he'd have trouble *not* eating the whole thing. I think I saw a bit of drool on his beard.

We kept going and saw some really lovely homes and buildings. We passed a museum and lots of businesses that were closed. We also asked at two different houses for a bit of yard to pitch our tent. This is really tough to do. The one poor lady looked so scared that she only cracked her door an inch and kept the chain on. I'm always afraid that they will call the police, but hey, maybe it would get us a room for the night.

The first place we come to is a chain budget motel. I cross my fingers that there is still a manager in, but I know there most likely isn't. The clerk listens and then says she can't make the decision for a free room. I would have to talk to the manager in the morning. I was also told they have the lowest price in town, so we blow the best part of the $50. my daughter has just given us for the room. It was total darkness at this point and we really had no other option.

Feeling sick to my stomach, but happy to get in a spot for the night, I start to get really down. My phone isn't getting a signal in the room and I stand at the door and talk to my daughter. I work on the edge of the bed to update the site. My face is covered with the grit from the road for the day and I'm shaking, cold, even though the heater is on full blast and Morton is saying that he's sweltering.

We eat our dinner and I get a shower. I feel a bit better and lay down as we watch the news. We are shocked and so very thankful that our story is the *LEAD* story! This has never happened before, not that we have seen anyway. It's also done so very well. They did a great job getting out just what we were feeling. Morton snaps some pictures of the screen and I decide to have one more look at my email before going to sleep.

It had only been a few minutes after the news and there were two wonderful emails. One from a person who wished us well and said she had seen us earlier and one from a woman who was offering us a room for Tuesday night. We only had to ride 57 miles. That's right....57 miles! If we can do it, it will be our best day ever. Morton discovers his flat that he fixed while we were being filmed just isn't holding. He has to use our spare to fix it. Now here is the situation. We have no spare, again, no food after we eat breakfast and just over $10. after we paid for the room. Cross your fingers that when I call the manager this morning they will be able to help us. It hasn't happened before with this chain, but there always is a FIRST TIME!

Day 72: March 13, 2007 - Tuesday - Motel 6, Wilmington to Virginia Creek Campground, Hampstead, NC

How do you describe a perfect day? There are no words I can type to tell you the feelings that were in our hearts and heads today. I think the saying that it is always darkest right before dawn, has to be true. This is one of those times in the journey that help you put everything into perfect vision. It was the worst of days, it was the best of days.

Last night when we had gone to bed we were hungry, almost broke and to tell you the truth, it was about the lowest I have felt on our journey so far. I kept telling myself that it would work out, because it always does. I was also trying to follow my own words of, *"As long as you are breathing, nothing else matters."* But I was scared. It is a nagging fear that is always hiding and comes out when it gets really tough. Last night was really tough. Calling the front desk, I spoke with Brenda, the assistant manager at *Motel 6*. She was so kind and wonderful and said they WOULD indeed sponsor us for last night! You can't imagine how great this felt. It had never happened before and last night I was hoping for the best, but expecting the worst. Someone has to invent a word bigger than just *"THANK YOU"* because it does not cover what we feel.

Being out here our senses have all really changed. Food tastes so great now, even our cans of tuna. We appreciate every second that we have together, we know how short this life is. We have been given a real gift being able to make this journey and the very best part is being able to share it with the people like you, who are watching and rooting for us.

We rode north on US17 on sidewalks, under a brilliant blue sky that was filled with trees that are pushing buds and blossoms. Spring, glorious spring! The feeling that nothing could be finer, was really in our hearts and heads. Then we spotted a dollar store. FOOD! Our bag was empty, except for a 1/2 bottle of lemon juice and some packets of sugar. While shopping I met this very energetic employee who had seen us on the news. She was really just the first of so many, dozens really, of people that we met today who are 100% supportive of what we are doing. It's odd...they don't think we are crazy at all!

Morton talked to a man from a tax office, who gave him a cup of coffee and offered the use of a bathroom. Morton was treated today, he had a cup of coffee as well as we were leaving *Motel 6*. Two cups of coffee, he IS spoiled rotten now! The sidewalk was great and before you knew it, there was a big chain store AND on the right side of the road. If we were lottery playing people, today might have been our day to get a ticket. But remember, Morton only has $1.25 in his wallet and we wouldn't chance it. I chat to some people who had seen the news. It is odd to have total strangers to ask me my weight after keeping it a secret for so long. I proudly shout it off now, even if Morton can hear!

Nicole, at *Fox News* in Wilmington, had really done a great job. I think they must have ran our story again in the morning because people were honking (friendly toots) and cheering us on all day. My favorite cheerleader we came across was a lovely lady from Shamokin, Pennsylvania. It wasn't because we shared a home state, but rather that she went to Morton, gave him a hug and handshake, then thanked him for supporting me. It was really moving. It also reminded me that I have the very best husband in the entire world. But don't tell him that I told you that!

This lovely lady also said something that was really sad. She told us that her husband would never support her when it came to dieting. He would tell her she was too fat. She then whispered his "short" coming to me and said that she never complained about that. She blushed a bit and told me not to tell Morton.

There was a sign up ahead and a wonderful smell coming from *Hamburger Joe's*. The sign said, 25 cent wings. Hmmm...we could afford four! We pulled in, Morton wondering why, then waiting with the bikes as I went in. They were doing a very brisk lunch business and our 1/2 cup of cold cereal had worn off ages ago.

The nice lady at the take-out explained they were only for sit-in, which I could understand. I went out to see if Morton wanted to take turns to go in and each have two wings...but we both felt like we would be the cheapest of the cheap, occupying a table for $1.00. Plus, Morton had a broken link in his bicycle chain. He was fixing it and I was sitting on an outside chair talking to Mari, my daughter-in-law on the phone. She was telling me that spring had came to Pennsylvania and we were just having a wee blether.

A man came over to Morton and was asking about where we were headed and I said bye to Mari and headed over to join the chat. Morton was speaking to him as he was tackling the chain and I know Morton can get a bit testy when he is working. I didn't want this man hearing Morton swear in Scottish either! It turns out the man is the owner of *Hamburger Joe's*. This location is his third, just opened recently. Just after a few minutes, he asked if we'd like a cold drink and wings and was off to get them for us. Our $1.25 still in Morton's wallet, this kind and generous person handed us a packed lunch fit for a king. PLUS, sodas with ICE! On this day that was turning so warm, this was pure luxury.

Morton had fixed the chain and we decided to head up the road for a place to eat our donated lunch. Again, on this perfect day, you KNOW we just had to find the most incredible spot. There was this large and lovely gazebo with benches and rocking chairs. It begged to be sat in and we did just that. It was surrounded by blooming trees and just a bit off the road, behind a medical type building. It is the kind of gazebo I would love to have in a backyard, if I ever have a backyard again. We feasted on the wings. There were celery sticks in the containers that tasted so delicious too. We are both starving for fruit and veg, since we really never get it fresh. We thought about saving half for dinner, then I worried about the heat of the day making the chicken go off. I ate nine wings and Morton ate eleven. With our starved day from yesterday, we needed this! Plus, we still had the ice left from our sodas, so we were able to make Morton's juice mixture was now ICE cold. Nothing beats a cold drink on such a warm day.

As we were finishing up, the phone rang. The lady who had offered us a stay was calling to say we wouldn't be able to because of rules on the base. It was at a Marine base. We had a chat and we completely understood. She was so apologetic, but on this perfect day, things are really meant to happen a certain way. We would have never made it the distance to her home anyway with the chain trouble we had been having.

A few miles on and we pulled into a gas station, again, on the RIGHT side of the road. A man was waving us down and Morton's chain had just done it again. The man is a person who bicycles all around the area. He gave us some great advice, told us about a bike shop about 25 miles in front of us and then wrote a note, offering to pay for the proper tires for our bikes at the shop! He had read on our website about all our flats and says there are tires that are tough to puncture. Wow! He also wanted us to get four inner tubes on him...as he knows we will need them on our journey. He was so supportive and kind, a perfect stranger.

Listen, there are the very most incredible people in the world. It is NOT doom and gloom. I am going to try my very best to never be a doubting Thomas again. Positive attitudes and SMILES are really the way to go through this glorious life we have. Use yours wisely! I sat in the shade as Morton was fixing the chain, when another incredible thing happened. These two ladies came walking down the same rode we had just been riding along. They were squealing and all smiles and said they couldn't believe they had ran into us. It seems that the had walked together before, but for one reason or another, had stopped for several months. One of them saw the news story about us, called the other and she had seen it too. They decided on the phone to start walking that very day and to NOT stop again! It was really fate that we all met up. These beautiful women are PROOF that what we are doing is so very important and WORKING! We will never doubt or worry about if our message is getting out to people. It is! It is really different to meet someone in the flesh *WHILE* they are out walking, then just reading about all the amazing things you all are doing now because you've seen us moving on this website. *KEEP IT UP EVERYONE!* We can all do this together and share this wonderful feeling of how great it feels, getting our health back! So, I hear you thinking, the day couldn't possibly get any better, right? WRONG! We were riding up a little hill, which I'm happy to say that my body can DO this now. The heat was really warm, we had drank loads of water, but I had on long trousers and a long sleeve shirt. My heart started to pound in my head and I pulled off into a gas station and mini store.

North Carolina is a really friendly state. All these places have rocking chairs or benches in front of them. I picked a big green rocking chair in the shade and sat down to have some water and cool off a bit, before heading out. Morton handed me a free paper from the area and I had a look through it for some clues as to where to stay the night.

People that were coming and going where all saying they had seen us, keep it up, we can do it and Morton was handing out lots of LittleChanges slips and asking them to watch it on the web! A vehicle pulled in with a mom behind the wheel and two children in the car. The mom said to keep up the good work and I walked over to have a chat with them. There was an instant click between us all and we were chatting away like we were long lost friends. The kids were asking Morton questions about Scotland.

Morton would answer and they would giggle about the way he pronounced words. I had asked the mom if they knew of a camp ground around. They did, it was right off the road, just a mile or two. They also told us to tell the owners, who are friends of theirs, that Emily and Walt sent us! We said our goodbyes and headed off. They promised to say hello on the site and watch our journey. We love it when people we have met out here keep in touch. It feels like home when I check my email.

The ride back to the campground was just beautiful. Coming off of the main road you hear all the birds singing as evening is just around the corner and things feel so much slower. The private road leading back to the Virginia Creek Campground was perfect for riding. Little gentle turns and wildlife everywhere. Talk about a nice private place. It is a hidden little slice of paradise that is about to get even better.

As we were pulling in to the office, a vehicle was just heading out. They turned in and pulled up to our bicycles and asked if they could help us. This was when we were lucky enough to meet Robert & Ann, the owners of this paradise by the water. We mentioned Emily and Walt and their faces lit up. They are really close to these special people and again, as if we were old friends that hadn't seen each other for ages, we were talking to them about everything under the sun. They told us where we could pitch out tent and then Ann asked if we would rather stay the night in a cabin. This would be great because it saves us two hours in packing up and setting up. Her husband went in to get the key and as they were showing us to the cabin, the vehicle with the mom & Emily & Walt pulled in! Talk about feeling all warm and glowing inside! They were here to ask what we were going to do for dinner and to offer to BRING us dinner. The last time this happened was back in Florida, at *Jonathan Dickinson State Park*, with Gary and Donna. It was a really odd coincidence that when I checked my email later, I had a message from Donna, the first I had since seeing them in Florida!

We all talked a bit more, got some pictures of our happy group and then Morton and I were on our own to get our gear in, the bikes and trailers tarped and to set the office up at the table and chairs that are in the cabin. Morton had given Ann one of our lucky pennies he had found earlier in the day. There is a Scottish saying that if you find a penny and pass it on, it brings luck and friendship forever. As Morton handed it to Ann, her husband Robert said he would make us a swap. He handed us a donation that would keep us in groceries for a few weeks! Morton and I were overwhelmed by these people. In this day and age, to think that we are really getting by out here on the kindness of strangers, is a powerful thing.

While Morton was putting the tarp on, I was making our bed for the next two nights up. Our feelings had gone from the lowest valley last night to the very top of the mountain. I called my daughter and tried to relate this incredible day. As she listened she was just stunned. She had been really worrying about us, but said she felt so much better now. We had a place to sleep and we were not going to starve. Sarah also said to tell Emily and Walt when they came back, THANK YOU for looking after my mom!

When they arrived back, the kids wanted to eat dinner with us so we all went into the lovely clubhouse here. There we shared this incredible meal, conversation, laughs and a friendship was made that will hopefully last our entire lifetime.

It feels like we are having a real family evening, what a wonderful treat.The places we are going and seeing out here are not the things that will stick in our minds in years to come. It's the people that we are meeting, both in person and on this website, that are making this truly the most amazing adventure we have ever been on in our lives. Falling asleep after a day like today is like being a child again. All the smiles from the day come back to you and I know I have a huge smile on my face as I'm falling asleep in a cabin in North Carolina.

Day 73: March 14, 2007 - Wednesday - Virginia Creek Campground, Hampstead, NC

Have you ever woken up far from your family, far from your home and still felt like you WERE home? That happened to me today. This great feeling of happiness and contentment washed over me as we woke up early and watched the sun creeping up over these two lovely ponds that geese and ducks float on. There was no need to pinch myself, I knew I wasn't dreaming. We had arrived yesterday to this piece of paradise and I can tell already, it is going to be very hard to bicycle away from here. Very hard indeed.

The computer is needing a lot of work, pictures need to be put in order and on DVD's...my computer is a bit lacking and needs all the free space it can get. Today I'm going to take advantage of it and get started. We have been invited to stay the day and we are going to do it.

Morton & I take turns going over to use the magnificent showers (great pressure, no hot & cold shocks and plenty of room) and he is suppose to write emails to his family when I am gone. Instead he gets caught on the telephone, on hold, with immigration. He is finding out the hard way about getting information updated via long distance. The office he needs to speak to does not have a telephone. Even though we had been in it last December and saw people on the telephone, there is no way for him to speak to them. He is getting frustrated with the system and I send him out to take a look at the bicycles.

The time floats away as I work with the windows in this tidy cottage open and listen to the geese play, the birds sing and the sounds of nature. Morton has been outside going over the bikes and trailers and about lunchtime, I decide to stretch my legs, back and feel the sun on my face. We head over to the large hall behind the office where you can find restrooms, laundry room, games, exercise equipment, books, magazines and the friendliest people on earth to chat with. We bump into Ann and Robert, the owners here, who are heading out for lunch. They invited us along and we head off out the lovely lane that leads you back into this oasis riding with them in their pickup truck.

Riding in a vehicle is now a rare occasion and it feels a bit special. We head to a place where the locals go. Sitting in the sunny room filled with wonderful aromas, we all have a look at the daily special menu. Morton and I decide to split a shrimp cake (think "crab cake" made with shrimp) and we order green beans and mixed greens to go with it. As we chat, the waitress brings out a basket of warm hush puppies. For anyone that doesn't know what this is, let me try to explain. My husband thought that hush puppies were shoes. Not this kind! It is cornmeal & seasonings, mixed into a batter and shaped into small balls, usually about as big as a golf ball. They are then deep fried until they are golden brown. They really range in taste, depending on the recipe. Some might have finely chopped onions in them. These ones were delicious. I almost had to sit on my hands to keep from eating more than just one. When our meal arrived, the waitress had brought a spare plate and I divided the food. It still shocks me that I do this. Things that I would have never done before are now taking hold and becoming habit. There were two shrimp cakes so that part was easy. I then slip half the green beans and the mixed greens, which were cooked veggies like cabbage, greens and other yummy things, onto the plate that will be Morton's. Fighting the temptation to take the bigger serving, I slide the plate over and after Robert said the blessing, we have our lunch.

I can't talk too much about it. It's late and I'm getting hungry thinking about it. It is fair to say that it was fantastic. We all said no to dessert. The waitress had told us earlier they had sold out of their chocolate cake anyway! Plus, I knew that we were not going to be the most active people today. There were still many files on the computer to be gone through. Robert and Ann treated us to lunch and then gave us a fantastic tour on the way back to the campground. We got to see the farm where they had grown peanuts and tobacco in days gone by. We also got to see some of their pets. Being on this farm, I was a little girl again looking at their miniature donkeys, miniature horses, llamas, peacock and even full grown horses. When I was eleven I fell madly in love with my first and last pony, Suzie. She was my world for a few years, until I got too tall to ride her and she was sold to a man with kids that were just 6 and 8. It was just like that feeling again. The lovely pony smell as Robert got all the miniature horses to trot over to the fence to say hello. There was one little frisky fellow that I really took a shine to. He splashed with his front legs right in the water trough, trying to either jump in or splash it all out. It was hard to tell. Ann told us that when a horse is born in May, it's said that they love the water. This little guy really proved that saying true. He was splashing away as I took a few pictures and even a video. He would stop once in a while to let someone pet his nose. I was enchanted and could have stayed all day. We rode back to the campground and the computer got a hold of me again. Morton did some reading on a Louis L'amour book he had picked up in the hall. It was a blissful way to spend the afternoon.

The evening came and we got another visit from Kathy, Emily and Walt. We told them we were going to stay for just one more night and had a bit of a chat. Kathy's mom had sent along a donation for our journey and once again, Morton and I stood in shock over the kindness of these people.

The water is excellent here, maybe there is something in it that grows the best people in the world. There is just no way, not even if I wrote for years, that I can relate how elated, relaxed, rested, at-home and wonderful these people make us feel. We really could just stay here forever and feel like there was no where else we had to go.

There is a Bible study group that meets on Wednesday evening and Morton and I had to say our goodbyes to the three special people and head into meet the group. It was this feeling of a close family again, only one that you really were welcomed into and felt part of. I didn't think about the fact that I was in a t-shirt and had sneakers on. That wasn't the point here. The pastor was very clear spoken and it was a great experience and fellowship. I asked for the group to keep my mom on their prayer list and after the study we got to chat a bit about our journey we are on. The evening had flown by, just like the day of pure bliss.

Saying our goodnights, we all headed off. Morton and I just had a wee walk to the lovely cabin we are in that is feeling like home. The air was warm and we sat inside talking for a while, then headed out to set on the bench on the front porch. It was another perfect day. We saw miracles happen, made friends that we will remember all our lives and we knew, without a doubt, that we are the luckiest people on earth to be here.

Day 74: March 15, 2007 - Thursday - Virginia Creek Campground, Hampstead, NC

Today the people in the campground are going to have a fish fry. Yesterday it was discussed and planned a bit and we were invited to come along. I was drooling at the thought of fresh fish, something that my dad always said was better then ice cream. Now I would have to agree with him.

A reporter from the *Sunday Post* in Scotland had emailed us about doing a phone interview. I had to get some of our images together for a story that he is going to be doing, so it was back to the computer. There is always something waiting for me to do on it. I do like to keep busy though.

Morton unties the tarp and attacks the bikes again. He is bound and determined to get my bike to actually go into high gear. It's good because it gives him something to keep occupied as I'm lost on the laptop. Again, hours breeze by as the windows and door are open on the cottage. I have the desire of sitting outside to work, something that I love doing. Today though, it's bright and sunny and the screen would be in glare. Morton had gone over and talked to some of the people in the hall. I was feeling very anti-social by being on the computer, but the interview and then all the photographs were taking my time. Chatting to the people here is something that I have really enjoyed doing. We are learning so very much about everything under the sun, you just need to listen! The local paper was sending a reporter out in the afternoon and the fish fry was happening at noon. The pastor had came for it and Morton and I had walked over to the pavilion with him. The pavilion was filled with so many faces and the food was smelling incredible. Some of the people we had already met, some we hadn't. We got a treat and met Kathy's mom and dad. You could tell in a flash just why Kathy and her great kids are so lovely! Again, we get this feeling that these are friends that we already know, just haven't seen before.

Dining at the picnic tables, eating this wonderful and homemade food, I nudged my knee against Morton's and hoped that he felt as great as I did. The sights and sounds reminded me of my dad's family reunion this past summer. Uncle Gene has a pavilion and loads of people turn up. You might not know who they are or how you are related, but a splendid time is always had by all. That was just like today. This past summer, the family reunion was the first one I had gone to in six years. I had been in Scotland and Morton had only ever heard the tales about the people, the food and the fun. He wore his kilt on a burning hot day (that is TRUE love!) and we took my mom on her first big car ride since her stroke. Three hours west of Gettysburg, Pennsylvania, through the tunnels and mountains, we rode talking away about the day. If I would have known for one second that would be the last time that my dad would make that journey...well, I don't know what I would have done. I did savor each second of that day. My son was along as well and it was very special. Mom did great, dad stayed right by her side and the "family" reunion turned into an extended family reunion as my uncle from my mom's side had came along for it. The more the merrier. It was brilliant. We laughed, hugged, talked until about six in the evening, then headed back for home. Mom was still on oxygen at night then and we couldn't stay over. My camera had been with me and I did take lots of pictures. The flowers were all in full bloom, the smiles all came easy and you know what, with all the kids that were there...no one got hurt! Always a good thing.

Today while we were eating at the long picnic tables, it reminded me so much of this precious memory. I remembered both my parents telling me that the one thing they both wished they could do is just talk to their own parents one more time. As a grown person I never thought that losing a parent would be so tough, but my dad was really special and he's left a big hole in a lot of our lives. Today I wished that dad could be here. He would have loved the people, the fellowship and of course, the fish that *were* better than ice cream. After lunch, Morton and I got our bicycles and helmets and sat in the office to talk to Ann and Mary. We were ready for the reporter and all my email had been sent. We talked about everything under the stars and before I knew it, the reporter was here. It turns out that the very day we happened to be at the gas station and met Kathy who directed us back here, he had been there too. He was buying milk and wondered about where we were headed on our bicycles pulling the trailers.

The interview went great and ended with Morton and I doing a bit of riding for his camera. It feels so different to ride the bikes without the trailers. I love it. I could go up any mountain without the 100 pounds of trailer pulling me backwards.

When he left we headed back inside. I think we get starved for conversation as much as we do for food! Robert and Ann were joined by lots of friends who were just chatting. Morton and I joined in and a few more hours slid by. The weather is calling for a 90% chance of thunderstorms in the morning. We agree that if it is raining, we'll stay another night. After all, I might get to brush the lovely miniature horses!

Making my evening phone calls to my mom, then my son and finally my daughter in Pennsylvania.

They are all well and they are all waiting to get up to six inches of snow tonight. Is it WRONG that I'm hoping for rain tomorrow? We have met this wonderful group of people who are treating us strangers like family...we feel like we are home!

Day 75: March 16, 2007 - Friday - Virginia Creek Campground, Hampstead, NC

We had our telephone alarm set for 6 am. It buzzed, we woke and the sky looked like it may or may not rain. We decided to pack and see. Both of us needed to get showers and when I came out of mine...it was raining. The weather forecast had said 90% chance of thunderstorms and they were SPOT ON! It was getting darker by the minute and about 8 am, we decided to stay another day. This proved a very wise choice. To say that it rained was a bit of an understatement. It actually poured. We were so very thankful we had a place with a real roof on it to hole up to avoid this bad weather day. Working on the computer, we spent the better part of the morning keeping busy.

Ann & Robert invited us back to the lovely pavilion for a real treat. Lunch was being served and shared and it was North Carolina barb-b-que on the menu. Morton had never had it before, neither had I...but again, Morton not only cleaned his plate, but had seconds. When it came to the fish yesterday, he had to sample a bit of this and then a filet of that. He loved it all. When we are all finished, Ann wrapped the leftovers up for us. That would be our dinner sorted! The rest of the day we spent in the office, chatting, while keeping the laptop on my lap. Guess what? I'm getting my LAP back to work on! After decades of having a belly that hung so far down on my legs, things are changing. Exercise works! We wish that we had someone who was techie to go with us and do this stuff, but it would take some of the closeness that Morton and I feel on this journey. We are getting a close as two people can get, learning what the other one wants or needs, before the other one even realizes it. I recall a line about a vacation in a compact car song, it was something like...*vacation in a compact car - in any sorts of weather, vacation in a compact car - will bring you close together.* I imagine a bike and a tent are about the same. We had our dinner and then Morton and I decided to get a candy bar to split from the rec room. They were only 50 cents and Morton only had his lucky dollar that came with the wallet that Sarah had given him. He didn't want to spend it, but the sweet-tooth won out and he was soon twisting to get the candy bar. We were laughing about the lucky dollar when the candy bar got STUCK. Panic set in and Morton gave the machine a shake. The bar fell, along with three others. Morton raised his eyebrows and said, "We are giving those back in the morning!" Of course we were, but first they had to make it through the night setting on the table. I'm happy to report, they all did.

Day 76: March 17, 2007 Sat *Virginia Creek Campground*, Hampstead to *Hampton Inn*, Jacksonville, NC

As we were loading up, Ann & Robert came over to say goodbye. It was going to be tough, but we all agreed we would see each other again. Morton and I would love to bring mom back here to meet these kind people and see this beautiful piece of paradise.

Almost forgetting, I grabbed the three candy bars that had survived the night. We explained what happened and guess what? Ann & Robert told us to take them along! Little did they know, that would be our lunch today!

We had a third bicycling with us today. Robert had gotten on his bicycle and gave us an escort out the road that leads you out of paradise. He was going to tell his friends that he was going to go all the way with us, but he didn't have a trailer! When I looked around and he wasn't there anymore, it was a little sad, but the road was really calling us. Waking up to such cold, we have on jackets and gloves. Today is a day for riding and for contemplation. So many things have happened that have led us to where we are right now. Things that had to happen to make it all possible. Things that shouldn't have happened to make it just Morton and I out here. Fate baby. There should have been eight of us. Mom, Dad, my son James, his wife Mari, my daughter Sarah and her husband Graeme. Sometimes I let my imagination run wild and think about how very different it would have been. But it wasn't meant to be. Losing my dad in September really set the wheels in motion to make it a two-person trip.

There are signs that tell us where Jacksonville is. The thing we are looking for is a bicycle shop that a man named Frank, told us about. By 2:30 pm, we found it. The owner wasn't in, but we were taken care of by a great bike mechanic, David.

He put our pathetic bicycles up on his bench and gave them a good going over. My brakes were about shot. He put new on and didn't even charge us for the labor. Soon we were on our way again and heading up the road. A hotel told us that they were all full and that all the hotels were booked full this weekend. We were freezing and figured it would be a night in the tent. Something, I can't really say what, made me pull into a *Hampton Inn*. I had never actually asked for a room from them before. After all, we are in North Carolina where everyone is so friendly. They could only say no. But they didn't. Holly said YES! We were going to be in a room tonight. A warm room with breakfast in the morning. Bliss, sheer bliss.

Morton and I were getting the gear into the room when a young Marine came up to us. There is a Marine base here and he was actually staying at the motel with his girlfriend/wife/not sure what she was to him/special friend. He asked what we were doing and we started talking about the journey. He was shocked that we were doing this. Listening, he told us that we will love Alaska. He was quick to smile, curious and a bit in awe that someone my size was taking a trip like this. He was impressed with the weight loss. Shaking our hands, he shocked me. He told me "Thank you for doing this." He thanked *me*. This young man, serving his country, said thank you to me. I was stunned. I felt very humbled. This young man then told us to be careful, stay safe and take keep warm when we tent. He parted by telling us that he was off to live in a fox hole. My heart sank. I wondered where he was off to and hoped he would stay safe and keep breathing. I thought about my son, at 24 and now married and living in Pennsylvania, much older then this young Marine. James had gone into the Army when he was just 17. My mind kept thinking of my own son all evening and missing his smile. He isn't in the Army anymore. He is far away from me right now and I remember how it felt to be the mom who came to see her son graduate from boot camp. I remember the feeling of joy when I would get a phone call or letter. To see his smiling face looking out at me from a photograph would make my heart soar.

Tonight we are thankful, once again for lots of things. We are thankful the bicycles were on their best behavior, thankful we are in the warm in a lovely bed, thankful for the new tires and tubes, thankful we had dinner at *Applebee's*, thanks to a kind lady named Charity. I'm very thankful that my son is at his house and not in a fox hole.

Day 77: March 18, 2007 - Sun - *Hampton Inn,* Jacksonville to *Holiday Inn Express*, Morehead City, NC

I'm Alive! That is usually the FIRST thing I think. It is a pleasure to wake up and feel so good and positive about what is in front of us. Today starts off fantastic with a hot breakfast that Morton is kind enough to bring up to me. I get breakfast in bed, with my laptop sitting on the little lap desk. The day is chilly as we leave. Holly waves goodbye to us and we get a few pictures. Then it's back on the bicycles.

Since David had gone over my bike, it feels so great. It is terrific to be able to stop when I pull ever so gently on the brakes. Before I would have to rely on running into curbs or putting my feet down to stop Fred Flintstone-style. My stomach has horrible bruises all over it from the lack of brakes on the bicycle. The bike is also a lot more tighter, easier to ride.

There are so many Marines in this town. Some have just came home from Iraq and there are banners and signs up welcoming them everywhere. It is bittersweet to see. I think of all the ones that are waiting to see their families again. I think of the ones that will never see their families again and my heart breaks. One banner sums it all up. It simply says, "About Time" and I stop to take a picture.

The sun wants to warm up but the wind, which is at our sides, is winter cold. The calendar tells us that spring is just a few days away, but besides all the blossoms on the trees, you wouldn't know it by the weather. My knee is really hurting today. I think it has to do with the cold, but I have learned to just keep going. It really does feel better when I can just keep going. If I can work through the soreness, without making it really bad, I can bear it. The secret is really paying attention to what is happening with your body. The water comes in to view as we pass a bridge. It's brilliant blue and we see men and seagulls fishing. There is a Jolly Roger that is flying on a ship. So many ships fly them now, I wonder if it has to do with *Johnny Depp* and the love of all things pirate. Yo ho, yo ho, a pirates life for me. A bicycle pirate?

There are no problems today with the bicycles. It might be a record actually. We have a full food bag, have spare inner tubes for all our tire sizes (there is three different sizes) and it feels so really good. Anything can happen now, we are prepared. Morton steps inside a store when we reach Morehead City, to just get one tube for our odd-size trailer tire. It is a big store and I'm out with the bicycles, in the shade and in the sharp and cutting wind. He is inside for what feels like ages. A few people stopped to wish us well on our journey. They have the common sense to get in out of this cold. I know my face is bright red from the breeze and I dream about getting warm. This morning I had put on my MBT boots, packing my MBT trainers away. My feet had been cold the last few days and I wanted to give them a try. *THEY WORK!* As I stood waiting for Morton, the only thing warm on me was my feet. Morton had been wearing his for weeks and weeks now. Clever Morton.

It was just a few more minutes, I think about forty in total, when Morton came out. He was telling me different prices on different things we had talked about getting. Mirrors, talc powder, warmer gloves...he had looked through the whole store! I said I had to get riding to get warm and we were off. This was one of those moments that I wanted to yell at him, but didn't. Killing Morton isn't an option, who would fix the flat tires?

Maybe it was because I had stood there for ages, but when I got back on my bike and started pedaling, both my knees went CRACK very loudly. They had gotten so stiff and sore, I was glad it was a bit of a downhill run to the road. 70 east was the new signs that we were looking for and we were on it.

There is a fork in the road, where 24 and 70 come together. There is a *Holiday Inn Express* on the other side of the road. Since they have always helped, I figured it was time to start looking for a room. It was nearly 6 pm. The lady at the desk, Amanda, really listened to my whole story. I do talk to so many different people about it, you would think that I get sick of saying the same things. But I don't. Instead, it gives me this fire inside me that makes me know we are doing the right thing. After listening and talking to me, Amanda asks if I can wait just a bit for Mike to come in. He would have to decide. It is nice and warm in the lobby and I think about Morton now standing out in the cold. Payback for my wait? I know Morton has shorts on and the wind had really picked up. I also know it hasn't been forty minutes yet. Hey, at least his feet will be warm and he has those new gloves on. Waiting just a few minutes, Mike arrives on crutches. He has blown out his knee. Just what I don't want to do, but both of mine are really sore just now. Mike listens while I give him the very short version. Without any hesitation, after checking that they had rooms available, he gives me the key. This means that *every night* in North Carolina so far, has been sponsored! This is so great. We want to see how very little we can spend this month, and every month. We never want to be down to our last $1.25 again and have hotels and motels to blame.

As more people see us on television, read about us in the newspaper and with each mile we go, people understand that we really are our here doing this. It isn't a game or contest, but rather a way of life now. It is something that will hopefully show millions that there are things you can do to change your body, change your destiny and change your luck! Get out there right now and start making your own little changes happen.

Day 78: March 19, 2007 - Monday - *Holiday Inn Express,* **Morehead City to Cedar Island, NC**

The best thing about waking up in a hotel room (or a house) is that you have indoor plumbing. This makes life so much easier and to think I use to have indoor plumbing each and every day. So many things now make us say "Oooooh & Aaaaah" that never would before. We have turned into wild sort of bicycle-riding-beasts, wild creatures, who underneath our rough interior actually enjoy toilet paper and a shower. Thinking that it was really early (4 am or so) I was shocked to see the clock said 6 am. The black out curtains on the window really worked well. Making a move, I got to the computer and start working. There are a lot of email, well over 100. We do love our email and thank everyone who takes the time to write us. Morton gets our gear packed and goes to do the breakfast. The *Holiday Inn Express* has lots of goodies that we enjoy, even oatmeal. It feels like it has been forever since we've eaten it. Morton does make the very best oatmeal, or porridge, as he calls it.

We had looked at the map and had a target set in mind of reaching Smyrna. The ferry, which is in Cedar Island, seemed a bit too far away at 51.5 miles. Today was one of our best rides yet. Not just for the stunning scenery, but the road stayed nice and level. Sure, there were a few tall bridges, but all things considered, we were riding through the set of a stunning movie set today. As far as your eye could see there were reeds and water. The sun was out and just dancing on the glistening surface, making you smile each time you saw it.

Timing was really good today. We met a few people by chance, that were very helpful with tips and hints about riding up through the Outer Banks. There were also a few people who stopped us just to say hello and take our pictures. It is such an odd feeling when that happens. We really aren't sure *WHY* they want to take our picture, but we are happy to chat with them about what we are doing.

Finally we pass a visitors center and pick up a map of North Carolina. We are shocked (sort of) to see that we are a lot closer to being out of the state then we thought. Maybe five days or so left here. What is happening with time? It seems to be sailing along at breakneck speed. Speaking of speed, with a nice tailwind, we were really cruising along today. Again, we made it through an entire day with no punctures. A good thing about this is, it means *LESS* people are tossing their beer bottles out the window. We saw a lot less rubbish beside the road then normal.

But now lucky pennies, they were a different thing. There we loads of them. Morton kept stopping and picking them up. In one spot he found 12! Today was going to be special, we could both feel it in our bones. We could also feel it in our sore knees. The sun was nice and warm for us, Goldilocks weather. Not too hot and not too cold, just right. The road had enough of an edge to keep us safe and traffic was very kind today. We had a lot of friendly waves, friendly toots, thumbs up and even some well wishes shouted out the windows in passing. Wide, sweeping floating fields of tall grass that was just swaying ever so gentle in the breeze.

Blue water behind it. Clear water pools that were beside the road and filled with thousands of little minnows. Birds everywhere, including a bright little bluebird who flew along from branch to branch with us for about a mile. Nature was in full bloom today. The sounds of the birds and the water could actually be heard, because as we headed away from the busy streets, the cars were far and few between. Morton and I even managed to have quite a long conversation while bicycling today. Miles and hours slid by as we kept riding. We didn't really stop for a proper break. The closest we came was when were indulged in splitting a $4.25 lunch at a Chinese restaurant. It was a plate that we would have both been able to eat one of in days gone by. Today we split this warm meal and had ice water with it. It really is about *LITTLE* changes people! Share your food!

We passed the point that we were hoping to get to while it was still early. We calculated the time and knew if we kept up the same pace we could reach the ferry by 7 pm at the latest, 6:30 if we pushed it. Riding up and down several big bridges, we had miles of sanctuary that we road through. My backside was getting tired, but it was so exciting knowing that we were going to go further today then any other. Just keep pedaling, was the thought that I kept in my head. Go the distance.

As we rode onto Cedar Island, we spotted a sign that told us the ferry was just three miles down this road. The whole day had been such a pleasure ride, this last stretch was just the icing on the cake. We did get chased by a big dog, but Morton in his loudest, gruffest voice told it to stop and it did. He has a way with animals. There were a group of kids out beside the rode who asked if they could squirt us with water guns. I told them if it was warmer, we would say yes. Still pedaling, Morton told me I should have stopped and chatted. Who knows, we might have been able to pop the tent up in their backyard. I asked him if he really wanted to camp by such little rascals, who knows...we might wake up to being squirted with hoses.

Finally the signs for the ferry were in sight. There was our campground we would be pitching the tent at. The sun was just thinking about setting and had painted the sky pink and gold. The white sand of the beach was piled in dunes that had golden clumps of grass dotting it here and there. The perfect vision after the perfect ride. Chatting to a man at the ferry, we were relieved to find the bathrooms unlocked. Morton joked about camping inside them. I thought this might not be a bad idea. We wouldn't have a tent to tear down and we would have indoor plumbing.

There was a man on a nice BMW motorcycle who chatted with us a bit, then we had to go set up camp before the sun went down altogether. There was a motel there but no luck in finding anyone around to get a rate or a room. The tent it would be. The campground was right beside the ferry and who knows, it might warm up this evening. Finding a place under the pine trees, I kicked all the cones and twigs out of the path of the tent. Morton set about doing his thing with the gear as I was shocked to see that we got no phone signal. YIKES! My kids are going to be worried. They always get a call at night. Oh well, there is nothing I can do about it. Getting inside the tent, I work on this page as the sky has turned dark. There is not much wind and I can hear a dog barking off in the distance. Morton has fed us and we are both ready for an early night. After all, we did cover fifty miles today.

Day 79: March 20, 2007 - Tuesday - Cedar Island to Hatteras, NC

The tent has gotten bigger. It is so much roomier with 100 plus pounds of me missing. We woke up early, still dark out, but being in the tent we had to wait until daylight to get moving. The tent is wet in the morning, so things just had to wait. We heard the whistle toot on the ferry and we knew we would have to get the 10 am one. It really was a lovely morning. Morton cut his orange noodle for the swimming pool that he found beside the road and stuck it over our poles for our orange flags. They do stand out so much better now. We packed everything up with a big day laying in front of us.

As Morton was digging around in the trailers I was sort of shocked to see the very heavy logging chain he had found beside the road in Georgia was now riding in MY trailer. No wonder it felt like I was dragging an anchor! When I asked him how long it had been in my trailer he gave me a sheepish reply. I swiftly took it out, sat it neatly on the picnic table and said that now someone else could have the joy of finding this treasure that we have never even used. Morton looked like I had just taken away his favorite toy, but he left the chain. I guess he knew that I would be checking my trailer for stowaway surprises from now on.

Heading over to the dock, we got in line with the bicycles and they called us to come up to the front. We sat straddled on the bicycles as the cars and trucks loaded, then rode our bikes on at the tail end. It was going to be a two hour plus trip and I was a tad nervous about getting seasick. There was nothing to worry about though. The sea was calm and we went on our journey, passing the time talking to other travelers. It was a great way to get to the Outer Banks without having the hassle of bridge traffic and a big diversion. Our bicycles are a real conversation starter. People usually have the same stunned look on their faces when they find out what we are doing. Morton and I really do love hearing about all the things that are working for other people too. It really is an incredible world out here. People let their guards down and really talk to you when you tell them how much you weigh.

Today we met this lovely couple with their little son on the first ferry. They are doing a tour to see the lighthouses on the Outer Banks. The man plays the bagpipes and was born in England, raised in Scotland. His wife plays the drums and they met through their music. There little boy is all smiles and is a real miracle, weighing less than 2 pounds when he was born. These lovely people tell us about a pub they are going to for lunch in Ocracoke and invite us to join them. We actually had beat them to the pub, not because we were going fast, they had made a stop on the way. It was so nice sitting and chatting over lunch. What an amazing family they are. We both had places to get going to and said our goodbyes and headed back into the town. On the way to the pub we passed a road that had a British cemetery on it. We also passed a lighthouse. They were both worth a bicycle backwards. The first stop was the lighthouse. We want to sleep in lighthouses along the way, but this one is not open for you to see. You can walk around it outside and enjoy the view, but we knew we couldn't spend the night in it. We wanted to check out the graveyard and then bicycle to the other end of the island to catch the ferry. First though, I had to get on the bike to make this happen.

Since we have started, I have gotten on my bicycle hundreds of times. I have only fallen once, the very first time we got the bikes. Today, it went up to two times. We were pulling out of the parking area from the lighthouse and had to turn left and cross the road. There was nothing coming and I led off. Something happened. Actually, several things happened. My knee (the bad left knee) locked, the other foot caught on the front wheel and in slow motion, I fell in the middle of the road on the my left side. It was like something out of a bad dream. I looked up and hoped that nothing came down the quiet road and Morton came to my side and picked the bike up off of me.

It was a bit embarrassing and I felt very stupid to have this happen, but it was something I didn't plan on. That is why they call them accidents. He asked if I was alright and I wasn't sure. My hand hurt, my knee hurt, my elbow hurt and my stomach hurt. It was a very ungraceful fall. Nothing was bleeding though and my knee didn't make the huge crack that I thought it might when I stood on it. I was more scared then hurt and got right back on the bicycle to head over to the graveyard for British soldiers. I was so lucky to have had it happen on a quiet street. How many times I have pulled out, when I should have waited, to beat traffic. It has taught me a very good lesson, WALK the bike across the road from a stop.

The graveyard was small and Morton didn't take very long. We both talked about staying in the charming little town of Ocracoke or heading towards the end of the island to get another ferry to Hatteras. We decided to ride. As inviting as the town looked, we do have a long way to go. The ride was remarkable. The sound on one side, the Atlantic ocean on the other. The traffic was very sparse for the 12 miles. We paused to see wild ponies, have a little rest and gander at the ocean. We both enjoyed being able to talk to each other too. Usually it's too noisy to speak, but not today. We were here before tourist season hit. There were so many people we talked to today, the day just slipped away. We soon saw the ferry in the distance, but there was a band of bicycles on the right hand side of the road and I just had to stop. These were real bicyclist. They had on bike shorts and jerseys and looked the real deal. They also had stunning bicycles. We quickly learned they were riding to where we had just came from on the other end of Ocracoke. They were with a college and were going to stay the night at a fire station. Morton and I shocked them with what we were up to. Again, when we tell people they look at us and then at the bikes and you can just guess what they are thinking...something along the lines that we are INSANE!

Morton and I waited again until the cars and trucks had all loaded, then boarded this ferry. The ride was a lot shorter and the sun was starting to make it's daily dive to the horizon. My telephone finally made a beep and for the first time in what felt like forever, I had telephone signal. Calling Sarah, she was relieved to hear from us. Actually she sounded a bit scared and a little angry. She said she was ready to call the police and report us missing. I didn't even think about using a pay phone, but I should have. You don't really think about parents worrying the children, but that is just what we had done. Again, I learned a valuable lesson today. I will use a pay phone if I can't get phone reception. Communication with our family is vital. There will be parts of our journey though, where there won't be a telephone. This will be really hard and hopefully we will find some way around this. Perhaps we could learn how to send smoke signals.

As we were getting off the ferry, the sun was huge and red and right above the water. We know how fast it falls, so we headed north to a batch of buildings that looked like one just might be a motel. Pulling in to a parking lot, a man asked us if we were there for a room. Since the sign had said they had rooms, we thought this would be a good place to start our quest. He said if we wanted one, we better stop that lady getting in her car and leaving. For the first time in a *long* time, I ran. Jogging or sprinting, I bolted to her car and quickly asked about a room. We talked just for a moment, then she took me back to the office and said she could let us stay in a room that hadn't been cleaned yet. That was fine with us. It was already getting chilly. She offered us clean sheets, but I told her we would use our sleeping bags. It is really so great to get a room, we really don't even mind if we have to clean it! As we came into the room and got set up, I was able to call home and let everyone know we were alright. Better then alright. I forgot to tell them about my spill on the road, but they can read about it on the website. It will also save me from being scolded by them on the phone about being careful out here. Morton sat out our dinner and there is a hot shower waiting on me. I think first I might check my email, it will be in the hundreds with people asking if we are alright. Not just my kids will scold me about not being in touch, some of you will have been worried too. Sorry about that and we promise to be careful! We just can't keep in touch when our phone doesn't get a signal. The Outer Banks have been so impressive so far, we are really looking forward to this part of our journey. Beating the tourist season might prove a bit iffy when it comes to places to stay, but we will see what is waiting for us up the road tomorrow. One mile at a time. *Email update:* Over 7,000 emails asking where we were and if we are alright. We are, thank you for asking and please don't call the police! We are alive, for now.

Day 80: March 21, 2007 - Wednesday - Hatteras Village to *Lighthouse View*, Cape Hatteras, Buxton, NC

This morning I woke up from a dream about ice cream. There was a big tub in a freezer and I was working my way through it. What started out as just one bowl was turning into another then another. The tub was empty and I had that feeling that I've been so familiar with over the years. Failing on a diet. There was light outside the window blinds and for a moment I was in panic that I had actually eaten this entire tub of ice cream. It wouldn't be the first time it happened. But I quickly realized that I was only dreaming.

My mind played over what all had been happening in our lives. There are many times that I can't believe I'm actually in control of my weight now. I had eaten everything I wanted for decades and hated every minute of it. The moment I would be eating the entire pie I would not really enjoy it, because I knew that I was slowly committing suicide with food. Morton had jumped into action and was busy packing our gear and getting ready to ride. I did the last minute things I needed to online and smelled something sweet. Morton was TOASTING cookies. He delivered them up warm on a plate, announcing these 4 cookies were weighing in at 300 calories. Today we would need them for the energy, but all the nights, hundreds of nights, maybe even thousands of nights, I would eat this many cookies and more. The entire pack wouldn't have been safe in the house with me. But not today. This morning I enjoyed these cookies. I didn't hate myself for eating them. I didn't cry and scream for more when they were gone. I just ate them and enjoyed them. Then we rode the bikes.

If our bicycles would have had wings, I think we could have flown today. Windy is a word that needs a certain amount of degrees to it. To say it was windy isn't enough. They said there would be gusts of winds that would reach twenty-five miles per hour. There were. Only I don't know about "gusts" it seemed rather steady and right into my red hot face. People are always telling me to use sunscreen and I do. It does nothing though when my face gets sand-blasted from the wind and grains that are blown into the sky (and my eyes) when a car or truck passes. Today it was windy enough that we were going uphill the whole 11.5 miles that we managed. The weather really does determine more than my muscles how many miles we can manage each day. It is tough when we get a north wind because not only is it cold, it slows us down. The sky had gotten very dark and gray. We also could tell by our map that we had a long narrow stretch to go through that might not have anywhere to stop to get out of the rain. There were other reasons we were wanting a short day as well. The phone kept ringing with various reporters who are doing updates on our progress. We like to send different pictures out to all of them, so it takes a bit of time (I'm thinking about 4 to 6 hours) to get all of this done. There is also this fear of no phone signal. I quickly checked my phone to make sure I was still in range and we decided to try to find a room.

There was a lovely place, on the right side of the road and I popped in to ask for a room...clean or dirty, full of furniture or not...just somewhere from out of the weather and where I could work on the computer. The two lovely ladies at the office were indeed able to help, but not with a room full of furniture. They left us stay in a room with a king size bed, microwave, refrigerator, spotless & shining bathroom and free wireless. Now I will work. Oh the updates I'll be able to get done here at the *Lighthouse View*.

Once inside the room, I quickly get to work on the computer and think about our very short day riding. It is good to be out of the weather and wind. Before long the feeling has came back to the tops of my thighs that had been chilled to the bone through my layers of fat and Morton is going for a walk to the local store to see if there is anything cheap and warm. He brings back a can of soup and a small frozen pizza. That is dinner sorted. As I do the pictures from our short day I see all the views we got to see today. Even though it was overcast, it was still lovely. There is a horrible picture on first of the bruise on my stomach. It doesn't hurt, but looks horrid. It is a combination of several slams into the front handle bars of my bicycle (it's base is too short for me) and then yesterday when I fell in the middle of the road, the handle bars hit me right in the stomach. I had held on to them the whole way down. I need to remember *NOT* to do that in the future. Thinking back to my uncle, my mom's younger brother, that I never knew, the name "Billy" pops into my head. He was just a little boy, four or five, when a motorcycle fell over on him. The handlebar hit him in the stomach and he died from this. Things like this make me worry when I look at the large bruise on my white belly. It doesn't hurt really and I make a mental note to tell Morton to mention it to the doctors if I should start being sick.

Thinking about medical care out here is something I try not to think about. Denial. My body usually has bruises on it, the legs, the arms and I really don't bruise easily. It is just a bit of the rough life out here sometimes. The camping, the riding, walking beside things that your foot can slip on or off, road hazards. But hey, there is a lot less of me to bruise now. Maybe I'm becoming more graceful.

As Morton goes over the gear for tomorrow and putting our clean clothes out, he switches the television on. I find it really distracting when I'm trying to send photo files, write emails and work on the website. But he has nothing to keep him busy, so I plug in the headset and switch on the Zen mp3 player. The first song on is Beethoven's *"Ode to Joy"* and my heart sails. It is one of the most refreshing and thrilling pieces of music on our little player. The emails are sending as I work on this, photos are being uploaded and Morton is happily watching *Star Trek*. It might sound one sided that I do all the computer work, and I do, but trust me, Morton is the man that is making the wheels go around on this journey. It was just a few miles back that we were snapping pictures of a flying saucer beside the road. Morton said his usual, *"That's BRILLIANT"* as he went over towards this little apartment. I asked him if he would like to spend the night in it..."Naturally" he replies. But not tonight. Tonight we are not in the tent. We are in a lovely room with a fantastic table to work at. I expect that you could just play cards, write postcards or have a bite to eat at this table if you were just here on a holiday. After the trip we hope to return to spend more than just one night in places we have fell in love with along the way...this is one of those places.

Day 81: March 22, 2007 - Thursday - *Lighthouse View Motel & Cottages*, Buxton To *Traveler's Inn Motor Lodge*, Nags Head, North Carolina

Waking up beside the ocean is a real treat. The blue sky peeking out of the haze was the icing on the cake. The wind blowing from the south was an added bonus. It was going to be a fantastic day, we could just feel it. The fact that when I looked outside and saw the weather was going to be on our side made my heart skip a beat with joy. Morton got everything downstairs, loaded and ready to roll. I worked right up to the last second, loving the wireless. My cell phone modem connection is so very slow...think "dial up" and you get the idea of just how slow it is.

How can we describe just how amazing the Outer Banks are? Picture this. The ocean is on your right, behind rolling dunes that rise to the bright blue sky. The sound of the waves breaking and the roar are what we listen to as we ride. On the left is what they call the Sound. It is the water is filled with fish, crabs and other things we don't have time to catch or eat. We are still waiting on our first fishing trip on our adventure. We have traveled over 1,000 miles beside the water now and haven't had a chance to get a line wet. Hopefully soon. A nice day of fishing would be a good break in our routine and would help me use some arm muscles to try to get rid of my flabby bat wings.

Morton has made a few custom moves on my bicycle. He took the big orange noodle he found, the kind that kids play with in the water, then he cut it up, stuck part on his flag on his trailer and part on mine. He still had a bit left over, so he put mine on my resting grips on the bike. They do make it so much easier to lean on as I cycle. After all, I'm gripping for eight hours most days.

My hands are getting quite tough. Blisters have turned to callus and I'm not going to win any awards for having soft, pretty, dainty little hands. But I can see my knuckles again, so there just might be a bit of hope for them. They day started out a bit chilly, but the bicycling soon fixed that. I was soon going into a bathroom to change out of my long black slacks for a pair of gray shorts. These had been stretched to the point they barely fit just a year ago. Now they are baggy on me. It is a great feeling and I'm dreaming of the day they are too big altogether and I have to get smaller clothing. We both plan on wearing what we have until we are finished or it wears out. Morton has a sewing kit that we are going to use to take things in. Of course our shirts really don't matter. Morton is also on the smallest notch of his belt and ready to cut a new smaller hole in it. This isn't a fashion show, so we don't mind baggy, worn clothes. Just so they are clean.   Hopefully my pants won't fall off of me when I'm bicycling for a news crew somewhere. That is what you *don't* want to see on the six o'clock news. We make very few stops today. There are big stretches of wild road in front of us. Traffic is almost non-existent at this time of year and I'm glad it's not the summer. There is a wildlife sanctuary we stop at that we *should* have filled the water bottles up, but didn't. We are really going through the H2o again. It is almost like being in the Keys. Staying hydrated is vital to us. Having a heat stroke is something we don't want. The heat shimmers from off the pavement in the distance and out of it I see what I *hope* is a mirage. It is a tall bridge. A large hump sitting in our path that as we get closer, we both know this must be the big bridge people have told us about. It will take us north and we have no option, other then swimming, but to bicycle across it.

It takes us two miles to get up to the bridge that people have told us is three miles long. It rises to cover the wide water below it and allow tall ships and tall boats to pass below. Before we tackle it, we pull off to get a drink of water. There are a few people there and we chat about the trip and the bridge. They have been over it in a car and tell us what to expect. After the rise and fall in the beginning, it stretches on, almost level. The big question is, will I be able to cycle up the tall hump? It is my steepest to date.

After a few pictures and water we are ready. We put the bicycles and trailer on the narrow edge that isn't wide enough. The left wheel on the trailers is hanging out in the traffic over the white line. The other tire is nearly pushed against the concrete rise on the edge of the bridge. Memories of getting my trailer bumped from the truck in South Carolina come into my head. These are scary thoughts that I push out of my head.

The one good thing is that traffic isn't bad today. It's actually sparse as we push off and start to climb. It is a gradual climb, then getting steeper. Morton had manually put my big gear into high earlier for our ride, now I was scared to lower it. I was in high on one side and low on the other. Pushing hard on the pedals, the sun beat down and the litre of water I had just drank, quickly became sweat. The top was in sight. Morton was actually shouting out encouragement from behind. Words like, "It's not far now, you are almost there" made me smile. I knew I was going to be able to do this. He could have saved his breath, but it was sweet that he was attempting to be a cheerleader. Nothing in this world can describe the feeling when I hit the top of the bridge. Pure joy and this sense of another big change coming from lots of little changes. It was something that I would have never been able to do just a month ago, but our daily riding is really paying off. My body is getting so much stronger after all the years of abuse that I gave it. This is what sheer bliss feels like.

They say you climb a mountain because it's there, well today I crossed this bridge because it is here and there was nothing else I could do. It was a brilliant feeling of not just being alive, but really actually living that pushed me over the top. When we were coming down the steep part, I tried to go as fast as I could. It felt great to get the wind in my face. Far below us on the beach, four young men were playing horseshoes. They were already tanned, wearing their swimming trunks and enjoying being outside. I left out a giant, "Yeeeee-hawwww" that would have made my girlfriend Karen smile. They all responded by letting out their own shouts of joy on this lovely spring day. Morton most likely thought I was crazy. They shouted and waved and I felt like *Mrs. Fitness America!*

Smiling for ages, needing another drink, we kept on a few miles before stopping. We sat our tarp down to sit for a moment in the small patch of shade that the trailer on my bike made. I drank another litre of water. Morton said he didn't think I was going to make it to the top of that bridge because I had slowed down so much, hmmm...little did he knew I had a secret weapon. Mentally I was already there, my body was just finally catching up.

Continuing north, we heard a shout from bicyclists behind us that they were going to pass. I kept well over and we all started talking as they were going by. We stopped for a few minutes and got advice on the road ahead and exchanged information with each other. They were both very fit men, real bicyclist and kind enough to stop and speak. We took a picture, I got a hug and a kiss and then they were on their way. Without any effort at all, they sailed off and were out of sight in under a minute. They must have been really moving. Morton and I were doing between 10 and 12 mph and everything does seem a lot faster at that slow turtle speed. One day we will be the ones riding fast and actually passing other people on bicycles. Who knows, maybe the day will come quicker then we think. The one man on the bike had mentioned a term we had heard before, *"Stealth Camping"*. Morton and I both scanned the trees and ground around as we rode on thinking that we just might see a spot where we could do this. There was water beside the road though, if it was tidal here (we really don't know) we might end up floating in our tent. We heard a story from a young man that it happened to not too long ago and it made us think twice of pitching up beside the water.

Soon, we couldn't really believe it, but we were coming into Nags Head. It was a place I thought we might make it to, but Morton had said it was too far to reach. Well, here we were, stopping long enough for Morton to snap my picture by the sign and then turning left to keep on Route 12. This feeling of going over our daily mark is fabulous and I love it! It gives you a real sense of achievement when you not just reach your goal but go beyond it. It also makes you want to keep doing it.

The very first motel we came to, the *Traveler's Inn Motor Lodge*, not only gave us a room with wireless internet, but Brenda, the owner, was kind enough to have a nice long blether with me. We talked about everything you can think of while Morton waited with our bikes. It was our longest break for the day and felt good to be in one place for longer then 10 minutes. Brenda handed me the key and we were off for the evening with the sun just thinking about setting. As I got to work, Morton went back to get a few pictures. The sound of the ocean is heard from the room and I know I'm going to sleep like a baby tonight, thanks to my wonderful bicycle. There is also the lovely shower. This one feels incredible after the long day, another million dollar shower. We also have a little kitchen in the room so we have a hot meal of chicken noodle soup mixed with a can of green beans. The beans overpowered the soup, or so said Morton, but it was great anyway. A warm meal, hot shower, cold water and wireless! I can't stay awake past 9 am, so I'm finishing this up in the morning as Morton is moving our gear outside. Blame it on the exercise and the salt air. Throw in the soft roar of the ocean and put it in a bottle and what do you have? The perfect combination for people who can't sleep.

Day 82: March 23, 2007 - Friday - Traveler's Inn Motor Lodge, Nags Head to Currituck, North Carolina
We are going to do something a little different for these next few days. Morton is going to fill you in on what has been happening. I'm having a tough time at the moment keeping up with the computer and trying to get enough sleep each night. As I get more physically exhausted, I get even crankier with Morton. He has offered, I said yes and here you go.

Morton: We left Nags Head about 9:40am and cycled along the coast road. We had to cycle on the road because about every twenty foot there was a driveway with steep ramps which play havoc with the trailer, always throwing the hitch out of position. After a little while Priscilla pulled into a little bench gazebo sending me off to take pictures of the beach while she rested and had a drink. The beach was an amazing sight running for miles and the beautiful breakers crashing in.

After a short break we set off again, moving up onto the busier road to accommodate our route better, again we had to stay on the road because there was no good foot-path. Kitty Hawk was a beautiful area and very blustery, we could see why Orville and Frank chose the area for their famous achievement. Lunch time was approaching so we decided to stop at a shopping centre that had a Subway and a dollar store. We shared a 6" sub for lunch and got some essential provisions from the dollar store. As we were about to leave I noticed a puncture on Priscilla's trailer. She then confessed to having ran over a cactus - what a surprise it's usually beer bottle glass! We set off into heavy traffic again.

Going over the bridge to the mainland was amazing, the view across the bay was beautiful. the ride down off the bridge was exhilarating. We zoomed down off the bridge and round the corner onto dry land unfortunately into the wind again. The Harley-Davidson garage we were about to pass had lovely benches so we had a breather there, the day had turned roasting hot. Our bikes got a few odd looks from some of the hog riders but they are usually very friendly giving us a wave as they pass. It was surprising with such a busy road that there was a huge lack of motels or camp-grounds, we had to keep cycling only stopping for a pit stop with a cold soda and to repair another puncture on Priscilla's trailer. Racing day light is no fun, a motel we tried was closed and no answer at a B+B, so we had to keep going. We ran out of day light about five miles from Currituck, fortunately the road edge was good and wide to keep us safe. We made Currituck about 7.45 Checking with the ferry office it was disappointing to find there were no campground, hotels or motels around. Checking in with the United Methodist Church we were graciously allowed to stay overnight in their church-hall. It was very kind of them to give us a safe place to stay.

Day 83: March 24, 2007 - Saturday - *United Methodist Church*, Currituck , North Carolina to
The Viking, Virginia Beach, Virginia
Morton: Rising early we made for the ferry only to find the first one had left at six not seven as Priscilla had been told. It worked out well though as she was able to take lots of photos of the sunrise. We had breakfast as we waited and I tackled some bike repairs.The ferry finally arrived and carried us over to the other side. We disembarked and headed off to find it was extremely windy and hard cycling. The scenery was amazing. We passed lots of people in red vests spring cleaning litter from the island. They were working like eager little beavers and had trailers-full already collected.

Passing through the wet-lands was breath-taking so many things to see on the way. We saw everything from snakes to turtles and loads of other animals including ferocious guard miniature wiener dogs.

Stopping for lunch at a campground Priscilla got online to check e-mail etc. Later on we stopped off at a library to get a Virginia State map. Luckily they had got some in for a summer kids project and were able to spare one because surprisingly libraries don't normally stock them. We finally arrived at Pungo. I again had to attack the bike, the bottom bracket keeps going slack. I don't know what's up with it and I'm scared to take it apart incase it disintegrates on me.

About three we couldn't resist some hot cooked food and got a delicious barbecued pork sandwich and cole-slaw to share. It was really cold and windy again so we plodded onwards to Virginia Beach, even though it had been saying we were there ever since we entered Virginia near the campground at lunch-time.

We finally came to a really good cycle path that took us into Virginia Beach, there was only one section of it that was dangerous when there was no signs to tell us to cross over onto the other side for the section past the aquarium. We were on the dual-carriageway when someone in a truck shouted to say it was there so we immediately crossed over to the safety of the pathway. We thought we had missed a sign until we saw another cyclist coming across that had made the same mistake as us. We arrived freezing where Priscilla had to phone round loads of places to find somewhere to stay, everywhere was full due to a soccer competition. We got into our room feeling like a couple of snow-men, it was so cold we could see our breath.

Priscilla got to work as I went out to get dinner from *Wendy's*. I got the value meal and Priscilla had the South West Taco salad. When you are on a budget the value meals are wonderful and as long as you don't get them all the time they are a good hot meal when you are hungry. I'm now going to pass back over to Priscilla. Cheerio the now! Priscilla & Morton - *The Viking* , Virginia Beach, Virginia

Day 84: March 25, 2007 Sunday - *The Viking*, Virginia Beach to *Super 8*, Norfolk, VA

Bicycling along the coastlines and borders of America sounds rather impressive. I can assure you that it is even better than our words can tell you on here. Waking up beside the ocean, hearing it, smelling the salt air...just amazing. When the sun is shining and the wind in blowing in the right direction, all is right with our world. That was how the morning started. I was working on the computer and trying to get in touch with the television stations we are going to be on in this area. The girls at the check-in desk had told me to give Neil a call in the morning and see about the room. I did, he said "YES!"

My memories of Virginia include a lovely trip when my kids were little to camp beside the shore where the wild ponies frolic on an island. I never really saw a lot of the state, but from what we see so far...we love it. The old advertising slogan, "Virginia is for Lovers" pops into my head as we bicycle down the boardwalk in sunny Virginia Beach, as we leave *The Viking*. Studying a map we opt to go out of our way a bit to stick to the coast. It also means that we will get to see the very spot that the British first landed, 400 years ago this year. We also avoid traffic this way. In the scale of things, what is an extra 5 or 10 miles when we are going thousands of miles?

Morton is talking about all the little energy gel packs he is seeing beside our path. This is a heavy travelled bike path and guess what....*SOME BICYCLIST ARE LITTER BUGS!!!* Now I know I usually moan about the cars and trucks whooshing past and tossing beer bottles out. I even had someone toss a cup of ice out at me the other day. But come on...*I KNOW* who is tossing these little packs of energy gel out. Me, I must confess, there was a time in my life I did litter. This was a taught condition. My parents and their parents didn't really think about litter. I had even joked in my younger days that it gave Girl Scouts something to do. But now I choose to pick litter up when I can and I never throw anything out a window, or off my bicycle now. These gel energy packs are a bit bigger than a pack of ketchup from a fast food place. They are made of material that will be here a lot longer than we will. They also need to be put in the garbage cans. Morton says that the people don't want to tuck them back under their bike shorts or in their pockets because they are messy from the gel. I'm shocked. That is not an excuse. Just as people take a plastic bag to clean up doggie stuff, take a plastic bag to put your used gel pouch in after you suck it up for energy. Sheesh! Enough of a rant now, it was just sickening to see. We counted over 30 in about a 2 mile period. Unacceptable.

When we came to the gate for the Army base, we had to check in at the gate. The guard told us that the marker was at the lighthouse. That was a bonus...a lighthouse and the landing place of the British. *Impressive.* He told us we would have to turn around and come back out this gate, not exit at the other end. We decided that we still wanted to go in, even though it meant covering the same ground twice. It would be worth it. As an afterthought, he told us we could go ahead through and come out on the bottom of the base. *Sweet.* Things like this, little miracles, we see all the time and now we are taking them for granted. I suppose after seeing we were willing to obey his rules, he made the correct judgement call that we weren't up to no good.

Getting closer to the big lighthouse, I'm smiling and bicycling in the sun. Even though I am wearing sunscreen, I am getting a very weird tan. There is a white line under my chin where the strap covers. My forehead is also white, my eye area that my glasses cover is really white as well. My glasses are for seeing in the distance (I'm blind as a bat with anything over 5 feet or so in front of me) and they darken when I'm outside. At first I think it is a mirage or a weird shadow. But no, there are two lighthouses here. We pull in and you can actually go up and visit the old brick lighthouse. Sadly, there is a charge to go in and we can't go. $4.00 is a small fee, but to us, $8.00 for the pair just won't work into our budget. That will feed us for two days. Taking pictures and having a drink of water, I notice all the ribbons hanging on a wooden picket fence at the entrance to the old brick lighthouse. I get chills on my arms when I see that there are both yellow and black ribbons hanging on it. The black ribbons have names written on them. They are the names of dead soldiers.

The only word I can think of is *"Why?"* This very moving spot, again seeing soldiers, young men, my thoughts turn to my son who is only a five hour drive from me. War isn't a necessary thing, not in this day and age. Why are we still sending lambs to the slaughter and killing innocent people along the way? All in the name of money.

When Sarah called me this morning, I could tell they were in their car. For a moment my heart leapt. I thought for a second that they were in Virginia Beach. Can you tell that I'm very homesick for my kids? They were just going out for the morning to meet one of her friends. I had asked if she was in Virginia Beach and she said, "Aww...I had thought about it." Maybe next weekend. My heart aches worse than my other muscles sometimes with homesickness.

Back at the lighthouse I try to think about happy things. The sun, the beach, the marker for the landing. Morton and I push off and go riding down the road to have a look-see. He takes a few pictures and we park the bicycles. There is a big wooden walk leading to the beach and he heads off while I sit guard over our gear and try to call my kids again. I know, I'm pathetic...but hey, I miss them BAD. A pickup pulls in and there is a couple who get out with their two little wiener dogs. Not only am I homesick for my children, family and friends...*NOW I'M MISSING MY GRAND-DOG!!!* Max, our furry little bundle of love, is just a five hour drive away...but these little pups are here right now. I go over and start chatting. The people are as nice as the dogs are cute. They let me pet their pets and take some pictures. Morton joins us and we talk about what we are up to. They tell us they are just out for a day drive and again, the conversation feels so good. I love Morton to bits, but it is nice to talk to other people too. It is just an added bonus when they have a cute little pup that I can cuddle! I'm hoping that James brings Max along when he comes to visit.

We get back on the bikes and turn to the left, putting the wind at our backs. We ride through this base. Morton is going ga-ga over all the "stuff" but I tell him not to take any pictures of it. I don't want to get in trouble and I really don't want to think about where we are. Instead I think about the next time my family will all be together. This is a place that pulls families apart as troop are deployed for our love of oil. Freedom has nothing to do with war, it's all about the money baby and for those of you who don't know it, oil *is* money. If you are near your family, *APPRECIATE IT!* Our lives are so short and even when you feel like your family might be a pain in the butt, trust me...when you don't have them around, you miss them like mad.

We exit the base and fight for our position on a road with no real edge to it. It's not too bad though, traffic is light and the sun is keeping us from freezing. Before long, we see a sidewalk and get on it. This sidewalk had several spots we had to get off and walk the bikes down off of the edge, where ramps should have been. We wonder to each other how a person in a wheelchair could ever really cope on these sidewalks. The answer is they couldn't. A small bridge shows us that the big Bay Bridge and Tunnel, is just in front of us. It looks like a bridge to nowhere. It is massive and we are not allowed to ride over it. We have decided to go up the Chesapeake anyway. We want to ride through Jamestown, Williamsburg, Washington D.C., and Baltimore. Then we can come back down the other side of the water. This adds about 500 miles to our trip, but hey, on a trip this big, what is another 500 miles?

The wind is whipping our faces and it's long past lunch. There are golden arches above, on the right side of the road and with a few tables outside. It's too chilly to face the cold tuna so Morton goes inside and spends $3. to get us each something from the dollar menu and a hot apple pie each. The warm food tasted fantastic and gave us each the energy needed to keep riding! Before long, the sun was hiding. It was as if someone had switched off the sun and switched on the freezing air. The breeze turned bitter and my face was red and hot from the wind. It still is as I put the back of my hands on my cheeks.

After our late night riding in the dark, I don't want to take any chances. We see a sign that announces we are in Norfolk and I know that we need to stop soon to hook up in the morning with a television crew.

We go on high alert for a room or campground. But first, we meet a mermaid. It just so happened at one of the parts of the sidewalk that we had to get off the bicycles. We lifted them down, lifted them up, then spotted this mermaid blowing in the wind. She was larger than life and I took the camera and asked Morton to go pose with her. I suggested standing under her outstretched arm. As Morton stood beside her, ducking under her arm, the wind spun her around. She hit him in the head and to steady himself, he grabbed ahold of her spangled boob. "Sorry" he exclaimed...and I cracked up. Morton was still laughing as I took the picture of the Mermaid and Morton, sure to become one of my favorites from this trip. I asked him if a mermaid had ever punched him before, but he was still laughing too much about it to hear me.

Riding on, we stopped at a group of motels. This was going to be night two in Virginia. They were all chains though and the person at the desk usually can't say yes about a room sponsorship. The *Super 8 Motel* was a bit different. The girl at the desk, Ally, listened to what we were doing. She called the owners and explained our journey to them. They were kind enough to say YES! Best of all, we are right in the backyard of the television station for our interview in the morning...AND they have free wireless and free breakfast. Maybe the slap of a mermaid was really lucky for Morton. Sanctuary and safety go hand in hand and getting out of the wind is an added bonus. We made our way into our room, which is just lovely. A really big television (all the better to watch the *Weather Channel* on!) a refrigerator, microwave, desk with a very comfy chair for working and plenty of room for Morton to work on his pedal assembly. He always puts a tarp down and never makes a mess anywhere we stay, but he does do bicycle repairs almost every evening.

Calling my kids, I let them know we are safe for another evening. After our time in the Outer Banks where our phone wouldn't get a signal, I don't want to scare them anymore. They worry about me out here even though I'm old enough and ugly enough to look after myself. After all, I have Morton too.

We both want an early night tonight, with an early start tomorrow. Hopefully we will find a way to cross a giant bridge that we aren't suppose to, then head north towards Williamsburg. I can't believe how far we have come...and Sarah, if you read this, you better come and visit us next weekend. Bring your husband, your brother and your sister-in-law...and don't forget Max the wiener dog.

Day 85: March 26, 2007 - Monday - *Super 8,* Norfolk To Newport News, Virginia

Last night we had the most incredible thing happen. Ally, at the front desk, had her mom, kids and hubby come in with dinner for us. The best part wasn't just the delicious food, it was the great chit chat that we had. It was really nice to feel at home, even though we were in a motel. We started the day off on a great note too. We had an interview first thing this morning with Wavy, Channel 10. It was right in front of our *Super 8 Motel* that we had been in. After the questions and answers, we left and were filmed riding off into the sunset...or sunrise.

There was something that was nagging on our minds as we rode beside the water. The map had shown us several bridges, none that we could go across on the bicycles. We knew we would have to fly, swim or hitch a ride...but we had nothing prearranged. Ally and her husband had offered to give us a lift over, but they had done so very much already, we didn't want to impose.

Since things are always seeming to work out for us, we just rode and enjoyed the bike line and sidewalks. The phone rang and we were going to meet up with Katherine from Channel 13. We are getting to be pros at threading mic wires through our shirts and clipping on the microphone to our necklines. We tuck the transmitter in our pockets and are ready to speak the words about getting healthy and taking control of your own life. Pulling the bicycles in, the camera was already rolling as we chatted about the journey. Again, after the questions we chatted a little and I wanted to ask one of the pickup truck drivers that were parked in the park for a lift. This was going to be a bit easier with a cameraman with me. Walking up to the pickup that contained an elderly gentleman, I explained what we were looking for a ride to Hampton over a bridge that bicycles and pedestrians were prohibited on. Sadly, the man wasn't going our way but was very friendly. We did some riding for the camera and then parted ways and kept cycling towards the bridge/tunnel that needed crossed.

Before we knew it, we were there. It was just after lunch and we were sort of loitering at a stop sign, hoping to talk to pickups that passed. A car pulled up, an SUV and the man got out, came over and asked us what we were doing. He had seen us being filmed earlier and was curious. He also had a special request. His grand-daughter was working on a school project where he was taking a stuffed fuzzy frog around the area and getting pictures of it. He wanted to get a picture of Morton and I holding the frog...so we did. Then we took a picture of me and the man who was on the mission...and of course the frog.

Since we weren't having any real luck at the stop sign, we rode to the end of the road. A lady who was cutting grass told us to try the other side of the highway. There was a marina over there and we might have better luck. We backtracked, went under the highway and stopped at the *Sunset Grill on Bayville Street*. When I walked inside there was a lady with the cutest dog who was so very helpful. Cathy listened to the dilemma and without even thinking about it, she arranged for a lift in a pickup right over the bridge. It was wonderful. Plus, the man who gave us the lift, literally lifted the trailers and bicycles up on the pickup bed with no effort. Morton jumped in to help with one trailer and before we knew it, we were going over the bridge and then down in the tunnel. Within just a few minutes, our obstacle was just a memory and a few pictures. The kindness of strangers will never cease to amaze us.Grabbing the map we try to get ourselves sorted out. We got out of the truck in a parking lot off the first exit after the bridge and really had to just get our bearing straight as Morton hooked the trailers back up to the bikes.

We needed to head across the bridge we were able to ride the bikes across and the sun comes out. The temperature starts to rise and we find our way to Route 60. Turning this way and that, we pass museums, old churches and lots of smiling faces. We are a bit like a circus coming to town I guess. The map didn't really show us that 60 runs into a main highway that bicycles can't go on. We take the alternative road of route 143, which will eventually go back into 60. Always a plan B!

We spot a patch of motels and try our luck for a room sponsorship. The first two say no, the third says that they can give us a special rate of $35.00. Since there is no way that we will make it to Jamestown before dark, we decide to get the room. There is never any real way to tell what is in front of us and I was really tired. $35.00 and breakfast in the morning...and maybe, just maybe, if we speak to the manager in the morning, we might get a refund and they will agree to become a sponsor, with me adding a link to our website for them and giving them our eternal gratitude. I'm not going to rule out that it will happen. I'll cross my fingers and hope for the best. Morton had gotten all of our groceries packed into meals for the next few days, so as soon as we up-load the new page we are going to take a little walk towards the water and then head for the shower. We are hoping that we get an early start tomorrow and make it to Jamestown in a reasonable amount of time. If you see us out here, please stop and say hello!!! It really makes our day when we meet people along the way who don't think we are homeless scroungers, though technically, I suppose we are!

A bit from Morton: Today another interesting day.......seeing how the news is made. It certainly is a job that keeps them busy. Driving out to interview us, then all the work setting up the cameras and microphones and filming. The trickiest part is when they are filming moving shots of us in traffic and from the back of their car. Fortunately today when they were filming us in traffic we had an understanding bin motor driver (garbage truck) behind us as we were filmed through a section of road-works, he kept the traffic in check until we finished filming and pulled over to return Priscilla's microphone. I got the chance to meet a Flat Eric frog that a gentleman stopped to have a photo taken with us to send to kids in schools. Thanks to the help of some kind people we made it across the bridge tunnel. When we were dropped of we decided to have a dollar toasted ham and cheese sandwich for lunch....it was so delicious.

After cycling for some distance I got sent in to do some shopping at a dollar store. I got some new things to try because tuna every day does get a bit boring. It's really hard resisting temptation to buy stuff but you have to remember the trailers can only hold so much. Our biggest problem is weight and also whatever we buy, will you have the facilities to heat the stuff up. Sometimes you have to improvise, like heating water in a soda bottle in a microwave to make hot chocolate and finding out that the bottles go soft and start to buckle as the water approaches boiling point......ooops!

Cycling through some areas we got some quizzical looks from the local residents, so hopefully they will see the news and realize who the odd couple cycling through were. Ending up on a busy four lane road we were surprised to find no-one was tooting their horns at us and apart from the pot holes it was a pleasant cycle.

Settling into a room for the night Priscilla got to work as I got dinner ready. Unfortunately cold stuff unlike the delicious hot meal we had last night prepared by Ally's mum. It was so much fun sitting down to a family meal and getting the chance to swap stories with everyone. I'll check out now and let Priscilla get back to work before she kicks me off as I take so long to type with two or three fingers and the odd thumb. Cheerio the now.

PS Thank to all the well wishers from Scotland. The print factory seems like ions ago hearing from the guys and I'm glad to hear you are doing OK. Cheerio again.

Day 86: March 27, 2007 - Tuesday - Newport News To *The Cedars B&B*, Williamsburg, VA

When you get the chance to go back in time, you always need to take it. This route wasn't on our original map, but we happen to be right in the midst of the Historic Triangle. The cities, Williamsburg, Jamestown and Yorktown, all are the belly of the birth of our nation. We couldn't just bicycle past it. We woke up this morning with no real plans in place for our fourth stop on our Must-See Cities tour. Something will turn up, it always does. We have found that some times the very best plans are no plans or *nae plans*, as Morton would say.

After sleeping in the motel room that wasn't sponsored in the morning (goodbye to the $35.00 plus tax from the monthly budget) I woke up with a horrible sore throat. I think it must have been because the room was actually a smoking room. The whole lower half of the motel had smoke hanging in the air and really was a bit like the smell you get when you are cleaning a dirty ashtray.

Last night the fire alarm had gone off for a good half hour and this morning I can't help but wonder if it was from all the people that stand about the hallways smoking. It is like the entire staff live at the motel in Newport News. It seems like a rather odd set up, but hey, we are only here for one night. The man who checked us in was really nice. I didn't want to go back and complain about the smell in our non-smoking room. He had also given us two coupons for a free breakfast, so I just kept quiet, did the work that needed done on the computer and looked forward to riding into Williamsburg. We got to see the reports that the news channels, 10 and 13, had done on us. We also got to get showers, always a good thing when you spend several hours bicycling and sweating even in the cold.

We head down to the breakfast room where another couple and their baby are eating. There is a man with the food who dishes up our plates for us. He said he never gets this many people in and we got what was left from the egg pan after he squashed the water out the side, a pancake that a knife wouldn't cut - we had to pick it up and crunch it apart and three wee sausages ...they were good.

Morton and I were pushing the trailers out our room door as a fight broke out between two female employees. There were no punches thrown, only threats. One was pregnant and one had two children with her. This brought all the other people out of their bedrooms to stare and smoke.

We kept our heads down and left as quick as we could. It was all a bit traumatic and my throat was really killing me as we rode west on route 143, Jefferson Avenue. This was one of the rare times we were happy to be leaving a place we had stayed. You never know what is going to happen and our life out here doesn't come with a set of instructions. We have to just ride and see. The scene around us changed. More motels. Darn. We *SHOULD* have kept going last night. There might have been someone in this area that would have been willing to help us with a room. This was the first real twinge of regret that I have felt in a long time on the journey. You really do have to go with your gut instinct and hey, at least we didn't get caught in the fight or have a "real" fire at the motel.

The day got hotter. The sun was streaming down on us and the wind that was blowing in our faces felt like it was coming right out of a furnace. We quickly went through our water that normally lasts an entire day. By lunchtime there were eight big empty bottles. Stopping at a *7-11* to eat our lunch in the shade of a tree, Morton went inside and got a *BIG GULP.* These things are huge, it might have even been a DOUBLE, it was a monster sized cup that he had filled with Gatorade. This was the first time that the sport drink was an option that we had seen. With our salty lunch, we also drank the entire vat of a cup. Morton said they do cheap refills. The cost was $1.49 for the first and .79 cents for a refill. I went back inside, added no ice and filled the cave of a cup, up to the rim. We poured the red liquid into our empty bottles and headed off.

As we got closer to Williamsburg, there was a bit of sidewalk with a man that had a tripod set up snapping pictures of us. We thought it might be one of the newspapers that we had emailed, but it actually happened to be this bicyclist and very nice man, Paul. He not only told us just which way we wanted to ride to get into Colonial Williamsburg, but offered us cold drinks of water and gave us his map! While we were all talking his neighbor came out. She had seen us on television and had a few questions about our journey. The best thing happened when she said that she was inspired and motivated and was going to start walking tomorrow! You have no idea how good it feels sharing this feeling that we actually CAN change the big and impossible feeling things in our lives.

We rode off towards this town that I'm ashamed to say I never visited before. We grew up just a five hour drive from it. I had thought about bringing my children before, but it was just a bit too far from Gettysburg, Pennsylvania to do as a day trip. Plus, like so many things that are almost in our backyard, we overlook them. When we turned left to head into the 300 plus acre living history museum, that really is a town, I regretted never coming here with my family before. There were old style fences with fluffy, fuzzy sheep grazing. It was bicycling backwards. People wearing period clothing, little boys running about in tri-cornered hats and my mind pictured how much fun my kids would have had here. We kept to the edge of the old brick sidewalks, cobblestones and had a surprise. Why don't we explore our own backyards?

Paul, the man with the camera, bicycle and great tips, had taken his evening ride into town. He was chatting to us as we rode, pointing out places and what happened there. It was like getting our own private bicycle tour of Williamsburg. When we got to the corner where William & Mary college sits, we said our good-byes. He promised to keep in touch on the website and we headed down Jamestown Road to find our home for the next two nights.

Spring seemed to be an afterthought now. This felt like summer. Warm sunshine, smells of flowers everywhere and the most beautiful buildings all glided by as we kept going. We only had a few short blocks and we were at *The Cedars*. This bed and breakfast is stunning, with lovely flower gardens in the front and the back. There is also a lovely gazebo with plenty of chairs that is in the very back of the garden, with woods behind it. It feels like you are in the country, yet you really are just steps away from the main heartbeat of the town. We pulled the bicycles into a parking area and were greeted by Bob, the owner. He is a man who has competed in the Ironman competitions, so he knows all about the benefits of exercise. We didn't need to sell him on the idea of getting 30 minutes a day to change his health outlook! We talked for a few minutes and then went inside to our lovely room that Grace and Bob have generously sponsored for us for two nights. Morton brought our gear inside, tarped the bicycles up and I did the bare bones of the computer work. We needed to get out and have a walk about town

. As we approached the shopping area, it was just getting dark. There were people coming and going, a store that sells kilts that caught Morton's eye and a movie house. It just so happens that the film showing was *"Last King of Scotland"* and Morton and I had both wanted to see it. We did our first real splurge since the journey began and I went on a date with my husband. We bought a small popcorn and small diet soda. As we waited for the movie to begin, we chatted to a couple who live in Massachusetts. The lady told me not to take it the wrong way, but I was even crazier then her son! He is going to bicycle across Iowa this summer. Sounds like a fun thing to do! When we entered the lovely theater with a real stage curtain, I was thrilled to see that I actually fit into the seat. The seats, or rather all the extra padding on my OWN seat, had kept me out of the movies for a long time. I couldn't bear to be wedged in the seat for two hours. But this was great. *I FIT!!!* I even had about an inch to spare. Wiggle room! Morton and I ate our popcorn, drank our soda and held hands as we watched this real-life drama play out on screen. The actor who played the Scottish doctor was spot on. There was a line about not having monkeys in Scotland, the Scottish doctor said if they did have, they would probably deep fry them. Morton and I both laughed because it was true. After all, where else but Scotland can you get a deep-fried Mars bar, or deep-fried pizza, or Morton's favorite, a deep-fried haggis or perhaps a black pudding! Walking the short stroll back to *The Cedars* we both felt as if all the stars were smiling on us. The moon looked on as we headed past the historic *William & Mary College*. There were some students out talking, walking and running. It feels like a place that you can relax and enjoy, with pleasant surprises around each corner. This is America at her best. Climbing into our fantastic four poster bed, I snuggle into the pillows. We are a million miles from a wet tent and thin horrible cheap sleeping bags. The stars were not only smiling on us, they must have all been lucky stars as well.

I think about the wonderful experiences that have been happening so far on our journey. Wondering why, after decades of battling obesity and depression did the light finally come on in my head to actually change my destiny. I fell asleep with the thought that it didn't matter just what made the light finally come on, but that it HAD, is the important part. Life can really be beautiful, when we let it. Who would have thought that finally getting rid of my fat would be so liberating?

Day 87: March 28, 2007 - Wednesday - *The Cedars* B&B, Williamsburg, Virginia

If you have never stayed in a Bed & Breakfast, you MUST do this. This needs to be something that you experience at least once in your lifetime. From the time you come down the drive at *The Cedars*, you know you are somewhere very special. The people here make you feel like you are family that have came home. We were given our keys yesterday and I forgot to mention the skeleton key for our room door. It reminds me of the keys in Scotland for the old fashioned locks. Some of the keys over there are several inches long. We have friends that have a key to their front door that looks like it would surely open a castle keep. The key is the first thing that reminded us of the "Old Country", the hospitality is the second. This place is incredible and every where you look, you see something else that catches your eye. Our bedroom, *The Martha Washington*, is so lovely, the famous first lady would have loved to stay here. There is a perfect wooden desk, four poster bed that is the height of pure comfort and the bathroom is spotless. It is going to be very tough to go back to the tent after this. This morning we woke up early, got the email and new page done on the website and then went to the most delicious breakfast at *The Cedars*. Bob and Grace were both there to chat with us. Grace, who had said *YES* to our visit, made the most delicious breakfast we have tasted in ages. As we were speaking about the journey, great tips from Bob who has competed in the Ironman (maybe I'll give this a shot someday!) time flew by and just as we were finishing breakfast, the newspaper reporter arrived. The interview was done in the loving living room here. Very comfortable and relaxed and then we headed outside to get some pictures with the bicycles. Now I almost forgot to mention, at breakfast, Bob took our picture. He does this for all the guests. He then went away and in just two ticks came back with two huge color portraits for us to keep as a souvenir. It is dated and has the lovely logo of The Cedars on the top of the picture. What a wonderful way to remember our special stay here. Morton and I were standing with our bicycles in the area behind the huge brick house. The reporter was having bother with her camera and Bob came to the rescue. He was able to use his, then email the photos to the newspaper. He also gave Morton and I these incredible brochures for *The Cedars* with OUR picture on the front! Talk about a really unique item! Even though Bob does the Ironman, we personally think he is a bit of a Superman!

Morton wanted to leave the trailers behind today and just ride with the bicycles. I wanted to take them, but since Morton rarely gets his way we left them behind. It felt like we were flying! I need to remember to tell Bob that it might be a good tip to train with the trailers fully loaded for the Ironman. Then when you take them off and are just on the bicycle, wooosh...you will sail! The weather couldn't have been nicer. We rode in the bicycle lane and up and down each street of this living museum of time and people and buildings. Horse and buggies are far less dangerous to a bicyclist than a car. It was quite relaxing. We found the tourist center and hoped that we could talk them into passes to get into some of the buildings.

They really only give the passes to the press, we were told. I tried to explain that we have hundreds of thousands looking online and it will hopefully increase to millions as our journey unfolds, but no joy. Oh well, we could still ride by the buildings. And that we did! We also found there is a free bus (with a bike rack) that will take you to Jamestown.

Hopping on board we road to the 400 year old place. There is an eight mile loop you can do around the island and we rode our bicycles around there. We didn't actually go in and visit the site for two reasons. The first being TIME...we never have enough. The second being bicycle chains. There was a place to leave the bikes, but would they be there when we came out? We can't chance losing our bicycles. We were also told that we couldn't take any photos if they were going to be published online, so it sort of put a damper on the visit. The bus ride and the bicycle ride were both great, we just wish we could have gotten a peek inside the gates. I suppose it gives us a good reason to come back again when we finish our journey.

When we got back to Williamsburg, we road around again. The sights and sounds are always changing and it did feel fantastic riding without the trailers. I had a little dream about what if we actually had a support vehicle that could carry our gear and we wouldn't have to pull our hundred-pound trailers that stop us in our tracks if there is a wind. Remember, it's FREE to dream and sometimes dreams do come true. Our adventure is proof of that! Who knows, a support vehicle MIGHT happen.

We had been given a list of places to eat in Williamsburg and I tried phoning some to see if we could perhaps have a restaurant sponsor us for our last evening. Dreams DO come true and Kristy at *Seasons Restaurant* said to come in and be their guests for our dinner. Delicious is a word that doesn't even begin to describe it. Now remember, even though we usually are eating cans of tuna, we still really enjoy the taste of them. They do get a bit old and tired, but we are happy for any food and exercise actually makes it taste better. The food at the *Seasons Restaurant* was simply divine. The service was incredible, even though they were quite busy, it was so fast and friendly. The setting was lovely with gas lights, candles on the tables and a real nice feel to it. Even though it was tempting, we were way too full for dessert, when our waitress asked. We have been known to split a dessert now and again, but we really didn't have any room to spare.

After dinner we took the most relaxing walk. We strolled through the old town for one last time, then headed into the grounds of *William and Mary College*. Talk about famous alumni...Thomas Jefferson went here! It is laid out in such a lovely way, with huge trees, brick buildings everywhere and the blooms all around the campus were in full swing. We watched squirrels run and play, watched the sun starting to set and then strolled back to our lovely B&B. Speaking of nature, I almost forgot to tell you WHAT we saw in the back garden at *The Cedars*. Now remember, this is just right across the street from the college. It is nestled between two churches and has been a B&B since the 1930's. Charming, comfortable, romantic and hideaway are a few words that spring to mind when you try to describe it. As remote as it feels, it is very much in the town. Just steps outside your front door is all of Williamsburg at your feet. But when you walk into their magical back garden, towards the inviting gazebo that is filled with comfortable furniture, something very special might happen to you. This is what happened to Morton and I. Right before we went to have our dinner, we had taken the laptop to the gazebo. I wanted to check my email, catch up on a few things and enjoy the beauty of this garden, that is bordered by woods. As we were sitting there, I heard something behind me in the woods. It sounded like footsteps and turning to look, I was right. More to the point, instead of footsteps, they were hoof-steps. There was a herd of deer, over a dozen, that had walked and ran into the lower part of the woods. Morton jumped to get the camera. They were just standing there, huge, still and so beautiful. Morton tried his best and if you look closely in the one picture, you can spot three of them. We were both really still because we just wanted to watch. In the distance a dog barked and the spell was broken. The deer all turned and ran back the way they had came. Morton and I were stunned to see a sight like this. Of all the lovely things we had seen today, this was the most unique. I would have never imagined that deer come in that close to civilization, but there they were. As we were walking back to *The Cedars*, I thought about the deer we had seen. Where do they live? What do they eat? There was really quite a little herd of them and hopefully they are all street savvy and keep to the woods. People were walking in to the churches on either side of *The Cedars*. Morton and I went into the breakfast room and played a few games of dominoes and then Morton wanted to get the laundry done before leaving in the morning. If you are within driving distance of Williamsburg, you have to come and stay here. Make sure you leave enough time to sit in the gazebo, be still and have a little rest and you might get lucky and see the deer.

Day 88: March 29, 2007 - Thursday - *The Cedars* Williamsburg to Saluda, Virginia

Imagine the distance of 30 miles. Picture a place you are familiar with. Do you think you could ride a bicycle to it? Today we had 30 miles in mind for our ride. Since we didn't want to backtrack, we took advantage of the free bus that would take us and our bicycles to Yorktown. Then we would have a little ride around, cross the bridge and continue north. It is an excellent way to get around the Historic Triangle of Williamsburg, Jamestown and Yorktown.

Morton and I were the only people on the bus. It's early in the season and fairly early in the day. The bikes on the rack on front of the bus and the trailers snugged inside, we sit and enjoy the view. The driver is friendly and has done a little chitting and chatting, but it is mostly a quiet ride. Something starts to scare me as I think of riding inland... the hills. We are going over some gentle ones now, easily climbed in the bus, but on bicycle it is a different cup of green tea. Especially pulling our heavy trailers. When the bus lets us off at the National Park Service entrance to the historic battlefield. Morton waits with the bicycles and chats to someone that had seen us on the television. I went inside to have a look at the map and use the bathroom.

Yorktown is really pretty, houses line the wide streets. Flowers are blooming everywhere. The grass in the lawns is bright green and very lush. We don't have time to do anything really except take a few photos and head for 17 North. We cross a bridge over the York River. There is a toll on the other side, but first a steep climb, which I make without stopping! You have no idea how hard this is or how great it feels to do. I get ahead of Morton and beat him to the tollbooth. I pull over and wait (he was taking pictures) and I glance down. There is a dollar bill laying beside the concrete wall. Picking it up, I hold it up to the tollbooth person. *"Finders Keepers"* she shouts over to me. *Wow!* I cross the bridge and get a dollar. I still have to go through the tollbooth and saw that motorcycles were 85 cents (I think) so I assume the buck will pay the toll. Looking behind to see where Morton is, I see something else. There is *another* dollar blown against the wall. I pick it up, hold it up for the tollbooth lady who is sitting almost across from me, where she gives me the thumbs up along with a grin. Now I really scan the area, but there is nothing else. Just Morton coming up to me. I hand him the notes and tell him that we can use them to pay our toll. With me in the lead, we cover the few feet that gets us to the tollbooth lady. She says, *"No charge for bikes"* and waves us through. What a great bridge to go over! When I asked Morton what was taking him so long, he had stopped to pick up 3 quarters and a two dimes. We almost wanted to cross back again to try our luck, but we kept going north. Our bicycles would now help us work off the excellent breakfast we had at *The Cedars*. They list their recipes online and I suggest making yourself some of their treats, you will love them. We came across a strip mall with a Chinese restaurant around lunchtime. Taking our money from the lucky bridge, we order a lunch special for $3.25 and split it. The food is good and even with splitting it, it is almost too much. I can't believe that I use to each this much on my own PLUS get an egg roll with it. Even though in both our pasts we would have never thought of splitting a meal like this, now it is habit. Riding through the lovely countryside, the names of areas were far and few between. There were a few signs for campgrounds and I thought about telling Bob at *The Cedars*, that now Morton and I were ruined. The tent would feel hideous after the lovely four poster bed. We missed saying goodbye to Grace, but our biggest *THANK YOU* goes out to the both of them for letting us stay at their lovely bed and breakfast.

When we hit the split for Business 17 to Saluda, we had to turn in. The campgrounds we were counting on were not open yet and the sun was going to do it's nightly disappearing act. There were a few businesses that we stopped in to ask about what was on the road in front of us. A spa, a retirement center and a mini market all gave no joy. There are two churches and we try to find a phone number, but again...no joy. Spotting the Sheriff's office, we venture in and I pick up the phone to talk to a dispatcher. The kind lady listens (it's a VERY good thing there are so many kind people in this world!) and then asks me to just hold on a bit. She takes the time to make several phone calls. Before long, we get the green light that we can camp right outside the office door!

Two deputies arrive and show us where to set up the tent, talk just for a bit and then are off on a call. There is bathrooms inside we are invited to use and we couldn't ask for anything more. Talk about a very safe place to sleep. Since we were riding uphill and against the wind ALL DAY, I was worn out. We made our bed up and I fell asleep within just a few minutes. I hoped I wouldn't snore too loud that the police would think that someone was being murdered in the tent.

Day 89: March 30, 2007 - Friday - Saluda To Tappahannock, Virginia

HAPPY BIRTHDAY MOM!!! I LOVE YOU :) We woke up early, before 6 am, but just talked about the day ahead. We knew it would be too early to pack the tent up because of the moisture, we have to wait for the sun. It was so cold we could see our breath and when we unzipped the tent and I got outside I couldn't believe my eyes. The tent was covered in a thick frost! When we got out and went inside, the same dispatcher, who had gotten off at 6 am, had waited around to see if we wanted a ride to the fire station to get showers! What a wonderful lady. It told you she was kind. There was also another dispatcher (another KIND person) who was there and soon we were all chatting away. They had to get to work and to bed and we needed to get riding, so as Morton tore down the frosty tent, I did a bit of updating on the website.

We had a clue that Sarah & Graeme might be coming down for a day this weekend. We have had our fingers and toes crossed. Sarah called to say for sure that they were coming. I was riding on air now. Sure my knees were aching and my hands were freezing, but Sarah was coming. It didn't matter that we were cold, tired, sore and hungry...I was going to get my homesickness cured for a wee while anyway. Her brother wouldn't be able to come along though. I was disappointed, but maybe next weekend. It seems like it has been years instead of months, that I have seen him. Focusing on all the good stuff, I just kept going.

There were hills, gentle and rather steep. I managed to get up them all. Then the phone rang again. It was Sarah saying that they were all coming. Four family members...Sarah and Graeme were going to treat us to a motel and it just doesn't get any better than this. Hopefully my son will be able to see that I really have been losing weight. We ride hard to get to the motel where we will all be meeting in Tappahannock. I want to make sure that I have time to get all my computer things done and there is another job I have to do before they get here. On the way to the room that Sarah has arranged, we are busy riding up a little hill when we hear a siren behind us. Surely we can't be speeding! Looking over my shoulder I can't believe that we are being pulled over by a police car. I shout to Morton that it is probably one of the officers we met last night. The man that parked his patrol car and then walked up to us was a stranger. I was smiling as he told me that this was a stupid place to be riding a bicycle. He was very stern with us, almost angry that we were on the edge of the road. Now up until a half a mile ago, there was actually a shoulder to this road. Right at this point though, there was none. Just a mere six inches and then the grass, which is impossible to ride on. He said he wasn't worried about us, but rather the cars that might get into an accident because of us. He said again that it was stupid to ride a bike on this road.

Trying to remain very positive and upbeat, I asked him how long the road lasted with no edge to it. I pointed out that we had just lost the edge a bit back. I also pointed out that this wasn't a road that bicycles were prohibited on and there really wasn't any other road we could be on. The officer said that there was no edge for miles. Told us to hurry and get off the road and then left. Within a half a mile we had the edge back and road in comfort to the room. I guess he never paid attention to the edge of the road.

When we spot the motel we go inside, get checked in and I set to work. There are so many things to be done before my family arrives, I want to just focus on them. I have clothes that I need to send home with them. These are things that had been tight on me and are now falling off. Plus, if I lighten the load on the trailer, the hills will be a lot easier. The pile is really tall. Four pair of pants will not work anymore and some things I never wear. It feels so good to get them out of my bag. The email I check is incredible. You are all writing the most terrific email, asking questions that really make me think and your words of encouragement are something that I just can't tell you how good it feels.

So with the computer work done, we are ready for our visit, we are going to explore tomorrow and do a bit of filming with a television station. We are also going to love every second of it and be thankful for family time!

Day 90: March 31, 2007 - Saturday - Tappahannock, Virginia

What a wonderful weekend. Perhaps the shortest in my life, but wonderful all the same. The company made it perfection. Our whole little group hit the streets and had a good walk around the town, down to the very interesting and free museum and down to the river. The town is filled with antique shops, friendly people and lovely historic buildings.

In the museum, we met another Priscilla, who phoned the newspaper to come and do a story on us. It was set up to meet back at the museum on Sunday morning, as we would be taking off with all our bikes, trailer and gear. It still seemed very far away on this Saturday afternoon and I tried not to think about the leaving part.

Seeing my son and his wife was so fantastic. It had been since Christmas that we were all together the last time. Three months and quite a few pounds ago. Time is going so fast out here, I know when I blink my eyes it will all just be a wonderful memory. Morton and I really do talk about that and how we need to just enjoy every second of this. Good, bad or ugly, we need to live in the moment. That was what today was all about. We did really nothing, but had a spectacular time doing it. We all lounged around (Sarah is having problems with her feet swelling if she's on them too much from being pregnant) in our room and talked about everything...well, most of us.

You know how Morton finds things beside the road? And the next part is, how he picks them up? A few days ago he stopped behind me and when he caught up he said, "I just got a gift for James". Now remember, for our anniversary, Morton gave me a tennis ball he had found for on my kickstand. The idea of the tennis ball is one he saw in Key West. People put them on their bicycles kickstand to stop it from sinking into the sand. My mind wondered for just a second about what he might have picked up for my son. "What is it?" I finally asked. Morton told me it was a video game for the computer. I groaned and told him to quit picking up trash. This is the man who asked in the Florida Keys if we could collect all the bottles that have a 5 cent deposit on them for Maine. True, we could have made several thousand dollars this way, but we would need several tractor-trailer trailers to carry them all. "It's in a case, it's fine, James will love it!" Morton fired off back at me. I recall all the little bits and pieces that he has found that have actually came in handy. The only reason his pedal is still hanging on to his bike is a bit of copper wire he found and shaped into a ring that worked as a washer. Maybe Morton was right.

To get ready for our low budget visit, we walked to the local store and bought 6 frozen dinners for 98 cents each. Morton stuck them in the refrigerator and made up some pink lemonade with the mix he had gotten. Given that gas prices are so crazy, I knew that they were already spending a fair amount of money to come see us, then getting our room on top of it, the 98 cent meals seemed very unfair. I can only say it is too bad that my daughter doesn't like computer games. Morton made the biggest hit with his "found" present that James spent almost the entire time playing it. It was alright though, he had twisted his ankle earlier when we were walking to the shops across the road. He was running to catch up with us and just misjudged a footstep. Over went the ankle and up came the swelling. Morton also pulled out a compression bandage from our huge medical kit. Mari and I squeezed his size 13 foot into it while he rested on his stomach, still playing the game. It was an easy and laugh filled day. I did a rare thing and had a 30 minute nap with my daughter while the room was filled with familiar voices talking about everything. I only woke up when I heard kids screaming and it turned out to be the yells from the computer children riding the rollercoaster on the video game Morton had found. We all felt like it was something that we do every day. In the past, it was. Our little group of six, seven counting Max the dog, were all home in the motel room. For a brief moment in time, my world, my family, were with us. This is all that matters in our lives, the people we know and love make it all worth living.

Sarah and Graeme headed for their room about nine. She does get very tired and needs her rest. We had all gotten up quite early and my eyes were getting heavy.
Morton had the good sense to switch the television off and for one last night, I slept with a smile on my face, knowing that my children were just a few steps away. You might say that instead of the empty nest syndrome, I have the empty tent syndrome. I miss them so much when they are not here. Talking on the phone is good, but it can't hug you.

Day 91: April 1, 2007 - Sunday - Tappahannock to near King George, VA

We had the tough task of saying our "Cheerios" this morning. It was lucky we had a big and challenging ride ahead of us, we had to keep focused on the road.

After meeting with the reporter outside the museum, we gave our hugs goodbye and are going to try to get together in the Baltimore area next weekend, if all goes right. They tooted and waved as they passed us and then called back to us on the phone to give us a report on the road ahead. This is a rare luxury of knowledge that we don't usually have. We usually ride totally blind.

All day long the sky looked like it could rain anytime. We were on 17 and had a really good edge to the road that kept us safe from traffic. There were bits of the road where we lost it, but it usually was good.

The only trouble was the hills. So many hills. Hills you wouldn't even notice in a car, but I managed to pedal over most of them. When I reached a few I couldn't make it to the top on, I got off and pushed, leaning on my bicycle. When we got to the town of Port Royal, we turned right on to 301 north. The sky just started to spit raindrops on us. We pulled into an overhang on a business and put our tarps on. The family had driven up this way to locate 3 possible churches for us to stay at. Sarah had even gotten the phone numbers for two of them. The trouble was, no one was home or answering their phones, so we had to keep riding.

Consulting our Virginia state map, we spotted a little gray road that might shave some time off. It was marked 607 and on the map looked straight and lovely. It would save a few miles and with any luck, we just might make it to the bigger town of Falmouth. The twists and turns were not the worst thing on this road. In fairness, it is a lovely drive and if we wouldn't have been worrying about the sun dropping out of the sky, it would have been a peaceful ride. Hardly any traffic, lovely things to look at, but the hills. They were very steep both down and up. Morton commented that it reminded him of Scotland. I think a bit of that might have been the way the sky looked too. Like rain could happen at any second. There were three or four hills that I could only get halfway up the other side of. They were just too tall and my knee has been sore since my fall down in the Outer Banks. I didn't want to hurt it, so I pushed the bike and heavy trailer uphill. Consulting the map again, I made a scary discovery. Maybe the straight line on the road was further ahead. Maybe we were on the little twisting road, just below it, that didn't take us to Route 3, but actually went west for miles and miles putting us out almost in Falmouth. There was nothing to do but keep going. Our speed was horrible because of the turns, hills and the pushing really slowed us down. We thought we might have about an hour left of decent riding. We both were looking at the woods to see if there were any places that we could sneak in and camp. We really don't want to do this though, it would be dangerous. There were signs of civilization coming up ahead. Through the fields and trees we could both make out a busy road ahead. This had to be our Route 3, which means we were on the right road. Whoever drew the map just made the line straight instead of putting all the 90 degree turns in it.

The tall steeple of a church had began to peek out at us and Morton and I soon came to the stop sign where turning left would take us to the town, still a few miles (maybe 12) away...or we could go right to the church. We decided to give ourselves time to get the tent up in daylight, we should head towards the steeple. Still under construction, we figured they wouldn't be having a night service. Instead we poked and investigated for numbers looking for someone who might be able to tell us that we could stay. We found the number of Ed, who was most helpful, invited us to stay inside and said we could even charge our phone up!

Morton and I set about getting our bed set up in what would become their main chapel, when the phone rang. It was Ed's wife, who had just made chili and offered to bring some out for us. A hot meal after the ride we had today sounded great, plus Morton and I both love chili and company. Two couples arrived not long after and they showed us to another part of the church. This part had heat in it and power. There Morton and I ate the delicious chili while our little group chatted. Lady, the fluffy dog, sat quietly at our feet and I couldn't think of a nicer place to stay for the night. When they had left, Morton and I slid three tables together. One of the guys had suggested sleeping on them to keep warmer and to make it more comfortable. It worked. It was very comfortable and we stayed nice and warm all night long. Sleep was very easy. The combination of the challenge of the hills, the weather and then the warm food and safe feeling, was just too much. I fell asleep within minutes as the rain was falling outside.

Day 92: April 2, 2007 - Monday - near King George to Stafford, Virginia

Waking up on a platform of tables was a bit unusual, but I didn't fall off. We didn't get as early of a start as we wanted today. We checked email and had things that we had to take care of before leaving the church. The men we had met before had came by and we got to get a picture of them with Morton and say thanks again, then set off. The weather was warm, the road was wide enough for us and we had an easy travel (minus a few hills) over Route 3. Morton and I were really excited, because we knew where we are sleeping tonight. There is a lady and her husband, who have invited us to stay the night. After a few email exchanges, the arrangements were made so we needed to get up the road.

We did lots of water drinking and before we knew it, our bellies were growling and we stopped at a farmers' gate to have our lunch. Spreading the tarp on the ground, we shared our dollar bag of tuna and finished two bottles of water. I could have laid on my back and watched the fluffy clouds floating over our heads. But we needed to ride, so climbing on the bikes we pushed off into traffic. My front tire sunk down and I jumped off the bike. It was flat and I didn't want to damage the wheel. Morton went to work and found this tiny wire that had found it's way into the tire. He was going to swap out the tire for one of our new ones that are suppose to be puncture resistant.

We ride and sweat and my mind thinks, just a few days ago I was wishing for spring, now here is summer in full bloom. The breeze is blowing in our faces but it's warm. I put on sunscreen over my arms, face and neck that just seem to be getting darker by the second. I also have the oddest tan lines on the planet.

Before we know it, we are at a split where 3 goes two different ways. I call the lady we are going to be staying with tonight and get her advice on which way we should go. I also let her know where we are and when we should be up in her area. There is a very busy junction she has told us about and suggests coming out to pick us up, rather then chance rush hour traffic coming home from Washington DC. She tells me that traffic is horrible then and there is no edge at all to the road.

Listening to locals is the smartest thing that we can do on our journey, so I say that we will call when we get there. As we are looking for US 1, we go up and down some BIG hills. The biggest we have ever been on so far, but just wee ant hills compared to what we have to go on later. We enjoy the sights and sounds, ride past George Washington's childhood home and talk between the traffic noise about the history in this area. Just amazing. There were a few hills where we had to push the bikes up them. The road was too narrow for us to take the chance of sitting on the edge of. This is deadly as you are coming over a hill. With cars going 50 to 60 miles an hour, we have no chance when the pass the top of a hill and head down on the edge. We even push down some hills because of the edge of the road, or lack of the edge of the road. My knee is so sore from the walking on a slant all day. The heat also has my hands and feet swelling and I wonder if it adds to the soreness of the knees.

We were within range of where the couple live that we were staying with. I called and we decided where the best place to meet was. Morton and I pushed and rode along, then were passed and tooted at by the couple. All our gear fit into the van and we set off back to one of the best evenings on our adventure.

In several emails, I had suggested Morton could make mince and tatties. This is a Scottish dish that is one of my favorite meals. Simple, cheap and Morton had ate it until it came out of his ears as a child. Now we were both starving for this dish. We got to chop and cook, me really just peeling the "tatties" or potatoes. The best part was the blether we had with this wonderful couple. They had been to Scotland and we talked until about 1:30 am about everything under the sun. It was just the best evening and we could have sat up until dawn talking. These are people that we feel so comfortable with and would like to visit longer. Hopefully, when our journey is over, we are all going to get together in Scotland. It would be excellent to show them all these places that Morton and I love and they didn't get a chance to see.

Morton and I were both a bit homesick for Scotland as we went up to what was one of the most comfy beds we have ever slept in. I hope that we actually CAN get together after the journey in Scotland. There is actually several HUGE places that you can rent by the week over there, maybe we should get 12 to 20 couples together for a LittleChanges tour of Scotland! Anyone interested?

Day 93: April 3, 2007 - Tuesday - Stafford, Virginia to Harrisburg, Pa

One of the things about the trip that we are LOVING...are the people we are meeting. You are all amazing and wonderful. Today we woke up in the home of two stars of our journey. They offered to take us to breakfast and then see us off on our way. We all could have talked for ages and had a great time at breakfast that was over too soon. We headed to a spot on the road where we unloaded our gear. They took us past the construction spot that was really a bit scary. It was good to have a lift past this potential hazard in the road, with no edge whatsoever. Morton and I said our goodbyes, crossed our fingers we would all get together again (for more than just a few hours!) and will always remember this couple as "friends". When we had been loading up, Susan handed Morton two 35mm film canisters and told him it was for our laundry. He said thanks, then discovered they were filled with quarters. He thought it was laundry detergent. He was over the moon with the quarters and kept going on about how the film canisters were a brilliant idea. He also reminded me that he had found one of these canisters that he wanted to pick up by the road to store his nuts and bolts in that he finds. We went down a hill and the edge of the road seemed to be holding up. We were crossing our fingers that traffic would be kind to us as we make our way into Washington D.C.

A phone call from Sarah changed our day. We needed to get up the road QUICK to get Morton to Philadelphia about his green card. Since he is Scottish, he has been going through the immigration process since June 2006. He is on the final leg of being allowed to stay in the USA, but we needed to get to Philadelphia like yesterday. We were calling to see if we could get a ride to my daughters, where all our paperwork is, but everyone was either working or had no car that would carry us and our gear.

Sarah found a car rental place that we talked to and they gave us a great rate and even brought the car out to us, just one mile south of Quantico. The gear fit in and we were headed north before we even really had time to comprehend this curve ball on our journey. My son and his wife have a spare room that we were going to stay in. Sarah and Graeme were picking his brother up from Scotland, who was going to be staying in their spare room, but we would all hopefully get to visit a few hours before we hit the bikes again. As I drove north on US 1, Morton and I were so glad we were in a car. The edge went away and the traffic was so busy. Why oh why can't there be edges on all the roads? Bike paths beside the roads would be better, but we would settle for a lovely little edge and I'm sure the car drivers would appreciate it too.

My mind went over everything that I needed to do while I was in the Harrisburg area. We can see my mom and say a late *HAPPY BIRTHDAY*. My driver's license needed renewed before May, so I might as well do that. We have also been wanting to have two banners made for our trailers in BRIGHT orange and I know a 24 hour sign shop in the area, there is a television station in our hometown area that wanted to catch up with us, so we might as well stay for the Easter weekend and get everything done that we need doing. I had talked to my sister on the phone and found out that she is going to be going to Cape May, New Jersey next weekend. We discuss catching a ride there with her, avoiding Washington DC and Baltimore and the traffic and roads. According to the map, we should have went that way, but we didn't want to miss the press in the big cities that were inland. We would have to talk about this and see what we were going to do.

Morton slept as I drove and it all felt like a weird dream. I was watching the mile markers fly past as I got closer to our destination. My mom's house was on our way, so we decided to stop in for a very fast visit. We still needed to get the car rental back to Harrisburg. We pulled into the drive and her car wasn't there. We were not sure if mom would be in, but went up on to the porch anyway. We could see the television on and mom was sitting in her spot, watching the news. I knocked and pushed the door open, singing happy late birthday. Mom was startled and so surprised to see us. She wasn't expecting us and started to cry. It was lots of hugging and just a quick five minute visit for now. We needed to get on our way to return the car, but said we would visit her tomorrow when we got back from Philadelphia and the immigration office. It was something that I have done thousands of times, waving goodbye in the driveway, but it felt like it had been a million years since I had done this. Mom looked GREAT, walked out to the porch and waved bye to us...we headed onto James and Mari's house. I telephoned Mari to tell her we were moments away and James had just gotten off of work. He had no clue that we were about a mile away.

We pulled to the stop sign at a t-junction and on the road in front of us, heading to their home, was my son. He was smiling and looked right at me, but didn't really recognize me. We pulled out behind him and he slowed down to about 5 mph as he starred in the rear view mirror. He turned into their neighborhood and we followed him. He still had his eyes glued on the mirror. He later told me that he thought he was seeing things. After all, there I was in a strange car when I was suppose to be on my bicycle hundreds of miles away. We got big hugs as we got out of the parked rental car. My son was asking why we were there, looking very shocked and I think half-afraid that something bad had happened. He was happy to hear that we were here for just a moment and we were both alright.

The sun was still shining on their lush green lawn, tulips were just getting ready to bloom and we got the grand tour of their new home for the first time. It is LOVELY! We stored our bikes and trailers in their shed and set off to take the car back. This was going to take us right by Sarah's house, where we were going to stop to pick up an air mattress to sleep on in the spare bedroom. What a day! Our night ended with loads of hugs, back at James and Mari's watching the first 5 minutes of *"Happy Feet"* before falling asleep. Morton and I both slept through the entire movie, then woke up to say good night and headed into bed. Our sleeping bags and pillows were set out and as we snuggled down, Morton said, "This mattress would be brilliant for in the tent". I was going to argue that it would be too heavy to put in our trailer, but I was too sleepy.

This had been a bizarre day and just the mental strain of it had taken it's toll on me. I was out for the count. Just as I was really getting into the sleep, Max came along in the room and hopped on the air mattress between Morton and I. We fell asleep with the furry little dog who had ducked under the sleeping bag and found his way to our feet. I hope that I'm not just dreaming.

Little Changes　　　**135**　　　*Priscilla Houliston*

Day 94: April 4, 2007 - Wednesday - Harrisburg, Pennsylvania

We are loving the family feeling, but missing the road. You know how they say, "The grass is always greener", true statement. This morning we woke up warm and dry with the sound of the rain pelting the roof and windows. It was great to be "home" with my son and his wife for a wee while. We had so many things to take care of today that were really boring, wait in line, get on hold, press 6 to speak to a live person, kind of day! At the end of all our needed work, we did get to spend some quality time with our family. When my son came home from work we all shared a meal together then headed off to my mom's house. It was going to be a short visit, so we could get back for him to get ice on his bruised ankle. Standing all day at his work doesn't do it any good, plus he has to get up early for work, but time slips away when you are catching up on the last three months of your life. My mom was happy to have a house that was full of family, then we said our good-nights and came back.

We decided that we can do all of our press in Baltimore, plus combine it into a "Must See City" stop. Morton and I have done a fantastic walk with *American Diabetes* there last fall and want to catch up with some people we met as well. Thursday we are going to catch up with one of the very first reporters who did a story on us, *Carrie Fairchild, with Channel 8, WGAL TV* from Lancaster. The forecast is calling for snow showers, so it is a LONG way from our 80 degree temps we were just bicycling in.

Day 95: April 5, 2007 - Thursday - Dillsburg, Pennsylvania

We woke up this morning to snow flurries. Cold wind was telling us that is was NOT a day for bicy-cling, but there were still lots of things to get done. We are only going to be around our family for a few more days and have to make the most of our wee stop!

The phone kept ringing all day and the good thing was, by 2 pm we had done two newspapers interviews, a television interview with WGAL, Channel 8, set up our television schedule for Baltimore and felt like it had been several days rolled into one! The weather stayed cold ALL day, we rode for just a bit for the filming, but my neck and throat are killing me. I had several cups of HOT chocolate to try to stave off sickness and took two aspirins. It might sound odd, but I have this dull ache in my jaw that I hope isn't a tooth ache. I didn't even think about not seeing the dentist for our two year journey. I suppose we will have to go to places along the way for dental and medical care, if needed.

Our little bit of riding in the snow was enough for us and the next time we get together with Carrie from Channel 8, it will hopefully be WARM. Just think, the other day we were getting ready to have heat strokes. Now snow flurries...the groundhog must have fibbed about spring coming. Of course we are excited about our weekend in Baltimore. Morton and I have been there several times before and fingers crossed, it looks like we might have a place to stay there. The weather has turned so cold that the thought of putting the tent up and sleeping on the ground is making my head spin, but things always work out.

Day 96: April 6, 2007 - Friday - Dillsburg, Pennsylvania To Baltimore, MD

Today Morton and I are going to have more car riding then we have had in the last three months com-bined. We have to drive to Baltimore, spend the day, drive back tomorrow & then REPEAT on Sunday. The reason for all this motoring instead of bicycling is because we don't have a place to STAY over in Baltimore and we want to spend as much time as we can with our family while we are right here. There is also a lot of press that we are doing in Baltimore that we will do along with our city walking.

Last fall we went on a great walk with American Diabetes Association, but today we stuck more to the Inner Harbor. This is a great city to walk in. There are so many things to see inside and out, that you will never get bored. Your feet might get sore, but you won't be bored. We met up with Sarah, Graeme and Martin. Martin is Graemes' brother who is over visiting from St. Andrews, Scotland. So as we were in our little group, there were 3 Americans and 4 Scots. We were outnumbered! It was fantastic though and we walked, talked, met people that have been following the site *(THANK YOU to those of you who came out!)* and did some video tap-ing and even had some professional photography done of us.

Even though we were all a bit chilly, walking and talking really warms you up. There is this horrible thing that happens called "TIME" and before we knew it, our day had flew by. Some of our highlights of Balti-more included *The USS Constellation* : James, Morton, Graeme & Martin explored and had a blast "literally" on this historic vessel.   306 The whole group went to the *Science Center* and played as if we were children again...some more than others (this would be Morton & James!) *Top of the World on the Trade Center*...what a view. Window shopped in the two great retail stores right on the Harbor. James wanted *EVERYTHING* in the Discovery store! Walked, walked and even did 8 flights of stairs....then walked some more.

After we all had an amazing day, we parted company and James, Mari, Morton and I got in the car for the ride back to Dillsburg. It's not really a long ride, but I fell asleep anyway. Max was at home, waiting in his big indoor cage. He was happy to see us and we all spent the evening talking and enjoying our time together.

Day 97: April 7, 2007 - Saturday - Dillsburg, Pennsylvania To Baltimore, MD

This was a **RED LETTER** day! It would have ONLY been better if Sarah, Graeme and Martin had been along with us. We left James & Mari's house *EARLY*, Max in his cage (don't worry, it's REALLY big and they put his water, soft cuddly bed and snacks for him) we head out for the day. We drive a different root and it takes me past a house I had lived in with my family as a child, the elementary school I had went to and sadly, the cemetery where my dad, brother, son-in-law, cousin, grandmother and grandfather are all buried. I am tempted to stop in, but we really do have to go. I will make it a point to go on Easter. They are all missed and all loved, but today I will not dwell on the fact they aren't here anymore. I will remember a smile from them and change the subject in my mind.

The sun is shining and in the car it's hard to tell what the weather is, unless I touch the window. I'm not sure if it's getting the extra weight off or it's just that it is that cold, but I'm freezing. Since Baltimore is not far away, we are there and parking before I know it. When you visit, shop around by having a bit of a drive for the best parking rate. There are many places to park and you need to plan on spending $20.00-ish to do so for the whole day. James and Mari not only got the gas going back and forth, they got the parking too. We couldn't have the weekend working the way it is without their help and assistance. Some times we take help from family for granted, but I really can't stress enough of how my children, sisters and nephew in Canada, have all helped me. The best part is that they barely think I'm crazy at all! After we park, we head to a dollar special early lunch. We know we are meeting up with a reporter at noon and the weather is so cold, we are all feeling peckish from the pancakes that seemed to be days ago now. The waterfront at the Inner Harbor is really a sight to see. The colors, reflections of odd angled buildings on the water, the movement of the water that holds various ships, boats and even bright green and purple, Loch Ness monster looking boats, all makes for the feeling of a very special event happening. This is a place that I would bring my children as they were growing up to walk, look in shops, visit dolphins and just enjoy.

Today I'm walking with my son and his wife, of course Morton, but also a very special treat. Cindy, a regular visitor to the website, has braved the weather and came out to meet us with her husband. We all meet up at the old wooden ship, *USS Constellation*, chatting and hugs passing around, until our cameraman arrives. We do the easiest interview ever, just talking like you would with your friends that popped over for a surprise visit. Cindy has gotten a pair of MBT's and has worn them (they are perfect for walking!) and she's brought along a permanent marker. This lovely lady wants Morton and I to sign her shoes! How incredible is that? We are flattered beyond belief and it is just the most dazzling feeling in the world to meet someone who is moved by what we are doing.

An hour or so flies by as we walk, chat and get filmed. We need to head off for a sightseeing that we are going to take in today and say our goodbyes to the reporter, Brad. There is time for a few pictures and I suggest Morton and I are supplied "Helmet Cams" if they want to catch some incredible footage. Each day we see things that are gone before we can get to the camera, good and bad. Cindy and her husband are heading back to their home in Pennsylvania and we walk off around the water. We parted ways in the shadow of the World Trade Center in Baltimore. A lovely building that has an observation platform where Morton had taken amazing pictures at the day before.

Everyone had agreed the *Maritime Museum* is something that we should see. Or should I say, sea? Sorry, my attempt at a pun, where there was none. We had looked on the map and knew it must be close to the aquarium, I just couldn't remember seeing it. A sign soon told us that this museum WASN'T in a building, but floating on the water right in front of our noses. It consists of a light ship, the *Chesapeake*, a submarine, the *Torsk*, a coast guard vessel and a lighthouse that I have always wanted to go inside. Best of all, you can get a pass to get you into all of them. This might be the best bargain in the city. We however, thanks to Anthony at the *Visitors Center*, had passes for these four parts of history, and boarded the light ship. Think of it as a floating light house. One of the things that I had just talked to the reporter about was all the things that I am able to do again that I hadn't been able to do for years. I spoke of using the regular bathroom when we were out instead of the larger handicapped ones. I wouldn't really fit in the regular ones before, now I can. We spoke of fitting into chairs better, putting on shoes and I even touched my toes for him...something that would have been out of the question last year at this time. Another thing that I'm discovering as I lose weight, I feel more confident to go out and DO things. Being in public isn't the shame that it once was. People aren't pointing and nudging their friends to have a look at the 400 plus-pound fatty. I am also happy about things that might have seemed like the impossible dream just a year ago. Climbing down the stairs to go below deck on the *Chesapeake* was one of these small achievements. First, I was able to manage, up and down and exploring this brilliant floating museum, second, I never got out of breath or tired. Just out enjoying my life. Oh exercise, why did I wait so long to pay attention to you? The real treat came as we were climbing through the hatches that are the doors that are on the 300 foot submarine. Even though I wasn't able to spring like a bunny through them the way that Mari could, I did FIT and manage all of them. A year ago I would have NEVER been doing this. It would have been an impossible task. Morton would have gone on and just showed me the pictures. I would have felt bad about myself and so upset I would have eaten whatever I could get my hands on. Comfort food, I think they call it. The truth of the matter is that it doesn't comfort us at all, only adds layers of fat to the problem. We just had time to see the two vessels when we had to head back to a tour on the *Baltimore Duck*. This is something you all have to do. Picture this, a big boat, part bus, past military vehicle, that not only gives you a city tour, but then drives right into the water to show you a duck's eye view of the city while you are bobbing along. Brilliant! When we collected our tickets at the booth (make your reservations EARLY, this sells out) they also handed us yellowish-orange bills on a bright green cord that we could blow in and make duck noises. Oh and did we! The four of us stood there trying to talk in duck, sing in duck and were merrily waiting on our duck billed chariot to arrive.

Since the weather was now spitting down snow, we decided to wait the 15 minutes inside the *Discovery* store. James could really live in one of these stores. He loves gadgets and even though he is an adult, he loves to try out all the toys. He and Morton were going to have a battle with electronic dragons, but they were both sorely disappointed when previous "children" had left the batteries flat. I took a few more pictures of this amazing pink poodle, Fifi, who was a bicycle, float and sculpture, parked outside the store. It looked natural sitting there and I was wondering what the rest of the entries had looked like. I also wondered if Morton and I would be able to build something like this to bicycle around on. No car or truck would say they didn't see us then! Walking back to the red tulips and yellow daffodils, flocked with pansies, we joined the others and climbed on board the *"Duck"* for the ride of a lifetime. It was a real hoot, or a quack. Our guide was a captain who first showed us the city. I learned things I never knew before, saw places that I wanted to visit and then, we were passing through *Little Italy, Fell's Point* and passing through a gate that took us to the water.

Driving into the water in a tour bus feeling vehicle is a bit odd to say the least. It was a very cold day and I didn't want to think about the life vests the captain had showed us how to fasten. Hopefully the craft was seaworthy. Fingers crossed and camera snapping, we were followed in the water by three real ducks. Talk about your special effects! This is the kind of stuff you just have to smile at. The view of the city from the water is just breath-taking. The afternoon light had the buildings glowing as we drove on the water. The wind was blocked by clear vinyl and it also added a filter to the camera that looked great as we were reviewing the photos later. Even though the tour was about 90 minutes, time flew by and we were soon dropped off back at the Visitors Center. We were all chilly and there stood *Phillips Seafood*, looking so very tempting. We decided to go have our dinner and then allow time for a good walk afterwards.

If I had unlimited amounts of time and space on here to write it all, I would describe this meal in great detail. There is seafood and then there is *Phillips Seafood*. It is just head and shoulders above the rest. They have several ways in Inner Harbor to taste their wares. You can have a buffet, which we did yesterday with our big group for lunch, they have a take-away service, which we didn't try, then there is the crown jewel of the spot across from the *Visitors Center*. Walking inside, a man is playing the piano and singing quite well. We are shown to a table with a million dollar view of the golden sun bathing all the buildings along the water. The waitress is lovely, explains the difference between a Chesapeake crab cake and a Ocean City crab cake. We opted for the Chesapeake's and fell madly in love. Little did we know, after the meal when the waitress brought around the dessert tray, there would be a wedding! Now I know what you might be thinking... *"Priscilla, you are on a diet, you are trying to lose weight...WHY ARE YOU LOOKING AT DESSERT TRAYS???"* But this is where the *Little Changes* comes in to play. We ARE getting dessert. I am going to have sweet and lovely things. The difference is, MODERATION and time and place. This isn't something that happens every day. Plus, we are going to have a nice long walk afterwards. No more will I eat a tub of ice cream, bag of potato chips, a whole pie and then drag myself off to bed. I will eat things that are delicious and decadent, but I will also do the work to keep the weight off. Don't worry...my mind has finally seen the light, my body has no choice but to follow. Back to the dessert tray...which, we were all talking afterwards and it would be nice to have "sliver" selections. You could try a thin slice of various lovely things, almost like a sampler platter.

Morton, James and I all got something different. Mari decided to have a cup of tea and just a bite of ours. That is why she is so fit. The platter arrived with our desserts on them. It was love at first sight for the newly married James. He quickly announced that the cheesecake was so good that he would marry it if he could. He held the plate up, looked at it lovingly and said, *"I do!"* Morton and I cracked up.

When we left *Phillips*, we were all enchanted with the clever projector game that had children waiting in line to stomp on the floor. Morton and James wanted to give it a go, but we all needed to walk. Leaving the waterfront, we crossed the road and started to explore this bit of sculpture you can walk through. It is a series of waterfalls, sculptures, flowers, various levels and all with the water from the harbor on one side and the city all around the other. There were a few signs here and there that said *"No Swimming"* and I could see why they would need them. There were waterfalls that you could walk behind, water that flowed at different speeds for various effects and this whole area was free to explore. We spent a good twenty minutes looking at all the clever aspects and the pure art of the work, then headed off to see the inside of a building that had captured Mari's attention yesterday. It is a large glass covered building that houses a mall and several other aspects of commerce. The mall was just beautiful. We weren't there to shop though, just look and in get in out of the cold to have a walk around. We went the whole way to the top and walked in and out of stores. Don't discount the benefits of mall walking. The trick is to not buy and remember you are there for the exercise. If you are a compulsive shopper, make sure you leave your credit cards and dosh at home! We really like to walk in a mall. The temperature isn't a problem and come rain, sleet or snow, you can always count on the surfaces for being very walkable.

After a few hours we made our way back to the garage and headed out of town. The lights in the evening in this magical city are as pretty as the sun dancing on the skyline during the day. We all agree that we need to come back here at the end of our journey and spend a few weeks seeing all the things that we don't have time for now.

Tonight as we drove back I managed to stay awake and talk. We really don't know if tomorrow night will be our last with James and Mari before we head off. We had been waiting on a phone call to see if we need to go BACK to Philadelphia.

Day 98: April 8, 2007 - Sunday - Dillsburg To Gettysburg To Dillsburg

Today was a FIRST since the journey began. My camera only took two pictures. Yes, that is right...just two for the entire day. They were of Graeme and his brother Martin walking off to go for a hike in Gettysburg. It was really a family day and just a quiet day in. I spent minimal time on the computer, although Sarah and James will tell you a different story, played a video game with them (something I never do) and it all felt like normal. Right now I just want to get through Morton and his seemingly never-ending saga on the quest for immigration. If we need to go to Philadelphia again, no problem...we just NEED to know what to do!

Today I designed a banner for over our trailers and we found a company that will have them to us by Wednesday. The forecast calls for the same cold weather the rest of the week and even though we need to get moving, we are thinking about making Saturday our jump off day. This all depends on what happens with Philadelphia. UGH...we both hate the not knowing! On Monday we can make calls, bug people and see if it is safe to set off again. We were lucky we were this close to Philadelphia and could do this, but what if we would have been out in Wyoming or Texas? If we have learned anything so far from our journey though, it is to roll with whatever punches that life chucks at us. No one has any chocolate today and I breathe a sigh of relief. I do not want to sit around and eat all day and manage to get through the day alright. My stomach is a bit iffy and Morton, Mari and I sit up until after midnight talking. I know I have to head to bed, but then once getting there, I'm wide awake. I am anxious to get moving again.

Day 99: April 9, 2007 - Monday - Dillsburg, Pennsylvania

An early shower started my day off. It was great but towards the end I started to get dizzy. Turning the water off and grabbing a towel, my head was spinning. I staggered into the room that Morton and I are staying in. As I fell back on to the bed my head swam and I asked Morton to get me something to be sick in. Thank goodness I wasn't, but he had a bucket at the ready for me. For the entire day I would feel this queasy feeling if I would stand up too quick, slight fever and really bad stomach cramps. My legs were really sore as well and believe it or not, as I was horizontal on Mari's soft leather sofa, I was doing legs lifts and stretches. The big wooden coffee table was pulled close and I worked with two fingers on the computer answering emails, arranging several interviews (that I will hopefully be alive for!) and spoke with my mom. I felt bad about not going out to see her, we wanted to ride our bikes the 10 miles or so to her house. But not today. I tried to sleep, but I have this thing about daylight. If the sun is up, so am I. My head was hot and then cold and clammy.

Morton learned, that at least for now, he doesn't have to go back to the immigration office in Philadelphia. Nothing is keeping us here now, we could ride tomorrow, on our 100th day, if my body is willing. We think things through logically. We still have a list of things we have to get done while we are in Central Pennsylvania. After all, we won't be back for nearly two years. Consulting a map we look at Washington DC and my body gives a bit of a shudder. I'm not sure if it is the sickness I have or the memories of the road. It had seemed like a good idea to leave our lovely coastlines and come in to our capitol, but in actuality, it was one horrible ride. Don't get me wrong, I love Washington DC, the thought of the tempting blossoms were almost worth the risk of riding on roads that were only made for cars and trucks.

My finger runs east from Washington DC and lands on Cape May, NJ. My sister is driving there on Saturday and has offered us a ride. I look at the little lines on the map that wiggle and squiggle from where we are right at this moment, back towards the coast. If I wouldn't know these roads, I would want to just cycle back to where we left off on our pit stop in Pennsylvania. The hills don't bother me. If they are too steep, we just push. There is a lot to be said for just riding down a road that we have no clue of what lies in front of us on. These familiar roads worry me. I remember no edges, construction and other things that are all obstacles when you are on a bicycle. We talk about the weather as well. It isn't bad riding in the cold. After all, 10 minutes on the bicycle and we are ready to take off our coats usually. While we are here we aren't spending any money. We aren't worrying about where we are going to sleep. We have electricity. We are also both missing our journey....bad.

Remember a few weeks ago when I was oh so homesick? It is really odd as to what a visit home can do for you. It fills you up with all this love and support and now I feel like I won't even have a twang of the homesickness for at least two or three days after we take off. Wanting to get our plans in place for when we are actually taking off (my sick tummy rumbles) we decide that Sunday, April 15 (tax time) is when we will begin riding again. Until then we want to ride our bikes to Harrisburg. See a few politicians at the capital building, do a few interviews from local press and SEE THE DENTIST! I don't fancy the idea of Morton having to dooberize my sore tooth in the middle of the woods in Maine when the pain is too much to take.

This stop has taught me a valuable lesson that I'm going to share with you...When you just sit still, your body gets hungry. Mine has wanted *more* food then when I am riding the bicycle for 7 or 8 hours a day. Remember this...it is why exercise is so important. It actually *CURBS* your appetite. We have also drank far less water while we are in the pit stop. Our bodies still *NEED* the water, we just aren't drinking it like we had been on the road. Max and I stay home after dinner, while the rest of them go to do the grocery shopping. I'm still not feeling well enough to manage a trip out to the store. Good thing Mari is an RN and has been helping Morton play nurse to me all day. I'm a quiet patient though. Give me a bag to be sick in, a bottle of water and a few animal crackers and that is me sorted! Access to the computer is always a plus too. While waiting for the group to come home, Max lays on my feet and keeps them warm. I have to figure out a way to dog-nap him and bring him out with us. My son couldn't live without his fuzzy little pup though. I'll just have to keep wearing socks to sleep in. I work and wait for them. It is 10 pm, then 11 pm, then midnight. When should I start to worry? You know the feeling, we imagine the worst and are then glad when it doesn't happen. I try to never do that much anymore though. There have been too many real tragedies in our lives that I don't need to worry about things that haven't happened. The music is playing enough to mute out the arrival of the car. Max jumps and barks his little head off when he finally hears it. In they come with all the "messages" (what they call the shopping in Britain) and they also have my nephew along with them. It is so good to see him that I give him a big bear hug without even thinking about passing my germs on to him.

They had all ran in to each other, talked and shopped at a store until the wee hours. Morton loves looking down each and every aisle, still fascinated with all the different American items on the shelves. Well, maybe not *MADE* in America, but you know what I mean. We talked for a while, with James heading off to bed first. He had to get up for work in just 5 hours, but then, he's just 24...so he can do that. I had to say good night as well, hugging Danny again (sorry if I made you sick!) and it felt great to lay down for real. Resting on a sofa isn't just the same thing. When I fall asleep I'm thinking about the road ahead. We will start riding on our big trip on Sunday, but if I feel better, tomorrow I will ride out to visit with my mom. Hopefully the germ fairy will come tonight and take away my bug, perhaps she will even bring her toothy friend along and I won't need to see the dentist.

Day 100: April 10, 2007 - Tuesday - Dillsburg, Pennsylvania
Feeling so much better after my lay-down day on Mari's sofa, I was all ready and raring to go this morning. Up early and tackling the computer, we had a lot of email. Usually with the harsh schedule of the ride, I just have

time to skim through, send a few lines and then save them in a special folder marked, "Well wishes" to be used for future reference. As I started reading all the positive things *YOU* write to us, I decided to share them with the world. You see, *YOU* are all inspiring us just as much, if not more, then we inspire you.

One of my emails was a proof of the banners that Barry at *Signs Now* in Hanover, is making for us. The banners are going to be so wonderful, but the one picture, a huge life-size vision of me in my bathing suit, is a bit hard to take. For the second time I have to make this picture huge to cut it out. My arms are so big, lots of folds and wrinkles in them. My legs, bare for the world to see, are like tree trunks filled with cottage cheese. My knees are almost invisible, hidden by the fat. This was all the night before our journey began. New Year's Eve, 2006, is one I will never forget. This image is one that will be a part of me forever. This image is also one that I never want to forget. Having it in full color on a life sized banner that will be shown to the world is terrifying, but it must be done. When I tell you that I am 100 plus pounds lighter and you look at me, you will still see that I'm almost 200 pounds overweight. This can be frustrating when I'm trying to make a point about little changes and people are just looking at me, not knowing how big I had been. Thinking about this banner is something that I had on my mind all day. It would come and go. I would get panic sessions now and then, *is this the right thing to do?* I dread even putting the bathing suit on in the room, let alone go global with it. It might bring harsh comments from people who just think I was a greedy pig that ate myself that way. I wonder if that is all there is to it. Could it be that simple, pure greed? I don't think so. Back to the computer, we set up appointments, touch bases that need touching and finally head off to visit my mom. Stepping in to her house I feel like I have never left. There are so many things there that remind me of my dad, it almost felt like he could just come walking in from the garden, his straw hat in his hand. But today isn't a day for gardening. It's a little cold for that. Instead we visit and catch up on the last three months. I know that our visit will be over before we know it. Mom has a special request to go for a walk up to the garden with me. My sister is on the phone with business as mom and I make our way off her front porch. Mom has really came far with her walking. She still uses her walker, but is getting so much stronger. Being away I can see a marked difference in her progress since her stroke in May 2006.

The path beside their pond is one that my mom and dad would walk each morning together. Mom got sad and we cried and hugged, missing my dad. She said she thought about moving, getting somewhere smaller. Easier to take care of. Dad passed away just two days before their 56th anniversary. We approach the garden. This was the real heart and soul of my father. He loved his pond with his fish that were more like pets then possible food. He did a lot of "catch and release", actually so much that I think he must have had names for all of them. The garden was guarded by a scarecrow dad had made last spring. As we got closer to it, my mom said, "It's his shirt." Dad had given the scarecrow the shirt off his back in exchange for scaring off the crows that wanted to dine on his corn. Raspberries need trimmed back, there is a fresh patch of dirt that has been turned over. Mom explains that my son, James, had done it a few months ago. It makes me miss dad more then ever. Our walk down memory lane was setting off all sorts of memories, all including my father. We kept each other cheered up as we talked and walked. I took pictures, gave mom lots of hugs and wished I had the time to help clean up all the limbs that had came down around the property during the winter. There are lots of friends and family looking in on mom but I still feel so guilty about being away from her.

With a twinkle in her eye that reminds me of her mother, mom tells me that when she is able to walk better, she will come and join Morton and I on the journey. I have no doubt in my mind that she will be able to come out and join us for bits and pieces of it. She is a strong lady.

Morton had been out with Mari, she's getting use to driving on the right side of the road. They knew that I wanted a visit with my mom and it just worked out that way. They pulled in just as mom and I gotten back to the porch. Climbing in the back seat of the car, I rolled the window down and stuck my arm out waving like mad. Tomorrow mom has a big day with doctors and a sleep study so I won't see her for two days. She is on the porch and waving and I feel like the worst daughter in the world as we pull out the driveway. Today has been a real rollercoaster of emotions. I was all worried about people seeing the BIG picture of me and lost sight of the much bigger picture. We are on this journey to wake up ourselves and the world that *exercise* is the magic pill. What I look like in a bathing suit at just under 400 pounds should be shocking. All our struggles, fears, soreness and hardships that we face while we are bicycling on this beautiful journey, are now in focus. There is nothing out there in front of us that is going to be as tough as what my mom had gone through over this last year. If she can do it, so can we.

Turning my thoughts back to the computer, when we arrive back to Mari and James' house, your words take me far away from today. I am focused again on the ride. The task that is in front of us is burning stronger then the feeling that I need to be with my mom and the rest of the family. They all want us to be doing what we are doing, just like you. I looked at the words that you have all been kind enough to write to us. There are thousands of the emails now, tucked away in our file. We are really not worthy of getting so much affection and support from total strangers. When we send you emails back and tell you thank you for your support and well wishes, we mean it.

April 11, 2007 - Wednesday - Dillsburg, Harrisburg, Camp Hill, PA

Morton and I parted ways today. He stayed at the house, while I rode with my daughter to her baby doctor appointment. She is 25 weeks now and can't wait for the big day to come. I knew this would be a special event. This is my little baby who is all grown up now, getting ready to have her own little baby. She and I are fiercely close and it's been hard missing so many of her firsts, I try not to think about all the firsts I will miss on their son. They have promised to come and visit us on the trail as well as to take loads of video. When we walked back to go to the room, the first stop was the scale. Oh how the memories hit me. This is the part I would dread, go into a cold sweat over and would be the real reason my heart would be racing and blood pressure soaring, when we would go a bit deeper into the visit. Remembering how I felt, I stood well back to give Sarah her privacy. The nurse wrote the number down and Sarah headed out of the room. I asked the nurse if I could step on the scales. Her jaw fell to her chest and her eyebrows met her hairline. I was the first person that had ever asked this question, she told me.

Stepping on I smiled. It IS working, the numbers are falling! This was Sarah's day and I didn't want to start talking about the journey we are on. It has a way of becoming the center of the conversation. I kept quiet and Sarah spoke up about my adventure and my weight loss. The nurse had the same reaction that everyone else has...disbelief & a bit of shock! She took Sarah's blood pressure and all was normal. Promised to have a look at the site, she left us alone in the room. It was finally all sinking in to me that my little girl was going to be a mommy. I know she really is 25, but in my mind she is just a baby herself. The doctor came in and was really fantastic. Even though we didn't get to see a sonogram, she did press the heartbeat detector, with a speaker on it, on my little grandson. His heartbeat is 147. Normal. I smile again...I now have a resting heartbeat of 52. Better than normal for me.

The appointment is over and Sarah is driving us back to her work, where she is letting me borrow her car to keep some appointments I have and to renew (finally) my drivers license. My phone just keeps ringing today and it is fantastic. We are really getting so many connections, work processed and the weather has been horrible, justifying our Pennsylvania pit stop. The drivers license place was a breeze. I recall the early days when it was crammed in a building downtown with no parking and lines that looked like they were selling the latest "must-have" toy on a Christmas list. You would wait for what seemed an eternity, only to come to a window to find you were at the wrong window, didn't have the right form and needed to start at square one again. But not today. Now the building has a huge parking lot with a man selling hot dogs. Inside there is a central desk that issues a number and dozens of windows, no lines, seats to sit and wait to see your number come up and before I could say "Speeding ticket" my number was up on the screen. There, in light speed (computers are delightful) I was issued a card to take to the photo room, near the exit. Again, entering, you get handed a slip with a number. Mine was 100. Walking towards a seat, it was called. The person that handed me the slip, pointed me to the counter where the man was seated to take my picture. I handed him the license that was going to expire at the end of May, signed my name, sat in the seat and smiled. The image comes up on the screen. It is just a so-so picture. I was expecting to see an image of Cindy Crawford. Instead I saw her older, fatter, big sister or aunt. Hey, we both have dark hair and a mole. I can dream can't I? The man says that he can take the picture again if I want. Jeesh, is it that bad? He must have seen the disappointment in my face. I really rarely see a picture of me that I like. There might be three out of my adult life that I can tolerate. I told him there was no need for a second photo, that is as good as it was going to get, for today anyway. He told me to take a seat and he'd have it right up. Just as I sat and started to chat a bit to Martin and Graeme, who were with me, the license was ready.

When I saw the two pictures, the one that had been taken in February 2006 and the one taken today, I broke out in a big grin. My big, giant cheeks are getting smaller. The head size was the exact same, but my face is much narrower. My chins are fading. It doesn't matter that I'm not as pretty as Cindy Crawford, I have a resting heartbeat of 52 and my drivers license picture is getting better with time.

The guys were dropping me off at a local mall. I'm meeting someone who is doing a story on us at the first mall that we started walking in. Being inside, it seems like just five minutes ago I was here and thrilled that I could finally walk three miles in a row. That was a real milestone for me and a moment of sheer joy.

After my meeting, I was going to walk. I was going for a donated massage from *Massage Therapy Associates* in Camp Hill. This would be my first massage since Savannah. A walk before the reward was in order. This is my home stomping grounds. I spent my childhood, youth and most of my adult life here. I have only lived in Scotland for several years, but I took a wrong turn and ended up being lost, on foot. Finally, too embarrassed to call for walking directions, I phoned Sarah. She looked online and told me which way I needed to go. I needed to have the exercise, so it was actually a bit of luck that I had made the wrong turn.

Even with my wrong turn, I still arrived about an hour early. I was hoping for someone to call me back from a local television station to come for a bit of a story. There are so many issues to be touched upon with massage therapy that would work in perfect with our journey. Beth, the owner and Karen, my therapist, couldn't have been nicer. We talked for ages about so many issues such as people being shy to get a massage. I know that in Scotland, where I had my first massage, I was so nervous about someone seeing my body. This is a fear that you *HAVE* to get over. If you never had a massage before, a proper massage, you need to do this for yourself. If you are in the area, come along to see Beth & Karen. You will thank me for it. Climbing on to the warmed bed, I wished that I could freeze this feeling in time. The blankets were so soft and warm. This was going to be my first *"Full Body Massage"* which I have always wanted, but have been too shy to go for. In Scotland I just had shoulders, neck, head, arms and once, legs. Today I was going to relax and enjoy this.

Karen began with my neck. I was on my back as she worked sheer magic over me. Miles and miles of tension just melted. I was silent and totally relaxed as my arms, legs, shoulders, and finally my back, were not just massaged, but this real feeling of rejuvenation was passed along. It was one of the most relaxing experiences in my life. They had offered a massage for Morton, but he didn't want to. He is nervous. Never having a massage before, seeing it as something only women do, he made excuses about wanting to work on the bikes. Maybe next time. When the massage is over, Beth has left two bottles of lotion for me that will go right into our medicine bag. We will come back here again in July we want to visit again. Karen gave me a bottle of water to drink and we said our goodbyes. I really wanted to ask her how she fancied being on a bicycle for two years and coming along with us. She is an expert as well as an incredible person.

Walking outside, the air had turned cold. Rain was coming down and my sunny walk to get there was now going to be a wet experience. My phone rang and it was my son-in-law, Graeme. He was just 1 minute away from me, offering to give me a lift to my next appointment. Joy!

So many things had happened today, phone calls from a magazine that want us to write our own story in 800 words, with pictures, that will be seen by millions of people, various press people catching up on where we are and then this oasis of well-being with the fabulous massage I just had. I slid into their back seat and wanted to just curl up and go asleep. There is still another set of pictures to be taken and then, a very surprise meeting. Actually two!

For the past several months, I have been getting the most incredible emails from a physical education specialist, Cindy. Today, after a volley of phone calls, we arrange to meet after school. She is bringing an associate and her daughter and we are meeting in a fast food spot. I have a quick bite (healthy as well) to eat before they arrive. These ladies are just BRILLIANT! We meet, talk for ages and brainstorm. We are going to meet again and hopefully work together to change the world. Don't laugh, we are going to do it. We need your help too, but we will fill you in later on all of that. Tonight they have to dash along and so do I. As they are leaving the fast food bit, in walks a friend of mine that I haven't seen for about six years. We were both shocked! We hug, talk fast and exchange emails. We promise to get together the next time I come back to town. Jeannie looks fantastic and I regret not having been quicker in thinking to get a picture of my friend. Next time.

It has been an incredible day and I still need to figure out how to get back to my son's house. Then the phone rings...or vibrates. It is my son telling me he's not picking me up. My daughter is. The plans for the evening had been changed and I just will just have a short walk before Sarah arrives. When my girl gets there I think of how lucky I am. I started my day with her smiling face and get to end it with the same. We have a quick peek around the baby department of the store that she has met me at. The outfits, blankets, crib sheets all mix together to make me feel very nostalgic about where the last 25 years have gone. Time doesn't fly, it travels at light speed. My shape and body really went south when I had my daughter. I tend to think of my body, "BC" --- before children and then the downward spiral. We walk and my knees don't click. My ankles aren't sore as we trek around the store. I am going to be alive to see my grandson in a few months, as long as the cars see me.

April 12, 2007 - Thursday - Dillsburg, Hershey, Pennsylvania

Being in Pennsylvania has been so very refreshing, resting, exciting and perfect. Even though the road is calling louder and louder to us each morning, this pit stop has been delightful.

Morton had said no to a massage offered by Beth at *Massage Therapy Associates*. Now this had NOTHING to do with their massages...they are perhaps some of the best in the whole wide world. You see, Morton was *SCARED* to try something new. He stayed home with the excuse of working on the bicycles...which he did do. We had a phone call from the people at *The Spa at Hershey* offering for us to come in, the very next day after my delightful massage from Karen at *Massage Therapy*. There were things there like a steam room, aromatherapy room, rainfall showers, chocolate baths and I couldn't say no...I am only human. Morton had seen how relaxed and wonderful I was feeling after my massage with Karen. He asked all the questions that a person who has *NEVER* had a massage before might ask. The biggest...what do I wear? Morton is modest. He is also breaking out of the normal comfort zones of his life and trying new things. We are more alive now than we have ever been...if he wasn't going to try a massage now, what could I do to convince him it would be the most enjoyable experience? Hmmmm...I turned to my friend and daily companion, the internet. Pulling up the page for *The Spa in Hershey*, he was able to see things. His roadblock still was the fact that he felt this was a "girls only" experience! He couldn't be further from the truth. The real factor though, I will always believe, that made him step out of his manly man comfort zone was the words....*Chocolate Massage*. Morton has loved our visits in the past to Hershey. He loves to ride the roller coasters, taste the chocolate and I think this whole Chocolate Town really has his attention. He couldn't say no, but as we were driving there he was so very nervous. I tried to remember the first time I had a massage and see if there was anything I could tell him to make him just relax and enjoy it. My big hang up had been my body. I hated to look at it, let alone have a *STRANGER* not just look at it, but *TOUCH* it! This was a worse thought than strutting up and down the street in a bathing suit. But my back was so sore and we had went with friends to a "Race Night" in a little village called Carrington, in Scotland. One of the prizes that night was a massage. Someone sitting at our table had won it, didn't want it and gave me the voucher! The person doing the massage actually came to your home with her table. Now I was nervous, this I promise you...but I had always wanted a massage. I was almost 40 at the time and it had been way too long to not have one. The health benefits of massage are proven and I think they should all be something that we do on a regular basis. The car got closer to Hershey and I shared with Morton some of the fears I had. He wasn't crying or clutching the door handle, but he was nervous.

When we stepped onto the brick path under the canopy, we could see the swimming pool and hot tubs through the massive glass windows. We wouldn't be doing these since we didn't bring our bathing suits. Things felt normal to him as we walked into the hall that led to the check in desk of the spa. It didn't seem out of the ordinary of what our life has been like these past three plus months, entering hotels, motels, campgrounds and all sorts of different places. The second we stepped into The Spa, I knew he would be fine. We had a brief sheet to fill out, were then taken to the changing rooms, there is one for men and one for women, then given the tour. Morton will have to tell you about what happened with him, I can only tell you about the women's side. A warm robe (I really would love to have a robe like this someday) that was a double layered robe (see the pictures) was given. This is a nervous spot for me. Would it fit? Would it wrap around my bulk? Then shoes were given out. My fat foot would hopefully fit, again...a needless nervous bit. The friendly girl gave me a tour of the changing area, lockers, showers, steam room, where all the bottled water is kept, all the goodies you can use while you are there and then left me to get changed, to meet up in a sitting area with plush chairs. Now for the moment of truth. Behind the curtain I am ever hopeful as I change into the robe. It fits! With room to spare.

The robe is so soft and lovely I could just enjoy the time sitting in it, happy the belt went around me. The shoes were slip ons and I have NEVER ever, ever, been able to just slide my foot in something like this. Not since I was a child anyway. Today, being another lucky day, my glass slipper was a perfect fit. They have real give in their wide strap across the top, so that was a help, but my feet ARE getting smaller. Not by length, but by width. Even WWW shoes were hard for me to wear. Could it be when I lose the rest of my weight that I will be able to finally shoe shop like normal people?

Going upstairs on the stunning staircase, there are huge windows that look out over the countryside and landscaped garden. All the people I see are in the same robe or are staff. It is very relaxed and calm. I hope Morton is doing alright. There are several rooms that you can just rest in while you wait for your person that is doing your treatment to come and collect you. The one I chose had a roaring fireplace, stunning views, delightful furniture, bowls of *Hershey Kisses*. Don't get me wrong, it just wasn't chocolate on offer. There was a whole array of fruits, baked goods, cold bottled water, coffee and tea of every description with proper china and the best, hands-down...hot chocolate I have ever tasted. Not wanting to have anything to eat before my treatment, I had a little walk around. Morton was just coming up the stairs and looked somewhat relaxed.

Being out in a robe in front of strangers was going to be tough for him...but he was coping nicely. We went into the room with the fireplace together to wait. This part is 100% true, no matter WHAT Morton might tell you. I didn't want to have anything before the treatment. I could say no to the little temptations around. I took a single *Hershey's Kiss* and that would have done me. But Morton...yes, Morton, got a cup of the hot chocolate and a slice of this nut bread. "Just have a wee taste" he cooed, holding the cup out to me. I do love hot chocolate. This was unbelievable. I don't know if they will sell the mix. I imagine this doesn't come from a powder. It was so creamy, delicious, just the right amount of chocolate...and I fell in love. As James wanted to marry his cheesecake in Baltimore, I thought about getting a job in this place JUST to have the hot chocolate near me. Thank goodness the person coming to collect me for my treatment came into the room and said my name. Now it was time for me to get nervous. I wasn't expecting, nor have I ever had, a male massage therapist. Yikes! Too late to panic or think. I gave Morton his delicious cup back and said bye, trotting off with this massage man.

Â Â Â Â Â Â The Spa is really busy, but it doesn't feel overcrowded. There are people we pass on the way to the treatment room and before I know it, I'm in the room, he is outside and I'm climbing on to the bed after shedding my robe. Every time I have ever had a massage I do a little chit chat. Today I rambled on and on. I have to apologize to this therapist. I know I was the most talkative person he must have ever had...but I was nervous, at first anyway. There is absolutely *NO DIFFERENCE* between the male and female therapist. It felt quite normal after the first two minutes and we did have a constructive talk about the journey we are on. I left feeling like I had no bones in me, from how relaxed I was, saying goodbye and back in the room with the hot chocolate waiting on Morton. The 50 minutes for the therapy had gone by in about 5 seconds of sheer bliss.

Â Â Â Â Â Â Morton came walking in just a minute or two behind me. The two chairs that faced the fire were free and we sat down with our bottles of water. He was talking to me about how his therapist was from Alaska. Morton said he really enjoyed it and it was so different from what he expected. I had just had a very unique experience. Never in my life have I had two totally different experiences like this, within two days. Both massages, both so very different and both so perfect and wonderful. I am pampered and spoiled beyond hope. My mind started thinking about how I could compare these two treatments, both donated by generous and caring places of well-being. Then I figured, I don't have to. Try this out for yourself. Totally different and totally perfect.

Â Â Â Â Â Â We could have lounged about this place of sheer luxury all day, but we were meeting a reporter that we have been working with since last autumn. After a bit in the steam room, a shower and saying thanks to the people that helped make this experience happen, we headed out to the car. James and Mari had left us borrow theirs. It was odd coming out of a place together and not looking for the bicycles.

Â Â Â Â Â Â Just as we got back to the house I had time to return a call from a newsperson in Washington DC. The NBC station there wants to do an interview, so we rethink our plans. We decide we will jump off from Washington DC, this will mean we are only 30 minutes north of where we left the road at. We can ride almost due east until we come to the Atlantic Ocean, turn left...and there we are! Sometimes things just work out right.

Â Â Â Â Â Â Morton gets our bicycles out of their shed and we head off, minus our trailers, to meet with Tim Pratt, from the *Hanover Evening Sun*. We have spoken many times on the telephone, but have never met. I'm looking forward to this. The bike ride feels so normal, but without the trailer, a bit odd. We arrive a the meeting point and have a fantastic interview. Tim is really different because he actually knows all about the journey. He reads the site and he is able to ask me the questions that aren't really explained. I know the article will be really good and their photographer is meeting us tomorrow morning to photograph us with our giant banner of me in a bathing suit. Saying goodbye and hoping that Tim can convince his paper to let him come out on the trail with us, we part ways. The importance of the press goes without saying on this journey. Reporters like Tim actually make it happen.

Â Â Â Â Â Â Morton and I ride back, having sat out a rainstorm as the interview was happening, the roads are wet and cold. I wonder where spring is. The fat robins grabbing the worms from the grass, thanks to the rain, are signs that it *SHOULD* be here. Walking in Mari & James' place, we are met with the delightful smell of a warm meal. Mari has made us a lovely dinner and after the massage, the second one in two days...the warm food, the bicycle ride and I am ready to go to sleep. There are things that I have to get done with the website. Now I actually have a deadline as well for an article that I am doing for a magazine. But the blow-up bed is calling me. This stop is getting down to the wire and we all know we only have a few more nights together. The cold wind is howling outside the window and I'm so thankful that we are inside and not facing the elements tonight. I'm approaching 44 and for at least 30 years I thought it was my destiny to sit on the sidelines and be the fat person out. I even got insulted once when someone compared me to being "fatty in the corner" but it was true.

I needed something drastic and BIG to happen to get me moving. Let me tell you, riding a bicycle thousands of miles is not only going to change *my* life, but it can change *yours* too. If you are the person who feels beyond hope, I'm here to tell you as living, breathing proof, there is *HOPE* and you CAN do this. Make this your day to start little changes.

April 13, 2007 - Friday - Dillsburg, Hanover, Harrisburg, Pennsylvania

The nervous feeling in my stomach today grew as we got closer to Hanover. I was excited to see this life-size banner of me in a bathing suit, then it dawned on me...the sight of me in a bathing suit on a little picture that is glowing on my computer screen is enough to make my belly flip, what would a 5'8" picture of me do? Mari, Morton and I pulled into *Signs Now* and my heart started to race. At least if I pass out, Mari is an R.N. and Morton has his first aid certificate, I thought. My face was red and hot. Thank goodness the air was cold outside the car and made me feel a bit better. Stepping inside the store, I got to meet Barry, who is the owner and made these banners for us. His wife and daughter were there, as well as Adam, who was the person who printed the life-sized me.

Apologizing to Adam for having to put us with a life sized version of a very fat me, we all have a little laugh. Even though it might be funny, I'm sure he's traumatized beyond belief, but he doesn't show it. He's a professional. Just as we are chatting a bit, the photographer from the *Hanover Evening Sun* arrives. He seems like a nice man, but I focus on the camera. Oh, the camera! Not only did he have one, two of our supporters from off of the site have came along to add moral support! It was great having them there, but I still felt very sick to my stomach from what I knew was waiting rolled up in the box. Barry was very kind. The first banner he pulled out was bright green and LOVELY! It says LittleChanges.com in GIANT letters and we will use this whenever we stop anywhere. Look for it beside the road as we are eating, talking, resting or taking a break. We want to let all the cars and trucks whizzing by know what we are up to! Everyone likes this banner. I love this banner. But I know what is waiting. Please remember that I *hate* being in my bating suit. Someone from this site once told me that she can't understand why men's bathing suits come to their knees and yet women's are cut sky high! Her wise words were sounding in my head, along with my heartbeat as Barry pulled the banner out. As horrible as the picture is, it is me. There is no airbrushing here. Just 343.5 pounds of me. A quick unroll of the vinyl banner and there I stood, in a bathing suit, in a room of strangers, with cameras flashing. This, without one doubt, was the most embarrassing situation of my life, with no one to blame but me for it happening. I gained the weight, I decided to do this journey, I asked Barry to make the banner and I had even ASKED the reporter to have the photographer come along for this. Now I didn't know if I could keep from breaking down
.   The reality of this banner was a real shock to my system. The tears were swelling up in my eyes and I was afraid I was going to cry like a baby. Always being the happy one, I covered my feelings as an expert liar can do and looked at the bright side of the moment. First, I'm doing something about this weight on my body. Second, there are people, real people, who care enough to watch us each and every day. There are also two lovely ladies standing here who cared enough to drive 50 minutes and 1 hours and 20 minutes to see us! Sigh....what a rollercoaster of emotion. It was the best of days, it was the worst of days, but I was alive to witness and be a part of it all. Any day I'm breathing is the best day of my life. This banner is something that I will keep until the day I die. I will never forget what had happened to me down to overeating and *NOT EXERCISING!* Moving is the key people...this is something that I never understood before. When I finally decided to quit making excuses and started moving, the most wonderful things began to happen in my life. After the banners had been put away and our deep thank you's had been said, we all decided to stop to get a drink and have a chat before leaving. It was really fun and as the five of us sat around a table at a fast-food place, I felt like the luckiest person in the world. Lucky to be alive. Lucky to be aware. Lucky to be one of the few people who get a chance to live their dream. It happens too fast and we all say our goodbyes. On our way home, Mari, Morton and I agree that we need to get something together in the form of a "meet up of littlechanges" for August, when we are back for Sarah & Graeme's baby.

The rest of the day I'm feeling a bit more relaxed. The trauma is over from the banner. Plus, we met my mom and sister for a late lunch. This was a real treat and again, as always, time flew by, never to be recaptured or ours again. James got off work EARLY today, so we all decide to go in to Sarah and Graeme's house. This is the first time we will actually have visited them since we have been in Pennsylvania. It is really odd, we have been busier this past week then when we are on the bikes! We need to get back on the road so I can have a rest! There were some things Sarah had stored for me and one is a bag of clothing my sister had given me years ago. Nothing had fit, too small.

Just for the heck of it, I thought I would try some of the clothing that NEVER fit me before. Most of them are sizes 18 to 22. Most of my clothing I wore at my biggest was the largest I could find, size 32 women's plus size, even then I had to be careful of the cut. Only the biggest and baggiest would go over my arms or around my waist. Tonight my heart soared. I pulled on a pair of size 22 jeans that my legs would not even THINK about fitting in just a year ago. Tonight, yes...tonight, they slid right on, somewhat loose (not baggy) and I could have faced 1,000 big banners of giant me's in bathing suits. The banner is a spectacular reminder of what was, never to be again. Joy, joy and pure joy! Sarah and I had a fashion show in the kitchen and I tried on lots of different outfits. Sarah was kind enough to snap some pictures, as we giggled into the night. It feels brilliant to wear sizes I haven't seen for decades.

My day of peaks and valleys is drawing to a close and I finish it up by flopping on Sarah's bed and talking for an hour about everything from baby to banners. I'm in the size 22 jeans and feel like anything is possible. Hey, if it feels this good at a size 22, imagine how I'm going to feel when I slide into a pair of size tens! In the morning we are going to NYC for a bit of the day....photos....maybe I'll wear these jeans. :)

April 14, 2007 - Saturday - Harrisburg, New York City, NY, Dillsburg, PA

The days of sleeping anywhere have begun again! We find ourselves waking up on Sarah's comfy sofa, the pair of us! Morton has taken the chaise part of it, I have the two cushion side. Our heads were jammed together on the pillows, cozy like, but a bit sore! Morton was covered with one blanket, I was inside a mummy-style sleeping bag that fit! They never have done before, they've felt like they had been strangling me, but last night I slept snug as a bug in a rug. We are up at 6 am for Morton to use Sarah & Graeme's telephone to call Scotland. They have a great free calling plan for it. Since the UK is five hours ahead, no one will mind getting a phone call at 6 am on a Saturday. Morton heads to the kitchen where his voice will hopefully NOT carry up the stairs to wake everyone else up. The first call is to his parents. He tells them what we have been up to, where we are and that we are heading off in the morning. They tell him they are going to Venice and I think about my missed gondola ride. Hopefully I'll get the chance to have a do-over some day. This conversation goes right into similar with his brothers, then on to other family and friends all across the Atlantic. I had told Morton to ask first if they read the website, because why bother telling them about places we have been and people we have met if they already know it!

Everyone in the house gets up and starts getting ready for the day. I guess you could say the light went on over all of their heads. Sarah had to stay home, friends afternoon party to go to, Morton had to go to the *Pedal Pusher* bicycle shop on Walnut Street in Harrisburg to borrow a tool to fix his bike (something specialized and actually, Ted at the bike shop was kind enough to do it for him! *THANK YOU TED!*) then he was going to bicycle back through Harrisburg to Sarah. Graeme, his brother Martin and I, were off to NYC. It was a whirlwind stop for photos before going to the airport to get Martin back to Scotland. The day was great for everyone and ended with Morton and I going back to James and Mari's place to spend our final night with the family. It felt like an evening to stay up all night, but my big car trip had me exhausted. Plus, I have another one to look forward to tomorrow, when we load our gear in the trunks of two cars and head for Washington D.C. and the lovely *Watergate Hotel*.

As sad as I'm going to be to leave my family, I will be over-the-moon and thrilled about getting on the bicycles again. I have been horrible for focusing on computer work and not the bicycle. I wish I would have gone to the gym with my laptop and worked while I pedaled. But I haven't.

April 15, 2007 - Sunday - Dillsburg, PA to Watergate Hotel, Washington DC

Saying a temporary goodbye to our family, the two cars that it took to get us here, left us in just a matter of minutes. At once our life back on the road began. We were standing outside the stunning *Watergate Hotel* in Washington D.C. Where had the last few days gone? The gear that we have with us now is strewn over the sidewalk. Cars that pull up in the valet area and drop off and pick up people have no clue as to what we are up to. I feel very thrilled to be back on the ride. Not even feeling a twinge of the homesickness, not yet anyway.

Since the time we got up this morning it has been raining. The drive to D.C. in the back seat of Sarah and Graeme's car was nothing but rain. We chatted and I felt bad that I hadn't got to spend more time with my daughter when I was back in Pennsylvania. We did get everything accomplished that we needed to though, that felt great. Wearing the size 22 jeans that Mari had been kind enough to let us wash at their house, I reflected on our pit stop we had just made. It was totally unplanned, as is most of life. Our plans of going through Washington D.C. and Baltimore looked like there were not going to happen due to traffic and location in Pennsylvania, due to Morton's green card. Now here we are, headed back to D.C., to head to the east and continue north on our fantastic adventure. Morton was telling some people the other day that the thing he hates about when I ask him to write something here, is that he sounds like he keeps repeating himself. We both use a lot of the same words, over and over, daily. These words like incredible, fantastic, brilliant, amazing, wonderful and similar. Really they don't lose their glow with us. When we tell you that we have had a FANTASTIC day, we mean it! We might even need to make it bold and put a few exclamation points behind it, to really drive our feelings home. I feel the same as Morton. We repeat ourselves but with fantastic reason to. There are feelings that we have about this journey that can't be summed up with words. It is so emotional, so unbelievable, so life-changing and to have this happening to little old us....it is completely overwhelming a lot of the times.

Overwhelmed is the way I feel as we are standing in the shadow, protected from the rain, of the lovely Watergate. The feeling just grows as I get checked in and get to meet Josh Graham in person. He is the gentleman who has emailed me that they can help, again, with a room! He is so very kind, knows why we are on this journey and yet again, a perfect stranger to us. He is willing to help and that my friends, is actually BRILLIANT beyond belief! All my life I have loved to travel. Starting at the age of two weeks until now, seeing the world, meeting people, having adventures, are all things that have been on my list of things I love in life. My weight had stopped me from being confident enough to do anything out of the ordinary before, now I find myself a little like a character in an Alfred Hitchcock film. He would take an ordinary person and put them into extraordinary circumstances.

This weather would send a shiver down anyone's spine and we are so thankful to have a room tonight. To have a room in a place like this is amazing! I take a bike through the lobby that is like out of a movie. Pushing the button on the elevator I glide up. Again, this feeling that all this can't really be happening to us, sets in. I have dreamt for most of my life of being a normal sized person, now looking back at me in the reflection on the elevator wall, is a person who is on her way down the scale as the elevator heads for the top. Our room is stunning. It has a huge king-sized bed, beautiful carved wooden headboard, a curved wall that has a ledge that is wide enough to work on, that follows the huge glass window that is more like a wall. The curtains get pulled back quickly to reveal this view of the world-famous Potomac River. The sight is dazzling and I have to force myself to go back downstairs to bring the second bicycle up.

Morton is chatting to Josh at the bike and trailers. We get a quick photo together, but in my rush I fail to notice that it is blurry. Later I'll find Josh and we can get a do-over picture. We don't want to ever forget the face of this kind man. Josh tells us to get room service or go to the lovely restaurant, Aquarelle, as his treat. Morton and I are stunned. We had been prepared by stopping at the dollar store and had planned on having a can of tuna for dinner. We will eat it, but not tonight. Today is one of those magical days that everything that happens to us seems to be glowing with the best luck ever known. Talk about your golden moments. We have to find a way to bottle this feeling up and give it to the world. We usually always have the same routine when we are going into a room for the night. Morton waits with our gear and I hoof it up. This only varies if there are stairs involved. Then Morton will do the climbing, lifting and grunting to get us in for the night. Today there is an elevator, so I make my next trip up and back. We both get a trailer and push it to the elevators. We have more stuff then when we took our pit stop. The worst part about that isn't the weight or where are we going to put it....it means now that I have weighed the trailers down, I can't complain when Morton adds "new finds" that he picks up along the road. I try not to think about it...who knows what he is going to pick up next?
Morton is taking the elevator behind me and I go down the lovely hall to our room, I can hear him giving someone the web address as he leaves the elevator. Our banners are going to really cut down the questions, but we are a rather curious thing to look at.

Inside the room, thank goodness it is HUGE, Morton tackles unpacking the trailers to repack them the "right" way. Just a few minutes ago when Sarah, Graeme, James and Mari dropped us off, their two cars were bulging. The huge trunk on James' car held our flattened trailers, one bike and odds and ends. His backseat was stuffed to the brim. Sarah and Graeme had gotten off lucky. They only had Morton and I and one bicycle. The menu for room service is full of lovely choices, but we settle on two meals that we will split in half and share. When it arrived on the tray covered with silver-topped platters, it was so delicious we couldn't stop saying "mmmm!". It was the first hot food we had today and our stomachs were really ready for it. This meal is a dream come true: Nicoise Arugula Salad with Seared Shrimp, Asparagus, Tomatoes, Fingerlings, Parmegiano, Balsamic Dressing & Aquarelle Burger on Toasted Sesame Brioche, Vermont White Cheddar, Lettuce, Tomato, Onion, Pickles served with house made Pommes Frittes, Raisin & walnut bread. This was the first time in his life that Morton had room service! We both loved it and sat at the window watching the Potomac River and the city lights. Incredible! This is a MAGIC MOMENT that will last for the rest of our lives. Once again, thank you so much Josh, you are *BRILLIANT*! I sit at the desk and start to work. How can I sum this day up for you? All the mysteries of being on the road start in the morning. We first will meet up with NBC and then hopefully the crew from the movie company that are making the documentary about our journey.

Questions start to pop into my head. Our daily questions again. Where will we shower, what will we eat, who will we meet, what will the weather be, will there be any close calls, will my legs cramp up from not getting used enough over the last couple days? Endless questions, ending with the biggest question of our day...Where will we sleep tomorrow night?

As the river flows in front of our room and the light is gone from the sky, I will resist and put my foot down when Morton wants to close the curtains...the view has gotten even more magical at night with reflections dancing on the water and the lights on the buildings throwing wet glowing lights on the river. Tomorrow is a whole night of dreams away. Tonight though, we know where we are sleeping. Our eternal thanks goes out to Josh and *The Watergate Hotel*. What a place to end our day and re-start our adventure.

April 16, 2007 - Monday - *Watergate Hotel*, Washington DC to *Howard Johnsons* Cheverly, Maryland

We are back in the saddle again. We woke up early to be prepared for the news station we were hooking up with. The wind was still blowing out, but the rain seemed to have stopped. Heading downstairs to the lobby, we met several people who were curious to what we were doing. The banners that we got on the trailers themselves are really conversation starters. One of the people that I began speaking with was from the hotel and offered to pack us a lunch. Amazing kindness! Just as we were leaving, the rain started ever so slightly. It is a bit cold but it feels so right to be riding. Since we semi-know Washington, we even know where we are headed.

The news crew is rushing around from the storm damage and are going to catch up with us later. There is another crew that we need to meet up with, so we head towards all the landmarks and take care of the first one. It was a lot of riding around, which was great when the wind was at our backs. There was one point that we were almost stopped still by the wind. It felt like we were in a cartoon. Washington is such a lovely city. There is way too much to see in just one day. You need many days to see it all. This visit is going to just be a very fast one. Even though we really want to see the sights, we need to keep moving because of the weather. The storm that has the east coast shaking and blowing is on us. We touch base with the news crew and learn about the horrible shooting at Virginia Tech. They are too busy now with the tragedy and we are told to call back tomorrow. We still want to keep riding though, towards the east and out of the city.

With the cherry blossom festival in swing and other things going on in town, there are no rooms tonight. Dwayne, at the Visitors Center, is trying to help us, but it doesn't look promising. We think if we move a bit east into Maryland, we will get lucky. We swing by Dwayne's office and he's put together a goodie bag for us. Two hats from Washington, DC, lots of information and much needed maps. As we bicycle today, we get keep getting stopped by the public. The banners are working! Lots of people are taking pictures of us, the banners. The wind is really fierce today. We are having a hard time going up hills and have to resort to pushing. We have gone down 7th to New Hampshire (US 1) and follow that east to 450, otherwise known as Annapolis Road. The side of the roads changes and sometimes we have a place to ride and sometimes we don't. It's a tough day of city riding with red lights and traffic. I feel bad talking about the press as it happens. It is usually the same thing and I don't want to bore you. We do another bit of telly and then we are really done for the day. It is all just so overshadowed by the unthinkable happening at Virginia Tech. There are a few churches we check to see if there is any chance of sleeping in. We have no joy and have to just keep going. We are worried about getting too far for the news crew tomorrow, but the bigger worry is the weather. It's now raining and the wind is just fierce. Last night's storm still seem to has some kick left.

At one point, both our trailers get shoved along so fast, we can't do anything but hold on. In just a minute it is blowing back against our faces, peppered with rain. My face is hot from the exercise and the rain feels like it is ice. It all leaves me asking Morton, "Are we there yet?" The wind is so loud he can't hear me. The trouble with our ride today is, we haven't been seeing any place to stop. No motels in sight. Then, just ahead on our right, there is a *Howard Johnson*. Morton waits with the bicycles as I go inside.

There are many people at the desk checking in and I get worried about space. Asking for a room sponsorship, Dan, Director of Sales, was able to help us. I have never been happier. Except for all the other times that strangers have saved us. Seeking shelter in a storm like this is a scary task. In a city we have no hope of camping. Morton was speaking with a man from Sweden outside when I went back to start shuttling the bicycles to our sanctuary for the night. We chatted a bit, then made our way into our room. It is huge, warm and within minutes, I feel like I'm going to thaw out now.

My feet were soaking and cold, I had worn my sneakers instead of my boots. My jacket was damp and my left arm was soaking from the rain. My face is so cold that it's hot. The room is just right and I have so many things to do online tonight. We are so grateful to have a room out of the wind. As I'm so very grateful thinking about where we are tonight I can't help but let my mind drift to our unknown future. Our journey will have much worse weather then what we rode through today. It has been a very tiring day, the wind, back on the ride and the feeling the terrible loss of lives with what happened at Virginia Tech. My heart goes out to all the families at this pointless loss of life. I can't even bear to watch the news tonight to see if our piece is on, it is just too hideous.

April 17, 2007 - Tuesday - *Howard Johnson*, **Cheverly to** *Country Inn & Suites,* **Annapolis, MD**

All day long I felt like the Wicked Witch of the West, pumping my legs up and down and feeling like I was going nowhere. You know the scene, as Dorothy was looking out the window and the house was carried on the wind. Oh the wind...every time there would be a break in the breeze and I would ungrip my hands slightly, it would only be for a second and the wind would hit us again, pushing our bikes around like toys. Good thing my trailer weighs about 5,000 pounds! It feels like that anyway. When we were in Pennsylvania I left clothes behind that were too big for me now and the things I replaced them with weigh a ton. Morton snuck heavy tools in to my trailer too, at least it feels like that. I'll have to investigate that later. It is a good thing though that I'm so heavy today, along with the trailer or we would have surely been blown away.

There are lots of hills and we do almost as much walking today as bicycling. It feels good to walk, but again, pushing my bike and the 10,000 pound trailer up the hill almost kills me. I feel as tired as when we walked on day one back in Key West. Today though, I don't have the high heat to deal with. It's cold, windy, cloudy and the sky looks like at any moment it could pour down on us. Joy! With lunchtime approaching I feel hungrier than I have in ages. The old "starving wolf" feeling. Scary, because I never want to be a bottomless pit again. It's so cold we can't face the cold food bag and there is a Wendy's on the right. Pulling in, Morton needs to wash his hands after a morning of putting my chain back on. We always go in one at a time and since I'm oldest AND a girl...I usually get to go first. It also helps that my bladder is the size of a radish and Morton knows I can't hold it. I like to wash my face as well as my hands. It's always covered in sweat, no matter how cold it is. The sweat makes all the grit from passing cars stick to my face and it feels wonderful to wash it. This is my beauty routine people, plus a dab of sunscreen and you are set to go.

Morton is going to get us a taco salad to share and a $1. burger for him after he comes out of his turn in the bathroom. I wait at the bikes, and wait, and wait some more. Obviously he is in talking to someone. He comes out, fuming. He had gotten a drink for us to share, ordered a small, instead of the one off the value menu (he thought that WAS the small). Instead of being 99 cents, it was $1.19. They wouldn't switch it up for him. He had just complained that there was no soap in the bathroom so I guess he wasn't on their list of people to please. As he's telling me his tale of woe, I'm eating. He gets to the part of the no soap in the men's bathroom, then tells me there was a guy in a Wendy's uniform coming out without washing his hands. Morton called him "manky", slang for "dirty" in Scotland. He didn't call him that to his face, but told me about it. Morton does have manners and always washes his hands, with soap. His mother trained him well.

Suddenly I didn't want to eat anymore. My stomach felt a bit sick, cramping from the hot chili in the cold temps. Plus I was getting all these visuals in my head. The guy not washing his hands, the health inspector that was coming out of the place with a swab kit in his hands and I just couldn't take another bite of the salad. Morton scored from this. He got 3/4's instead of 1/2 of the salad AND his burger. We both decided the food bag would have been a better bet. I think it will be a while before we stop for warm lunch. I also won't eat anymore if he tells me there is no soap in the gents.

Once we leave civilization a bit and we are in the woods. Not sure where this was at, but it was so peaceful, bike lane for most of it and the views are of my childhood. We are only one state away from where I grew up, so it's natural they would look a bit similar. The trees, waking up after winter, are all pushing their leaves. They are having a hard job seeing the sun today though. It just isn't there. The sight and sound that really takes me back is the little creeks running beside us. They would be called "burns" in Scotland. These little rushing waters show the signs of the rain that happened during our night in Washington D.C. They flow fast, little waterfalls here and there and being on a bike I feel just like I'm ten again. My little brother and I would spend our entire days outside in the summer. Each and every day really. We would ride our bikes down to this little stream that had us totally under it's spell. We could wade in it to cool our toes, lay on our bellies and observe nature up close and personal and find countless ways to entertain ourselves. My mom wouldn't see us again until dark or if we got hungry.

When Morton and I take a break for water on a piece of guard rail, I get some pictures of the sun just peeking out for the first time today. It is lighting a bright green soft carpeting of moss. It is also showing a bank of soil that suddenly looks like a little village sculpted out of the dirt. I'm ten again and laying on the village that my brother and I discovered, that looked a lot like this erosion. Ours was made of a clay and was beside big flat rocks, ten and twenty feet across. We would start the day in shade, using little sticks and twigs to carve roads in our village. We would be in the full sun during the day while we worked. I can remember spending the better part of a month shaping our village up.

Imagination and the playful heart of a child. Can you imagine what would happen now if you told your bored 10-year-old to go play in the mud? Maybe they would like it, but I somehow think that something is missing. We have been ruined by technology. We are recapturing that joy, the simple pleasures, that we knew as a child. I tell Morton why I'm looking at this eroded side of a bank with such fondness. He likes hearing stories from my childhood and always searches his memory to share one of comparable value with mine. Today though he had nothing for me.

We are halfway up a hill that we are having to push the bikes on. I feel one drop of rain on my face and it snaps me back into our journey. Pulling our weather gear on we hope to stay dry. The rest of our ride is filled with chains jumping off tracks and Morton having to get his fingers mucky putting them back on. I'm really feeling tired, sick to my stomach and missing my little brother. The good old days. Heading up a rather steep hill, my gears drop as they should and my chain stays on. I am climbing, about halfway up, when it feels like someone has tied a rope around me. I have learned quick that when something doesn't feel right as you're riding, you have to stop at once. Otherwise the damage can be too severe to fix easily, sort of like with the gaining of all my weight, only I never listened to my body before now. This time it was a flat tire on my trailer. It wasn't because I loaded it up too heavy, it was because of a broken piece of glass that someone chucked out their car window. I'm sure it was once a bottle. Morton went to work and we were both trying to remember our last flat tire. I think it was right before Stafford, Virginia. He finishes, then does his walk around check where he squeezes all the other tires while he still has the bike pump out. His tire on the back of his bike if flat.

Turning the wheel he discovers a big piece of metal, not glass, that was once a nail sticking out of the tire. As he pulls it out with the pliers, it is over two inches long. It is the same color as a twig and neither of us saw what we had rode over. I was just glad I hadn't got my flat while coming down one of the steep hills. I know my speed has to reach 25 to 30 mph. A blowout at that speed could be fatal for us. He fixes the puncture and we are off. It is nearly 5 pm and we just come back into civilization and Annapolis, Maryland. At a stop light we see a *Country Inn & Suites.* We pull the bikes to the overhang, incase the sky lets loose with the rain that it has been threatening us with all day long. We know when to take advantage of overhangs that block the dreaded sun and the dreaded rain. Steve at the front desk, gets Richard, the General Manager for me. I explain what we are doing and they are kind enough to help us with a room. We also get a picture with Richard, just before he heads home for the day. It was lucky to catch him and as usual, we appreciate being inside on a dark and rainy night. Morton and I are thrilled we have a room so close to the front door and he chats away with people as I cart the things back and forth. We are told there is a pool and hot tub and you can even choose DVD's to watch in your room. We decide to get a movie, have a swim and then spend an evening actually resting. After today, with the wind and hills, we really need it.

My big purple bathing suit with the bright pink flower on it, that I wore in my banner picture, has been left in Pennsylvania. It is *too* big at the legs now and hangs down about 3 inches or so. I have opted for a black bathing suit that is about 10 years old and had only been worn twice before. It is a size 22 and I figure, if I can get into the jeans, the bathing suit should be a snap. It fits like a charm. The only trouble is my fat arms and legs. I'm happy with my stomach and how it is going back to where it needs to be, plus, it's covered by the material. But the arms and legs are a shocker. Plus, I have a dodgy tan on both of them. My calves are the only part on my leg that is tan and just my forearms. I look so odd.

But tonight I have the feeling that it doesn't matter how I look. People can look away if they don't like it. My body is aching and the sounds of the hot tub are too good to resist. My dread of being in public in a bathing suit is leaving. The pool and hot tub area are wonderful. There is a lifeguard and I have a bit of a chat with her as I'm getting ready to get in the water. She tells me the temperature on the pool is 90 degrees. Ahhhh....Morton gets a few pictures as I'm getting in and I don't even freak out about it. I want them now to remind me. It's also good to look at pictures because they see things that my mind doesn't see. The water is so perfect. At once my muscles start to feel better. I swim around using just my arms, my legs get enough of a workout all day. It is delightful. Morton joins me and we could have stayed in there all night long. I would have been happy to sleep right beside the pool! As the hot tub bubbles away beside us, I climb out of the pool and walk over to it, passing under the shower I had used before swimming. It is a perfect set up here. The hot tub is warmer, nice and deep and really big. We climb in and soak for about ten minutes, before saying goodbye to the lifeguard and going back to our room. Talk about a great ending to a really tough day. I think I won't be able to stay awake to watch the film, but I manage. I fall asleep right before the end for about five minutes. Morton fills me in on what I missed. As usual, when I put my head on the pillow, I'm asleep within a few minutes. Sweet dreams are made from days like these.

April 18, 2007 - Wednesday - *Country Inn & Suites,* Annapolis to *Best Western, Kent Narrows Inn*, Grasonville, Maryland

For the most part the food we are eating out here comes out of our red food bag about the size of a reusable shopping bag. Standard fare is tuna, peanuts, crackers, trail mix, pretzels, raisins, anything that isn't perishable and is kind of on the light side. Today though, our meals are a bit different thanks to some amazing people. **Breakfast**: omelet with cheese, blueberry bagel with cream cheese, fruit & yogurt, milk

Lunch: BEAUTIFUL lunch at *Galway Bay* in Annapolis courtesy of the lovely people at the *Annapolis Visitors Center* : We had oysters in a Guinness batter on a bed of homemade coleslaw, plus, we split the BEST corned beef and cabbage we both have ever tasted. The best part about the meal was getting to chat with Fintan Galway, the owner. His accent made me miss Ireland!

Dinner: 1/2 bag tuna, 1/2 bag microwave popcorn, 1/2 apple with peanut butter

Late night snack: none | Today we bicycled 17.5 miles

   I started out by checking my email. There were 122. None of them were spam...all from you lovely people out there watching and following our story on here. It is odd, but those of you that write on a semi-regular basis, we are really getting to feel like we know you. It always is a great way to start the day. It's a sheer joy and we love it...keep them coming. I read fast and type fast. Unless something drastic happens, we will always answer. We were uploading some files and decided to grab breakfast while the computer was still doing it's thing. *Country Inn & Suites* feels more like you have came home, then to a hotel. It's a nice feeling as we head into the room where this lovely breakfast is laid out. Morton offers to make me a waffle, but I go for the omelet. It was lovely. The routine of getting our gear out and ready was a bit easier. All the practice.

   We were soon loaded and heading into Annapolis. I'm ashamed to say that I have never visited this historic place. I know nothing about it really, just that there is a big naval academy there. We still need a map of Maryland and the answer to *HOW* we are going to get across the Chesapeake on a bridge that bicycles aren't allowed on, but it will all happen. We have the sun trying to shine and no wind. It is a great day to be out here and I'm *LOVING* our banners on the trailers. They really explain it all. I think it makes people a bit more tolerant of us out here on their roads too. There is one spot where we have to go very slow through a giant mud puddle. There is no choice. We take it easy and it's not as bad as I thought. Plus, on the other end there is a lovely patch of tulips I get to look at. We get the idea that maybe we could ask a car dealer for a lift over the bridge. We soon learn this isn't a good idea as we get three "NO'S" in a row. We keep riding, what will happen, will happen. If we aren't interested in buying a car, they don't really have time for us. The streets are lined with lovely buildings and the sidewalks are turning into lovely brick paths. It feels like we are riding back in time again. We have no clue where we are going, but we stick to 450, ever hopeful we are on the right path.

   At an information center for businesses, Morton learns where the Visitor Info center is. It means turning off our main path (THAT is the lesson to be learned, don't be afraid to turn off the main path!) and heading down another road. We need a map, so we go for it. Little did we know, stepping inside and up to the desk, our whole day was going to change in a big way. First things first, I visited their ladies room. Then I made my way to the desk. There were a lot of people in and I signed their visitor book as I was sort of just waiting for my turn. A gentleman asked if he could help, then gave me a map. I asked if they knew a way for bicycles over the bridge. Suddenly, they all sprang into action with ideas, brainstorming, phone calls and before I knew it, they sent Morton and I off for a proper lunch (which was so delicious) and had us coming back at 3pm to get a ride over with two of the women that work there! They also called the newspaper and had a reporter and photographer turn up to do a story on us! My *ONLY* regret is that we weren't staying in Annapolis. We are making Annapolis one of our first places to visit when we finish our journey. The town is just lovely, easy for walking and very friendly for bicycles. Big, wide, brick paths are everywhere and the trees were all in bloom. It felt like we were dreaming. Morton and I rode down the lovely sidewalks, smiling, feeling so great about meeting these living angels who were helping to change our lives and destiny. Perfect strangers who are indeed perfect.

We are blessed and we know this. How can I ever complain about a flat tire or the weather when there are such kind people in the world? We bicycle on Maryland Avenue and see *Galway Bay*, where we will eat lunch at. The owner, Fintan Galway, comes out to tell us the bikes will be fine there. He's right! He takes us inside and I feel like I'm actually in Ireland. I remember our trips that we had to the Emerald Isle, when we had lived in Scotland. There weren't enough, we were always working. The Irish and Scottish people share the same smiling ways. Fintan also has a lovely accent, I could have listened to him all day! Funny, that is what a lot of people we meet say about Morton. We talk about what we are doing, the route we are taking, then we have the most delightful lunch. We share a starter and a main course and Morton has a Guinness along with his. This is the first time he's done this and I tell him jokingly that he better not get a BUI, *biking under the influence*. He also has a pint of water along with the lunch, so I'm sure there is "nae danger" of Morton swerving on the bicycle. As we are getting ready to leave the lovely *Galway Bay*, a group of women come over to our table. They know what we are doing and are all offering their well wishes & support. We chat and get a picture and again, I feel like this can't be happening. We have met several people today who tell us they are so moved by what we are doing that they are going to not only watch the website, but start getting their daily exercise. *SUCCESS!* We want to motivate you, NOT nag you...into doing what your body wants and needs. Only you can change it, remember this.

There is this feeling in the air here today that spring has arrived. The trees are all blooming, people have their layers of coats off, lots of people are out walking and everyone seems to be smiling. I suppose that is because a giant smile is on my face almost all day. Perhaps it was the hot tub last night. My body is feeling like it's in the spring mode too. No cracks or pangs in the knees today. It is almost time for us to get our lift over the bridge. With full bellies, we pedal.

We head back to the *Annapolis & Anne Arundel County Conference & Visitors Bureau*. Maura and Mary Jo pull in and we load up the trailers and the bicycles. Morton and I each ride with one of them as we head off across this modern marvel of a bridge across the water. Maura and I talk about how Morton and I met and before I know it, we are there. We unload the bicycles and both our new friends tell us they feel bad about dropping us off. It is a tough feeling out here when we meet new people. Saying goodbye to someone that you have just met and connected with can be as tough as saying goodbye to your best girlfriend. Consulting the map they had given us (& a bicycle map too!) we wave and ride off. Not quite into the sunset. Thanks to daylight savings time, we have an extra hour and then some.

The road has a bike lane. How we love bike lanes, no matter how narrow they are. It feels like a bit of the road that we are actually allowed to be on. Plus, as we move closer to the coast, the hills aren't as steep. If there is one thing we would love to have, it's cameras for our helmets. We would love to be able to capture what we are seeing that happens. Ducks flying and landing on the most beautiful water, a lighthouse in the distance, green fields that a hawk is flying over, things that happed too fast for us to get the camera out for. But for now, we just have to stop once and a while. Usually Morton shouts, "Go slow!" and since I'm already just going fast enough to keep the bike upright, I know this means he is either going to pick up something he's found or...he's going to take a picture of something that caught his eye. This is where all the pictures of me from behind "riding slow!" comes from. Today he takes photos of the beautiful pristine landscape.

With the clock approaching 5pm, we think about a place to stop. We know we haven't gone that far, but a good part of our day was spent on the crossing of the bridge. Now, with the headlights coming on the cars that were all heading home, it seemed like a good time to seek lodging. The *Best Western* was on our left and before you could say, "Lucky Day" I was inside talking to Marc, who helped us with a room for the night! The world is wonderful and we won't have to put the tent up tonight! Not that we mind doing that, it's still really a bit cold in the evening and so far we haven't really been sick at all. Plus, camping takes two hours off of each day with set up and tear down. Time is the one thing we can't ever seem to have enough of, right behind drinking water. We head to the room, with an outside door, where ducks are just walking about. Morton has taken a load of pictures of them and Marc tells me they also have deer that visit in their adjoining field. There are turtles in the lobby and the wildlife abounds. We love it! There is a pool and a sauna. We should go but I have emails to answer and over 20 of them are interviews for newspapers. We are happy to do this, but it is time consuming. Besides, if my body gets to go swimming two nights in a row, it will be spoiled and expect it every night! We make our nightly phone calls of letting my kids know that we are safe and sound. I talk to my sister with my mom in the background. It is like a three-way call. Mom's speech has improved so much since her stroke, but she really doesn't like the telephone. Even though I can understand her, she gets flustered on it. I try to tell her as long as she is breathing, nothing else matters. Anyway, I speak "mom!"

April 19, 2007 - Thursday - *Best Western, Kent Narrows Inn*, **Grasonville to** *Best Western*, **Denton, MD**

      We started the day off with meeting Bryan McBournie with the *Bay Times* newspaper. He came to our room to hear our story and see us off. It was really a great interview and we appreciated him seeing us on virtually no notice. Bryan took pictures outside our room and then as we were bicycling off with a "Share the Road" bicycle sign, almost as if on cue. We waved as he passed us and we were off and riding for the day.

      The weatherman had been spot on with his forecast of "sprinkles". We spent the entire day in various degrees of dripping skies. When we were ready for lunch, there really wasn't anywhere to stop. Just lovely fields, trees and miles of the best road we have ridden on for a long time. The edge was so wide, we loved it! Every road in America should be like this. Level again, the riding was simple. It left plenty of time to enjoy the sights, listen to the silence when there were no cars and feel the rain on our faces.

There is a lumber yard and the rain had just gotten heavier. Time to stop. We decide to pull in and have our break in the dry. It's a bit off the road. We get off the bikes and two of the men that worked there both said they passed us earlier on the road. Everyone passes us! We had a bit of conversation with them and then ate our lunch while sitting on a stack of plywood. The smells made me want to do a bit of remodeling, but we don't have anything to remodel. Our tent does need a bit of sewing on it near the zipper, but other than that, we are fine and dandy. Our goal is to get to Delaware today, but as we get back on the road, we discover with the help of a local that Denton is going to be the only place with a motel and camping. They are both off the same exit and I go to the *Best Western* first. It's still raining and the thought of putting up a tent in the rain isn't a pleasant one. My right ear has been aching all day and I'm getting a bit of a sore throat again. I've also been cold since lunchtime. Inside, the girl at the desk listens to what we are doing. The manager is gone for the day, but she offers to call him. She does a fantastic time explaining everything and Jay, the manager, agrees to sponsor us for a room for the evening. A huge thank you to both of them. When people take the time to listen to us they usually help. We get to the room and my face is hot but the rest of me is cold. I take two aspirins and get a hot shower and then set about on the computer. There are calls to make, emails to answer and the task of updating the journal. I wish that Morton knew how to do it, because nights when I feel like this, it would be great if he could. Maybe with a bit of time he could be doing it, but then he might expect me to fix the flats and the broken bicycle chains. We are going to try to make it the whole way to the ferry tomorrow, but it is 47.5 miles. HOPE-FULLY I will wake up feeling better with the ear ache gone. The temperature is going to be in the 60's and the sun is going to be out.

April 20, 2007 - Friday - *Best Western*, **Denton, Maryland to** *Hotel Blue*, **Lewes, Delaware**

      When you wake up in a different place everyday, it's hard enough to get your bearings, but when you wake up and have no clue as to the time OR where you are, it's even worse. Typically my body wakes up early, always. It always has and I can't seem to sleep in. The latest I've ever slept in, in my almost 44 years on the planet, was a Sunday morning in Scotland. I had been out with Morton at a little local pub in a tiny town called Lasswade. There were lots of people that he knew there and when the pub shut, everyone walked over to Lee's house to continue with their chatting, drinking, laughing and merry-making. Since I had never been to a party like this in Scotland (or the US) I was wide awake, enjoying it all. There were lots of different people that had came along. I had just moved over to Scotland and was fascinated by all the things that were so different than to what I was use to. After hours of talking, people started heading off, the three of us heading back to the little town of Bonnyrigg. Morton's good friend Graeme (not my son-in-law) was along and the two of them nearly had to push me up the steep hill. It wasn't my weight that was doing it, but the fact that it was 5 am! I slept in that day until 2pm and felt like I was going to hear my dad yelling at me to get up out of bed or I was going to sleep the day away. That would have been a trick, since dad was 3500 miles away at the time.

      This morning felt the same. I woke up so tired, feeling like it had to be 2 in the afternoon. I think it was a combination of lots of things, the weather, my throat, being on the bicycle all day. It was a surprise to see it was only 6 am. I felt like I just had the longest sleep, but could have continued for about 5 or 6 more days. My body clock was set spot on though, up I rose to jump on the computer and Morton packed the gear and made us each a waffle for breakfast. It's really nice to be in a place where we can get something hot to eat in the morning that doesn't come out of the food bag. I had done a phone interview with a local paper earlier and wanted to get some shots of the *Best Western* in Denton where we had been staying. It is one of those things that we are learning as we go along. We want everyone to watch our journey and be a part of it. This means lots of interviews. I have lost track now of how many I've done. You've read this here before, but they really are all different. It is odd how that works. You would think there is only one way to say we are going thousands of miles by bicycle to lose weight and spread the message that movement will change your life. We know the cure for obesity, moderate what you eat and move more. With exercise being the thing that most people neglect when they are dieting it is surprising to see how effective it is.The photographer from the paper isn't able to make it out, so our photos will have to do. Morton takes maybe perhaps the most hideous pictures of me that I have ever seen. These are the pictures that will scare the mice away. Sigh...I see my body changing when I look at it, but in some of these pictures it's enough to make me ask..."What did I look like 100 pounds heavier?" The day is a complete opposite to yesterday and the "sprinkles" we got drenched with all day. The sun is out and very warm, almost hot. The road is something we dream about...super wide edge for us and almost 100% free from glass! It is going to be a great day to push on for Delaware and then the ferry. As we cross into Delaware, I learn a lot. This is the first state. I knew this, but I didn't. Morton and I talk a lot about what and where we are going through and I usually let myself down by not knowing things I should. Being American he expects me to know everything about our country, which I don't. We do stop and read the signs and plaques along the way. The road, if it is possible, had gotten even BETTER in Delaware. It's wider on the edge, not a lot of traffic on the road and we just chat away and pedal.

As lunch time approaches, we stop by a "No Loitering" sign in a small town. We have our lunch in the sun sitting on steps to no where. I call to talk to my mom but she's busy with someone who has came to see her. My sister and I chat for a bit and then we head off. Even though our lunch was good, we had it sitting in smelling distance of the local pizza shop. *Torture!* The smells were so lovely.

We really are making good time and have been called by someone who has been following the site in Cape May. She has invited us to spend the night and we are thrilled. We figure, if we get to the ferry and can't find a place to stay in Delaware, we can just head over and pop up the tent in her backyard! I am a big believer in "PLAN B" but to tell you the truth, we usually don't have one. This journey is teaching me the phrase my dad would say, "Flying by the seat of your pants." He had been a pilot in WWII and in his days, they really did fly that way. Instinct was a key factor in decision making. It has became a way of life for us. Dad would be proud and a bit amazed I think, at just how far we have come with not much of a plan to speak of, other than "ride the bikes and walk!"

Fate, Karma, Destiny, Luck, Providence and words like this, really wrap up our days. Sometimes, most of the times actually, things just work out. We have both learned to NOT worry about things, because they always seem to work out. We meet some incredible ladies outside a little shop and chat for a bit. We take a picture then head inside to use the bathroom and treat ourselves to a 25 cent popsicle. I have a frozen root beer flavored one and Morton has a *Banjo*. It's vanilla ice cream, covered in a chocolate shell and they are both just 25 cents each. On a warm day like this, it is a real treat. The town is filled with Victorian looking mansions and houses. We bump into a lady on the sidewalk and stop and have a chat about the health van pulled into the library that is giving free mammograms. Morton tells me I should go in and I give it a pass. First, where would they send the results to? Since paying hundreds of dollars for his physical for his immigration last summer, he has learned that things that are medically related in America are always expensive. He thinks that because this if free, I should jump right in there. But I had one right before we left Scotland, so free or not, I keep riding. There are such lovely sights along the way and smells to match. We see buffalo, Arabian horses, shaggy ponies, birds of every description, and lots of cute dogs that bark at us. A few just watch, with their heads cocked, but most can't resist the temptation of barking. The smells of fresh cut grass, flowers blooming and just fresh air, work wonders for us. Even the smell of my sunscreen mixes with it all to make it feel like this is just a ride in a lovely park somewhere. We ride without a care in the world, perhaps because we do have a "Plan B" tonight.

As we come in to Lewes (pronounced Lewis) I do something I have never done before. We sit in a parking lot and I check my email. I had written to a place to ask if they would be able to help us with a room and I just have this feeling. Usually I feel nervous about taking my laptop out in a parking lot because I don't want to become a target for robbery. With the numbers rising on my incoming email, I see one that looks like it might be the one. I click on it, under the tree and sitting in mulch, then let out a squeal of joy! We have a room. We are near it right now. It's actually so close to the ferry that we will be able to not be in such a rush in the morning. Joy! Morton was worried about me opening up the computer outside. He does worry a lot sometimes, but I have a feeling after this journey, it will be a lot less.

Packing our link to the world away, we head out towards the heart of the town. As we come down the street leading in, we catch sight of a huge lovely old church. I'm saying to Morton lets stop to get a picture as I first hear the pipes. There is a lone piper on the steps of the church squeezing out a tune on the bagpipes.

Morton and I watch and listen and I almost get a picture of him. He's practicing for an upcoming wedding. I hope they have a day as lovely as the weather today. Morton and I were going to speak to him, but there were some people that came out of the church and started talking about the upcoming wedding and what got him interested in playing the bagpipes. Mel Gibson in Braveheart was what did it! To think that he would have the patience to learn. Everyone thinks that Morton plays the pipes just because he is Scottish. But he doesn't. He does wear his kilt for weddings and special occasions though. That is as Scottish as it gets.

We keep riding through this charming town. The houses are just picture postcard perfect. It would be great to spend a few days and explore, but we really want to keep heading on. How are we ever going to get back to all of these amazing spots? We need to live several lifetimes to fit it all in. Passing the main street, we stay on the road leading to the ferry. We cross a lovely canal and then turn left on to the road that our hotel for the evening is on. Pulling in to *Hotel Blue*, we both sort of are a bit stunned. It is stunning. Morton gets a picture from the outside, which is lovely, but when you walk inside, you are just bowled over. Their lobby is so very chic, yet not the kind of chic you can't be comfortable in. Even though it looks like it is right out of a magazine, I don't feel out of place in my bicycling helmet. The lovely lady at the front shows us to our room...again, we are bowled over. This isn't just a room. It is a place that I could live forever and ever and always be stunned when I walked in. From the carpet to the chairs to the use of size and space, this suite impresses us. I am very fussy now with Morton, we leave the bikes and trailers tarped outside. I have him take his shoes off. This place is just so lovely I call Sarah to tell her about it. I know that she would love the color scheme and the way it looks. There is bathroom of my dreams. A huge walk in shower, a huge soaking tub that Morton falls asleep in for about 40 minutes and attention to detail that is spot on. There is even a REAL fireplace. I want to stay in Lewes, Delaware for weeks and weeks. Did I mention it is RIGHT on the water too...with a private porch! Stepping out on our porch I see that it has a real pond with fish and a waterfall on it. Wow! The chic interior and the way they bring nature right up to you is amazing.

I work like mad on the computer. Wireless internet with a strong signal and there are tons of emails to read. One is from a producer that we have been trying to connect with. She puts the magic words on, "Call my cell phone no matter what time it is!" and I see that it is 7:30 pm as I dial her. We are getting together with the crew, finally, that we were suppose to meet in Washington DC. They are going to cross on the ferry with us, follow us around and we are all going to "act natural" as the camera follows our movements. "Acting natural" is a lot harder then you think. First, I feel compelled to make endless chatter and say things I would never say to Morton. Morton is MUCH better at this, he is quieter by nature and isn't really bothered if there are cameras or not. He will still stop to pick up a penny he sees or a piece of "treasure" like a broken screwdriver.

There is one catch...they really want my kids to be here. Sarah and Graeme are in, so are James and Mari, they can carpool here to split the turnpike tolls and gas. They can't stay the night, due to budgets and I rush like a mad woman to find a place to stay in Cape May that we could all stay in. I know the filming is going to take longer then the 4 or 5 hours we are told. I also know that being pregnant, Sarah gets tired so easy. My children are so supportive of what we are doing and I really wish I had the money to splash out and just spring for a motel...but we don't. Instead I start calling, late in the evening, from a directory I find on the internet. There are a lot of machines I get, or places that are not open for the season yet. My spirits remain high as I keep calling. I think about calling the girl that has invited us to pitch out tent, but I don't. I would never impose on her kindness in that way. Putting up with 2 strangers in your backyard is one thing, but 6 is a whole other game. Sarah calls during my phone calls to tell me to not stress out. If it doesn't happen, they will still drive down. She tells me that I should enjoy the day and not be in a panic. She jokes that they can always sleep in the van, but again, her being pregnant, this isn't something I find comforting. It is different trying to look after someone else out here, not just Morton and I.

There is a call that I make, where I feel the person on the other end can actually understand what I'm going through right now. He takes my details, promises to call back and I keep calling, watching the clock as it becomes borderline "too late to call" and I still keep at it. Then my phone rings and it is a number I don't recognize. As I answer it is a newsroom that is trying to catch up with us in the morning, in addition to the people that we have to "act natural" with! We go over the details of getting together and there is a call coming in. I don't know how to put someone on hold and I have to miss the number.

Dialing it back, it's a lady who says that she would like to help, but they are not open yet. Sigh. As she is telling me some other places to try, a number pops up. Again, I miss taking the call, but I'm returning it in just a few minutes. It is a voice of the person I had spoken to earlier and he is going to be able to help us. We, all six of us, are going to be staying at the *Palace Hotel* in Cape May on Saturday night!

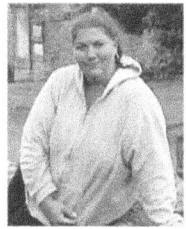

Scotland, September 2001
Weight 250 pounds

Morton, my future husband, had no clue as to what I weighed here. I felt good, healthy and happy but that was pre-moving in and getting married to one of the best cooks in Scotland.

In my five years spent in the UK I gained an unhealthy 190 pounds, more than I should weigh in total.

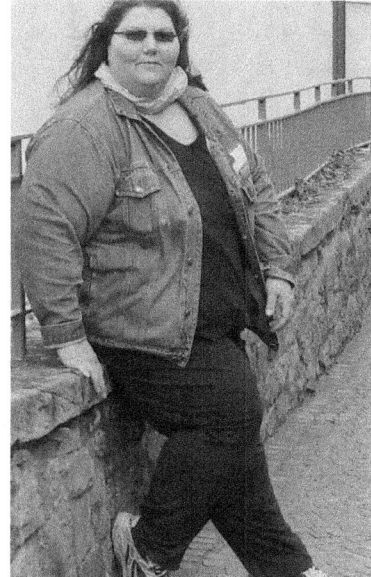

Germany, April 2006
Weight 440 pounds

My weight was stopping me from living a normal life. This road led up to a castle at the top of a steep hill and I had to take many "breathing breaks" along the way.

Of course I would lie to my husband and tell him I was stopping to take pictures, enjoy the view and many other creative lies I used over the years that really fooled no one but myself.

Italy, April 2006
Weight 440 pounds

Italy is one of my favorite countries in the whole world and I have to say I had one of my most embarrassing moments here.

While walking into a store, two little boys were coming out. They both got scared when they looked up at me, then began laughing. Since I didn't speak their language, I have no clue to what they said.

I've never told my husband or family about that. It wasn't enough to make me change though, we went right to this location and ate lunch. I had dessert.

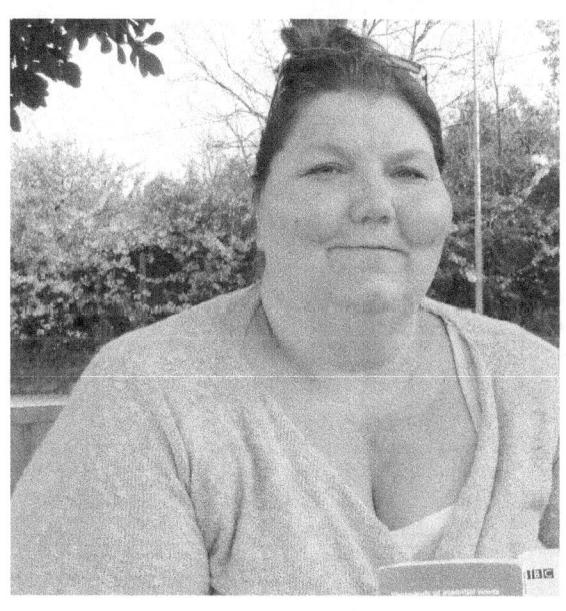

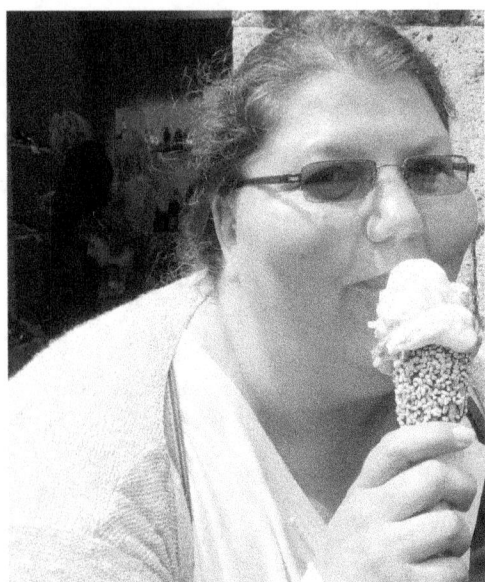

Sienna, Italy May 2006
Weight 440-ish

<<<

Since I was two weeks old I have travelled, logging up visits to over twenty countries and forty-eight states. As my body clearly shows, I love ice cream. Without one little doubt, Italy makes the best.

In this picture I'm actually trying to hide behind the cone while Morton captures this moment. I can remember trying to suck my cheeks in while licking and hoping that he wasn't getting my whole body in the picture.

Dressing in layers I hoped to blend in with normal-sized humans, but alas, I was the fattest person I saw in Italy.

Pennsylvania, May 2006   >>>
Weight 447

Sitting beside my dad in the stroke rehabilitation center where my mom spent almost two months, the chair doesn't fit me. Notice how I have to sit to the front while the arms dig into my hips.

The smile on my face is trying to cover the real fear I was feeling when I finally realized after decades of abusing food that my weight wasn't just my problem. It was hurting those around me. If I didn't take care of me, someone else would have to.

When the light went on over my head, the answer was so simple I thought that I had to make it my goal in life to share this secret with the world. Moderate what you eat and move for at least thirty minutes each day.

Exercise is the secret pill we have all been looking for!

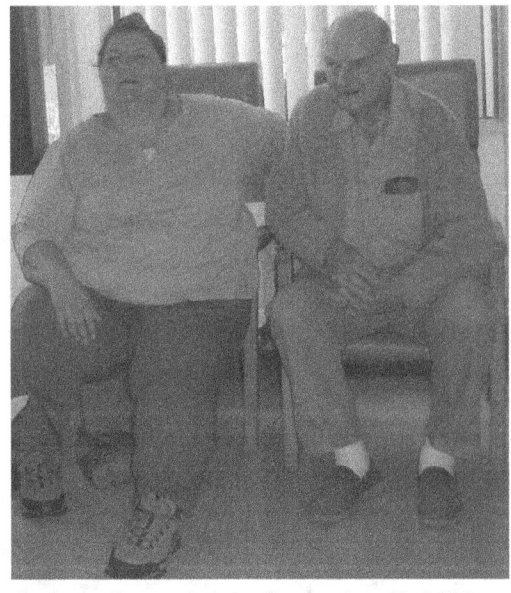

Gettysburg, Pennsylvania September 10. 2006
Weight 372 pounds

The day after my dad's funeral, we had a scheduled walk in Gettysburg. I almost didn't go, but I knew my dad would want me to get healthy.

My backside is the one on the right, my daughter Sarah is the small backside, by my side.

Sarah has been a constant help with my battle against obesity and my hero.

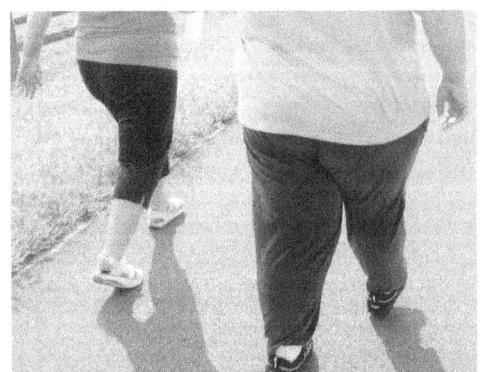

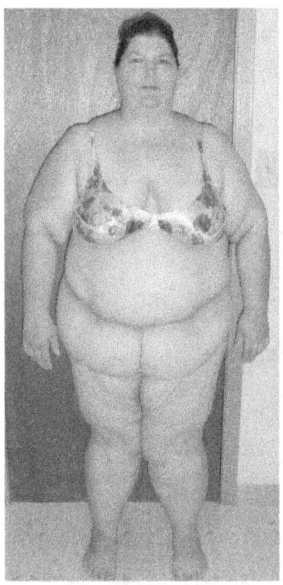
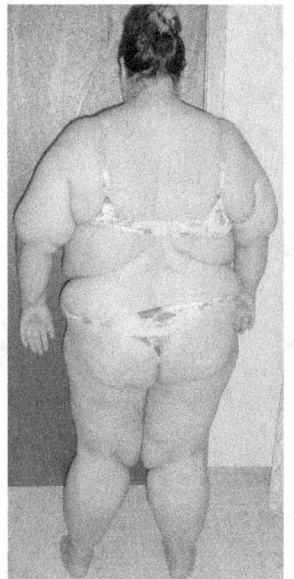
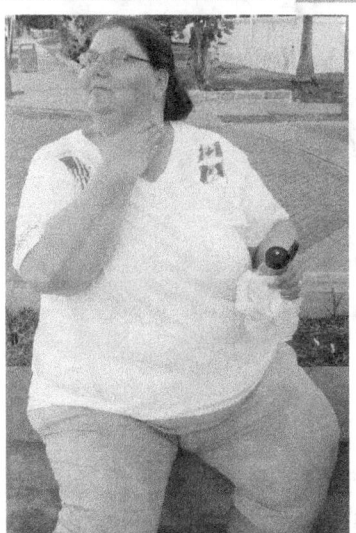

Pennsylvania August 2006
Weight 384

The rolls and the outside of my body look so bad here, I can only imagine how that fat is choking my heart and clogging my arteries.

After just a few months of walking though, there has been one of my belly rolls that have left and the fat wrinkles on my right arm have went from three to one.

The really wild thing is that from the front, it looks like I'm not wearing any underwear, though I promise I am! My arms also stick out all the time, unable to lay flat against me because of the layers of fat.

Key West, Florida
January 1, 2007
Weight 343.5

I'm still not sure how I made it through that first day walking in Key West. Lots of sunscreen, water and breaks.

>>>

Notice the tarp on the ground to stop the fire ants from feasting on me.

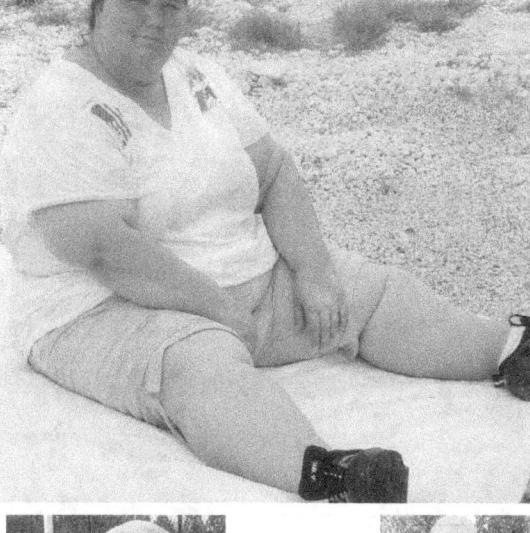

<<<
The sight of guardrail would make me happy and serve as my sofa for the next six and a half months of living on the road.

Our wheelchair waits loaded for Morton to push.

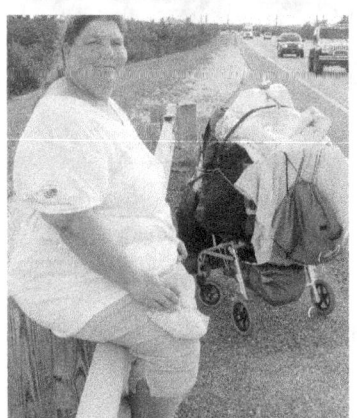

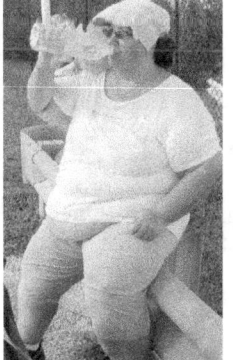

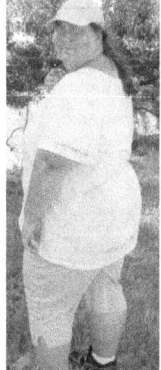

Does
my
butt
look
BIG
in
this?

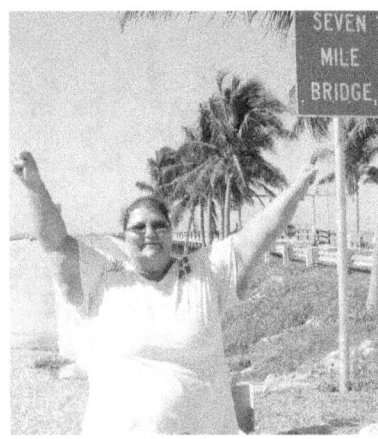
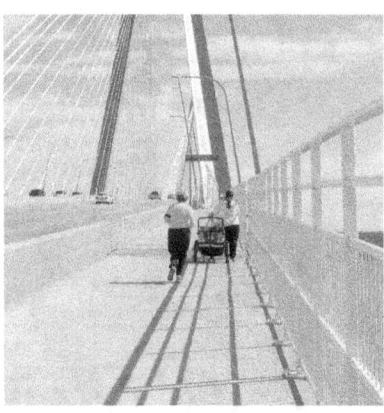
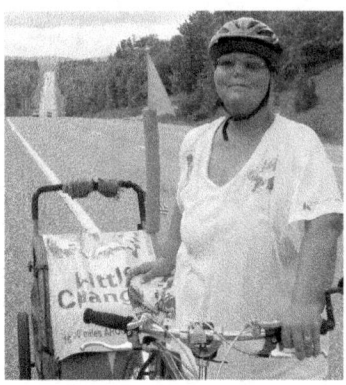

Crossing the 7 Mile Bridge on foot
The feeling was BRILLIANT!

Pushing the bike over a perfect
bridge in Charleston, SC

The mountains of Maine tried to
kill me, but didn't.

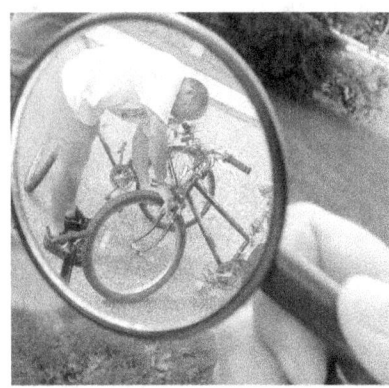
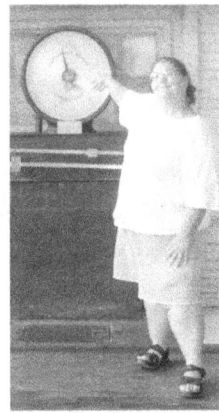
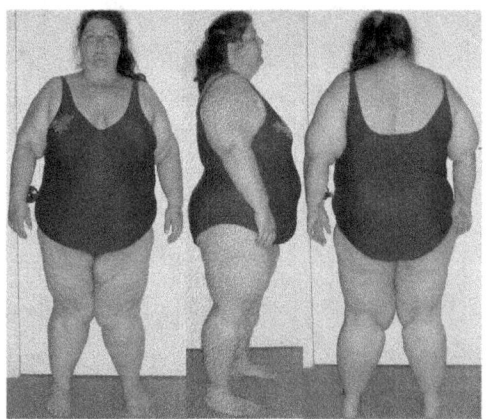

Morton was forever fixing flat tires,
wheels and being my hero on a daily
basis. Dooberizer extrodinaire!

No longer afraid of
scales.
Cheyenne, WY

Key West, Florida December 31, 2006
Weight 343.5 The night before the journey began.

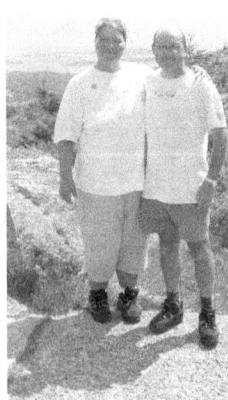
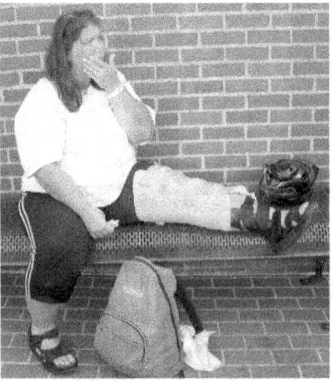
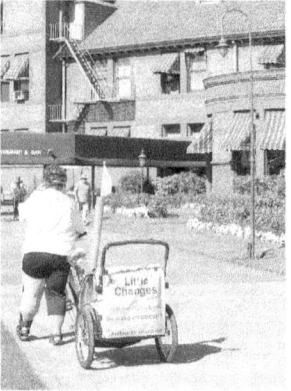
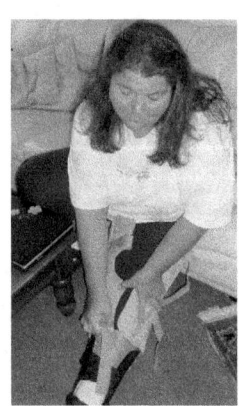

MDI, Maine On top of
the world with Morton.

Portland Oregon September 2007
After the injury, I'm eating lunch
while crying.

Using my bike as a crutch I limp
to the train station while pushing
a 100 pound trailer.

The knee stopped the
journey, but not me.
I will not rest until I'm fit!

April 21, 2007 - Saturday - *Hotel Blue*, **Lewes, Delaware to** *Palace Hotel*, **Cape May, New Jersey**

The day was really great but emotional. We were in route to Cape May as our family heading there from another direction. We bicycled for *Fox News* all around the Hotel Blue in Lewes for a while, then rode to the ferry. It was going to be a day of "acting natural" in a situation that is really not a natural one.

The ferry ride was about 80 minutes and in the middle of the crossing, the sea was really rolling. My stomach was so sick and I just had to lay down on the bench on the top deck and try to sleep. It was one of those times that you wished you could just be on dry land, but much like us on the bikes, we had to just keep going! On the other side we met up with the people that are doing a documentary. It was really a different experience and the hours just disappeared.

Before long we were pulling into the *Palace Hotel* and it was like finding an oasis in a desert. It is so lovely and we get to meet Bruce, the incredible man who arranged at very last minute, for all of us to stay. We chatted for a bit and then we headed for our room. It was great having extra hands around to help get our gear inside. It took us only 1 trip! Then we were back out for more filming combined with the practical exercise of shopping. It made a real difference being in a car where we could cover the 10 miles in 10 minutes. Morton and I got about 5 days worth of food for $19.00. It was great and we have some different things on our menu coming up. We also all had dinner at KFC. James, Mari treated us and Sarah & Graeme shared a biscuit and an ear of corn. It was really tasty.

After a day of odd surprises, again, we didn't even know any of this was going to happen until Friday evening, we headed back to our lovely place at the *Palace Hotel*. We are in a room where there is a living room, balcony looking at the ocean with nothing in front of us but lovely sand dunes, a kitchen, table & chairs, 2 double beds, 2 televisions, 2 bathrooms and the feeling that you are really all just in a lovely home on the beach. Being that we were all tired, the snores started happening about 9 pm. I had good intentions of making my way to the desk to have a chat with Bruce, but I just couldn't stay awake. I had to head for bed and I think I might have been asleep before my head hit the pillow.

April 22, 2007 - Sunday - *Palace Hotel,* **Cape May to Ocean City, New Jersey**

This has been, without a doubt, the most grueling day of our journey. I am emotionally wiped out, we were caught out after dark and getting to see my kids in such a weird way...I just need a shower and to go to bed. Sorry, people. It has just been the longest day of my life and I'll give you the full details in the morning. I'm crying like a big baby right now and just need to rest Priscilla

Monday morning - The sun is out. That is good. Last night I was just exhausted. Mentally, physically, every which way you can be. I think the correct term is "shattered".

The day started so great. My kids and their spouses were with us. We were going to do a bit of nothing in the morning, sit on the beach at Cape May right across from where we had slept the night before in the *Palace Hotel*. There was still the job of "acting natural" for cameras, which now seemed like a terrible intrusion. These were my last few hours together with my family and I didn't really want to show the world what a bad mother I am by saying goodbye and riding off into the sunset. My kids are 25 and 24, but remember, they are always going to be my babies. We got all the gear lugged across the sand to a platform of some sorts, almost like a deck on the beach. It was the perfect place for us to lounge about for a bit while the guys all played in the surf. James and Graeme had a game of standing on the shore to see who would leave the cold water first. As waves splashed up on them, they held their ground as we watched from 100 yards away. It was light-hearted fun and the first time since we started, that we actually just laid on the beach. Even though we have been walking or bicycling beside it for almost four full months, it has never happened before.

Sarah was resting on the wooden deck and I found a pale orange, transparent shell for her. We had a little cuddle and I didn't say my usual of how much I was going to miss her and her growing belly, but she knew. The four of them were going to stop at a place they had seen on the other side of town and have lunch before driving back to Pennsylvania. Morton and I quickly ate our lunch, since it was noon, on the mystery deck, while they looked on. It made me feel odd, eating my lunch in front of them. This wasn't how food worked in our family. Food is a very social thing with us. We would have big plates of it on the go whenever we got together. We got together a lot and the food always flowed like wine. Today it was different, me eating my own lunch and not offering to share any. It was also odd knowing that our days of free-flowing food were over, as was our time together.

We hugged, they headed for the car and Morton and I headed off on the bikes. We had turned right to make our way to Ocean Drive, which would run us up the beachside way to Atlantic City. I thought that they wouldn't come past us this way, but they did.

I was alright until I heard the friendly, "toot, toot, toot" and spotted their car. My heart gave a flutter and with them still in my sight, driving away from us, arms still waving, I was hit with the biggest case of homesickness I have ever felt in my life. Why didn't they stop for one more hug? I have had too much of *saying goodbye* lately and can't take it.

The urge to just follow them was overwhelming. Haven't I learned enough of controlling food portions and getting exercise? Isn't it time to go home, live in a house with indoor plumbing, refrigerator with ice cube trays and sleep in the same bed every night? I thought about this for the next couple miles as the coast of New Jersey passed by. Dialing my sons phone, he answered and I said, "I miss you" to which he told me he missed me too. "I want to come home" I continued. He thought I was joking, but I wasn't. I would have gone with them in a second if they would have turned around. The trouble is, I would have regretted doing that for the rest of my life. Instead, I just bugged him with a few more phone calls, made while I was riding, trying to find out if they would be sneaking up behind us again after they ate their lunch. But they weren't. My heart felt like it had gained all the weight back that I have lost over this past year. Suddenly I felt very heavy, tired and old.

The sights to see were stunning, but I was only halfway even seeing them. Thank goodness the traffic and broken glass were both at a minimum, again, I wasn't noticing anything. Then something caught my eye. It was in North Wildwood, walking along a sidewalk. A dear elderly man, with his arm out and around his wife. She looked like she had suffered a stroke, her one leg was dragging a bit. They were out for a walk, as slow as it needed to be, but together. I tried to remind myself of how good it is to be alive, they are living proof of this. Visions of my dad walking my mom in their garden came into my mind. My homesickness for my children lessened as I was missing both of my parents so bad. Mom is in Pennsylvania and I will be able to visit with her when we go back for Sarah and Graeme's baby. But my dad has passed away. Sigh... I think it's just a day to be sad. There are a few bridges with tolls on them to get around these places that I have never been before. Wildwood, Avalon and heading north, even Ocean City. All in New Jersey. They are places that would be packed if it was just six weeks later, but today, they are almost like ghost towns. Signs in windows announce the places that are closed for the season. The houses all seem to be for rent, with signs on them, but when I try a few numbers to see about sleeping in a garage or backyard, no one answers. We keep riding, hoping to come across a motel or campground that isn't shut. I miss my chance to ask for lodging in a backyard when a lady we are passing tells us she has seen us on television. It turns out she is from Pennsylvania, near WGAL, who do updates on us. We chat a bit and I pet her dog, but we keep going. Five minutes later I tell Morton that I should have asked to camp in her backyard.

We still have two good hours of daylight left and with a little luck, we might make it to Atlantic City. There, worse comes to the worst, we could sit in a casino all night and try Sarah's plan of sleeping on the beach by day! She had suggested this in Miami where we could find no room and had to kill our credit cards with expensive lodging on South Beach. Our ride is going to take us through some incredible places this summer, all in peak tourist season. This is why it's so important that everyone watching please get involved. We are glad to camp wherever! Our needs are very simple and for most parts, we are housebroken. There are a few churches. I call the numbers on one in Ocean City to find out it's just seasonal. It's winterized and the man on the other end of the phone can't give us permission to stay. The sun is really falling quickly now and we pedal for all we are worth. Around 8th Avenue, there are a group of other churches. I ask Morton to go investigate for phone numbers since I have to go to the bathroom very bad. He thinks I'm saying, "Go beg for a place to stay!" which he will never do. He goes off on this big deal about how he isn't going to talk to people about staying there. First, they can't understand him with his thick Scottish accent. Second, I'm better at explaining what we are doing. Suddenly I think about how many times Morton has arranged a place for us to stay on this trip. It has been one time. On day three I think. With Captain Steven in Summerland Key. Actually, he offered for us to pitch out tent in his backyard and Morton happened to be closest to him in distance to accept his offer, so he didn't even have to ask. Feeling like I'm the only one that can do anything for the PR side, computer side, arranging rooms side and EVERYTHING side, I get very upset. Combine this all with the night setting in, cold coming on, having to go to the bathroom so bad it feels like my back teeth ARE floating and missing my family so bad and I start to cry. I burst out in waves of uncontrollable tears. Morton takes action at this point and goes to try to find a number on one of the churches. No joy. He tells me there is a pizza place on the corner I can use the bathroom in, but it's closed. We just head back around where we had been and try to ask at all the hotels that look like they might be open. Again, no joy.

By now, my tears have somehow taken away the urge for the bathroom a bit. We pull into a place that has a VACANCY sign lit up. I think about the movie that is out right now with the same name. I hate things like that, they put terrible images in our minds when there are so many nice things out there. Just as I'm getting over my fear of Norman Bates, along comes the film *VACANCY*. That's entertainment, I suppose. This place is neither like the Bates Motel or the dump I see in the commercials for the new film. It looks like a family beach-side motel. The lady says the very best she can do is $49. She would have to talk to the owner, who may or may not help us. At this point, all the street lights are on and it is dark. We have to just bite the bullet and get the room. The bathroom is worth the $49. I suppose. I get the hottest shower I can stand and get all of my cry-ing out of my system behind the pulled curtain. After I get on the computer. I can't really write about today right now. There are too many tears in my eyes and I am ready for sleep. My body and my mind has reached the breaking point today and sleep is my only hope. This morning I find so much email from all of you. I pull a real strength from it. You are all so kind with your words and I feel very weak and silly. I am out here because I choose to be and I'm lucky enough to be alive and doing this dream of mine. Morton shouldn't be asked to go in and ask strangers for a place to stay, he's just tagging along for support of me and he *does* do so much.

We each have very different roles out here, while on this trip. I just have to remember that some days will be a lot tougher than others, but the end result will be worth all the struggles.

April 23, 2007 - Monday - Ocean City to *Caesars*, Atlantic City, New Jersey

Timing is everything. It helps us get in to a room before dark, it helps us talk to people and this morn-ing, as we were going to just start riding for Atlantic City, timing made my day. Looking a the clock, I knew that we had about 15 minutes to leaving, so I made a phone call to see about a room. The *Atlantic City Convention and Visitors Center* had helped us by sending an email to some potential room sponsors. I had no idea who they had sent it to, but I called *Caesars*. Quicker than you can say "I'm on a roll!" I was on the phone with Chris, who had gotten the email and told us the excellent news that *Caesars Atlantic City* was going to sponsor us a room for two nights. This will be the time we need to do our press, speak with people, see some sights and ride the world-famous boardwalk.

The bad night we had just had was now a far away memory. Our luck had changed for the better and we rode under the sun to our destination that was just a short ride north. We also had a south wind that pushed us right along. We looked over to the ocean and saw the boardwalk begin, while Atlantic City was now in our vision. Heading towards the boardwalk, we experienced the joy of riding free from red lights and cars. It was brilliant.

Just as we were coming in to the city, the newspaper called us to do a story and to find out where they should send the photographer to. We made our arrangements and kept heading to Caesars. Soon we were riding for the photographer in the shadow of what was going to be our home for the next two nights. After-wards, we met up with Chris who got us settled into our room. He had also arranged for us to go see the show, *Dancing Queen* this evening. We have to say, both the room and the show are grade A, top-notch, wonderful and our huge thanks go to Chris and all his help. He made these two crazy bicycle riding health freaks feel like a couple of VIP's. Not an easy task, but the surroundings are just so superior. We went to the *Visitors Center*, took a walk on the boardwalk, did a live radio interview and then got ready to go see the show. We re-ally don't have dress clothes, so I wore a pair of SIZE 22 capri jeans and a white top. I also let my hair down, literally. It was odd not seeing it in a ponytail or under a helmet.

The show was better than we had hoped for. Singing, dancing, songs that we all knew and we were seated by these two great ladies who were on an adventure of their own. They are driving across the country on a girl's road trip! It was as if fate had seated us all together at that big semi-circle booth. One of the ladies had just lost 100 pounds and felt fantastic and was trying to talk her friend to lose her weight. She confessed that our story was just what she needed to hear to quit making excuses and start making changes. It was music to my ears! Afterwards, we started to think that maybe, just maybe, since we are perhaps the luckiest people in the world, we should have a go at the machines on the floor. But then, checking funds, Morton sees that we have just $7.00 in his wallet. We decide to save our gambling luck for our next visit to this wonderful city and to focus on just enjoying the sights and sounds tonight.

In the morning, from 6 am to 10 am, you can ride your bikes on the boardwalk. We are going to do a couple interviews, ride our bikes, visit a few places and then set north again.

April 24, 2007 - Tuesday - *Caesars*, Atlantic City, New Jersey

The day began with us taking advantage of the bicycle riding times on the boardwalk. If only there was a boardwalk all along our way. Sigh...one can dream. It is the best feeling in the world to ride and not worry about a car or truck wiping you out. There also are not any hazards that are going to give you a flat tire. We had spent the morning chatting to people who saw the story in the paper or heard us on the radio. We also had a bit more press to do, which went well.

We found ourselves with a very full day, already over and it was only 11 am. This is what happens when you wake up before 5 am! I got the chance to do some painting on the boardwalk. It was too tough though to get focused on what I was working on. People were chatting to Morton and he was talking as if I wasn't there, since I was concentrating on the painting bit. It was really pleasant though. Perfect weather, great location and there were even some people who asked if the painting I was working on was for sale. I think they thought I was a street artist, though I use the word "artist" very loosely. It was really just a bit of watercolor and trying to paint how I was feeling at the moment.

We put our bikes back in our lovely room at Caesars and set off on foot. We had forgotten to pick up our NJ map in the tourist office, so we went back to get one. We sat for just long enough to give it a good look over and then trotted up the boardwalk to *Ripley's Believe it or Not!* That place is really something you have to see. I love looking at his cartoons, reading about where all he went and looking at the oddities. My favorite thing in there was the gypsy wagon. I have always wanted to have one since first reading *The Wind in the Willows* as a child. Mr. Toad traded his canary yellow gypsy wagon on a motor car, a mistake I would never make. There was a couple that we seemed to end up looking and laughing at the same things. They were so cute and she would giggle like mad every time he would jump from a surprise or try to walk through this twirling tunnel. They were just out for a lark, today felt the same for us.

One of the tough things about stopping in a place as exciting and always on, such as Atlantic City, is to just take it easy and have a look around. The good thing about Atlantic City is that you have the excitement of the casinos at your disposal 24 hours a day, but you also have this rich and colorful history of this seaside town to explore. We did a bit of both, though we didn't do any gaming at all. I really wanted to play roulette, but our budget doesn't have one spare cent in it. We returned to our room and I got to work on the web for about four hours. There are so many things to be done and getting all the things lined up for NYC is a tough task.

Tonight we had the most amazing meal at *Phillips Seafood*. It is actually in this wonderful shopping area that is right on the water and connected to *Caesars*. It was just so tasty and fresh. It was even better because we were both so hungry after our day outside of walking, talking, interviewing and breathing in that lovely ocean air. I felt ready for bed when we got back to the room at just after 8 pm. I knew tomorrow will be back on the bikes and trying to make some mileage before the rain comes. But the computer is calling and I end up working until 1 am. So much for an early night!

April 25, 2007 - Wednesday - Caesars, Atlantic City to Tuckerton, NJ

There are so many things that happen each day, I don't want to bore you with all the details...but we meet some really incredible people. This is an everyday fact. As we were checking out of Caesars we chatted to a few people who were curious to what we were pulling in the trailers. They did look a bit odd being pulled through the casino. Sadly we can't tell them it's bundles of money we won because we didn't get to play!

Once out on the boardwalk, I wanted one last picture of us in front of the place that had been so kind and generous to us. A really nice guy offered to snap a rare picture of Morton and I together, then was a bit amazed when he found out what we are doing. It really doesn't seem like anything unusual to us anymore, but it is great seeing peoples reaction. Their excitement and questions always astound us.

I have got to sit down with Morton and come up with our *TOP TEN* questions that we get asked....as soon as we have a bit of time on our hands, we will do it. Today we ride with the wind at our backs a bit, but then in our face and sides. The breeze coming from the ocean is seeming to change direction however it wants to. The boardwalk isn't going to last long and before we leave it, we see a familiar face. A bicycle ambassador that we met on our first day in, is the last person we see and talk to before heading off back into the land of cars and trucks. He had told us the best way to get where we wanted to go and we had to do a little switching around, but before we knew it we were on 9 north. Today we faced a bit of a problem. 9 runs with the turnpike for about 2 miles and our bikes aren't allowed on the road. We decide to worry about it on down the line and keep going. The beautiful thing about our journey is that it really does seem to have a life of it's own. It also has the most friendly people on the planet watching and helping us along the way!

As we ride we are getting lots of the friendly toots. The press was kind to us in Atlantic City and it shows. There are waves, thumbs up and lots of kind words. There is also a nice, wide side of the road. All is well with our world. There is a small town we come to that has a park that looks like the perfect place to eat our lunch. Again, remember how timing is everything...this is what happened next. As we leave, we meet a man who is a bicyclist and gives us advice on which way to go and how to get across the bridge that is on the turnpike. It is as simple as giving a phone call for permission...yipee.

When we get to the part of the road where 9 joins up with the turnpike, it was very scary getting on it.

Not only were the cars and trucks whizzing past us, there was a sign saying NO bikes. We worried about what happens when a police car stops. I didn't even have a name to give them of the person I spoke to about getting permission, but I would cross that bridge if it came. There was two miles that we had to go like mad to get back on just 9 north. These were the most two very frantic miles of our ride. The road was plenty wide and we hugged the right tighter then ever. Morton says he was hoping not to get a flat tire and I was just hoping to not hear a police siren behind us. When the exit appeared, what should be going past us but a police car. My heart raced as he ignored us completely. I think that he knew we were getting off the turnpike. I think he also had to know that there really was nowhere else for us to go. Coming up the ramp I almost jumped out of my skin as a lady screamed out her car window that we should *NOT* be on the turnpike. We did no harm whatsoever, had plenty of room and I don't know why she felt compelled to scream at us. Maybe she thought we did this every day. The road, 9 north, was just beautiful. Lovely towns, wide surfaces that were free from litter and the traffic wasn't too hectic. It was getting cold though, the forecast said rain was in our future for the afternoon and we wanted to make it to a town called Tuckerton, where there were campgrounds waiting! Just as we came into the town, I started to worry that our day was suddenly going to go very wrong. The girls in the dollar store told me the campgrounds were shut. There was a B&B ahead they told us, then it was a good 15 miles until a motel. Since it was about 6 pm, starting to rain and getting colder, we were going to try our luck at the B&B. As I knocked on the door, the couple who ran it said they were full. They told me that ahead was a motel, but it was about 15 more miles. Yikes! Panic still didn't sink in though, we are getting to be experts at staying calm. We just got on our bikes and rode on.

There was a church, but no number and no answer when I called the number that Sarah had looked up for me via telephone calls. I got an answering machine and we knew that we just had to keep going. Worse comes to worse, we could always push our bikes if we lose the light. Then on our right, was another church. This one had it's phone number on a sign *(all churches should do this!)* and as Morton went to investigate if anyone was inside, I made a phone call. I got a recording, but on the recording was a number to contact the Vicar. I had to call back to get the number and was quite surprised when the Vicar himself answered.

The Vicar told me they were inside the church, having their first community meal. He invited us in, where we dined with several dozen people on the most delicious *HOMEMADE* food, then got a tour of the lovely building. We also got to pick out which room would be our sleeping quarters for the evening. Best of all, it was all unplanned and yet perfect! We chose the library, but then switched to the nursery. There is a soft play mat on the floor that Morton has put out our thin sleeping bags on. Morton also got out the laptop and to our surprise, we got wireless! Talk about great luck or being in the right place at the right time. As the rain comes down on this lovely town, we will sleep tonight in a warm, dry, comfortable place. Our dinner was going to be cold tuna and instead was a wonderful home cooked meal and getting to share it with the friendly people was just the best we could hope for.

April 26, 2007 - Thurs *Holy Spirit Episcopal Church*, Tuckerton to *Hershey Motel*, Seaside Heights, NJ

If the early bird gets the worm, then we should be able to go fishing! We were awake at 6, leaving on the bikes a bit after 7am, and heading north. Ernie came out nice and early to lock the door behind us as we rode off on the nice wide shoulder. This part of the country is certainly lovely. There are so many beautiful homes, parks and the trees are all in full blossom. Spring is sticking right with us, has been since January! But we won't complain of the cool temperatures today. It is a lot better than roasting. We can always put a jacket on, but there are only so many clothes you can take off and not get arrested! With the early start, we were sort of riding with the commuters and people heading off to work. It was a hustle, bustle feeling but we didn't get any mean HONKS of the horn...only friendly ones accompanied by waves and smiles.

Before we knew it, it was 9 am and we were outside a lovely library. I went in for the bathroom and to have a look around at the book sale they were having. I love to read but don't really have to time to on this trek. If I'm not riding the bike or walking, I'm working on the computer. I was tempted to get just one book, but then thought about my rule for Morton "If you pick it up, it goes in YOUR OWN trailer!" and thought otherwise. My trailer seems to be gaining all the weight I'm losing. Today was a day for spotting tulips in full blooms, seeing seas of daffodils and becoming intoxicated by the many garden centers that have various blooms out beside the road. There was one garden center we passed where a lady was working with tubs of flowers. I really wanted to stop and volunteer our services, mine anyway, for the day. It would be lovely to work with the flowers and plants all day. One of the things I miss being out here, is the garden. There is something so satisfying about weeding, dead heading, planting and watching things come to life from a dried up seed from a packet. The next big garden we come across I am going to throw out the anchor and stop for the day. We have often eyed up greenhouses and commented that they would make a good place to stay the night. Before the trip is over, I imagine we will stay in one or two. Today we got confirmation from the *Hotel Pennsylvania*, in New York, that they are going to sponsor us for our stay there. This is such a big relief! We need to be in town for three days for press. They have even offered us space for doing an actual press conference. How exciting is *THAT*? The hotel is amazing and in a perfect location for us while we are in Manhattan. It is right across from Penn Station and Madison Square Garden. We can't wait to get there and we have to say a giant *THANK YOU* to Jerry for all his help in making it happen.

We are so excited about the time we are going to be in NYC. It is going to be Sunday morning when we get there and today while I was riding, I was mentally going over all the things that we have lined up press wise. My mind usually just focuses on the day at hand, but a stop as big as New York requires a bit of forward thinking. I try to think if there will be any moments that we can squeeze in a trip to this place or that...hopefully we will be able to. Like much of our trip so far, we blink our eyes and it's history. The road is great again today. I love seeing the woods that is growing by 9 north. Trees that are just thinking about getting their leaves out, some with blossoms on them and the smell of spring approaching is in the air. There is more traffic which means that Morton and I don't get to talk a lot. I always wonder what he's back there thinking. Talk about seeing America!

To think that five years ago he had never even been to our country before is pretty staggering. Now he's getting to see and do things that he's only seen in movies. We said it before and I'll say it again, dreams do come true if you are willing to work at them. My son calls at lunchtime and he's still sick. His wife seems to be getting it too. I hope that Morton and I both keep healthy. We do get plenty of fresh air and exercise, so we should be alright. It's good to hear James, even if he is all stuffy and congested.
I start to think of my kids as we are bicycling along. There are moments when I imagine, "What if?" our trip would have been the 8 of us instead of just 2. Mom, Dad, Sarah, Graeme, James, Mari and Morton and I...but we will never know. It might have made us all get on each others nerves. There are many times out here that it is so stressful and scary.

My sister Cindy is giving a baby shower for Sarah. Again, it's hard for me to think about the baby, because I want to go to Sarah and spend the last few months of her pregnancy rubbing her back. Instead, we live on the road now. I have an invitation to the shower that came via email. It's lovely and my sister is doing an amazing job organizing and doing the other million things she has in her daily life. People are coming from far away for the shower, which is next weekend, but I don't think I'll be able to make it. We should be in Connecticut or even Rhode Island and the logistics is going to be tough. Miracles do happen though, we'll see. If not, Sarah will understand. She is this brilliant person who has always been wise beyond her years. She knows, better than anyone really, why I'm on this journey. She is the shoulder I cry on when I've had a bad day and she is the little rock that reminds me why I'm finally changing my life.

There are two temperatures we see today. One says 51 degrees and one says 53. *Brrrr,* either way. There is also a cutting wind in our faces, but we ride along at a slower pace. Morton is complaining that his knees are sore. He thinks it might be the cold or wind. Spotting a little Chinese place with a $4.00 special sign up, we stop and split something hot. It is so tasty and really hits the spot. The owner comes outside to chat with us about the journey. Morton had been carrying around two gold chains and his first wedding band from his *practice* marriage. This isn't due to sentiment, we have just been meaning to sell them. They are only 9 carat gold and when I go in to a shop today, find out that they are worth just $24.00. It is better than nothing though, will pay for food for a few days and help keep us moving, so we sell them in a shop in New Jersey. He wonders how much he would have gotten for the scrap gold in the UK, but there is no way to know. It's gone now and we are $24.00 dollars richer.

When we reached Toms River we started thinking of a room. The first six places all say "no rooms" or "not open" so we just keep heading east on 37. There is a big bridge (oh the bridges!) that we have to cross and it is more than just a little bit hairy. We loose the edge, but on the good note, there are 3 lanes going east. There is a bit of a blind spot at the top, which is always scary. Before we know it though, we are finished with it and have no edge at all. Riding right in traffic I hope we live to see the night, no matter where we have to sleep. Morton took a few pictures and we then had to make our way across the traffic to head north. Lane switching on bikes is tough, but we do it. There are lots of motels, some open for the season, some closed. One gives us a rate of $45. for the night, but still out of our budget. We keep heading north. Maybe we will be lucky enough to come across another church, fire station or a place that is able to help with a room. Then our daily miracle happens. We see a sign for a church and what a church it is. Historic and right beside the beach.

We dial the number and talk to Dennis. He is worried about our comfort of staying in the church and suggests that if we go find a room, he will come along and pay for it for us. This is a perfect stranger, with the emphasis on the word "perfect". Can you believe it? This kind man drives down and meets us at a nearby motel. We have a little chat and then he is gone. In the morning, we will stop by this church and get some pictures for you. It really is lovely and would have suited us just fine. But instead we are in a room. There is a shower (LOVELY) a kitchen, two bedrooms, great workspace for me catching up and even a sofa for Morton to sit on to fix the slow-leak puncture on his trailer. We have a warm supper and I have to now just read and reply to the 323 emails we got today! At just 30 seconds an email, it means about 2 1/2 hours should do it. Things are shaping up well for our ride in Central Park on Sunday and we will keep you posted on our day. All of the people who are out there thinking about our journey and how it can happen that we are on it, the answer is easy. Take any challenge with the first step. After that, it's gets easier.

April 27, 2007 - Friday - *Hershey Motel*, Seaside Heights, New Jersey

Things were very wet today. It started early and the forecast called for 100% chance of rain, saying it was going to last for the entire day. They were right. We were really dragging our feet and our wheels. We were loaded and ready to ride nice and early, the rain was just so heavy, we kept hoping it would slow down a bit to encourage us to leave the sanctuary of the room. Check out time had come and gone and I needed to speak to the owner, Ann, about the *Hershey Motel* sponsoring us the room for the night in our safe & dry retreat. The trouble wasn't the rain, it was the phone! We kept getting so many calls yesterday, most from the press and things were just really happening. The lovely girl at the front desk popped by to say that Ann was going to be leaving soon, so I had to make a dash, with phone in hand, to the main office to ask for a sponsored night. Ann was just wonderful and said they could help. I had this great load of worry taken away and the phone rang as I was saying goodbye and thanking her. Making a dash through the rain back to the room, I told Morton he could take off his rain jacket and get the laptop back out. Whew...it was going to be a day of working, not riding.

Morton and I have been learning PR as we go along. We are not professionals out here and I just don't want to pass through NYC without really getting to connect with the press, then in turn, with more people watching the site, the better. The method to my madness is this, more people watching is SAFER, plus, more people watching means there is a better chance of back yard camping along the way. But the biggest things is, we really do want to make a difference in your lives. Today flies by faster than any other. The phone never really quits ringing and things are really shaping up for NYC. We have a lot of big milestones coming up as well. Tomorrow, Saturday the 28th of April, we will cross our 2,000th mile. This is something that is really staggering for me. To think a year ago I was eating myself to death and getting Morton to put on my shoes. Like the old ad says, *"You've come a long way baby!"* Morton is lured with the thought of a grocery store just a few blocks away. There is a break in the rain and he makes a dash for it. Poor Morton is really bored and a bit restless. He can't really do anything to help with the computer work or phone calls so he decides to see if there are any bargains to be had at the store. After about an hour passes, it dawns on me that he has been gone for ages. I know he likes to look at all the aisles, but even for Morton, it's a long time. Looking out the window I am horrified to see it raining buckets. This is really a bad storm and he has most likely held up, waiting for a break in the weather. Seeing our bag hanging open that we keep the camera in, I panic for a second that he has it with him. It will be soaked and ruined!!! Then I see it sitting beside the bed. Picking it up, I get some pictures and then catch a glimpse of his bright yellow jacket running down the street, carrying bags. Turning the setting to video, I get Morton on film coming in from the fierce rain. He has with him three soaking plastic bags stuffed with bargains. "I spent all the money" he exclaims, with a pause as if he's waiting on me to scold him. "I think I still have $3.00 or so left" he adds. He is safe and he does have three bags of food. So he spent sixteen dollars, it wasn't as if he traded our cow for magic beans.

Worried as he was unpacking the goods, about where we were going to put all of this food, he pulls out a soaking wet paper bag with fast food. It has 2 "dollar" chicken wraps and 2 (for a dollar) apple pies in it. He tells me that he thought $3.00 for lunch was alright and it was warm. Morton has to hang up his clothes by the heater because even the raincoat didn't save him from the rain. The water had soaked right up his t-shirt, his shorts were wringing wet and his socks on the tops were soaked. The only dry thing really, were his MBT boots. Quality shows. I got back to the computer and Morton set about getting all our gear packed for a second time today. In the course of the rainy day, we managed to move no where, but got so much accomplished. I was on a roll with our upcoming NYC visit and kept working until Morton was fast asleep on the couch with the telly on. It was almost midnight before I shut the laptop off and woke him up for bed.

The last thing I did was check the forecast, *SLIGHT* chance of rain...far better than 100% chance. Tomorrow we ride over 40 miles and will cross our 2,0000th mile. It does seem like just yesterday we walked away from Key West, now here we are on the north east coast of New Jersey, ready to cross into New York. See what you can do if you are willing to make a few little changes?

April 28, 2007 - Saturday - *Hershey Motel*, Seaside Heights to *Nauvoo Cottages*, Highlands, NJ

Did I mention how the toughest days out here can be some of the best? That was today.

There have been smells that I have told you about on our journey, some good, some bad. Today we came across the worst, ever. The last thing I do each morning before we leave is switch the camera on to make sure I have the battery in it. It is a little thing we do, because one day we *did* forget and had to go through the panic of the feeling of having lost our one and only camera battery. Pushing the button down, nothing happened. The motor didn't make it's little buzzing noise, pushing the lens cover open. Nope, nothing, nada. I thought the battery might not be in it, but Morton assured me it was. I handed it over to him to sort out and kept working last minute style, on the laptop. Morton said, "Do you smell that?" I sniffed the air. "It's like someone has lit a match." he added. Jumping up to smell the camera we both groaned at the same time. There was this horrible, burnt smell coming from the camera. "That will be the motor fried." said Morton. I stared at him in disbelief. Not the camera! Anything but the camera...well, not the computer either. What a time for it to die on us. Right before a glorious ride into the town called Highlands. Right before passing all these incredible mansions beside the beach. Right before getting on a ferry to head into Manhattan on what will be the chance for a hundred lovely pictures....not now!!! But it was dead, fried, finished. This was our first real taste of what happens when something you rely on every day fails. It is the bad part of not having the finances behind making this journey.

Something that would be easily solved if we had things like cars to go to the store and money to get a new camera, are now like dreaming the impossible dream. But I'm not going to let it ruin my day. We have the camera in the phone...that will do for now. Groan. Money can't buy happiness, but it could buy a camera.

We head north, hugging the coast and saying "Ooooh" and "Aaaaah" a lot. There are such pretty sights and the day is just wonderful weather wise. We can see some of the leftovers of the flooding they got yesterday. Stones and grit washed by the water at the edge of the road. It was all the proof we needed that yesterday wouldn't have been a good day to bicycle here. Canoe maybe, but not bicycle. The ride felt like it flew by. We did talk to several people but I was too shy to use the camera phone on them. I knew the picture quality was going to be rubbish. Places that I had never seen before flew by and we got quite a few friendly toots and thumbs up. We are always so thankful of that. You can tell in an instant a nice toot on the horn as opposed to an angry one. Short and sweet means *good luck, safe journey.* Loud and long means, *out of my way or I'll plaster you to my hood.*

When we rode in to Highlands and I spotted their amazing twin lighthouses, they remind me of castle towers, I felt the pang of not having my camera. I didn't miss any photos of flocks of flying pigs or dancing unicorns riding unicycles, but there were tons of great scenes. The town of Highlands really took us by surprise. It is really lovely, right out of a story book. Since we are meeting a reporter first thing in the morning, we decide to bicycle to the ferry so we will know where we are going. We start to think about places to sleep. Since tomorrow there will be a marathon here, the town is full up. I call the police station to see if they can help. A wonderful dispatcher, Mandy, listened to our special request and said she would make some calls. In the mean time, we were going to keep trying to find somewhere ourselves. We knew the B&B's in the town were full, we had tried to contact the churches but had only been able to reach someone at one. There was another church the pastor we spoke with had recommended trying, but we only got a recording there. We decided to go back into town and visit the church in person.

Highlands is named correctly. This is a very hilly bit that is right on the coast, flanked by these amazing twin towers of lighthouses. The church we were looking for was at the top of a very steep hill. I opted to wait at the bottom with the bicycles while Morton went upon foot to investigate and inquire if there was any room at the inn. He came right back down to tell me he heard music inside. It was about 5:40 pm and I asked him to please go back up to speak with the people as they were coming out. Someone might have a solution to our safe-sleeping problem. Morton had taken along the phone camera and called me to tell me the priest had said we could sleep in the basement! Joy! Quickly I called Mandy to have her call off the search for a place for us to stay. We then had to push the bikes up this steep hill, only to face our second big disappointment of the day. While we were waiting outside, the priest had called another priest who said no. The reason he told us was that they didn't know us. I offered the card of the vicar from a few nights ago who could vouch for us, but it was words spent on ears that weren't hearing. Our hearts and spirits sank as we walked away.

It might have been our lowest moment so far. Pulling my phone out, the battery fading on it, I called Mandy at the police station and told her the basement of the church had fallen through. We were back to being home-less tonight. She promised to call us back and we decided we better hold tight at the church. It was going to be dark before long and we didn't want to go back down the hill, only to have to come right back up.

We were both really hungry, shared some water and an apple. Sitting on the steps of the church I felt like crying. It was really feeling hopeless. If a church can't help you, especially one called *Our Lady of Perpetual Help*, what hope did we have?

Back at the ferry we had spoken to a lady that had a one bedroom place. She told us to come back if nothing turned up and I was thinking that we might have to do that. Then my phone rang. It was Mandy. She gave me details about a person who was going to meet us at these colorful and marvelous cottages, that aren't open yet. They were going to let us stay in one, courtesy of Bill Weber. Our contact person was Carla, whose name I was writing on the palm of my hand while taking directions. Just as I was phoning Sarah to tell her the good news, a car pulled up in front of us at the church. Out jumps Carla who is just brilliant! She leads us right to the cottages, along with her sister and her sister's son. Before we know it, there are so many people there to wish us well. They are asking questions and are excited and supportive of our journey. Even Bill, the owner of these wonderful cottages, comes out to show us around and make sure we are comfortable. The highs and lows of just a space of five mere minutes had my head spinning. It is scary when you think you might have to find a place out of the wind and sit up all night, but that is what we had been feeling before our turn of amazing luck. The journey is a miracle in itself, but the people that are helping us, looking out for us and being so very kind to us, are the real miracles. It is just amazing and we are truly blessed. Tonight we will sleep safely in a lovely cottage, painted bright colors with a lovely courtyard behind it. There is a big ginger cat on the porch and Morton is already sleeping. All is right with the world, yet again!

April 29, 2007 - Sun - *Nauvoo Cottages*, Highlands, NJ to *Hotel Pennsylvania*, New York City, New York

Waking up at the cottage early, we headed through the town of Highlands and made our way to the *SeaStreak* ferry. It was a bit cold out and we got there in time to just sit for a moment and look across the water. You could just see the world-famous NY skyline in front of us and behind us were the hills that rolled up, with the lovely twin lighthouses setting on top of them. Soon we were met by Sarah, the photographer from the paper. I had forgotten to warn the paper that there were roads that we closed and slow because of the marathon that was being run. Carly, the wonderful reporter we had been speaking to by phone, got caught right in the thick of it. As we waited for the ferry, Heather from the *SeaStreak* public relations department arrived. She had helped arrange for us to have free passage on this fast ferry that would save us from having to climb several dozen stairs to cross a bridge into Manhattan.

Carly had called to give us an update on where she was and Sarah snapped pictures as we loaded our gear onto the boat. We placed the bikes and trailers on the very front deck and then sat and had a chat with Heather, other passengers and were watching the clock. We had this feeling that we were going to miss Carly, as the boat had to go at a certain time. We waved goodbye to Heather and Sarah and later I found out, Carly had just arrived as the boat was indeed, "streaking" across the water. The interview still happened, by phone, so we have to make it a point to stop back in this area to meet Carly. She had done a brilliant job on the story. I had told her about the mix up in with the church, actually, the big NO we got from sleeping on their basement floor and it was in the article. I hoped that it would serve as a wake up call to churches to become more stranger friendly.

Morton and I were really enjoying the ferry ride. I have been to Manhattan by bus, car, train and even truck, but never by water. The ride ruined me and now I can't imagine any other way to go. No traffic, no tunnels, no red lights, just the sight of this city getting closer. The ferry also felt less bumpy than being in a car. Just a smooth glide on a sheet of glass. Cruising under the bridge was just wonderful and we were both so giddy with our visit to the biggest city in America right around the corner.

When we landed in midtown, right on 42nd Street, the crew helped us get our gear off the deck. We were right in the heart of the legendary city. The streets were so busy we stuck to the sidewalks for a few blocks. The trouble is, even though they are so wide, the streets were very busy too. Becoming very brave and bold, we headed off down the street with heavy, never-ending traffic. As with many of the things we have been the most afraid of, they turn into a experience that we feel really good about. We found the drivers to be great with bicycles, though it was very busy and crowded. You had no time to gaze upwards at the buildings, you had to keep your eyes on the road. When the lights turned red, we would stop and get some pictures, smile and look around. This will be an exciting stop, we can just feel it. We are not far from our room, but we need to go to Central Park to meet a reporter. We have the thrill of not only riding in Central Park, but also, riding through Times Square. Talk about the thrill of a lifetime!

After our ride in the park, we went back to the Hotel Pennsylvania to check in. The location just blew us away. It is right across from Penn Station and Madison Square Gardens. It is also just a few blocks from Times Square. The hotel is massive, incredible and have great handicapped ramps for us to bring our gear in like a breeze. The room was huge, we love the doors. They remind you of a train, which is why this hotel is the Hotel Pennsylvania. It's from the days of the Pennsylvania Railroad, which my grandfather and father had worked for. Being a Pennsylvania native, I felt right at home here, in the heart of this very big city. We had another telephone interview with a reporter and headed off to Times Square. We were going to get to have dinner at *Bubba Gumps,* courtesy of the lovely Monika. We had a long day and sitting in this fun place, above the lights of Broadway, felt like we were in a dream. The dazzling dream of NYC. Brilliant.

Having a walk around the bright lights and taking the best pictures we could, we headed back to our lovely room. We were so thankful to have a fantastic room and headed for bed. I had the laptop out and was on my belly working on it until after midnight. There is so much involved with the behind-the-scenes side of the trip that we have to learn as we go along, but what a fantastic way to learn!

April 30, 2007 - Monday - *Hotel Pennsylvania*, New York City, New York

This is the only place in the world that you can have a day like we have had today. It started at the *Today Show* at Rockefeller Plaza. There were balloons everywhere, tons of people and the entire cast of Spiderman 3. We were starstruck and while poor Morton had to stay with the bicycles and trailers, I got to see the cast, get their pictures and get their autographs on a lovely Spiderman mask. The morning and afternoon whizzed by with photos, interviews and lots of walking. Our bikes got put back to the hotel and we headed towards the Ed Sullivan Theater, where David Letterman is filmed. Again as if caught in this odd world between reality and television, we chatted with people we had only ever seen on the television! We really enjoyed ourselves, saw Kirstin Dunst for the second and then third time today, gave one of her publicists a LittleChanges slip and then laughed our way through the taping of a show with David Letterman. It is odd not having the bicycles to worry about and we stroll like tourists on these streets of a city that you feel like you know, because you have seen it a thousand times in the movies and on television. When we were at the *Late Show*, we had gotten a call from the PR person at the *Hard Rock Cafe* in Times Square who invited us to come for a meal tonight. We didn't really have much of a lunch so we were starving. In Times Square we saw a *Tasti-D-Lite* and went in to get some pictures. They are a sponsor of our journey and the people inside were so nice! They made a phone call to find out about us and then even gave us each a dish of ice cream. Morton and I found a place to sit right in the middle of Times Square and ate our ice cream while enjoying the view.

We talked about the incredible day we had just had. It was full of pleasant surprises and thrills, laughs and the nicest people you can imagine. We are mortified that we don't have a real camera, but we are going to get a cheap one tomorrow, too bad when we saw all the celebs we just had the phone camera.

Morton and I had never been in a *Hard Rock Cafe* before and I looked at all their very cute shirts and things that I want to wear when my weight is gone. The next time we are back here, I will be able to actually wear things like this. It is a thought that seems not like a dream, but rather a fact. The food is just incredible, the music, the sounds the memorabilia will just bowl you over. We had the best time here and then headed back to our room. Again, it was well past midnight before I fell asleep. We were also on a real excitement buzz from the story Carly had done in the newspaper. It was the ENTIRE page, top to bottom of PAGE TWO! It was a great article and we can't say thanks enough for it.

As the city played on outside our 12th story window, we fell asleep with no problem. After all, we had to get up at 5 am and have another day like this.

Day 121 May 1, 2007 - Tuesday - *Hotel Pennsylvania*, New York City, NY

Today I am up early and a bundle of nerves. We are holding our very first press conference and I now know why people have publicists and press agents. It is a lot of work and has my nerves wrecked. We have emailed dozens of newspapers, television stations, radio stations and the Associated Press have been kind enough to put us in their date book. *Hotel Pennsylvania* is kind enough to let us have space in their amazing ballroom with the most fantastic view of New York that I have ever seen and the morning rushes by as Morton and I prepare for something we have never done before.

The biggest fear I have is, what if no one comes? I have talked to people who say they are most likely coming, but can't promise anything. We are happy news and any disaster or shooting, fire or big news story will make then not come. The morning is spent on the telephone calling to confirm and not getting anywhere.

I understand that news just happens and if something is going on live, it takes the place over a scheduled conference. My stomach is flipping and twisting as we put the bike in the elevator and head for the top floor. I had a call from the *Associated Press* and they were there. I breathed a big sigh of relief. At least there would be someone and anyone who knows anything about the press will recognize that the *Associated Press* is one of the strongest forms of press, if not *the* strongest in the world. This was a giant weight off my mind.

It turns out, there were only three members of the press there. Two from the papers and one, the cameraman and reporter with the Associated Press who was videotaping the entire conference. This was not a huge affair, even though we were in this amazing setting. This was a really casual and nice interview. My fears were all melted away and then Morton started to unroll the banner. Oh no, not the banner. It never really gets any less shocking seeing this creation. It is a hard cold dose of reality to see me at life-size, 343.5 pounds. I know the only way I could even be semi-pleased with this picture, is if I had ANOTHER banner of me at over 400 pounds. There is a picture I have that we have to save for this book. It's just too shocking for the internet. Be warned though that it is an image that might make you never want to eat anything again.

We did a bit of filming in this ballroom that overlooks the *Empire State Building*. There were pictures taken and then we were off. Again, another fear has been faced. Stepping far outside my comfort zone, it is comforting to know I'm stronger than I thought. We need to go get a camera, as we are bicycling off tomorrow. We also need to do another interview with someone who couldn't come to the press conference. We leave excited to get the word out. Move it and LOSE it! Make the impossible happen, it's easy.

We had been in town a few days now and still hadn't seen my niece, Angela. She's an incredible writer, actress, singer and all around amazing person who I have been very close to since the day she was born. Tonight we are going to finally get together. Her boyfriend Adam comes with her as they come to the hotel and we chat for a while before heading off to get something to eat. Morton and I split a hamburger, fries and diet coke and hours slip away as fast as they usually do when we are with family. We get some great pictures on our REAL camera now and again, we stay up way past midnight for our last night in the big city. Where has the time gone?

Day 122 May 2, 2007 - Wednesday - *Hotel Pennsylvania*, New York City, New York to New Rochelle, NY

Last night we were up way past our bedtime....again. New York is not the place to get extra sleep in. There is way too much to see and do. This morning we get a semi-late start. We have the big job, or I really should say Morton has the big job of packing up the trailers. He has a system and after a bit of pushing and pulling, we are setting off.

The time flew by so fast and we were so busy with press we didn't really get a chance to see any of the things I had hoped for. Next time. The other thought dawned on me that I didn't have a map of New York City. We decided to bicycle through Central Park and pick one up at a visitor place. No joy, only maps of Central Park. Bicycling in Central Park is something you never want to miss. Do it when you come to this place and you will never regret it. The sights and sounds were just sheer quality and it was hard leaving this bit of paradise. We headed past a bicycle shop and got a bicycling map of NYC. This was going to see us off of Manhattan and into the Bronx. Wait a minute...the Bronx? I got this chill of fear down my spine. I recalled a movie with Paul Newman about the Bronx...it was a dangerous place. I hope that time has changed it for the better as we head towards it. Passing tulips blooming on Park Avenue the thought of a bad neighborhood within bicycling distance seems like an impossible thought. There is nothing but rich here, 300,000 dollar cars, real estate that would feed a village in a third-world country. How could anything bad be lurking right around the corner?

As we rode the traffic was just crushing. Literally. I was bumped, but not knocked over three times. The worst came however, when a lady who didn't have a spare two seconds (the time it would have cost her to let me pass her turn) came wheeling around the corner. I knew I had no chance of avoiding her besides slamming on my brakes. As I did this I screamed and she gave me a unintelligent hand gesture, the middle finger salute. As my bike ground to a dead stop from me pulling the brakes and planting my feet on the ground like anchors, my stomach hit the handle bars. "That is going to leave a bruise, but I'm alive!" I thought. I wondered where she was going that she couldn't spare two seconds. Somewhere terribly important, I suppose. Morton said that she swerved into the other lane as I screamed. I didn't see this, but the thought that she might have hit me, hit another car and who knows what kind of chain reaction would have happened...all for two seconds. My nerves were fractured as we hit the Bronx. Getting over the bridge was a nightmare, two attempts led us to dead ends and turnarounds. Why oh why am I here? Why didn't I plan ahead and have a route figured out instead of living so hard in the moment? There were lots of people and cars out. Plus, the big trucks, buses and emergency vehicles, the whole part of our ride became a blur of fear. I was scared I would get hit, scared I would get mugged and scared I would never get out of the Bronx.

Morton was giving me grey hair by the second by talking to guys are red lights who were asking him things like, "How much is that bike worth?", "What do you got in there?" and other things that were code for, we are going to take it from you. I told him to not answer, drive on and run red lights if he had to. Just keep up and keep yer trap shut! He is naive and has to be reminded that lots of Americans have guns. But like so many other things I have learned on this journey, miracles happen every day. Today my miracle was not getting hit & killed. Several times really. There was also the miracle of the Bronx. I have no idea what I imagined, but it wasn't the case. The people were friendly, lots of waves and smiles. The shouts of "We saw you on TV" came from all ages as we made our way north. Besides a few shady characters at a few random red lights, my fears were completely unfounded. Sure I was bumped by a couple cars, but nothing that hurt.

We were looking for Boston Road. This is actually our old friend US1 from Florida. It was good to see the black and white signs with the number 1 in the middle. Like spotting an old friend, we were both smiling as we got on the road. There was a point on this road where you leave the Bronx. It is a bridge, one side city, one side suburbs. It is an unusual thing to see the changes happen so fast. There are lawns again instead of parking lots and high-rise buildings. Spring is really happening here and we smell a fresh cut lawn. I start relaxing at once. We made it through safely. As I said, the people on the streets were great. It's the ones in the cars that were just not getting the concept of "Share the road" that scared me. But we did survive, all in one piece. A bit bruised, but very alive. There were few stops today, just lots of serious riding. I did a few interviews on the phone, but when we pulled into New Rochelle, we hadn't gone as far as we wished. The sun told us it was time to find a place to spend our last night in New York.

As I was inside asking about places ahead of us, Morton met a lovely lady from Nigeria who is opening a healthy eating spot, right across from the police station in New Rochelle. We talked and I asked if we could sleep in her garage. Rather odd, but we didn't want to put her or her family out. Instead, she took us home with her and spoke to her husband. The two of them agreed that they wouldn't let us sleep in their garage, but we were welcomed to the living room. This family opened their home to us and gave us one of our nicest nights yet. Their three children were so nice, polite and all smiles. They must have wondered about these strangers with sleeping bags about to camp out in their living room. The oldest son put on a movie for us to watch and relax as his mom was in her kitchen working magic. She is one of the best cooks on the planet and we will go back to visit her cafe when we are finished with the trek. The food kept coming and just the whole hospitality experience was overwhelming. After our long day, her husband must have noticed how tired we looked and told us to get some sleep. We were off to sleep, hopefully NOT snoring, as the sounds of family could still be softly heard in the lovely home.

Day 123 May 3, 2007 - Thursday - New Rochelle, NY to Riverside, CT

Staying in someone's living room, we want to be as good of house guests as possible. When my phone rang at 4:30 this morning, I was scared! Hoping I hadn't woken the house, it was the television station and I talked in almost a whisper. The voice on the other end said there was a note that we would be starting early. We made arrangements to meet outside and Morton and I set about getting our gear together and out to the trailers. The bikes and trailers sat in the garage that we had offered to stay in. The house was a lot better, as there was a beautiful bathroom for us to use. Quiet like mice, we headed outside to wait on the news crew. They arrived and we were in the perfect spot for the filming. It was a breeze (we are getting use to this now) and the people *News 12* had sent out were top notch. *Lisa LaRocca* was really clever and asked us lots of great questions. They really knew their stuff and made it a fast process. Thank goodness our kind hostess came outside. I was really hoping they would speak to her and they did. She was brilliant.. I also can't sing her cooking skills loud enough...she is one terrific cook! I love Nigerian cooking, fresh and delicious! If you are in New Rochelle, eat at her cafe for a real taste experience.

We got an early start, but when I took another call from the press. It's going to only get busier, but I never expected as much press as we got today. The end count was one television station, one radio station (in person) and three newspapers, two sent photographers out to meet us. We didn't get a big ride in today. What did happen though is we got to speak with so many people. All the press recently has lots of people stopping to talk to us. Morton was passing out our LittleChanges slips fast and furious today and had to replenish his stack of them from the trailer. He has handed out thousands and it always makes me smile when I get an email from someone who has gotten one of the slips. The weather was so good, almost too good. I rode in a t-shirt with my black jacket packed away. Maybe for good, but I have a feeling I will wear it again.

We wanted to cross into Connecticut and after some amazing parks, blossoms and people...we did! It seemed almost at once that the hills started. Why am I so out of shape? I'm not going to lie to you, I pushed the bicycle today like MAD! The trailer HAS to go on a diet, I have to figure out a way to lighten it's load. That was my biggest thought today as I was riding. It is weird, but we really do need every thing that is inside our little trailers. This is either going to kill me or cure me. With aching muscles, I pushed and shoved up one hill and then sailed down the other side. Talk about your cardio workout!

As we came into Greenwich, there was a library. I had hopes of having a peek at a map and reassure myself that we are indeed going in the right direction. You don't want to get lost on bicycle, trust me on this one. The library is huge, filled with computers that speed my search and show me that the whole way (nearly) in Connecticut, we just need to keep on US1. Simple and easy. I don't even have to write anything down. There are benches that sit outside this library and Morton and I decided to eat our lunch there. We ended up staying for over three hours and doing many interviews. We were not in a hurry to leave and people kept asking us questions. We love it when this happens. Between the hills and the press, we had a bad day of mileage, but it ended on a great note. We came across a church right before stopping for the evening that helped us on our journey. They weren't able to offer us a room to sleep in, but they actually offered to get us a motel room. (This is what I posted on the website)

What *really* happened was that I went in to the church, spoke to a lady who said they couldn't put us up anywhere in their massive buildings. I was polite when told the lady who could make that decision for the day had left. It seemed a fair comment for me to ask if there was any way the lady in front of me could call the decision maker. I was told that the lady had left at four o'clock and had a really tough day, she didn't want to bother her. Thanking the lady I walked out, very sad, but feeling like there was nothing I could do. No is no. We rode for about a mile or so after I told Morton there was no room at the inn. He has gotten use to churches that say no. But something wasn't setting right with me. I stopped my bicycle and called my daughter, asking her to find the phone number on her computer for the church that had just said no. I called and without really even thinking before I spoke, I just started talking to the lady that had sent us off without use of their sanctuary. It was a talk that was emotional and straight from the heart. I cried real tears and Morton just stood there watching, a bit in shock I think. The fact that we could go on and find somewhere else was apparent, but what if we would have been at the end of our rope? What if we had been angels traveling in disguise (we aren't) but what if we were? I also told her that now I know how Mary and Joseph must have felt. She listened to my endless words of all the things I had wanted to say to every church that had said NO to us. Why were they doing that? Are they not there to help people? We didn't want money or food, just a safe place to sleep. I thanked her for listening, though through my sobs I had to wonder if she could understand me. I told her I just had to say that and sorry if it was upsetting to hear. Hanging the phone up I leaned over on my handlebars and continued to cry. Being a former student of a Christian school, I had read the Bible. I knew that there were only ten commandments, but I thought somehow these churches must have been seeing an invisible 11th commandment. Worse yet, they seemed to be practicing it.

The 11th Commandment must go something like this. Collect lots of money from your people who attend your church, build huge buildings with expensive materials, then only open your doors for a brief time each week, leave no contact number for people to call you who come to the church and most of all, refuse to help strangers. Of course we know there isn't an 11th commandment, but the churches that have all said no to us seem to think differently. We even had the private number from the vicar in Tuckertown, NJ who said that people could call him for confirmation that we were alright...talk about a good reference. We didn't want to do any harm, we only wanted to sleep. A simple request really.

My phone rang back and it was one of the vicars from the church. The lady that had said no and gotten to hear my emotional wrath on the phone had passed along the message. She had said earlier that she had looked at our website and I wondered if she read the article that was linked to it about our bad luck with the church in Highlands NJ. The vicar asked where we were, I was still semi-sobbing and told him I thought we were a few miles north of him. I'm not sure why, but I expected him to ask us to turn around and they would welcome us for the night with open arms. Instead he told me if I kept riding about ten miles, there would be a hotel on the right. He would drive up and pay for the room for the night for us. My mouth fell open, but I heard my thank you coming out on the phone to him. This man drove up and met us, paid for the room, said he was sorry that we couldn't stay with them and wished us a safe journey. The money he spent on the room could have gone for food for the poor, towards something that was more important than our journey. We just wanted a bit of floor. But what could I do, I wasn't going to say no to a free room.

Day 124 May 4, 2007 - Friday - Riverside To Bridgeport, Connecticut

Today is the first year anniversary of my mother's stroke. She was sitting at her kitchen table crocheting, then her life changed forever. It only took a second for her world to be lost. My dad called my sister-in-law, Melissa, who acted fast and got mom off to the hospital. The outlook was not good and it was going to be a long, hard road ahead of her. At the moment it happened, Morton and I were in France. We were going to start a new part of our life and actually work in a laundry service. It was going to be a big change in our life and for the first time in three and a half years, I wouldn't be working 7 days a week, 12 to 14 hour days. With the phone call, our whole lives changed. We headed to America and to help my mom and dad. The rest of my life, my mother's stroke, will always be something that I am thankful for. First, mom's legs were to the point where she wanted them amputated from diabetes. She wasn't following her diet and they were hard, swollen and purplish-black. They hurt so bad she would even cry in her sleep. Mom was also smoking several packs of cigarettes a day. This all changed with her stroke. She had to get her diet right as she was spending the next two months on her back in the hospital. My mom is amazing. She worked very hard, got her speech back, got her moving back and is now healthier than she has been in decades. She still has a long road to travel, but she's going to make it. I think of mom and all her struggles when we are having a tough day.

Today was one of those "best of days, worst of days" days. We encountered all the hills in Connecticut at once, or at least it felt like that. They are so thrilling to ride down, but a tough climb up. We are doing it though and happy to be alive and having the chance to do this journey. We got a taste of fresh watermelon today and I think if there would have been the chance to eat a WHOLE watermelon, I would have. But at $3.00 for a slice, it was a luxury that we could only afford one of. Morton and I were sharing, I was tempted to eat the rind too! Morton was complaining about the cost and what all it would buy and I told him I CRAVED the watermelon. True, I'm not going to have a baby, but I am going to have a grand-baby! Not long after our watermelon splurge, we were pushing the bicycles & their 100 pound trailers up a hill, when a lady stopped and gave us $5.00! It was just incredible. She told us to keep up the good work. This is one of the miracles that I tell you about on here. I made sure I told Morton that was for the watermelon! Plus, with the extra $2. we have enough for 4 cans of tuna!

It seemed like we had only just started bicycling when it was time to start looking for a room. We thought that we would bump into lots of motels being on US1, but there really weren't a lot. As it got later, all the same old daily fear set in. "Where would we sleep?" After much searching, phoning, walking in and trying to find a place, we just kept pushing on. We found ourselves on top of a big hill in Bridgeport, Connecticut with no where to go. It was dark. The sun set fast and we saw the big blue "H" showing us there was a hospital just over the hill. I knew it would be safe to pull in there and try to use a phone book to locate something. The lady there was helpful and agreed that riding the bicycle after dark was the sure way to wind up in a bed in the hospital. The crazy law-suit society that we live in prevented various fire stations and churches from being able to help us tonight. We need to re-think what we are doing America. If we are living in a society where two people riding their bicycles to save the health of the world can't be let sleep inside for fear of a lawsuit, something is REALLY wrong! We got a local hotel to help us with a ride, but they were not able to offer us sponsorship for a room. It meant almost $70. from our budget for May is gone. Sigh...sometimes there is nothing else to do though. We had made over 30 phone calls and sleeping in the hospital wasn't an option, though we gladly would have. By the time we got into the room, it was 10:30 pm. Morton took a picture of me that I really don't like, he said "smile" but I was actually too tired to. I only had strength for a shower and then sleep. While I was taking my shower I was thinking of my mom and how far she has come. She still has a long way to go, just like us, but we are all going to make it. We just have to all remember to enjoy the ride.

Day 125 May 5, 2007 - Saturday - Bridgeport to Branford, Connecticut

We are getting fitter in hilly Connecticut. Today we didn't have to get off the bike and push so much. It was amazing with the difference between the days, but we have decided to get our load lighter. As we ride we talk about what all can go from our trailers. We agree to get rid of the pillows. Instead we will just keep two of the pillow cases, which will become our clothes bags. We are also going to get rid of half the things in our medicine bag and tool bag. I know I'm in for a shock when I finally see what is in the bag. I plan on keeping the camera handy and showing you just what Morton has been picking up beside the road.

There are so many honks and waves today. The press in this area have been fantastic and lots of people know why we are riding. We have people stop to say that they are going to be watching. We even meet one man who saw the story in the paper and pumped the tires up on his bike and was out for his first ride in over a year! Brilliant!

Since we only managed to sleep about five hours last night, I'm going to make this entry short and sweet. It was a great day of riding and the hills were a lot easier. As the night started to come, we tried for a room to be sponsored, but with no luck. We have a card that we have credit on from so many nights stay, so we got a room about 7:30 pm for a reduced rate. We are calling it an early night and have to go early tomorrow, with over 45 miles to ride.

Day 126 May 6, 2007 - Sunday - Branford To *Mystic Hilton*, Mystic, Connecticut

This was the day that we will never forget. It challenged us as we have never been challenged before. It stripped us down and showed us what we were really made of. It picked us up and carried us further than we ever imagined on our dream. We started with a bit of backtracking over miles we had already been on, then set about following US1 along Interstate 95. It is a road that is old, very old. Parts of it is called "Boston Post Road" and we have been on it since we left NYC. It is one of the most scenic highways we have seen so far.

Connecticut is the start of New England and also the start of the hills. We aren't complaining, just stating the facts. We will get up all of them, no matter how long it takes or how many times I have to lean on my handlebars and gasp. We rode harder then we have since starting. We also felt like we were going uphill the entire way, with a gale force wind in our faces. The elements were tough.

As tonight was a bit unusual, in that we know where we are sleeping, we need to get to Mystic. The *Mystic Hilton* is sponsoring us for a lovely few nights and it is the first Hilton we will be staying at. The thought of a warm bed is a comforting one, but I have to be honest with you...I hit my wall today. Several times. The thrill of coming down a hill was replaced by the fear that there would be another one waiting for us. Why is my trailer so heavy? If I make it to Mystic, I'm chucking out half the stuff or more in my trailer. Maybe I'll have a yard sale! Several calls to Sarah throughout the day keep me posted on the baby shower. In all my excitement about Sarah's special day I had forgotten that it was my sister's birthday. Yikes! After all, we both feel the same about birthdays. We like to just keep having them, but forget about them.

There were several train stations we passed on the way and I told Morton we should take one. We had a long way to go after all. It was going to be really tough, even the wind was pushing us back. We really did have to even pedal going down hills. Morton thought I was joking about the train and I suppose I was. It was tempting though. The road criss-crosses interstate 95 several times. It also joins up to it at points to cross water. We have to go over one bridge that has an amazing foot path for bikes & walkers. The next one we aren't so lucky with. It has to be crossed, but the sign says no bicycles or pedestrians. We grit our teeth and pedal over. It actually is really good. Wide edge, great view and we are only on it for about a mile. Then it is back to the up and down of the lovely hills. About 10 hours into our day, we knew we weren't going to make it in time for our meal at *Riverwalk Restaurant*. I called to reschedule and we kept going.

Morton had spotted a man who was holding up a sign near a gas station we stopped at for the bathroom. There was no bathroom, but Morton did take action from the sign. It said, "Hungry, will work for food" we didn't have any money to spare, but we did have a bag of pretzels. He took them over to the man and we were back on the bikes. It was the last of our food and I have to admit, I was afraid the man really wanted only money. We still had miles and miles to go and no food at all now. I'm ashamed to say I scolded Morton for this. Shouldn't I know to expect the best in people?

As the hills kept coming, we kept going over them. They were getting tougher, longer, steeper and my body was wearing out. I drank lots of water and tried to focus on just the next bit of road in front of me. Just a little bit further, I hoped. The sun was setting and I felt helpless and angry at myself for not starting earlier. We did take off at 8:30 am and calculated that we should reach Mystic at 5 or 6 pm. It was now 8 pm. The sun was fading quick and there were still hills to climb. Just after we came down a super steep hill, I was mortified to see another right in front of us. I broke down and started crying. I was physically exhausted, mentally finished and forget hitting a wall, this was hitting the Great Wall of China. Morton offered to push my bike to the top of this hill, but I knew that I needed it to lean on at this point. My arms stretched out to the handle bars and I leaned on the seat. One foot after another, I crept slowly up the hill. I tried to think about all the things that I needed to that would help me get through this.

We have come so far, but maybe I shouldn't be out here. Maybe I am too fat to get fit. Maybe I should just call it a day and get off the bicycle. As both strong thoughts and very weak thoughts were creeping into my thoughts, I looked around to see that we were at the top of this hill. Surely it had to be the last. Surely the twinkling lights at the bottom had to by Mystic. Since it was dark, I would have no way to know until we reached the bottom. We went slow because in the dark *(DO NOT TRY THIS AT HOME)* it is so dangerous. You can hit a stick, bottle or hole that just might kill you. A car that doesn't really notice you during the day has an even great chance of hitting you at night. We had reflectors, but no lights on our bicycles. Crazy and stupid. But it was our lucky night. It was the last hill and we sailed into Mystic on our bicycles that were making creaks and moans, they were tired too.

We called the *Mystic Hilton* for directions and before we knew it, all the things that had been a struggle, were completely gone. Met at the desk by the smiling face of Jessica, she gave us a big basket they had for us. In it was a giant bag of pretzels. I was thinking of the man who had held the sign about being hungry. Hopefully he had a warm place to sleep tonight. Going upstairs to our room, Morton and I reflected just long enough that it had indeed, without a doubt, been the toughest day of our journey. After today, we know we can get through anything.

Day 127 May 7, 2007 - Monday - *Mystic Hilton*, Mystic, Connecticut

Have you ever dreamt about visiting somewhere for a long time and worried that it might not be all that you hoped for? You see, I have been dreaming about Mystic since I was a child. Looking through *Yankee* magazine it seemed like there was always an article with photographs that looked like the perfect place to visit. I'm pleased to tell you that Mystic was everything I dreamed of, then some. Morton was equally impressed and we had a day that took away all our aches and pains of yesterday. There is the first look we had, in the dark, of Mystic by bicycle. Today was a bit different. We rode our bicycles across the street this morning to see the *Mystic Aquarium*. The sun was out and we were lucky enough to get to see all the wonderful creatures that live here. The aquarium is way more then just an aquarium. There are so many things to do, you have to visit them or their website. I was really in love with the penguins and whales. We really enjoyed our morning and could have stayed the entire day.

My email needed seeing to, so we decided to come back to the room and download the camera. After my lovely Samsung had gotten fried in New Jersey, I contacted Samsung who were kind enough to send another one out to my daughter's house. Being able to record a journey like this is a must and I wish that I had my Samsung camera here. The quality of the pictures is just stunning.

After a lunch made by Morton and hot water, we headed off to *Mystic Seaport*. This is really the heart and soul of the town. It is also a place that you have to see when you come here. We had the thrill of seeing it with Michael. He really knows his stuff and didn't even seem to mind all of Morton's questions. Again, time flies and we were doing an interview with the paper, "The Day". Michael had shown us the highlights in this historic village, but we knew that it would take several days to really get it all. The interview was great and soon we were finished and left to have a look around the *Mystic Seaport*. We had been onboard the only wooden whaler left on this planet, we had also heard a bit in the life of a whaler. I will never again think that WE had a hard day. The kind of life those men led was just grueling. There is a long standing rumor that history is boring. This is not the kind of history you learn for a text book. A place like *Mystic Seaport* brings it alive. You can not only see it, ride on it, walk the streets of it, peek into all the houses and buildings of the historic seaport, you can also smell history. When we stepped inside the long building where the rope was made, the smell is just something to be experienced. You see all the machinery, see the huge stacks of rope and can only wonder about the people that made the product that tied so many lives together. The smell of the wood from the building and the rope were just like really being back in time. It is hard to explain but as I looked at the spools of twine that would be wound into rope, Morton and Michael walked to the other end of this long building. All of a sudden this story, not just an idea, but an entire story popped in my mind about this building, or more to the point, the people who worked here. When we sit still for a few days, I will write it down.

My parents would have loved Mystic. When this journey of ours is finished, I'm bringing my mom back to see it. I know she will love it. Anyone would. There is this learning theme through Mystic. You can learn at the *Mystic Aquarium*, you can learn at the *Mystic Seaport* and I only wished that it wouldn't have taken me thirty years to get here.

As our day wound down, we strolled to the place we would be having our dinner. The restaurant is right at the end of the *Mystic Seaport* and we were soon looking at *Seamen's Inne*. Once inside, we got to meet the fantastic chef and were treated to the incredible menu. The food was just so fresh, creative and tasty. We are going to remember it for ever. Morton really did want to lick the plates...he kept raving about the lobster bisque and we both really had a great time. A can of tuna is going to fall way short after this. Since it is usually just a steady diet of tuna, trail mix, cereal bars, canned fruit and veg and the occasional dollar menu item from a fast food joint that we consume, let me tell you about the meal at *Seamen's Inne*. Believe it or not, lobster creme brulee, 1/2 cup New England Clam chowder & 1/2 cup lobster bisque, scallops & seafood pie, finished with 1/2 key lime dessert that was just like a dream come true! This is the kind of food I would love to eat every day for the rest of my life. And I wouldn't gain weight. I'd gladly ride my bicycle all around the magnificent Mystic to burn it all off. After dinner we walked back to the visitors center to get our bicycles. Riding them without trailers, we head back to the *Hilton Mystic* for the work that awaits. There are just 244 emails, so hopefully, it won't be a LATE, LATE night.

Day 128 May 8, 2007 - Tuesday - *Mystic Hilton*, Mystic, Connecticut

Food in Mystic...FIVE STARS!

Lunch: Courtesy of *RiverWalk Restaurant* : Rhode Island clam chowder, chicken salad with cranberries, walnuts and FRESH VEG!!!!, 1/2 apple crisp with ice cream.

Dinner: Courtesy of *S&P Oyster Company* : Artichoke dip with crisp chips that were warm, seafood platter that was broiled with scallops that were huge, fresh and shrimp that was so very tender & tasty, then we split a piece of NY cheesecake with an Oreo crust!

We woke up this morning early and I started right on the computer. I thought a 6 am beginning would be enough to get through things before we set off into town, but as usual, I underestimated the amount of email. We found out that the article that appeared in *The Day* said the wrong hotel that was sponsoring us in Mystic. We are at the **Hilton Mystic**, as you all know. It is a frustrating typo for us and we feel bad about it. Not just because we are enjoying the fantastic room (I could write a whole book about how comfortable the bed is) but the *people* at the *Hilton Mystic* have just treated us fantastic. From the very moment we arrived it has felt so special here, to have the paper NOT give credit where credit was due, was just gutting. Calling the paper, they said they would print a retraction, but it just had Morton and I feeling terrible. I know it wasn't our fault, but I really was so sad about our lovely sponsor in Mystic not getting the mention they should have. Kerry and the other people at the *Mystic Hilton* were really good about it. They did this out of kindness, not for press.

After meeting so many of the *Mystic Hilton* people downstairs we got some great pictures and headed out to explore Mystic. Remember, I have never really been here before and for years have imagined it. The town, I'm very happy to report, is everything I hoped for and more. The people in Mystic are lovely and very lucky. Some of the best food on the planet is right here. We have been eating the most delicious seafood. Today are food journey was starting at the *RiverWalk Restaurant*. It's in a lovely building and the menu was very tempting. I actually went for a healthy salad that was scrumptious and good for you. Even our dessert we split was healthy...apples, spices, ice cream. The building is right beside the *Chamber of Commerce*, so after our bellies were full, we went in to see if we could get a map. Inside we met these amazing ladies. Tricia, the president, gave us long sleeve t-shirts (think of all the chilly New England nights we are going to have ahead of us!) and Mystic potato chips, some lovely spritzers and an invitation to a get together happening in the town that evening. Morton and I were thrilled!

We said our goodbyes and headed off to watch the drawbridge do it's thing. It opens and closes (if there is a boat waiting) at certain times. I have been over lots of drawbridges on bicycle and on foot these last several months, but this one is really special. It has real character and is world-famous. There are shops of every description along the streets we are bicycling, but they don't look like the typical tourists shops. Again, they seem to have this certain charm and character. These are shops that the locals use too. One of the tough things of our journey is seeing all the lovely things and knowing that you can't even think about buying any. The day is perfect and we chat to so many nice people. Some on vacation, some that are lucky enough to live here, but all of them are friendly. Morton and I explore, take time to sit on a sunny bench as I do an interview, then something pulls us back to *Mystic Seaport*.

Yesterday when we were in, our time was way too short. It is the sort of place that you can stroll for hours, days and I think even months and never really take it all in. It is right on the Mystic River and is alive, vibrant and bustling with activity. It, like the *Mystic Aquarium*, is focused on education as well. Today we call on Michael again for help to get in and he comes through like a trooper. We get to go through the doors that lead us into this world from the past, that you can walk down the wide dirt streets and just take it all in. The value for money for the admission ticket is just great. You get to go in every building, on board incredible ships and there are also so many people around to really help you understand what it is that you are seeing.

Morton and I stay as long as possible, trying to take it all in. There really is just so many things to do, plus, there are these incredible people there who can tell you anything you want to know about the place. Morton was in his element and asking loads of questions. It was a place we could have spent several months explore, perhaps even years, without getting bored or wishing to be anywhere else. Mystic is like a beautiful rare pearl that catches the light and glows different colors, depending on how you look at it. We headed over to the lovely courtyard on the other side of the river, where the *Chamber of Commerce* get-together is happening.

It's lively, fun meeting lots of people and the weather is just beautiful for it. Morton and I chat with lots of interesting people, but there is one person that really stands out & I connect with...Susan. Susan works with *American Heart Association* and we just fall in to this conversation that we are both on the very same page with. We exchange ideas, promise to keep in touch and before we know it, we are heading off from a very special enchanted evening.

Morton and I are having dinner at *S&P Oyster Company*, but alas, we have a very flat back tire on my bike. We do have the puncture repair kit with us, but no pump. We decide to just go to the restaurant, have our wonderful meal and then worry about the tire. We push our bicycles all the way there. We did have a terrific meal, in the candlelight, sitting right beside the Mystic River. The food was lovely and afterwards, we set out to the bike problem.

We thought maybe I could wear the backpack, ride his bike and he would carry mine back to the room. It was about a mile that we had to go and I knew this would work. I forgot though, Morton's bike is a lot longer than mine and it felt very odd riding it. I ended up just pushing to keep pace with him and we were all set to have a nice walk back. The weather was great and we were chatting away, when a van pulled up. It was Susan, who I had met earlier. She was in a replacement vehicle while her car was in the shop and was able to offer us a ride to the gas station for air. It was just another case of being in the right place at the right time. When we got to the gas station, our conversation continued for a while before we said goodbye for the second time that night. We have this feeling that we will meet Susan again.

Morton and I finish the night back in our lovely room. It is going to be sad to leave here in the morning, but the trip is waiting. We will be back to Mystic, hopefully again and again. Who knows, perhaps one day we will call it home.

Day 129 May 9, 2007 - Wed - *Mystic Hilton*, Mystic, CT to *Shelter Harbor Inn,* Westerly, Rhode Island

Everyone of our days that we actually wake up, is perfect! We have a feeling today that is a bit sad. Leaving a place like the *Hilton Mystic* is tough and not knowing where we are going to be again tonight is exciting, but scary. Plus, the people here are just amazing. *Amazing* isn't even big enough to cover it. We have a delicious breakfast, say our goodbyes and head off. There are so many people that we come across that say: hello, ride safe, keep up the good work...it's a great day. Just before leaving Mystic, we share a light lunch in a part of town we were near just the night before. It feels like we have been here for just two seconds now. We really did need more time to visit Mystic. I suggest a week, minimum.

Sunny and warm, we feel just how heavy the trailers are. Why oh why didn't I chuck half the stuff out of them? Oh well, we push when we need to, stop to do phone interviews and gradually make our way to this bridge that runs over the river that divides the lovely state of Connecticut, with the equally lovely state of Rhode Island. New England is really one of the friendliest places on the planet. We love it.

Kerry from the *Hilton Mystic* lives in Rhode Island and had invited us to stay at her house. She had already done so much for us, we didn't want to impose. We would keep bicycling and see where the day led us.

We got a call from a photographer who was going to meet us from a newspaper in Rhode Island. We met up at a Chamber of Commerce where we were picking up a road map. The photographer was riding ahead of us and then we just had the easy job of bicycling past him.

He was using an amazing lens, 400x - incredible! We were in mid-stride when my phone rang. It was Kerry. I have gotten very good at answering the phone and still pedaling. Maybe not safe, but there was a man on his stomach, beside the road, taking pictures, I had to answer the phone...great action shot for the paper!

Kerry asked where we were and I tried to explain. She said she found us a room, at a lovely place and they are willing to help us for the night. My mouth fell open and I couldn't believe what I was hearing. The camera was still clicking, so if my mouth is hanging open in the paper tomorrow, it is all because of Kerry! Morton is asking what has me shouting, *"WOOHOO"* and I try to explain to him over the noise of the road. He can't believe it. This is a first. It is the very first time that someone else has called to ask a stranger for a place for us to stay. Did I already say, *"WooHoo!?"* I was so overtaken with joy and disbelief, even though I knew I was suppose to just cycle right past the photographer...I stopped. We had been chatting earlier about how things just seem to work out on this journey. There is no real way to explain this feeling of what is happening, it just does. I had to share this brand new experience with the photographer. He was amazed as well.

The clock had ticked away and it was almost 5pm. We have no idea how time goes so fast, but it does. The *Shelter Harbor Inn* was just ahead and it was just about the time that we start our daily quest of a safe place to put our heads down for the night. Timing and great things! We pulled in off of US 1 and it was like coming on to a movie of a classic New England inn. A long drive, blossom covered trees, a huge historic house that is perfect and inside...well, lets just say that the people in New England are as amazing as the scenery. We are standing in front of this lovely place and Morton is snapping away with the camera as I go inside to meet Brittany. The furniture, the windows, the feel...just lovely. All right off the pages of a magazine. But the people are the real story. We all chat for ages about the journey, the twist of fate and about how this night will be a first on our journey. Someone actually doing MY job (not that I mind at all...I LOVE IT!) of securing a room for us and to think that we are going to be staying here when we had been thinking about pitching the tent in a park that is just up the road. Morton sits in the sun on a lovely chair, waiting for me to finish talking. Inside we all talk about a whole range of topics, then we head off to our room for the evening. It is as lovely as the cherry blossoms, it has queen-sized beds, a real fireplace, period furniture....perfection. Plus, there is breakfast in the morning. Morton and I are both still stunned. "WOW" is the word you should have heard us saying, no matter where in the world you are! We were that blown away with what Kerry did for us and what this wonderful place is doing. BRILLIANT!

After we got our gear inside, we walked over to the reception area to take a few pictures. Morton hadn't been inside and he wanted to say thank you as well. We were asked about dinner, which we had a bit before with our packed lunch. They made us up a lovely tray with salad, fruit and even iced tea and sent us on our way. The computer got cracked open as I ate this fresh veg and fruit. Joy, there is free wireless internet here. I only hope that I don't wake up to find this is a dream. The luck of our journey isn't luck at all. It is all down to finally being positive. Finally smiling and looking for good. Finally deciding that my health is something that I can do and the best part, pass all of these wonderful things on to others.

Our first night in Rhode Island is one we will never forget. We have came so far, with still a long way to go, but just *THINK & IMAGINE* what might happen tomorrow - anything! Remember as well that for the first time in my life, we are living in the moment and enjoying every second of this dazzling ride.

This day would not have happened like this if it hadn't been for the kindness of Kerry at the Mystic Hilton. She is this amazing person, actually everyone we met there was as well, who really make a difference in the world.

Day 130 May 10, 2007 - Thurs - *Shelter Harbor Inn*, Westerly to *Narragansett Cafe*, Jamestown, RI

Today started off so lovely, with a wonderful breakfast in a beautiful dining room overlooking the mist that had came in from the sea. We ate, said our goodbyes and headed east. We had a delightful ride in the clouds that looked like they were on the land. I was feeling so light from all the weight I have been losing I wonder if perhaps I'm floating instead of bicycling. Today is a beautiful dream. We had our lunch on a picnic table in the sun, met several new friends along the way and even made a pit stop in Wakefield for a special chocolate that someone had emailed us about! It was great. We didn't know how it could get any better.

There was a big bridge to cross to go on to Jamestown. Earlier in the day Morton had called the state police to see if we were allowed. He learned we could cross the one to Jamestown, but not to Newport.

Just before we got on the road that took us to the bridge, we stopped right before a red light. I just happened to look down to see that we were standing over a mound of pennies...lucky pennies. Morton made a mad scramble to pick them all up, happy to see some silver coins mixed in. Over the next few yards we found more and more. It was quite bizarre. Morton was dodging in and out of cars grabbing these coins that must have just fallen off the back of a truck. We were both saying that something very lucky was going to happen, after all those lucky pennies of course. We kept on going though, it was really warm out and we still wanted to make it to Newport before nightfall. We still had a big bridge to cross that we weren't allowed on, so we were going to have to get a move on. The urge for a bathroom had hit both of us when there were none to be found. We just kept going towards the bridge, hoping the other side would hold a place to stay and a bathroom. There is always the woods and even though we are getting quite wild out here, we like to stay as civilized as we can. The temperature on the bridge was so much colder. It didn't help with the bathroom calling. We just kept pedaling as hard as we could for the top of the bridge. We were almost at the summit when the police pulled in behind us and talked to us over their loudspeaker. Mentioning something about being in violation of homeland security, I was relieved we weren't getting a speeding ticket. They gave a *whoop-whoop* blast on their siren and had our attention. The first thought that crossed my mind is, *I'm not pulling over until I reach the top!*

. At the other side, after a police escort down the bridge where we were told to get off of it as quick as possible, we explained what we were doing and that we did call the state police barracks. The officer was really great and told us where to go to find churches and perhaps lodging. Seems someone had called them. They thought we were going to blow the bridge up. We said our goodbyes to the nice officer and I hoped that I wasn't going to wet my pants as we kept riding.

Not long along the road, there was a little pull off area where a pickup and a car were stopped. We could just tell the guys were there to talk to us, so we stopped. One, James, gave us each a bottle of cold water and a powerbar each....sweet! The other, Danny, offered to give us dinner at his cafe in Jamestown and a place to stay....told you those pennies were lucky! We headed down the road and before we knew it we were bicycling past lovely fields, pastures, even a windmill and Oreo-colored cows. Then came Jamestown and finally, the place that Danny owns, *Narragansett Cafe.* What a warm welcome we received! We pulled our bicycles right in the cafe that reminds me of a pub from Ireland and I make a mad dash to the bathroom.

Lynne was tending the bar and made me a special drink...delicious, but not sure what it was...and they treated Morton to a pint. Then we were cooked a lovely meal, able to use the free wi-fi, then Danny and Lynne invited us to stay over at their house.

We ended the evening sleeping in their bed (we wanted the sofa, but they insisted on it) and before we turned in we listened to a beautiful version of *"Fiddler's Green"* that made me get a lump in my throat. I love that song and the person singing it was brilliant. We drifted off to sleep with this incredible feeling that my last night of being 43 was a day I'll remember for the rest of my life. Thank you to all the people we met today, who stopped and talked, who gave us tips and directions and thanks to whoever lost the 100 lucky pennies!

Day 131 May 11, 2007 - Fri - *Narragansett Cafe,* Jamestown to *Las Palmas Inn,* Newport, Rhode Island

Everyone has heard the expression, "We will cross that bridge when we come to it" right? We are actually living that way today. There is a BIG bridge that we can't ride over, but we have a great new friend, Danny, who borrows a pickup from a friend and takes us right over it! We said our goodbyes to Lynne, she is really fantastic, then Danny drives us over the massive, tall bridge. It looks like the bridge from *Brigadoon,* as it disappears into the morning mist. Just as we get unloaded at the *Newport Visitor's Center* and before Danny has even pulled out of sight, our phone rings. It is Annie from *Las Palmas Inn.* She invites us to stay the night in Newport! So now, instead of just having a bicycle along the coast and then heading north, we get a chance to see this seaside town. Morton and I are overjoyed! We get to the lovely inn, just a few blocks from the visitor center & right in the historic district. Annie is something else! She did a nine-month trip around America by train and is the mother of nine children! The twinkle in her eyes tell me that she knows the secrets to a happy life. I wish we had more time to chat, but she is heading out and Morton and I need to do some things as well.

We had gotten another call right after our call from Annie. It was from the people at *Rose Island Lighthouse.* They didn't have space to have us stay on Friday or Saturday night, but we could stay in a REAL lighthouse on Sunday night, right off the coast of Newport! If only we could get a room for another night sorted. Annie took care of that. She invited us to stay for Saturday night too and I was on my way to the BEST birthday of my life. Now I can get going on setting up our "accidental visit" in Newport. There is press, contacting the visitors center to get help with passes and while I was doing a telephone interview, a local press person asks my age. I tell her today is my birthday and Morton overhears this. He cringes and starts trying to apologize for forgetting while I'm still on the phone. I knew he'd remember sooner or later.

Morton is actually very sentimental and never forgets my birthday or anniversary. He treats me to hand-made, heart-felt cards with a special message from him and is way more romantic than I am. I smile that he thinks I'm upset that he didn't start the day by giving me a birthday kiss. The lady on the phone tells me about a local restaurant that gives you a free lunch on your birthday. After the call, we decide to head over there. We don't want to spend money on a meal out, but we can handle FREE! Hopefully they will let Morton and I share.

We head out to the *Newport Visitors Center* where they don't just give us passes to see things, they also give us lovely golden pins shaped like starfish and they make us *AMBASSADORS* for Newport! Morton and I are thrilled and it is now our pleasure to invite you to visit Newport and be sure to tell them that Priscilla & Morton sent you!

There is such a thing as a free lunch. At our free lunch, where the waitress is kind enough to let us split it, she chats easy with us. She is from Pennsylvania as well and even tells us to keep the tip we were going to leave. People can be so kind and generous that if I spent the rest of my life saying *thank you,* it wouldn't cover it. I have to spend the rest of my life passing on this feeling to pay them all back. We are meeting Grace, the photographer just outside the seafood place. We do some pictures, share some stories and are then on our way. Grace had told us about a lovely bicycle ride, where to see the church that JFK was married in and we rode off without our trailers. I had also forgotten my glasses, which wasn't smart. Not only was it tough to see the road, but on the way back to our room, I misjudged a curb. I fell off my bike like a ton of bricks. It wasn't pretty. My wrists, left knee and the side of my face got roughed up. My body felt sore almost at once and I knew it was so stupid to not wear my glasses. I can assure you it wasn't a vanity move, I just forgot them! We were parking the bikes for the evening and headed off on foot for a ghost walk tour. Almost on cue, there was a fog in the harbor and our party of ghost story hunters were off to hit the streets. It was a great way to spend an evening and although we didn't see any ghosts, we still had a great time. As Morton and I walked back to our lovely room, I realized just *WHY* this has been such a great birthday. It is the first time in my adult life that I haven't felt horrible about my weight. I know it is in control now, that I am doing all the right things to live to see another year.

Day 132 May 12, 2007 - Saturday - *Las Palmas Inn*, Newport, Rhode Island

It is always the same. No matter how late I go to sleep, I wake up early. Turning 44 didn't change anything. I still woke up early, before 6am and started on the email. I hoped to get all the pictures uploaded, but there just wasn't time. We needed to get going if we were going to see Newport today, so the photos just have to wait. Email always comes first since it is my lifeline to the world! Please don't take it the wrong way when I talk about how much email we get. I love it and will always answer, as time permits. It might take a day or two, but I will answer.

We leave the bikes and set off on foot towards the *Newport Visitor Center*. I'm a bit sore after my fall yesterday, but no worse for the wear. The visitor center is great, with the transportation hub right there too. We start our day on a trolley and get a real education of Newport. What an incredible story, set in such a beautiful setting. Morton and I then try out the city transportation and take a public bus to *Green Animals Topiary Garden*. This is one of the most amazing gardens in America. It is a good haul away, then a big walk down a hill, but was it ever worth it. This garden is not to be missed. The topiary of animals and the grand house overlooking the water makes you want to just live here. The only thing we are missing is a ride back to Newport. We can do the bus again, but I really don't want to.

As we are walking around, we start talking to a mom and daughter. Morton shows the mom how to use her Samsung camera (it's just like ours!) and then I ask them if we can get a ride back to town with them. Not only do they take us, they drop us off right at *The Breakers*. If you visit any mansion while you are in Newport, you can't go wrong with *The Breakers*. It has it all. The history, the stories, the lavish decorations that make your senses spin. I can hear my dad in my head saying, "How would you ever keep it clean?" and smile. When we are finished, we visit a supermarket to get our food for our day on the island and then our night in the lighthouse. Then it's back to the room to get all our gear sorted out. We had another amazing day, loads of walking and now I hope to hit the hay before midnight. After all, we all know I'll be up early tomorrow.

Day 133 May 13, 2007 - Sunday - *Las Palmas Inn*, Newport To *Rose Island Lighthouse*, Rhode Island

I am writing to you from the kitchen table of *Rose Island Lighthouse*. It is the morning after our night spent on this enchanted private island. There is hustle and bustle of the island variety going on around me, but what I want to try to do is capture a bit of it for you. Annie at *Las Palmas Inn*, set out a lovely breakfast for us. We chatted for a bit, then headed off to the pier where we would catch the private boat going to the island. Anyone can do this, you can even play lighthouse keeper for a week! We had a bit of time for one last ride around part of Newport, but then went to Goat Island, named that because in the olden days they kept goats on it. Makes sense. Morton and I were wondering what we were going to do with our bikes and trailers. There was a hotel right there and I thought about asking them to store it, but it feels odd letting all of our things out of our site. After all, it isn't like a car you can just lock up. Our trailers are just canvas and could be picked up and carried away. Even though they just hold clothes, medicine, sleeping bags and a tent, it would be terrible to try to replace them. I can't even begin to think of life without trailers, even though they weigh a ton. I telephoned Charlotte, the lady from *Rose Island Lighthouse*. She suggested just loading them on the "*Starfish*" and taking them to the island...perfect! Morton and I got this done very fast and painless. We were a bit nervous at first that we would let a heavy trailer fall into the water as we were loading it on the boat, but there were no accidents.

The morning was cloudy and I thought about the graduation that was happening at the college in Newport at 10 am. The mother and daughter that had given us the lift back from the gardens were going to it. The same time that we would be setting sail for the island. Hopefully the weather would brighten up for both events. It did. We met the people on the dock who are going to be the lighthouse keepers for a week. The man, Chris, had made this clever item that is going to separate the salt from the sea water, so they will be able to water the garden at the lighthouse. You need to read about this place, then come and discover it for yourself. Nothing really can encompass how special it is. You feel a million miles away from everyone and everything, yet right across the water is the beautiful seaside jewel that is Newport.

When we landed on the island there were a group of people leaving. I tried not to think that in the morning that would be us. *Live in the moment*, my new motto, is something that we all need to learn to do. The island is home to so many things, wildlife, birds, geese and the ever-passing humans in boats and ships. You could spend years sitting in the bright white wooden chairs and watching it all. As I'm enjoying just sitting in the sun, I realize that about a year ago, this chair would have been uncomfortable to sit in. Now it fits with room to spare. Sheer success. As Morton and I explored the lighthouse, from basement up, I climbed the steps and didn't run out of breath. My knees don't go "Snap" and "Pop" anymore. My body is recovering from decades of over-indulgence. For that I am so thankful. My life is now something that would have been just fantasy a year ago. Now I know that there is no limit to what I can do, with a bit of hard work. There is a flag flying under the stars and stripes here. It says *"Hope"* which must be the motto for Rhode Island. It sums up perfectly how I feel for the first time in my adult life. There is indeed *hope*.

Morton and I explore, talk, sit quietly, look at the water, see the bridge, think about what a perfect day it has been and the time just glides away as it should do when you are stranded on an island with someone you love. We had brought pasta and sauce for dinner, but as Morton was brining in wood to the Fog Room (maybe my favorite room!) he said that Mike & Tanya invited us to eat with them. They had grilled the most amazing food and the four of us sat in the sun, sipping wine and just talking. It was really special and hopefully, we will be able to keep in touch with them on our journey and beyond. I had been down in the Fog Room when I got a phone call from a rather special place. I knew we were going to be riding near Fall River, Massachusetts, so I emailed a very unique bed & breakfast. To my pleasant surprise, I got a call from the owner saying that we could stay with her. It is pure magic when we know where we are going. We chatted for a while, discussing the history of the house, our journey (I rambled on and on about it, but I feel very passionate about what we are doing!) and then she asked me the question..."Would you like to sleep in Lizzie's room or the murder room?" not the typical question we get asked! After consulting with Morton for 2 seconds, we chose the murder room! Of course the house I'm talking about is the infamous Lizzie Borden house. Wow! Anyone who has been following our journey so far knows that we like to go on the ghost tours, hear the stories of the history of where we are, but this house is just something that I never thought you could stay in. Especially the murder room!!! Can you imagine? It is going to be a very fun evening, but I have to focus on getting back into the moment here. Our trip is just so big and we are in such a unique spot right now, the murder room will have to wait. Plus, I read an entry in a log book here about people spotting a ghost right in this very lighthouse. The sun was setting and Morton had a fire going in the Fog Room. We were surrounded by the water on three sides, the waves lapping the stones and it was one of the best sunsets of my life. If you look out the one side, you see the Newport Bridge, just starting to twinkle with the lights. You look out the other window and there is the sun setting on the horizon and the lovely town of Jamestown. The other window offers you a view to the wide open water, just beyond the harbor. Anything could be out there. It does wonders for your imagination to look at a sight like this.

We talk for a while with our new friends, then my body suddenly realizes how early I had gotten up. We say good night and head for our lovely bedroom, overlooking the twinkling bridge. There are a million stars out and for once, Morton actually lets me keep the curtains open. I suppose he isn't scared about a seagull peeking in to catch him in his underwear. It has been a dream-come-true sort of day. We will never forget it and now have yet another place on our list of *"MUST COME BACK AND SEE AGAIN!"* that is just growing and growing. I would love to get to play lighthouse keeper for an entire week. It would be great, except leaving that final morning when the good ship "Starfish" returns to take you back to the mainland.

Day 134 May 14, 2007 - Monday - *Rose Island Lighthouse*, Rhode Island to *Lizzie Borden B&B*, Fall River, Massachusetts

We woke up early today, about 5 am. Light was just pouring in the windows and the view was just stunning. We were looking out over the bridge we had crossed in the truck with Danny from Jamestown. Today we will leave the lovely *Rose Island Lighthouse*. Knowing that you just have one night in a place like this is hard, but thank goodness the boat doesn't come back to get you until 10 am. Five good hours for us.
I set up office in the old kitchen, surrounded by items from the past. The window looks out over the water and it is still-blue. Morton sets about getting our gear to the dock, after a quick breakfast of pop tarts that was made nicer by fresh strawberries courtesy of Mike & Tanya. The couple who are staying on for a week as the lighthouse keepers are up and at it early. They are painting, cleaning, raking and doing all sort of things on this amazing island. Morton shouts to me from the dock. He checked the lobster pots and there was one in it. We decided he was way to cute to munch and he wasn't that big. He was left go and Morton kept at getting the gear sorted while I typed away at my email.

The morning whisked by and soon the *Starfish* was heading back to us, with Joe at the helm. We were so thankful we had Mike (very tall & strong helicopter pilot!) who gave Morton a hand loading and unloading the trailers. My heart was wanting to stay on the island, but I also knew that tonight we would be sleeping at the infamous *Lizzie Borden Bed & Breakfast*.

As we were heading out of Newport, we caught up with Channel 10, NBC and did a very FAST interview. It was excellent timing and we kept on pedaling. There was a big bridge that we came to that bicycles were not allowed on. I didn't want to get slowed down by the normal quest for bridge crossing, so we called the state police. They were great, switched us over to the local police and within a few minutes, we had permission to cross. We have learned this a bit late in the game, but better late than never!

On the way over we had a toot from Grace, the photographer we met in Newport who took our picture for the weekly newspaper. She gave me a quick phone call to say hello and goodbye. That is the only real sad side to this trip. We meet so many nice people that we have to say goodbye to, way too quick. Before we knew it, after several hills which I rode up ALL but one, we saw a sign that said Fall River. There had been no "Welcome to Massachusetts" sign (or I missed it) but a local confirmed that we were indeed, in Massachusetts. Yippee, another state AND in the home town of Miss Lizzie Borden.

Before we knew it, we were pulling in front of the lovely green house, meeting Lee Ann, the amazing lady who was good enough to sponsor us a night in this legendary place. We chatted for a bit, stuck the bicycles in the barn (where Lizzie *said* she was, eating pears, when the murders happened) then, we went inside to meet Lizzie. The house is incredibly beautiful. Anyone who appreciates houses that have character, style, history and are tastefully decorated, would swoon for this one. They would also swoon when they found out just what has happened here. The tour started in the kitchen, into the dining room, then the living room where Mr. Borden bought the farm, then into the front parlor, then...past a dress that had belonged to Lizzie, then up the stairs. The staircase is all original. The hands of the killer, whoever it was, would have glided over it, just as ours were now doing. It gave me a bit of a chill as that thought crossed my mind. After all, Lizzie was found "NOT guilty" so if not her, who? At the top of the stairs, all the bedroom doors were opened. The light just pours into this house and it really is beautiful. We walk right into the room in front of us, the guest bedroom when the Bordens lived here. It was also the room where Mrs. Borden met her horrible end. It was also the bedroom we were going to be sleeping in. *Welcome to the murder room.*

In the corner, there is a dress on a dummy that was worn by Elizabeth Montgomery, when she portrayed Lizzie in a film. It is a lovely dress, with photos of Elizabeth herself, wearing it. My mind was drawn to the other photos however. As you are standing beside the bed, looking at the wall, you see a crime scene photo, one of the first ever. It is black and white, thank goodness. You notice at once that it is the EXACT location of where you are standing. You also notice Mrs. Borden, face down, right where you are on the carpet. It makes you want to jump back a bit. Me, I decided that Morton was getting THAT side of the bed tonight.

We were dying for a shower, so I jumped in first. There is a trap door or something in the bathroom that sounded like it was wiggling and I tried not to let my imagination run too fast. The shower was perfect, better than perfect and I was out of my normal clothes, so I had to put on a long-sleeved shirt from Mystic Connecticut, long pants and then head back to the bedroom. As you come out of the bathroom, you are looking right into Lizzie's room. This place is really amazing because you can actually walk around and see everything, from the attic to the basement. I walked into Lizzie's room, my hair in a towel and had a little peek around.

Her bedroom is beautiful. It is just as she had it, except for the placement of her bed. It had blocked a door that is now open. From Lizzie's room, you can go into Emma's room. Emma was the older sister who was off visiting friends when this horrible double homicide happened. I step into Emma's room, my stocking feet silent on the floor. It feels a little like they just stepped out for the day and I feel a bit like some sort of peeping tom. I've seen a lot of things in this world and have been in over twenty countries and forty-eight states, but I have never seen anything like this before. I'm stunned.

There is a card for a sister on the dresser, it is from Lizzie. There is also a dress on a dummy that belonged to Lizzie. These are the real feeling ghosts that you will see out of the corner of your eyes here. Pieces of the past making you catch your breath in the present. Deliciously spooky stuff. If you go through the door that Lizzie's bed had once blocked, you are in the parents room. This is a somber place to walk in, at the very back of the house. Since Mother's Day has just past, it is not a surprise to see cards on Mrs. Borden's dressing table. It is a surprise to see they are from Lizzie and Emma. The people who run this place has a wicked sense of humor that will make you smile, nervously and then look over your shoulder. I loved it.

Back in our room, Morton had been setting up my work area. He chose to set a chair right over where the body is in the picture. My back was going to be to the bedroom door and he was going to get a shower. I felt very odd, tried not to look at the crime scene photo and switched on the computer. As soon as it booted up, I was back in the present. The mystery, murder and history were all replaced by a real *shocker*! I had over 2,700 emails. Not one of them was spam. Many of them just say "well done" "keep going" and offer your kind words. Others offer places to stay, the majority asking about the Lizzie Borden house and they are all read. I promise you that. The stories have really been running on us now and we are shocked at how many people are visiting the site. Millions of people from all around the planet are discovering LittleChanges.com I get stuck into work and barely notice when Morton comes back from his shower.

Lee Ann has been kind enough to let us use the washer and dryer in the basement (poor Morton) and he goes to do our wash as I continue with email. There were diabolical things that happened in that basement, still glowing with blood under special lights from a former investigative filming crew that was here.

Later, we get a great tour of the house by Dee. She was a real expert and we learned more from her than I can remember from the book I read so long ago. She also explains how the door handles are all original. Door knobs we are turning, Lizzie would have turned. I think back to my thoughts about the banister and re-mind myself again that *MORTON* has to sleep on the murder side. There are other people in the house, experts on the history who write about this unsolved crime, another man who has been coming back to the house and doing photography. Jay shows us some VERY unusual photos of a face, where there should be none, that looks like Mrs. Borden, face down. I get chills as I think of the photo in the very room I am sleeping in tonight.

Even though we sleep in different beds every night, I always have "my" side. This is the murder side. As we go to bed, I am on "Morton's" side. He asks why and I tell him I want to be close to the bathroom. This is a lie. I want to be close to the door in case I need to make a fast escape. I also want to be further away from the murder side. I'll tell him the truth in the morning. If he survives.

Morton is kind enough to rub my back as I quickly fall asleep. He doesn't even have a clue as to why I wanted his side tonight! The bed is so comfortable though and I'm so sleepy, I fall asleep quick and my eyes don't open again until it is daylight. Even if Miss Lizzie herself would have sat down on the bed last night and sharpened a hatchet while sitting on my feet, I wouldn't have heard a thing!

The bed is perfection and the room actually reminds me of sleeping in a haunted room at my grandmothers house where a murder had taken place over a hundred years ago. To me it wasn't scary, unless I let my mind wonder. Tonight I was too sleepy to do that. Thank goodness.

Day 135 May 15, 2007 - Tuesday - *Lizzie Borden Bed & Breakfast*, Fall River to *Captain Haskell's Octagon House*, New Bedford, Massachusetts
Breakfast: Traditional breakfast at Lizzie Borden Bed & Breakfast + something very special! We ate in the dining room (if you know your history, you will know why this is WILD, it is where the bodies were laid out on the tables) and had delicious fresh fruit, warm bread with nuts, eggs with cheese, home fries, johnny cakes and DELIGHTFUL conversation!

The smell of coffee came creeping up the staircase and right in the bedroom. The soft light of an overcast sky came in the shuttered windows. We had survived the night in the murder room! Morton was packing as I was frantic and working on the computer. The experience here is one we will keep with us forever. It has been a great time, great people, great tour and now comes a great breakfast. The cook is brilliant and the food is so delicious. Morton and I are so thankful for a good breakfast. It really sets you up for a great day. Conversation at the breakfast table revolves around Lizzie and then house. Morton and I aren't experts, but we have really enjoyed hearing the experts speaking and asking them questions. It really is fascinating. I guess we will never really know who did it.

There is a reporter and photographer coming and we get back in the riding mode. We say our good-byes, go out to the barn to hook up the bikes and there is a flat tire. Was it Lizzie playing a prank or planning to hitch a ride? *Hmmmm....* The house really isn't scary at all, but quite beautiful and a bit haunting. For me it was also nostalgic feeling. The interview is fantastic. You can just tell when someone really understands why we are doing this two-year trek. We get a few photos, Lee Ann gives us these fabulous t-shirts stating that *"I SURVIVED THE NIGHT"* and I decide to NOT tell Morton why I wanted his side of the bed. It seems silly now. It will be something that he will tease me about. The photographer tells us how to get out of town and goes ahead to take some action shots. Lee Ann also gives us a map of Massachusetts. We are so thankful that she had us stay...I want to go back on a night that I don't have 2,700+ emails!

For now we ride. I replay all the events in the last few days, then months. This journey keeps surprising us, as do all of you. There are so many people now that are tooting and waving! It is great to meet people out here who are making their very own little changes too. Never forget and never stop doing this. If any of you fancy something really different, please tell Lee Ann that we sent you when you go to Lizzie's. Trust me, you will LOVE it! It is fantastic, fun and a real-life who-dun-it!

Morton and I see the signs for New Bedford. A James Taylor song plays in my head as we follow the signs for our road. There is a bridge that says a bicycle isn't allowed over it, so we head for the visitor center. Sure enough, they help with ideas and a map. They also tell us about a free 22 minute movie at the whaling museum. As we pull in and I go inside to find out about storing the bikes, Morton meets a reporter from the local paper. This is all accidental, but fantastic. We arrange to call him to do the story after we have got a place for the night and do the interview in the morning.

For now we want to see a bit of New Bedford, but again, we consult the visitors center for brochures. The very first bed & breakfast I call, *Captain Haskell's Octagon House*, I get the owner, Chuck. I relate our trip and make the request for room sponsorship for this evening. Chuck says come on over at 5 pm and Morton and I now have a good look around with happy hearts.

There are cobblestone streets, brick sidewalks, very old and beautiful buildings and of course, the busy port. We know that we haven't ridden far today, about 20 miles, but we are both so very tired. It is a very tiring thing and waking up so early, then staying up late takes it's toll. We have both celebrated a birthday now living on the road and we aren't getting any younger...well, perhaps we are.

At 5 pm we are at the most lovely house and meeting Chuck. He shows us where to stow our bikes and trailers, then gives us the grand tour of this grand house. Fantastic interior and exterior. Outside there are lilacs blooming, inside there are cactus blooming in a greenhouse sitting room. It is just lovely. Morton does his shower and is asleep by 8 pm. I am at the computer, ready to tackle my email (just 125 today) and try to catch up on the ones from *Lizzie Borden B&B*. Tonight I will be sleeping on MY side of the bed and hopefully be there *BEFORE* the witching hour!

Day 136 May 16, 2007 - Wednesday - *Captain Haskell's Octagon House*, New Bedford to *Rosewood Motel,* East Wareham, Massachusetts

We started our day early, 5 am for me, 6 am for Morton. I needed to do the computer thing. If only I could find 4 to 5 more hours each day. At breakfast we had the most amazing chocolate chip & black cherry sconces. Have a look at their website, maybe Chuck will share the recipe with you. They were so moist and amazing and made with healthy things. After, we met in the loving living room of the house with a reporter, Don Cuddy, from the local newspaper. It was lovely chatting with him. He is from Ireland and got a chuckle when I told him that it was great luck that he had bumped into us yesterday at the Whaling Museum, it saved me from having to flog our story to the press. The word "flog" is one that he hadn't heard for a while. Even though I never picked up a Scottish accent when I lived in Scotland, I did pick up a lot of words they use over there. It was easier to fit in and communicate.

Morton and I head out to the bikes after a great chat with Ruth to get our picture taken before heading out. The camera man is a bit surprised that I am holding a camera as he is taking pictures of Morton. I get to tell him what we are usually told, *"Just act natural!"* It was good fun and I can't wait to read the story. Turns out it made the front page!

We ride over the bridge and get a great view of New Bedford. Morton snaps pictures and we then decide to ride through Fairhaven. The reporter had told us how lovely it was and he was right. All the flowers blooming, all the people honking and waving...it was really great. It added a bit on to our mileage, but worth it. There are people out working in their yard, cutting grass, raking their yards. At first it doesn't dawn on me, but suddenly I realize why my heart is getting so heavy. There have been a few older men in their gardens and I'm missing my dad. This is our first spring without him. I see the blooms on the fruit trees and think of how he would take such good care of his plants and trees. The hole that is in my heart will never forget him. His words are in my head often. He had sayings for so many things. I wish I would have recorded some video of his stories. I think about Sarah's baby coming along and never knowing his pap. It is so tough. I know that time is suppose to heal things like this, it has been since last September and I still can't stop being reminded of him everywhere.

Today is so lovely and I think that the spring time is about re-growth, hope and new life. Dad wouldn't want any of us grieving and being sad about missing him, but I can't help it. Dad was about smiles, not tears. When he was just a boy his nickname was Hap, because he was always happy. That is what I try to be today.

We ride and ride, my mind on my family and I start getting dizzy. My head is pounding and I stop at a park, with Morton pulling in behind me. I realize that I haven't drank any water since breakfast and my body is dehydrated. We sit at a picnic table and I feel like I'm going to pass out. Morton has the camera out telling me to say "cheese" and I just have to put my head down on the picnic table for a while. The word I want to say to him is nothing like cheese.

Sarah calls on the phone and hearing her works magic. I start to feel better. We also get some food in our bellies. Stretching out is fantastic for relaxing. Sarah is having trouble with her feet swelling, poor little Sarah. Am I a bad mommy for not being there for her? I am just a phone call away, but it isn't the same when you are as close as we are. After our break we get back on the bikes. There are two telephone interviews, one for a magazine, one for a newspaper. I realize that our lives are really changing with the trip and again I wish I had several more hours in each day. I'm still missing dad.

We go grocery shopping at a dollar store. I pop into a chain store to see if they have protein powder. No joy. We need a GNC or something like that. Kerry from online, has given us money for protein powder and we really need some! While I am shopping in a store, I hear this sad song on the radio. It is about one person dying and waiting at the pearly gates to go in, until the other one gets there. A lump comes in my throat and I finish getting our cans of tuna and head back out. Who writes songs like that and WHY? Maybe to make us think that life is so short we shouldn't take one single second of it for granted. Calling my mom, we talked for about 15 minutes. She tells me one of dad's beloved fruit trees has died. She starts to cry as we miss him together over the phone. Losing a parent is really harder than I ever could explain.

The day presses on and I try to focus on nothing but good thoughts. Thinking of Sarah's baby, Alexander, coming at the end of July. This is a testament that life does go on, but it is always and forever changed. My mind is taken off missing my dad when I try to push off from a red light. It is an uphill bit and somehow I twist my back as I start to pedal. The pain makes me pull back and I barely make it through the light. We stop a little down the way and I try to get Morton to push really hard on my back where it hurts. It does nothing for me. As we get past the 20 mile or so mark, we start hunting for a place to stay. Into a few motels and hearing no, we keep heading east. We just keep bicycling and my sad thoughts of my dad are replaced by finding a place to stay and this sharp pain I have in my back. There is motel just ahead on the right. I go in and the lovely lady asks her husband to come and speak with us. I explain what we are doing and ask for their help with a room. Sunil says yes and we chat for a bit about cricket and football. He is really nice and makes sure I have the code to the free internet access. When we get our gear in the room I'm exhausted. I get the computer out and start putting in my 5 to 6 evening hours of photos, downsizing them for the web, doing the web page and the endless enchanting email.

Just as I'm starting, sitting cross-legged on the bed, the button that I have pushed a million times under the mousepad, comes off! I am terrified. What if my computer died on me? I moved it around a little and miracle or miracle, it clicked back into place. There is already a screw missing from the back of the laptop..

Tonight as I finish this entry I'm going to count my blessings. I'm lucky that I had my dad for 43 years. I'm lucky I have a place to sleep tonight. I'm lucky I have a wonderful family who I dearly love and I'm lucky that little piece fit back into my computer or I couldn't have made this post.

Day 137 May 17, 2007 - Thurs *Rosewood Motel*, **East Wareham to** *Nautilus Motor Inn*, **Woods Hole, MA**
The only "rain" we saw today was a shower of pink petals falling off a cherry tree. Spectacular! This morning I was thinking about how to squeeze more time out of our days. I was doing lots of last minute things and thinking about the time. Never enough of it, is there? Then I went over all the time in our day that we could trim down. It dawned on me for the first time that our days when I have a place organized for us to stay at, I save at least an hour or so by going place to place asking. It might be worth a try to see if I could email some places in Woods Hole and see if anyone could help us with a room.

With the help of the lovely internet, I soon emailed all the places you could eat or sleep in Woods Hole. You NEVER know unless you try, right?

We had just bicycled towards a big bridge we were going to be meeting the photographer from *Cape Cod Times* newspaper at, when my phone rang. It was Arne from the Nautilus Motor Inn in Woods Hole. He said he would be happy to sponsor us with a room tonight. I shared this great news with Morton and a huge load was lifted off my shoulders. We knew where we were going today and where we would sleep.

Before long the phone rang again, it was the owner of *Pie-In-The-Sky* inviting us to come in for dinner when we got into town. This was just amazing! They were the only calls we received from Woods Hole, but they were all we needed. Food and a place to sleep. The stuff our dreams are made of. It meant a shower at the end of the day, a place to work on the website and at least an extra hour. We could see a lovely bridge in our near future, I thought it must be the one that the photographer was waiting on the other side of. There was a car that had pulled over and a man and woman got out smiling. They had read about our journey in the paper and stopped us to say "good for you!" We also discovered that Dick, Barbara's husband, ran the only thermometer museum in the world. He has a collection of thousands of them! Chatting for just a few minutes, we kept going towards the bridge, only to find that our bridge was further ahead. We still made decent time until we got stopped going up the hill approach towards the bridge. It is great to chat with people though and we never will miss the chance to do so. Taking off on an upgrade with the bicycle is one thing, but when you try to do it pulling a 100 pound trailer, it is nearly impossible. We opted on pushing the bicycles and I really had to lean into mine to climb the steep grade. Right before the top I climbed on the bicycle. My legs pushed down for all they were worth and another miracle happened. I was able to ride to the crest. The feeling of coming down a bridge, a hill or anywhere that you can't keep up with the pedaling, is quite a good feeling. The wind on your hot face, the sense of another bit of the "impossible" conquered. I take incredible joy out of these times. At the bottom of the bridge, I could see the photographer and another person standing with him. We had quite a few honks and toots going over the bridge, so it was a bit of a mystery on who it could be down there. We pulled in to see the smiling face of Dick, who had went home, got us a lovely lighthouse thermometer and then met us on the other side of this landmark to give it to us. It will forever live on my refrigerator. Earlier, I had told Dick about our early days in the Keys as we were just starting our journey. It was so hot and in the 90's. I wished we had a thermometer so I could tell everyone JUST how hot it was. After Morton and I talked about getting one at the next dollar store one night, the next morning we had a little miracle happen. My father who had passed away last September loved a good thermometer. To him they only had to have a two things to be a good thermometer. One...Numbers big enough to read from his kitchen window, looking out to see how cold it was. Two...Made in America, he was a big believer is this thought. His thermometer needs were simple. A few years for Christmas or his birthday, I would buy dad a new one, making sure it met the two rules. Dad would always find a place to retire his old one to. Out by the garage, in the stove room or another spot. This day back in the Keys, just after Morton and I decided we would spend a dollar to get a thermometer the next time we passed a dollar store, we found one on a fishing bridge. It was sitting up, beside the edge of the concrete, just waiting for us. Bending down to pick it up, my heart swelled as I saw the big numbers and in big letters, Made in the USA. Dad would have approved. The thermometer was only with us a short time. Morton killed it by stepping on it. It was quite accidental and just before we got out of the Keys. It wasn't his fault. We were rushing to get our tarp over our gear as we were pinned down by a terrible rain storm. His foot stepped just as the thermometer slipped and a loud "crunch" followed. Even the fact that it was *Made in the USA* couldn't withstand the weight of Morton. It had taken us through our soaring temperatures though. Now, here we are standing in Cape Cod, so far north of where we began this journey and a kind man is giving us one that will live in our pouch on the bicycle for the rest of our trip. Hopefully it won't get squashed by Morton or me.

The photographer got some great pictures of us. Not that we are a great subject matter, but it is rare that I get to see a photo of the two of us riding together. His choice for the pictures was great, setting wise. This massive bridge, then the shrubs in the shape of "Cape Cod", very nice indeed. The reporter, Amanda, told us about 28A. The road that runs beside the noisy, busy, 28. We were going down the road all the way to Woods Hole. As we rode I felt like I was inside the glossy pages of *Yankee* magazine. I felt like some of these houses and buildings, decked out with tulips and blossoms, had been gazed at by me while reading the magazine for years and years. The back road was a bit tougher riding because the edge wasn't as wide, but it meant that Morton and I could chat away. We could also hear all the birds singing and chirping, see cranberry fields, the sounds of a drill coming from boat works shop and say hello to people outside their homes. Timing does play a big role in our days now. We don't really eat lunch at any certain time. Usually when we can find a place to stop, a bit of guard rail to sit on or a curb, it is where we eat our lunch. Rainy days we look for cover to eat under, but today was sunny and nice. There was a picnic table sitting beside a group of store and we pulled our bikes onto the lush green lawn. I called Amanda to let her know where we were and Morton broke out the water and the tuna. There were a few other calls I needed to make and just as I was finishing with my last, our lunch already eaten, Amanda pulled in. She sat and chatted with us for ages. It felt like talking to a friend and not an interview. Very nice and relaxed. It would have been easy to just sit there for the rest of the lovely day, but we had a room waiting for us. We should get there about 4 pm, I thought and this meant that I just might get to sleep before midnight!

It was a beautiful ride until I noticed that I had lost Morton. Something made me look over my should and see him *NOT* there. He must have stopped to take pictures, who could blame him? This road is so scenic, it's a wonder he wasn't stopping every 10 feet. I rode as slow as I could go without falling over.

Looking behind to catch a glimpse of the orange flag, I saw nothing but the trees and flowers. About 10 minutes had gone by and I started to get scared. Surely he would use HIS phone and call me if he had a problem. He must have gotten caught chatting with someone. Just then a car slowed down beside me. *"Priscilla, Morton broke a wheel."* the man said. Here it was the very man I had spoken to earlier on the phone that was giving us the room for the night. He had met up with Morton pushing his bicycle behind me on the road. I told Arne that I would just pull over and wait for him. Arne said he would go back and let Morton know. Pushing the bicycle well off the winding road, I sat on a sandy bank and waited for Morton. Times like this really lets me feel how alone the two of us are out here. Why hadn't he shouted that he had a problem? Why did I keep going when I knew he wasn't back there? We need to set up a better system (this is where headsets would come in handy) to keep in touch out on the road. Rather than panic or beat myself up over things I SHOULD have done, I called Sarah. We talked for a short time before I saw Morton coming. I hoped that he just had a flat tire, ripped tire or something that he could fix. What he had is two broken spokes on his back wheel of his bicycle. Impossible to fix, even if you are a great DOOBERIZER! There was nothing to do except push. We just had two miles or so to go, which should have been fast.

But we were on a hilly, twisty, narrowish road, lovely, but hard to push a bike pulling a heavy trailer on. Morton told me to ride on ahead to the motel, but I wasn't going to leave him. Sometimes people can't understand his thick Scottish accent and I need to translate. Plus, it is better to stay together. Safer somehow. Soon enough, we came into the town of Woods Hole. This place is really lovely and has a ferry that takes you right across the water to Martha's Vineyard. All new territory to Morton and I and we looked around and tried to take it all in. My eyes focused on the sign for *Pie-In-The-Sky*. The owner had invited us to stop in for something to eat and my tuna had worn off several hills ago.

The motel was just right up the road from it, so we just got a salad to share and a sandwich to share and the girl made them both to-go. We carried the brown bag up the hill, pushing the bicycles and trailers towards the *Nautilus Motor Inn*. Once inside I could set about trying to find a bicycle shop, but it was after 6 now. I wrote down numbers and would have to wait until morning. We are learning to be patient and while Morton did his nightly ritual of taking care of the gear, I worked away on my falling apart laptop. He was soon snoring and I thought about my extra hour in the day. I fired off some emails to people on Martha's Vineyard hoping for a room, perhaps a meal and then went to bed. It was midnight.

Day 138   May 18, 2007 - Friday - *Nautilus Motor Inn*, Woods Hole To *The Red Hat B&B*, West Tisbury, Martha's Vineyard, Massachusetts

This day is going to be my hardest day to write about. It will be difficult to sum up and I will fall way short of telling you just how we felt. I will try. It started with rain. Lots of rain. That kept up all day, it's still going now with a nice howling wind from time to time. The weather, however, isn't today's top story. We began the day with this huge hunk of trouble on our plate called broken spokes. It meant pushing our bikes (after all, I can't ride ahead and LOSE Morton!) until we could get something sorted. I was thinking backwards and trying to get in touch with shops that were already behind us. The solution however, was waiting just across the water on Martha's Vineyard. I hadn't thought of looking in that direction yet, but I would get to it. Morton braved the rain to go out to buy a *Cape Cod Times*. I had read the article online and really wanted one, because it mentions Sarah and our up-and-coming new grandson in it! I thought it would be nice to mail home to her. I meanwhile, kept working on a solution to the bicycle problem. The time was early, we had been up since 5 am, me working on the emails and Morton working on the bike, trying to have a miracle happen that he would be able to fix the unfixable. No joy though. It was a thing that a professional would need to see to, or it was broken beyond repair. As Morton came back with the paper tucked under his raincoat, he was beaming and all excited. He was going to get us each a danish for breakfast, but didn't have enough money. Odd, I thought...that shouldn't make him so excited. He told the girl that he was sorry, he'd just have the newspaper and skip the danish. As he was paying for it, the man behind him in line, who had read the paper already, paid the $5.50 for the two breakfast treats. *Brilliant!*

I hadn't had any joy on the phone, so I decided to check my email. There were so many wonderful emails from people all up and down Cape Cod to come and stay along our journey. We will be able to take up three or four of you on your generous offers, but sadly, we would have to stay over 700 nights to take you all up on it! We are just thrilled about that. It looks like our whole trip up to the very tip of Cape Cod and back down, will be spent with people from online who have read about us in the paper! BIG JOY! This put me in such a positive frame of mind I just thought, lets push the bikes to the ferry and see what happens on Martha's Vineyard. After all, we have a place to stay over there, it will be dry inside and something always turns up.

We do like walking and we weren't really bothered about having to shove the bikes all around the island. How tough could it be? Then something told me to check my email again. We get so much of it and I really do answer all of them, but I was shocked to see about 40 new ones come up between the 10 minutes that I had just hit the send & receive button. One email (remember that ONE is all it takes) gave me the number of a bike shop on Martha's Vineyard. The man told me that Craig is the person to see about bike repair. My hand dialed the number and Craig himself of *Craig's Bicycles* answered. I explained our dilemma. Craig listened and then said something along the lines of, "I have two bicycles that you can have, I think they will be perfect for you." He explained they are from the 80's, in great shape, barely used and a matched set. He has gone over them, given them new tires and they have thousands of miles in them. Unbelievable but very true! Hanging up, my hands were shaking. Morton had been picking up bits of the conversation. He knew something big was happening, he just didn't know what. I told him what Craig had just told me. All Morton could keep saying was, "You are joking, aren't you?" But I'm happy to report, it wasn't a joke or a dream. Craig was the ultimate in good samaritans. We floated with our bicycles down the streets that were running with water, on the little fluffy clouds of hope. We knew that we wouldn't be pushing our bicycles for long. At the ferry, a huge ship was pulling out, full of cars. Another was being loaded with trucks as we sat in line at the check in booth. Our clothing was soaked and the rain was dripping off both our noses. It was cold, but I really didn't feel it. My plastic .99 cent poncho was failing and we did look like two drowned rats, pushing bikes, waiting behind a line of cars. Although, even when things seem bleak and dreary, there really is always some bit of hope to hold on to. We knew that just across the water were two bicycles waiting, then on another part of the island, warm and dry beds. These are the things you think of when you are soaked to the bone, seeing your breath in the air and waiting on your ship to come in. The people at the little check in booth knew about our journey. They suggested we go check with Kevin to see if we could get on the ship that was loading up, rather then waiting in the line for the next boat. After all, our bikes will fit where cars and trucks won't. Kevin had seen the paper. He was smiling in the rain and we chatted for a moment about the journey. He gave us each a handshake, well wishes and sent us to board the boat! *QUALITY!* He also promised to watch the site, which we gave him a soggy slip to direct him to it. The ride across was a lot of up and down. It really wasn't bad, except I get seasick easy. A man offered me a pill for it, but I just put my head back. We met these amazing ladies who we were chatting with. The daughter of the one lady has been bicycling all around Michigan since she was just seven-years-old!

We got off the boat in Martha's Vineyard. Again, this is the stuff that dreams are made of. I picture James Taylor sitting in a very chic place, chatting away, warm sun, smiling people and of course, lots of fit people on bicycles. Today however, JT is no where to be seen. It's wet and dreary, but still lovely. The weather actually gives it this air of mystery. Morton and I push the bikes up the hill to *Craig's Bicycle* shop. When we go in the door, soaking wet and dripping all over his floor, Craig is very friendly and smiling. He chats with us for a bit and shows us our lovely bicycles. I want to ask Morton to pinch me, but I don't because I know he would do it. They are a dream come true. A matched set (I called dibs on the GUY bike though...I still outweigh Morton, but not for long) and I like them so very much I'm even going to give them names. They are constructed like tanks. The parts on our old bikes that are plastic, are metal on this pair. These bikes will make the journey. No problem at all. Craig has a busy trade and flurry of customers and Morton and I ride the bikes around the raining parking lot. They ride like we are flying. I remember that it is because we don't have trailers on them. But soon enough, Morton is hooking the bikes up to our trailers.

There is a place that Craig is hopefully going to keep our bicycles. We want to go back to the David Letterman show when we are all finished and throw them off his roof. I would love it if Craig would come along. After all, he's playing a huge part in keeping our journey going. We wave goodbye and head off. We still have a ways to go to get to *The Red Hat Bed & Breakfast*, where we are going to be staying the night as guests of Harriet. We are all set with directions and I start pedaling in the pouring rain. Guess what? The bicycles PULL like a dream too! The are like going from tricycles to the very bike that Lance Armstrong rides. They are so superior to what we had been on, there is no comparison. It is just amazing. The gears shift like butter, rather then our old bikes which crunched, clunked and always felt like the plastic cog was going to snap. They were toys, what Craig has given us is bicycles. JOY! As we are riding along it doesn't matter that we are soaked. It doesn't matter that our hands are numb with cold. It doesn't matter that the cars and trucks that pass us spray us with water that is puddling up on the road. We are 10 again, with new bicycles. We ride with happy hearts that are getting healthier with each passing mile. The weather can't stop us on bicycles like these. Nothing can. We come to a fork in the road. There is a couple ahead who have pulled over and are now standing out of their car in the rain. We pull in to chat and they tell us that they had just seen us on the news.

Little Changes **189** *Priscilla Houliston*

These people are locals who live here until it is too busy in the summer for them. Then they go to Maine. Who knows, maybe we will see them up there! Saying our goodbyes, we head towards our home for the evening. The side of the road is wet, but the smells of the trees being so damp are just delightful. Meeting Harriet at the door, we talk as Morton shuttles in our gear to the porch. It is still raining. Real rain, not sprinkles or drizzles. This is the proper stuff. Wind blows it around a bit, but it is the kind of rain that makes flowers grown and trees sprout leaves. A soaking, steady rain. We get inside, get showers, get human, get warm and now with my toasty laptop I get to share this day with you. I'm sitting cross-legged holding my laptop on a lap that wasn't there a few months ago. It was hidden with my fat roll that hung down so far it is a wonder I never tripped on it. Our plans are to sleep early (Morton is already there) and tomorrow, ride this magnificent island that has a real pull to it and a real magic. It is also home to the best bicycle shop on the planet, thank you Craig!

Day 139   May 19, 2007 - Saturday - *The Red Hat B&B*, **West Tisbury to** *Oak Bluffs Inn*, **Oak Bluffs, Martha's Vineyard, Massachusetts**

Today we were staying on the island. We knew where we are staying, so it was no real push for time, like we usually feel in the morning. I was able to linger over the email (700 plus people wrote to us from Cape Cod & area offering us a place to stay!)and make a plan up for the next few days and I discovered something. You know a few days ago I said I wanted to try getting at least one day in advance organized to save time from trying to locate shelter for the night? Well, Massachusetts has done better than that! With all of your emails and invitations to stay over, we now have the next *WEEK* sorted! How incredible is that!?

That means that for the next whole week, we can happily bicycle the day away, knowing we have a place to put our heads down at night! We could get use to this. It also means that we should have saved 7 hours, since we spend at least an hour each night seeking shelter! Woohoo! The smile is plastered across my face as I go down to have breakfast at *The Red Hat B&B*. It is almost like an island, on an island. Very private and even though you are not far from everything, you feel quite remote. It has a wonderful feeling to it. The house is beautiful and it feels like a real home.

Morton and I fall into conversation with two lovely women who are visiting as well. The conversation and coffee flows (for them anyway, I have never even tasted coffee!) and before long, we notice the time. We want to get on the bicycle trails and have a ride, but there is still the soaking wet packing to do. Packing wet things is a horrible task, but it must be done. Since we had arrived drenched, we had a load of wet laundry that Harriet offered to wash for us! I saw it as the chance to get more computer work done and Morton could get the rest of the gear loaded. Then before we knew it, Harriet was offering to have us stay for lunch. She made beautiful blue fish that was out of this world. It felt so comfortable there we could have stayed for weeks. If only we didn't have to bicycle away from paradise daily. Looking out over the lush green lawn, there sits a fire ring with chairs. I pictured how the place must look in the summer with people sitting and talking about the things they did that day on this magical island. Morton and I are soon heading off, Harriet getting some pictures of us by her lovely red hat that hangs on the street number, marking her long drive.

We hit the bike trail and we are loving it! It is wide, paved and even the hills on it are fun. There is only one big one that I don't manage. The trouble was, I slowed down at the top, while pedaling. The weight of the trailer actually started pulling me backwards! My trailer *HAS* to lose weight...no question about it. We don't take a direct route to Oak Bluffs, we meander around a bit. I really wanted to ride every inch of this island, but there just isn't time. Again, Martha's Vineyard will get tucked in our book that is ever-growing, of places that we *MUST* return to.

Reaching Oak Bluffs, it is hard to miss the *Oak Bluffs Inn*. It is huge, very huge, pink (a lovely shade) and sits at the top of the main street in the town. The first thing I fall in love with is the big, wrap around porch. It is loaded with lovely furniture, perfect for sitting out on and enjoying life. Walking inside, it's hard to take it all in. The place is just so lovely, but it feels very welcoming. Not like a big museum house, this is a place to relax and live in. There is a note on the phone with instructions on how to get a hold of someone if no one is around. I follow them and get to talk to Eric. He tells us *WELCOME* and that we are just up the stairs. He will be back soon and we get our things in and go for a walk around the town. A photographer we worked with in Rhode Island told us to be sure to see these houses that make up a camp here. All brightly colored and just amazing. She tried to explain it to me, but my mind didn't take it all in. Seeing is understanding. I knew as soon as we walked back a side street that we found the spot. House after house, gingerbread houses, sitting and waiting for the visitors. Only a few showed signs of life, but they were all lovely. We are here just one week before it blossoms into full summer life. Today we get a peaceful stroll, pictures with no crowds of people in them and just a wonderful day. Chilly and a bit damp, but wonderful.

As we are getting back to the house, there is a rush of activity. People all around, getting to meet Eric, then Rhonda, who are having us as their guests. The time is too short, as usual, but you still feel that you have just met really amazing people. We also have a great chat with Laurel, a lovely lady that is on the radio here. Too short again, where are the days where our hours seemed endless? I guess that is called childhood. Morton and I just sort of hang out in the living room. It feels good to look through magazines, see a bit of what is going on in the world around us. I had intentions of getting the laptop out there, but it didn't feel like a spot for working. It felt like a spot for relaxing a bit.

When we went up the stairs after a bit, the lovely room with the unusual arched window that you get to sit out in, was the perfect area to get down to business on the computer. But again, there was a shower that was calling to me. After that, I couldn't resist the look of the bed. The sheets were soft as a dream and I fell asleep while looking at the lovely glass house in the room that holds a miniature garden in it.

Sounds from the people below floated up, soft and muted. Before I knew it, morning had came and my computer was still patiently waiting. If I could talk I'm afraid it might have scolded me for neglecting it. It only seemed fitting to relax on this island. It runs on it's very own time. The people are easy to smile and no one seems shocked that a man named Craig, gave us bicycles! Instead they smile and nod and say, "That's the way it is here." Put it all down to the magic of Martha's Vineyard.

Day 140 May 20, 2007 - Sunday - *Oak Bluffs Inn*, Oak Bluffs, Martha's Vineyard to Marstons Mills, Massachusetts

We *hated* to leave Martha's Vineyard. This is a strong statement, but very true. Our time on this island has been just incredible, but today we have to leave the shelter of island life and set off to the mainland. This is a place that we will come back to, minus the heavy trailers and ride every pass trail going. It was a short ride down to the ferry after a delightful breakfast at *Oak Bluffs Inn*. The water looked calm and I hoped I wouldn't see my breakfast again on the boat. You know I don't do the ferry well and get seasick. I would be a poor excuse for a sailor.

On board we start talking to loads of people. Some knew what we were doing from the press, some were shocked and before we knew it, it was time to get off in Woods Hole. I had gotten to cuddle a lovely puppy who was huge, black and very fluffy, just 13 weeks old, named Ben and it had been a great crossing. The rain started when we got back to the mainland. It was just a drizzle first, nothing much really. We just peddled a bit before we felt the need to pull over and break out the gear. Now here, I have to explain, the word "gear" is fancy-talk for Morton's raincoat that was given to him in Florida by real bicyclists and my 99 cent plastic poncho. They are seriously lacking and we hope to beef it up one day in a charity shop when we get lucky enough to find rainwear that will BREATH. Since the story came out in *Cape Cod Times*, we have had a real outpouring of email with offers to stay on the Cape, with people, in hotels, cabins and everything you can imagine. We had over 700 emails of offers and literally just got out our map to determine where we were going to stay. Tonight, we were heading for Jane & John's house. Now this is where it gets a bit odd. You know how things just sort of "happen" on this trip? Well, Jane & John had just by chance, seen the paper, then decided to contact us. They normally don't get it. After a few emails and a phone call, we were sorted with the directions and we had our first night of staying with someone who had contacted US!!! There is a whole week of it in store for us and Morton and I are thrilled to bits.

The ride was just beautiful. The countryside and the towns were begging to be explored and photographed, but the weather stayed steady with the drizzle, so the camera stayed in the backpack. We hoped it was waterproof, tucked under Morton's bright yellow rain jacket. My poncho flapped and kept me almost dry on the top part of my body. I was just having the thought of, "At least we won't arrive as soaked as we were at Harriet's place", when we pulled in to *The Red Hat B&B*. I had that thought too quick though. We were just a couple miles away from our sanctuary for the evening, when the heavens opened. It didn't rain, it waterfalled on our bicycling butts. Just drenching and non-stop. My glasses had to be taken off, they were useless. Since I can't really see five feet in front of me without them, I was bicycling blind. Morton followed, getting splashed by my wake. Puddles and little rivers were running down the road. Lovely road beside a lake. Actually, it might have been a bit drier if we would have went right into the lake. The water hit us from all directions. It stung our faces, then the wind blew as we let the bikes rip down any hill. It was almost too painful to take but I figured the faster we got there, the faster we could get out of this weather. The twenty minutes lasted at least 22 hours....or so it seemed. Then we saw a sign. Actually, a car. An outstretched arm pointed the way and I knew that we had just met John. I shouted to Morton that I hope they have a garage. I was dreading having to meet our hosts with soaking wet bicycles that we had to tarp up. As the car pulled in the drive, the garage door opened magically. I swear I heard a choir sing! *Hallelujah!* It was brilliant. We rode right in, said our hellos, got out of as much dripping wet gear as we could in the sanctity of the garage and in just an instant, were in the house, smelling our delicious dinner-to-be and I was getting to take a hot shower. I have said before that a shower after a hard and hot day on the bike is like a million dollars. This was a hot shower after a freezing cold, rainy ride and it was worth at *LEAST* 2 million. Easy. Jane had us in a lovely room that overlooks the beautiful trees and wildlife. It was warm and dry and I was the most thankful person on the planet. I could hear Morton talking downstairs earlier, now he was upstairs for his turn at the 2 million dollar shower. I hoped that he would appreciate it too! John and Jane are just wonderful to us. We sat and talked away the hours, ate incredible food and even though we were strangers, this felt like visiting friends that we had known our whole lives. They are just fascinating and have such a zest for life...just incredible people. They are both United Kingdom natives and it feels a bit like we are back across the water on our lovely island that is Britain. Wide awake, with the clock telling us it was way past midnight, I didn't want to, but I knew I had to go to sleep. Tomorrow would be here too soon and we would go again. This gypsy life is tough sometimes when you are really enjoying yourself so much and have to just go, but we are getting use to it. The bed was worth 2 million as well, just right, the temperature was perfect and we fell asleep safe, dry and I think that both of us can agree, with two new and delightful friends. Hello and goodbye.

Day 141 May 21, 2007 - Monday - Marstons Mills to *Ridgewood Motel & Cottages,* South Orleans, MA

The morning came too quick. I could have slept in, but most mornings I do wake up so excited about starting to ride, that it is tough to even think about sleeping in.

There were sounds of the other people in the house, up and about, so Morton set about getting our things downstairs all packed and to our laundry, which Jane had been kind enough to let us do. Clean clothes are a must out here. We had a wonderful breakfast and I hope Morton took notes on Janes' oatmeal. The walnuts, raisins and apple were just great in it.

Pushing our bikes out into the sunshine, we snapped a few pictures, hugged and I hoped we would meet again. We rode off with a snack that Jane had given us, following the directions that John had given us. We passed the lovely lake, on the other side of it and had to stop for pictures. The water was so clear that you could see out into the deep part of it. Morton stood looking and wondered how cold it was. Today he wasn't swimming though, today we are riding. The people we are meeting out on the streets are ruining us. When you toot at us, it's to say *HELLO!* Some of you clapped, some stop us and tell us we are motivating you *(WE LOVE THAT!)* and some of you give us thumbs up. No one shouts angry words or blows the horn in a mean way. It is just incredible. Tonight, again, we know where we are staying. It really does take a load off your mind as you are riding along. Plus, it buys me the precious time I need to work on the website. There are so many things that I NEED to do, hopefully over the next two days, it will all happen. The sky is so blue today. It is also very *fresh* out. There is this certain smell in the air that can only be explained by the rain. We ride happy today, very happy. After our soaking yesterday, Morton and I agree we have to start stopping in thrift stores to try to find real rain gear. We also need to look for a smaller coat for me. I get lost in the one that was snug on my belly a year ago. I'm not complaining about that one...I'm thrilled with it!

Ahead on my right I spot a thrift store. This one has some bonuses as well...there is a health van parked outside that is offering free screenings on blood pressure, cholesterol and blood sugar. We want to know these numbers! Morton waits with the bikes as I go in first. The ladies inside take my blood pressure, 115/88, pulse 72 (remember that I was just cycling, my resting rate is about 52), my blood sugar is 95, my cholesterol is as follows : TC 196, HDL 69. The nurse said it looks great! Woohoo!

Now it was Morton's turn. As he disappeared into the van, I went into the food bank. A person we had talked to about our budget, the journey, etc., had suggested stopping by food banks. Perhaps they could help. The ladies inside did help! They gave us tuna, peanut butter, Cheerio-s, soup, cans of some fruit and veg and their well-wishes. This will really help us along. It is a bag full and I head back outside to wait on Morton. He will be so shocked at the free food he might fall over. He comes out, a bit worried. His blood pressure is 117/64, great, blood sugar is 90, also great, his pulse is 57 (remember though, he was resting longer than I was before going in) but his cholesterol was TC 235. His HDL was 52, but he was really stuck on the higher number.

The rest of our ride, Morton kept chirping up about what he can do to get this down. He wondered how high it would be if he wasn't exercising so much. Just earlier, we had stopped at a nutrition store and bought a $20. giant tub of protein powder thanks to our friend from the website, Kerry. Morton said he was going to cut all his red meat out now. He is going to get serious about lowering his numbers and without medicine. As we ride on, I think about everything. How our trip is just showing us the prettiest things on the planet and the most wonderful people. Each day I tell people that the world is really a lot better place then we think, if we just take the time to look around. All along the way today, we are talking to people. We love it when you stop us...it is *NEVER* a problem and we really do love to talk about what we are doing. We also want to bring the whole world along on this adventure and you can help us do that. Our journey really is your journey too.

Morton and I meet a special group of people right before we stop. There are several ladies waiting for a school bus. We meet them, talk for just a few minutes and then are gone. It is one of those chance encounters that will stay with us always. One of the kids who got off the bus and met his mom was Ben. Ben is just amazing. This lad and him mom visited the site when they got home and when I checked my email, one of the first ones was from Ben's mom. She said that Ben had just emailed us money, with her help of course. He wanted the money to come from his piggy bank. This is just so moving, we can't ever sum up what it means to us. Ben wanted us to be taken care of and was afraid that we lived in "the wild" - - - he also wanted his mom to invite us to stay over. With children like this on the horizon, the world is going to be alright. It really is a beautiful thing, kind and compassionate and so young. Thank you Ben, your donation is going to go to get a mirror for my bicycle. I really need one and every time I use it, I will remember our very short meeting that changed my life.

It wasn't too long after this, that we were pulling in to *Ridgewood Motel & Cottages*. It is just like off a postcard. Picket fence, flowers, lovely cottages that are spotless and fresh and best of all, the people. Our host tonight, Stan & Agie, were the very first place that we will stay that we didn't have to *ask* them for the room! Agie emailed us and *offered* it, as did so many other wonderful Cape Cod people! This is just so amazing! We stand with our bicycles on the corner, getting some pictures, talking to people who live around here and just counting our lucky stars. What a day today has been. Beautiful people and weather to match. You have no idea how wonderful it is when someone tells us that they are inspired by what we are doing. Those words you give us, those kind and moving words, are what keeps us going when it isn't sunny and lovely. You are really helping to drive this journey and I hope you realize that.

Without all of you, this wouldn't happen. Without the kindness of strangers, we wouldn't stand a chance of having this dream come true. Don't believe it when someone tells you how bad the world is. It's just not true. The world is what we chose to make it and *YOU* have made our world beautiful. My faith in mankind and myself is restored. My health is well on the way to recovery. My husband, even though he is a bit worried about his cholesterol, is so supportive and giving in making this journey happen for me. Best of all, we are making friends that I feel we will always keep in touch with. Connections, no matter how we make them, are things we want to keep forever. In the cottage, I am going to catch up on several things that I should have already done. There are pages that need work, people that need emails answered and I will get to them all this evening! I still have four hours to go until midnight and there is wireless internet here...anything is possible! My day ends as almost all of them do, just me and my laptop. And of course there is the smile on my face.

Day 142   May 22, 2007 - Tuesday - *Ridgewood Motel & Cottages*, South Orleans To *The Inn at Cook Street*, Provincetown, Cape Cod, Massachusetts

Today we got the rare chance of riding without cars. When we left the lovely *Ridgewood Cottages*, it was just a short ride to the town of Orleans, where the Main Road took us right to the trail. We have been on some other trails, but this one is just outstanding. It is wide, new, places to stop and sit (which we did) and it was a lovely, uneventful yet totally amazing ride in surround safety. Before jumping on the trail, we did a surprise interview. There was a store front, with a post office and a newspaper. While I made some needed phone calls, Morton popped in to see if they wanted to talk to us. They did and before we knew it, we were doing an interview in the parking lot, with people stopping by to say hello. It was really a good time, lots of questions by the reporter *and* the people who stopped to watch it happen. Back on the trail we talked to a few people. Mostly we just rode, enjoyed the day and put on lots of sunscreen. I could feel my face getting hotter and hotter. I am not quite sure why, but my sunscreen doesn't seem to be cutting it on my face. My eye area is all white from my sunglasses, but across my nose and cheeks it is red. Before we knew it, the trail had ended and we were on Route 6. People had emailed me, told me in person and had a really worried look on their faces when they said to be careful on that road. We actually found it not bad. It had a wide edge and we stayed right on the edge of it, far from harms way. The ride was lovely, though there were a few hills that I thought I was going to have to get off the bike and push, I was able to climb all of them. The bike really flies down the hills, but climbing them is tough. There is a real difference between our old bicycles and the new ones. Each day I enjoy them more and more. We arrive in Provincetown at a decent hour. It is filled with houses that have been here for ages, art galleries, incredible shops, charming streets and on one street, looking down towards the water, is *The Inn at Cook Street*. Lisa & Doreen have been kind enough to let us stay for the evening. We are shown by a very wonderful man to the most lovely cottage. It has a loft room, is decorated like something out of a magazine and is oh-so private. The bikes are parked, we shower, eat and head out on the streets, walking. It is a great way to end our day, but I know I have to get on the computer. There is always something to do. If only I had a twin that loved the computer.

When we get back, we get a phone call from my son. My Uncle Abe, my dad's younger brother, has died of a heart attack. I think about his smile, the way he always liked to play jokes and the last time I saw him. It was last summer at my family reunion on my dad's side. Uncle Abe was smiling and had shown us this toy wind-up monkey that did tricks. He was just in and out of my other uncle's house, too fast. We never think it is going to be the last time we see someone, but there always is the last time. There was a big hug involved. It was a good hug. Uncle Abe was out the door and that was that. Out here on the road, I think about missing his funeral. I feel bad about that, but I think that he would have understood what we are doing. I try not to wonder if he was seeing the doctor about his heart. The heart was the thing that gave out on my father last September. We will get up tomorrow morning, the sun will come out, but now I have the news that I'll never see my uncle again. Life is so short, so very short. This death underlines that for me and almost screams it into my face. We have to do the things we want to *now* and we have to take care of ourselves *now*. It is the only course that will lead us to our futures. Tomorrow as I ride, I will remember my uncle's grin, his great sense of humor and his kindness. I will also hope that a few people that are reading this will take a minute to think about their hearts. 30 minutes a day friends, we all need it.

Day 143 May 23, 2007 - Wednesday - *The Inn at Cook Street*, Provincetown To *Sandbars*, Truro, Cape Cod, Massachusetts

Waking up to soft light coming through the high windows on the lovely cottage was a gorgeous way to start this perfect day. When we went inside for breakfast, we met the most amazing people from all over. I love breakfast at an inn or B&B, you never know who you are going to meet and it's always fun. It forces us in a wonderful way to mix with our fellow-people. The food was incredible, then we all did a lot of picture taking, then before we knew it, we were heading out the door with some delightful homemade muffins. What a very special place this is.

We leave the lovely *Inn at Cook Street*, heading down to the radio station, WOMR, where I got to do a fantastic 30 minute chat on air with Char *LIVE*. It was just incredible, talking to a friend, with lots of other friends listening. Morton, waiting outside with the bikes, missed it. Poor Morton. But while he was waiting, he was chatting away. There were two ladies that stopped and Morton was saying to one of them, in his Scottish brogue, that even *FIT* people like yourself, need 30 minutes of exercise daily. The conversation went on a bit, the lady he had been speaking to getting very quiet. She suddenly told Morton that she had put on a bit of weight, but he wasn't going to make any friends by calling people *FAT*. Morton was appalled and embarrassed. Thankfully, the other lady with her had understood that Morton did indeed say that she was *FIT, not FAT*! Hopefully they went away not thinking Morton was a lunatic! This is one of the reasons that he likes to stick together. Sometimes people have a hard time understanding him and he really never would insult anyone (except a few close friends & family members back in Scotland...you all KNOW this!) and it would be as a joke.

We head down the busy Commercial Street, so very alive with people, galleries and the light. There is such a glow to this town that I just want to stick an easel in the sand and stay here. Painting the countless ships and boats, tails of whales you see in the bay and the endless stream of beautiful people. Most of who are smiling. How can you come here and not smile? Bumping into someone on the street that we know from the website is a treat! Her husband and herself are out for a bike ride. It feels like we have came home, though we have never been here before. This is an odd mixtures of the buzz and excitement, but yet the things we all love about a small town. This lovely lady has offered to give me a free haircut, but the timing isn't just right. Besides my hair stays tucked up and under my helmet from morning to night. I do a telephone interview for a newspapers somewhere out west, in a state that we aren't even going to pass (on this journey anyway) that will lead to more viewers. I know that when people discover this journey, it makes them hungry for their own. I want to help them find fitness.

We make our way to the *Chamber of Commerce*. We are picking up a map, saying hello and fall into wonderful conversation and an unexpected delight. People often ask questions about what we eat. Usually canned this and that...lots of tuna. When this question was asked and answered, the lovely ladies face lit up and she asked us if we would like to have a meal tonight. *Yes, please!* She treated us to a meal on the water...just incredible. I just wish that she would have been along so we could have chatted and got to know each other a bit better. I feel at a disadvantage out here when we meet people sometimes. I have nearly my whole life history on the website. The wild thing is the number of people reading it! We have more people tagging along then most published authors and newspapers readership and the pressure really feels on a bit for my writing. Some of you are kind and generous with your email, telling me that you enjoy reading our journey. I am really just writing what I know, as it happens. This diary, log, journal...call it what you will...is just simply my notes on the day. We don't have enough time to give it justice, but someday, somewhere, I'm going to sit (still biking each day though) and fill in all the blanks. There is time for that, perhaps. But now, we are living in the moment. Really feeling like there is no tomorrow, just enjoying each second of our lives.

Morton and I go to our next stop, where Pattee, at the *Sandbars*, had emailed us with an offer to stay. Morton and I did the easy cycle out from the town to this room with a view. This has actually been our best ocean view so far. The room is *RIGHT* on the beach. We meet Brian, the lovely dogs and I just have time to check a few email before we need to bicycle back into town. Pattee invites us to have a glass of wine *AND* do laundry when we get back! Without the trailers holding us back, we made it to town and the place we were having dinner in just 10 minutes. Bicycle Ptown when you come here...you will love it!

The meal was incredible and we can't say *THANK YOU* enough to the lovely *Chamber of Commerce* for the delicious taste of the town. We split a dessert, since we were bicycling back. Remember, *MODERATION* (as in, we *SHARED* the dessert) and *MOVEMENT* (as in, we bicycled afterwards) are the key to a healthy lifestyle.

Tonight was a night for bonding by the fire. We all gathered on the beach, Brian and Morton got a great fire going, we had watched the sunset and it was all just so perfect. The stars came out, the lights from Provincetown reflected on the water and Brian brought us all blankets to take the chill off. This was a very special night. Pattee's daughter was there for a while, but then went inside, leaving just four new friends on the beach.

Cairo, a big lovely blonde dog, laid in the sand at Morton's feet. I kept feeling my cheeks ache from smiling so much and while there were just a few dozen stars in the early evening sky, I counted them all as my lucky stars. Morton and I will never forget tonight, the new friends, the laughs and the view....one of the prettiest on the whole planet.

Day 144 May 24, 2007 - Thursday - *Sandbars*, Truro To Provincetown To Eastham, Cape Cod, MA

It was a perfect night last night. I actually ignored the computer and chose to watch the dying embers of the fire on the beach from my belly on the bed. The sky was inky blue and these orange sparks that would just catch the wind and then disappear, were the perfect thing to fall asleep to. The view out the same window in the morning was just stunning. The "window" is actually huge glass doors that opens on to the decking that walks you right to the water. You can also just go right in the sand and get to the same blue water with a million dancing lights on it. This is the sort of place that you can paint, read, sit quietly, laugh with friends and never forget. When you get Cape Cod in your system, I see it becoming a way of life. The Cape is a state-of-mind and a place you want to return to. One trip is all it takes and you will never be the same.

Today we are heading out to the *Cape Cod Lighthouse*, or the *Highland Light*. I ride with Pattee, holding the lovely Luna on my lap. She is a little black wiener dog (just like my grand-dog, Max, only he's red with long hair) and I fell madly in love with her. She has such a little lovely personality. Luna's best friend is male, but isn't a man...it's a dog named Cairo. He is a gentle giant who she uses as a pillow sometimes. He is in the car with Morton and Brian and It's a treat to go for a drive, covering the distance that it had taken us a few hours to ride in just a few minutes. The jury is still out on my mode of transportation, but my new-found love of bicycling may be a bit slower, it is so much more cost-effective and healthy for you, it has to win. The lighthouse is setting in the perfect spot. It has been moved, due to the shifting sands, but it stands tall and lovely, looking out over this view of water and beaches. We get to go for a hike in the woods, with the new friends of the two and four legged variety, then wind up on the beach. I could have stayed there for at least a lifetime. It was just perfect. Morton and I had to ride back in to Provincetown though. We were doing a bit for the local television station that was really a treat. The best thing about doing a piece for television is that we never have to worry about hair and makeup. The odd thing about this part of our trip is, that it was the only place (that we know of) that we were going to have to ride down a road we had road already. It wasn't a long distance, but it was still the only place, besides the Florida Keys, that this would happen.

Since we were going to be a bit tight for time in getting to Eastham, our destination for the night,

Pattee had offered to give us a lift down, hence we DIDN'T bicycle backwards, well...just a bit. It meant that we could enjoy a morning with Pattee, Brian, Cairo and Luna and still make it to our stop tonight on time! We were going to visit Melissa at *Little Capistrano Bike Shop*. She had emailed us back when our bike was broken and offered her help. She was glad when we got the new bikes from Craig, but still invited us in to see if there was anything that we needed. The shop is just a *LITTLE* bit off the bike trail and it is really worth going and seeing them. They are just amazing people. Melissa told us to have a shopping spree on her for anything that we wanted. It felt very wonderful and strange and I just couldn't do it. Our needs are simple and we really do have the bikes under control now, thanks to Craig. Melissa had read about our desire for mirrors and her son, Josh, a great mechanic that we want to kidnap, put two on our bikes. She also gave us bottle carriers that will come in so handy. They have this amazing big tree that is growing beside the shop. People toss tires up on it, blown inner tubes and it is quirky and very clever. It looks like a Christmas tree that is wishing for a new bike. I had a shot, after Morton got one of our old tires up on the first throw. I throw like a girl, it was embarrassing. It took me three tries to get my tire to find a spot it liked enough to stay. Needless to say that Morton had the camera rolling for all my disappointments. We rode back on the trail to Kate's house, where we were in for a real treat. Lots of real treats actually! The first treat was meeting Kate. The next treat was getting an *outdoor* shower! Wow! This was a great experience. It was a hot sunny day, combined with my daily beauty routine of sunscreen, sweat, sand and the occasional bug that gets caught in my hair. The shower felt amazing! If I ever live in one place again, I really would love to have one of those. Before I knew it, we were having a first. There was a reporter from the *Provincetown Banner* who came out to the house for an interview. It was fantastic, he was really great and I babbled on and on. I can't help it and I really do feel bad about doing it every time I get around anyone that will *listen*, but I feel so passionate about this journey, five minutes just won't do it! People started arriving, friends and neighbors of Kate's. The party was really starting when I finally shut up and the interview was over.

The pictures that were done are actually the first that we aren't standing by our bikes, sweaty from the day of riding. Instead we are with our hostess in her lovely back garden, in front of all these people who came along for a great night. Morton and I had a small time to chat with our hostess at the end of the evening out on her deck. Everyone had left and the sky was so clear you could see millions of stars. It was just a wonderful experience, that like all our other evenings, is over before we know it.

There are several volumes of books worth of stories we have encountered so far. It would take many lifetimes to realize just how this adventure we are on is working around other people's lives. From the emails you are sending to the people we are bumping into out here, taking their first walk or bike ride because of our journey, it fills my heart and soul with this wonderful feeling that I have never really known before.

There is something different with me now. I am changing before my own eyes and I learn things about me I never knew. I discover that I LOVE to motivate people. It feels great to pass on a wonderful thing and the funny part is, the more motivation I try to give away, the more I actually get. Brilliant!

Day 145 May 25, 2007 - Friday - Eastham to West Yarmouth, Cape Cod, Massachusetts

How many PERFECT days can we have??? Right now, we are up to 144 of them. Make that 145 in a row! If you look at a map, West Yarmouth, it actually isn't west of Yarmouth, it's south of it. The place we were going to stay tonight was in a direction that we weren't really going to be heading, but the lady we had been emailing back and forth with, Stella, just seemed to be a person we needed to meet. This really happens out here, we meet these incredible people that just raise our spirits and send us sailing. Stella is one of them! This also meant that we got to stay on the bike trail for the whole distance of it. Blissful riding! Plus, this morning we had one of the people from last nights party going to bike with us down to a forest where our friends Judy and John had just stayed a few nights ago. It will feel fantastic and familiar. Judy & John had both commented on how beautiful it is and we really wanted to see it. We also wanted to stop back by Melissa's at *Little Capistrano Bicycle Shop* and get a picture of her lovely sign.

We said our goodbyes, then set off. There were three of us together on the trail, chatting and going nice and easy. Soon, there was a big bang. I knew this sound wasn't a drive-by shooting. Morton had a blow out on his trailer tire. He put the spare on and when we got to the bike shop, Josh told him to go easier with the tire pressure on that trailer. The rims are plastic, not metal (hey, it was what we could afford!) and they are subject to blowing out easier. Great advice. I tossed the blown out tube on the tree and it stuck the first time. We hugged and I asked Josh for the second time what he was doing for the next year and a half. Who knows, if Morton keeps learning how to fix our bikes as we go, we just might settle down on the Cape and Josh could take him under his wing at the *Little Capistrano* shop.

The rest of the ride was just lovely to the forest. You pass these lakes made by glaciers, people out getting their 30 minutes of exercise and then some and the weather was sunny and hot. Soon we were hugging another friend goodbye at the forest and Morton and I kept going on our own. The bicycle trail took us all the way in safety and mostly shade. Brilliant to ride in any sort of weather. As lunch approached, we sat on some big boulders to eat our tuna. I realized that my legs are becoming so much more flexible. I can almost get my knee to my chin now! This is something I haven't been able to do since I was a teenager. There was a lake with a beach that tempted me to take off my shoes, roll up my shorts and walk in to my knees. The water was cold, but I would have swam if I would have had a bathing suit on.

As I was drying I sat on a bench that had a dedication plaque on it. It was in the memory a person that had passed away in their 20's. They said the person always brought smiles. Life is so short we need to smile more. I don't know the person, but smiled as I remembered others I have known who have left too soon.

My uncle who recently passed away was one of the smilers. The sad thing is though, he was just a few weeks shy of his birthday that would have got him the golden ticket of Medicare. He was afraid to go to the hospital for fear of the bills that would follow. If he would have gone in earlier, he would most likely still be with us. It makes me angry and ashamed that a country as great as the United States can't take care of her citizens health. We need a major reworking of our medical side of the way we run things. It shouldn't be a business, but rather a service. Living in the United Kingdom for several years I can tell you that their medical for everyone plan DOES work, regardless of what you read in our papers about it. We need to all get involved and not let one more person die because of their fear of the doctor and hospital bill. It is really shocking and I have to change my thoughts.

Today wasn't a day to be gloomy. It was perfect weather, not a cloud in the brilliant blue sky and the smells were just intoxicating. There are lilacs, blossoms of every description, pine and I was able to just really enjoy this moment. As we rode into Stella's house, we met this angel that lives here in West Yarmouth. If you know her, you will know this is true. Wow! Morton and I are never, ever, ever, going to forget this moment. Her dad, Dustin, has this wonderful apartment (the penthouse!) that joins the home. He stays in it when he is in Cape Cod, living mostly in Florida. They just really rolled out the welcome wagon and we were shown the washer & dryer (JOY!) then the penthouse. Stella had a bag of things for us, she said to take what we needed. She also had a gift box for us. We were left to get our showers and I had a peek in the bag.

You all know that I have been looking for an ORANGE rain jacket, so you know my joy when I pulled one out. This is a lovely one, but the size on it is XL. I held it up and told Morton that he could use it until I could fit in it. He went down to bring up our other clothing bag and I tried it on in privacy. Even though Morton knows my weight and size, I didn't want to try it on in front of him. I had a feeling the arms would never hold my fat arms. But guess what? It fit! And, not like a glove! It *ISN'T* skin tight. I flew down the stairs to hug Stella who was giving Morton a lesson at the washer. She will never know what that jacket means to me. First, because she gave it, second, because it is proof positive that my body IS changing! There were so many goodies in the bag, all I can say is, Stella is a mind-reader. In our gift box that she had thoughtfully made up, I found something that made me cry. They were lovely postcards, stamped and ready to send, just needed a message on them. I had this twang of guilt for not sending my kids, my mom, loved ones a card. But we do talk each day. These are going to get written with messages of love and sent on their way, thanks to Stella. Did I say WOW?!? The other items in her gift box included new toothbrushes (I had just been thinking we needed to replace ours, it has been almost 6 months of HARD living!) lotion, vitamins, good treats, little flags for our bikes, a *BLINKING* light that Morton will wear when we get caught out after dark (you know we will!) and just one thoughtful thing after another. I'm getting choked up right now thinking about it. Until just a few minutes ago, we were strangers. Now we are friends. Smile world, it *IS* a beautiful place we are in, just look around you.

The evening was so special. The food was healthy, delicious and made with love by Stella. Her husband and father are lucky men to have this lady in their lives. She is pure brilliant! Stellas' dad goes out of the room and comes back with these two beautiful t-shirts from Cape Cod. Now I know where little Stella gets her kindness from. What a night! I don't want it to ever end and I want to buy the house beside Stella.

Morton and I headed to the penthouse for the night before midnight! I knew I had a lot of email to do and this site. I did however find the time, to put that orange XL jacket over my head just one more time. It will soon become looser on me. Then I'll be able to do an "L" and maybe even an "M" someday. But for now, I'm happen in the moment, loving my life, my husband and all our new friends.

How do we stretch more time and more moments like this into our lives? Why don't we take the time anymore to socialize with people around us? I wonder and wish.

Little Changes   **197**   *Priscilla Houliston*

Day 146 May 26, 2007 - Saturday - West Yarmouth to *Sandollar Bed &Breakfast* Sagamore Beach, MA

Today was one of those memories that we are making every single day out here, that would take me about 20,000 pages to describe to you. We began with Morton packing, me holed up in the penthouse doing the computer and the rest of the house doing the morning things. I was going to go with Stella to her work for my first ever bra fitting. Since I have lost 140 pounds, I'm in serious need of this. My undergarments are in a real state now, two of the bras have several knots tied in the back of them to have them fit at all. They give no support at all and Morton has even offered his hand at helping by taking some in by hand with his little sewing kit. Bruce drove down with us, so I could get a ride back and Morton stayed behind to get the bikes and trailers ready to roll. Stella is really good at what she does, the very first bra she gave me to try fit better than any other I have ever worn. I couldn't believe it was *ME* in the mirror. No wonder Marilyn Monroe even slept in a bra, this looked great. I would have to fight the urge to bicycle in just this wonderful bra. Dusty, Stella's dad, was going to treat me to this new bit of lingerie. Actually, Stella told me that I need two of them. It's a bad thing to wear your bra day in and day out, you need to give them a rest to return to their shape. Wonder if Marilyn knew this? So for the first time in my whole entire life, a man bought my lingerie. It was so unexpected! Morton take note. *I loved it.*

Stella and I hugged goodbye and I felt so sad to leave. This is one of those painful things about this journey. We meet so many kind and wonderful people that you bond very fast with, then before you know it, morning comes and we ride off. The dreaded morning after. I keep hoping that it will get easier to ride off into the sunrise, but it really isn't.

Today we head off for Sagamore Beach and the *Sandollar B & B*. This is the very last night we know where we are staying. It has been a new thing to us, getting more invitations than we could accept and trying to keep a time schedule. We did *FAIRLY* well except for a few missed connections here and there. I am so sorry we didn't have the chance to meet everyone that had emailed us. But that would have taken a fair amount of time, at least two years. For today though, we just rode and enjoyed the day. The lilacs are every-where. The dark purples to the pales, even snow white ones with their lovely dark green leaves to contrast. These blooms won't last long. They fragrance our ride that we are loving every second of. It is a rare and in-toxicating smell. We find our way to 6A without any problems. This road is one that is more for cars, but there are a fair amount of bicycles too. The sun is hot, our sunscreen disappears as we sweat and we drink so much warm water I'm sure we will drown. For the morning we just ride, gentle, easy pace, letting the trailers dictate how fast we go. They still weigh 100 pounds, so says Morton, but I put their weight at at least 120. The next set of BIG scales we see, I will weigh them.

As lunch approaches, I spy a gazebo. A *Golden Gazebo*, outside of a gift shop of the same name. We pull in and take advantage of the shade and a bench. BLISS! As Morton is over beside the road draining our cans of tuna that Stella had given us, the owners comes out to offer us cold water. She is kind, has a lovely cat and we chat about the weather, the ride and the lovely setting we are enjoying. Remember when times were simpler? People would stop and chat, offer strangers a cold drink of water and do things that seemed of an-other place and time. Well, *THAT STILL HAPPENS!* The world is such and amazing and beautiful place, this is true, but the people...the people are just beyond belief. Cold water to hot bicycle riders, walkers, or just a neighbor across the fence, turns back the hands of time and connects us. Nostalgic and nice. After lunch, with REAL tuna (there is a big difference...the cans that Stella gave us are name brands, ours...are not) fruit cups, again, the name brand and we can really taste the difference...we head off. We have had two bottles of *cold* water, more sunscreen on and away we go. Riding along, I think, "The term 6A must mean, 6 AMAZING!" This road is just lovely. Houses that are so old, tidy gardens that are blooming, picket fences...with still gravestone's standing every once in a while with dates from the 1700's. The people here seem to really take a pride in their places. Each home we saw on 6A was lovely and I wanted to stop and take pictures of each. Never enough time though even though my camera can hold 500 images.

Morton had a look in a Coast Guard museum while I waited outside. I called a few people that I needed to and just enjoyed the cold concrete steps for a seat and the slice of shade that I was lucky enough to be in. It was a hot one! We passed through Sandwich and I got a call from Margie. Her sister and two friends were going to ride out to meet us at the bridge. We were also going to get in touch with a news crew that was going to film us coming over the bridge. We rode as fast as we could wanting to get there and not keep anyone waiting. My bladder was in need of a bathroom and right before the bridge is this lovely bakery, a half mile away maybe, that not only let me use the restroom, they *gave* us a bottle of icy cold water each. My face was bright red and hot, hair sweated to my neck and I was shiny all over. The tan I have, dark brown from the hands to the elbows, the neck and face and from my knees to my ankles, was all wet with the heat of the day. The bathroom was a cool oasis and I washed my face. It seems like the only thing my sunscreen seems to do is to get in my eyes and burn them. The grit, heat, sweat and most of the shiny-red, get washed away with the cool water. When I get back to the bikes where Morton is talking away, I feel like a new woman with my clean-ish face and new bra on. The ladies tell us that we have only a half mile to go before we hit the big bridge that takes us off of our precious Cape Cod. They are right. Soon we are pushing our bikes up one side and down the other.

Since we have began, bridges hold a special place with us. Even though some are scary, we really do love them all. They are exciting, breezy and the views are the best when you are standing up there. This one is very special, because as we are coming off of it, there stands Cindy, Joyce and Cricket, waiting to escort us back to the lovely *Sandollar B&B*. They are just so bubbly, smiling and lovely. I feel bad hugging them, since I'm all hot and horrible. My shirt is wet and it's not because I splashed water on it. At least this morning I had been clean and did have deodorant on.

The ride back to Margie's place was so much fun. We chatted as we were going, staying in a line of sorts. It gave me a taste of how fun it would be to ride in a group bigger than just two people. We were pushing up a very big hill and before we knew it, we were pulling in to this lovely huge B&B. We were all taking pictures, while in the driveway, parking the bikes in the garage. Morton wanted to line us all up for a shot of the sign on the mailbox. Someone said, "Wait until you see inside!" so we did. We walked in through this lovely home and were hit, head on, by this view. The house sits up on a cliff, though you can get to the beach easy enough. The view is just astonishing. I think I said, *"OH MY GOODNESS"* for at least five full minutes. Every times my eyes would look to the east and that view would come in, I would say it just one more time. They have a massive deck that you can sit on, rock on, eat on and just live on. It looks over the water, where Provincetown sits, right across this blue body of movement. We all made the deck home and talked to lots of people, while Margie brought out trays and platters of food. Shrimp, cheese, crackers, bacon wrapped scallops...plus, glass after glass of ice cold water. This was beautiful, but was just an appetizer!

The waves lapped the shore, the occasional laughs and words of people on the beach floated up to us, but we were all in our own little magical world. This was so very special with the feeling that an evening such as this, as all our ones before, will never come again. Enjoy the moment while you are in it. People think that we have good stories, but what we are finding is that *your* stories are far more interesting. As we chat, some people leave, some people come over...like Margies' mom, a lovely lady who we had a great time speaking with. Margie has told us that we are all going to have a go at the hot tub. It's on the deck, huge and waiting. She did not have to twist our arms. Before that though, we eat more salad, chowder and I have a 1/2 glass of wine. It is just so delicious, delightful, dear and my mind tries to get a hold of each and every memory.

After sunset, which was golden, we get our bathing suits on and head for the hot tub. My bathing suit is baggy in the butt...I LOVE IT! I won't be able to wear it much longer. We all get in, Morton, Margie, Cindy and I. After about 20 minutes or so, we all decide to call it a wonderful night. Morton and I discover our lovely room, off on it's own. I little retreat to paradise. So lovely, living room, bedroom and a deck overlooking the hot tub and the water. The big glass door gets pushed open and the air is scented with the lilacs that are in the room and waiting for us to enjoy. There is also a bottle of champagne on ice for us. I have two glasses and Morton has the rest. The bed has a skylight over it and we can see the moon as we fall asleep exhausted, smiling and thankful to be alive and well in the hospitality of Margie!

Day 147 May 27, 2007 - Sunday - *Sandollar B&B* Sagamore Beach To *Christ Church*, Plymouth, MA

Good morning world! What a wonderful day to be doing what we are doing. After a breakfast that was so delicious we had SECONDS of this scrumptious oven omelette, Morton and I did our daily thing of getting ready to go. As we said goodbye and thank you to Margie in front of her lovely home, Cindy, one of the lovely ladies who had escorted us in, rode with us for the first five miles of our ride. We parted ways at a little cafe by the road, then Morton and I headed in to Plymouth on our own.

There was a hill, no, maybe it was a mountain. Whatever it was, call it what you will, we rode as hard as we could up what seemed to be a never-ending incline, then had to give it up and walk the bikes. It was our toughest one yet. So steep and long and the sun came out strong and hard on cue. At the top however, the whole world looked different. Through eyes stinging with sweat and sunscreen, Morton took some pictures that are seriously lacking. They don't grasp the joy I was feeling at the top. It was incredible and getting to the top of Mt. Everest can't feel a lot different. As I'm pushing, pedaling, walking of even just sitting through a tougher time, I now have so many words to carry me through. I will think about everyone that is really on this journey with us, all of you who have reached out and helped us with a place to stay, food to eat, something to wear, a shower...all miracles and all appreciated. You are all at that top of the mountain with us, but I don't think the picture he took will show that. Instead, there are beads of sweat all over my face and I know that the ride down is going to feel cool...even chilly. That is the payoff for the hard climb. The treat of letting the bikes just roll, trailers pushing us and hoping that we don't hit a bump, stick or rock that will knock us down.

Just before the very top of this hill a car slowed down beside us. The lady at the wheel asked a few questions and then with cars stacking up behind her, she wished us well and drove away. Morton and I both commented on the fact of her kindness in stopping on the hill, the fact that not even one of the cars behind her got mad about it.

In just a bit, there was a little pull in area, where we considered stopping for our lunch. Something made us both keep moving though. We are really learning to just listen to each other, how we feel and I think that we both felt the urge to just keep heading up one hill and down the other towards Plymouth. About three miles shy of the town, the same lady that talked to us on the steep hill, came walking out a driveway. She was with some other people at a lovely house, where there was a party happening. She waved at us and invited us to come in. It was a graduation party, in a wonderful location, with lots of people that were NOT red and sweating. Her inspiration to invite us in came from a graduation speech she had heard the night before. The person speaking said that we *need* to be curious, find out things...our trailers and our just being there had made her curious. So she did what most of us do not do, she got involved. Turns out that we had a great conversation there with a few people, cold water, lovely sandwiches and then this lovely lady invited us to come to her house for the evening about 20 miles still up the road. We had wanted to go to Plymouth to get some pictures, so we thanked her and said *perhaps* and we parted ways at that. Curiosity is good.

The last time I was in Plymouth, the only time actually, I was a teenager with my mother. It was this trip that I still can't really figure out how it happened. We went to the Plymouth Plantation, the Mayflower II and saw this movie where my mom fell asleep. We stayed at a little motel with a pool, which I'm sure we bicycled past, ate a lobster dinner and then, went back to Pennsylvania. It was the only time that my mom and I ever did anything like that.

Today, riding through things that sort of looked familiar, I tried to remember if all these hills had been here. Of course, the last time I was here it was in a car...a lot different. Even just riding a bicycle on it's own would be different. Our trailers however, are so heavy that if we stop on any sort of hill, no matter how slight, they start to pull us backwards. When we came into town, we headed for the water. There was a tourist info booth still open, with bathrooms and we took a break there. There is a wall that provided us a place to sit and we tried calling around for a place for the evening. I told you before that we were spoiled rotten with all the offers of places to stay, from your houses, your b&b's, your cottages...now we had nothing! After a week of knowing each night where we were going to be, I forgot how desperate it can feel as you see the sun setting and have no idea where you are going to sleep.

Morton is really no use when it comes to this. He lets this part of it all down to me. He says I do the computer and the shelter, he does everything else! Sigh, I know this...it has been this way since January...but all you kind people, Craig, Lee Ann, Arne, Harriet, Rhonda, Eric, Jane, John, Stan, Agie, Lisa, Doreen, Pattee, Brian, Melissa, Josh, Kate & all her friends, Stella, Bruce, Dusty, Margie, Myles & just everyone that has gone so far out of their ways to help us...*you have RUINED US!!!!* True, it was in a very good way, but still...I'm left sitting here in Plymouth with this feeling of "HELP" and not quite sure what to do.

Trying all the places that are listed in the tour book, no one can help. I call the police line and the officer tells me that the campground is about 5 miles away. I don't have a number for them and don't want to run the risk of going there and being told there is no place to pitch the tent. I start calling numbers for churches in the area. Most churches, when they are not open, have an answering machine. This is great if you are in the area and will be here for a few days, but when you are a stranger passing through, it really doesn't help. We get to the *Christ Church*, dial to get the recording, only on *THIS* clever recording, they go on to give you alternative contact numbers. My pen writes the numbers down, four of them, which gives me great hope. I have a good feeling about this. Plus, it's the same denomination of the church in Tuckerton, New Jersey, where the people were BEYOND kind to us. This church proves just as helpful. The pastor is going to meet us there, which she does, lets us in, invites us to make ourselves at home for the evening and Morton and I are sorted for the night! We use the music room for my make-shift office and I let out a quiet squeal for joy when I see that there is wireless here! There is also water for washing our faces, brushing our teeth and a super clean toilet. As I start to just work at the computer, which I usually spend the minimum of 6 hours a day on now,

I get so tired. I am having to wiggle around, stretch my arms, drink water, anything, to try to stay awake! This has been a long and physical day. We started out with saying goodbye to new friends, always tough. Then saying goodbye to Cindy, who had ridden with us, tough again, then meeting more people we say goodbye to, then the BIG hill/mountain/Mt. Everest of Massachusetts, then the EMOTIONAL stress and strain of *WHERE ARE WE GOING TO SLEEP???* I forgot, in just one short week of knowing where we were sleeping, just how tough that it. No wonder I was exhausted! Morton had made the sleeping bags into our bed on the carpeted floor. Our thin foam mats were under them. Our pillow cases were stuffed with our clothing (the pillows stayed in Provincetown) and these were all in my line of vision. No matter how hard I tried to focus on the computer and mountain of work that was before me, my eyes would lift to see the lovely sleeping bags...calling me to come and rest. Since I am only human, I gave in. But I'm going to tell you a bit about...what happened next...usually I don't do this, but this is a very special one!

In the morning, getting up at 6 to get on the computer to work, my email had an invitation to come to Boston for a very special meeting at the State House. It is tomorrow, 1 pm, which means that we won't be seeing Plymouth. We will ride to cover our 50-ish miles today, by the coast, not the main road. We feel rested, ready to go and thankful for a place so nice to spend our only night in Plymouth.

Day 148 May 28, 2007 - Monday - *Christ Church*, Plymouth To North Weymouth, *Arbor Inn Motor Lodge*, Massachusetts

You know you were tired when you can wake up after sleeping on the floor and say that you have had a good night sleep. That was me this morning. I worked away the morning trying to get things in order for our very fast visit to Boston. So many things to try to arrange...hopefully they will all fall into place. Just before we left the church, we met a man who was outside watering the plants. I told him this was the way to make it rain. If that failed, wash your car. Forget rain dances...just get the hose out. As we pulled away, the first couple drops started to fall. Morton and I groaned a bit, but it wasn't bad. We decided to not dig the rain gear out and it was soon all clear...for a bit.

6A is the road we will stick on all day. It is pretty, but busy. It also doesn't have a lot of edge to it in places, but it is a lovely ride. We are really getting a work out with the hills. I had to push up only two today though. The map shows that there is a ferry that will eliminate two bridges that we may not be able to cross. We still have to go over 30 miles to get to it, so we don't do a lot of stopping. We had gotten a late start as it was. Morton and I are both suffering from all the pollen that is floating around right now.

Our eyes are watering, our throats are scratchy and I am coughing. I have never been bothered by allergies before and hopefully it just goes away. I suppose it is to be expected when you are living outside. There are punctures today, two of them. We also have one good rainstorm that makes us hold up for shelter under a roof. There are many honks, claps and thumbs up. One guy actually scared me by giving me two thumbs up, out the window, while driving!!! Keep at least *ONE* hand on the wheel. When we got to the place where the ferry will leave from, we couldn't get any churches to answer. I was shaking a bit from not eating and had to use the bathroom at a grocery store. I got a tub of seafood salad and told Morton I just had to have a few bites before heading off again to search for shelter.

There is a motel ahead and just as it is really getting dark, we get there to find that it has just rented out it's last room over the phone. The next motel is six miles ahead, so we need to call the police. They get us to the fire department, who try for about 40 minutes with no luck. The entire time, we have been sitting in the dark outside the motel on a bench. Just as we are contemplating sitting up all night at the local pharmacy, the man at the motel walks out. The people that booked the room called to cancel. He was *GIVING* us the room for the night. The moral of this story is, Morton and I stayed calm. I didn't panic or get upset. No tears were shed and I didn't curse at Morton and beg to go home. We ate the seafood salad, chatted with some people and even had our photo taken a couple times. We made it through another day, the rainstorm and the flats.

Tomorrow we land in Boston and with a bit of luck, I might even get to speak at the State House. Anything in this life is possible. It's midnight now, we are getting up at 5 am and heading towards a city that I have never explored. We have no plans for tomorrow night, anything goes.

Day 149 May 29, 2007 - Tuesday - North Weymouth, *Arbor Inn Motor Lodge*, to *Omni Parker House, Boston*, Massachusetts

Could the sky be any more blue today? As we get ready to go, I slide the windows open to breathe in *SPRING*! We all know at this time of the year, as the day heats us, it starts to smell like *SUMMER*. Something about warm pine needles smelling like days filled with camping, kids home from school and long evenings, seem very far away on a sunny, cool morning. This is a day like that. Checking my email, I fly through it.

I'm getting better at this! I love reading and writing to you all who care enough to take the time to comment, ask questions or just say hello via EMAIL. It is also nice to hear from people that we have met along the way. It always makes us smile, even Morton!

We have just a short ride to the ferry we are taking into Boston. It is a commuter variety, very affordable (only $6) and will solve the question of getting over bridges that we aren't allowed to ride on. We *HIGHLY* recommend trying this service for a lovely ride to Boston. The boat we sailed on today was super fast and super friendly. The gangplanks were wide enough for us to drag our gear on with *NAE BOTHER*! Plus, when the people on the boat found out what we were doing, they put together a delightful and healthy lunch for us to take away. This is the kindness of strangers in action. I had only ever driven NEAR Boston and had never had the chance to explore it. Approaching by boat you sort of feel like you are coming into Venice, there *IS* a lot of water around it. There is an arch as well, that caught my eye. It had the biggest American flag that I had ever seen, hanging in it. Spectacular! Talk about a grand way to enter a grand city.

When we were ashore, there beside us was a steamboat called, *"Samuel Clemmons"*, my sister's favorite author and I had to get a few pictures of it. Morton and I rode under the arch, pushed the bikes actually, then ventured out into the city. People told us to be careful for the traffic in Boston. We found it to be fine and dandy for bicycling.

Things are at a slower pace on a bike, you can take it easier and not feel that you *HAVE* to make the green light. Plus, we have no horns! Always friendlier. This city is just lovely. So historic, so friendly, everywhere you turn you see the old and new buildings, mixing together to bring you this enchanting skyline. Picture perfect. We made our way to the historic State House, stopping at the General Hooker entrance. There is a statue of him on his horse, but I couldn't tell you what he did. I will have to look it up I suppose. My mind was set on more current history. Today we were invited to come along to the State House. A person who has been watching our journey in Pennsylvania, contacted a person in Massachusetts, they are both involved with physical education in the schools. This is the BEAUTIFUL part about our journey....people are telling each other about it and incredible, remarkable things are happening.

Maria, who I got to meet inside, along with lots of dedicated people who are trying to make a difference, was just wonderful. We talked, connected and then, inside this huge, historic, State House with a golden dome, we both gave testimony as to *WHY* physical education should be a part of a child's education. *WHY do there have to be laws like this?* Why, when the budget gets cut, can't people see just HOW important physical education is? What good is it to teach a child how to read and write if you aren't going to teach them how to take care of themselves physically? We are condemning the children to get into lazy habits, neglect their body and don't say the PARENT will do this. Look around you people ...things NEED to change. So, for three short minutes, I got to speak my mind about our adventure, my personal experience with exercise and the fact that I am living proof of what happens when a person *DOESN'T* exercise. I was the last speaker on our panel and people actually clapped, even though they had been warned earlier NOT to, due to time! It was so extraordinary! Wow, this has to be right up there with the top ten moments in my life. It was unexpected and the good news is that I wasn't really prepared, but rather just *talked by the seat of my pants* while wearing my helmet. Nerves were taken over by the passion of what I feel, though I have to tell you, sitting at that table before a committee of senators and representatives, my heart was pounding in my head. I looked at the other people that were going to be speaking and they all had note. I had nothing. Except of course, the helmet strapped to my head hiding my sweaty hair. My feet were not even touching the ground as we left the room. We took a quick photo and then I was off to find Morton.

He had been sitting with the bikes and trailers outside the State House for several hours now. I felt bad about this. Poor Morton, always sitting and waiting on me. Today though, he had the phone with him and did he EVER take care of business! He had handed out loads of our little changes slips, did an interview and best yet...talked to the people at the *Hilton Mystic* to see if they could help with finding us a room tonight. I had no idea how long I would be and we came in to the big city, last minute and without a place to stay. It was very cheeky of me, but I had called Kerry and left a voice mail. Kerry and the rest of the people there really came to our rescue. *YOU HAVE TO STAY THERE* when you go visit Mystic....these people are so special and really care about what we are doing. The call had came through and the people at the *Omni Parker House* were going to give us a room for the evening. It was right around the corner for the State House, in the oldest hotel in America! It is also the prettiest in Boston.

First though, we rode to the visitor center where they gave us some passes to see some of beautiful Boston. Remember, we weren't expecting to be here yet. There were so many tempting things to see and do,

Paul Reveres house, boat rides, tours and we could really do any of them. But today, we decided to just ride. The city is great to bicycle in, or walk. When we got to the *Omni Parker House*, the place was really like something out of a movie set. Huge, grand, elegant, historic and just incredible staff.

They had given us a junior suite that was enormous, we had enough room for 10 bikes and trailers! I got lost on the computer and Morton set about doing the things that he does that keeps us running. Morton will never tell you about all the things he does, so I will. He takes care of *EVERYTHING* except the computer, room planning, route planning and the media. Other than that, it's ALL Morton. The thing is, with the computer ever growing, he always is done before me and I'm left clicking away to his snores. Tonight was going to be different though. Tonight, there was a huge moon. The kind of moon that begs you to walk under it, so we did. We heading towards Beacon Street, passing the golden dome of the State House and my heart gave a race of pitter patters. This street borders the Boston Commons, the lush green carpet that rolls out towards another garden. Trees that are so enormous, statues and people everywhere walking under the street lights. The perfect evening in Boston. The evening is warm and Morton comments about if only Scotland had warm evenings like this. He is discovering a whole new world of weather here, as well as cultures, sights and sounds. Soon we are to the sign that everyone around the world knows. *Cheers.* We walk down the steps, into the bar and I expect to hear, "Norm!" but nothing. We sit down and Morton has a pint (he HAS to, this is the most famous pub in the world) and I have a glass of water with lemon in it. The place is busy and there are a lot of other tourists there, seeing the similarities, but discovering that it doesn't look like the tv show. We just stay for a bit, then head off to walk on the other side of the street and through the Boston Commons.

My sister Cindy told me about the hotel we were staying at. She had been there several years before and loved it. There are so many famous people who have stayed there, historical, literary and even theater people. We feel very posh as I sit at the lovely desk and work. Morton sleeps, I type on, excited by the day and still not able to believe just how much my life has changed. Not just my face that stares back at me in the mirror, but my whole life. I am doing things that I would never have been brave enough to handle before, whether it's riding my bicycle in Boston, or speaking at the State House. So many big changes in me all thanks to lots of little changes.

Day 150 May 30, 2007 - Wednesday - *Omni Parker House*, To *HI Boston*, Boston, Massachusetts

Where does all the time go? Last night I closed my eyes and this morning, just a few seconds later (or so it seemed) I jumped awake with the thin glow of morning peeking through the only little gap in the blackout curtains that really work. It was day, but what time? Morton told me it was 6 am, so I was up and off. I was worried that I had overslept, but this doesn't really happen to me. My body knows 6 am and doesn't like to miss it. We were meeting a news crew this morning and without a place to stay tonight in the city, we would bicycle away from Boston. I had to try to get caught up on my email and Morton got our gear in order as I let my fingers race over the keyboard. We need to get another clock that has a few extra hours on it...this one with just 24 isn't cutting it. Before I know it, the emails have to stop and we pack to meet our first interview of the day in the lobby. As usual, it is fantastic. If I live to be 100 I will never get tired speaking to the media about what we are doing. It is an honor, a thrill and a privilege and there are always different things to talk about. After all, no two days are ever alike in our world, or any. We ride, smile and laugh through this sunny Boston morning. My mind thinks of other interviews, in the snow with Carrie, almost dark in Wilmington North Carolina, getting on a ferry to go to Manhattan...so many people taking the time to help us get the word out about our journey. The press are fantastic, they are really making our journey a world-wide event, not just a crazy fat lady on a bicycle trying to pedal off the pounds.

As we finish with the first report at the State House, our second media date is there. It is also GREAT, we don't have the lovely Beacon Hill to ride up, so we don't break such a sweat. Thanks again guys for making this so fun for us. It really is good to smile sincerely for the camera. There are a few people we talk to on the phone for interviews. It does get a bit boring for me to tell you about the interviews, I'd rather just share the links with you and let them speak for themselves. Google me and you will read all the interviews you want. Earlier in the day we discovered that my photo had made it's way to the *Boston Globe*! Very exciting indeed. The picture, or should I say the *subject* in the picture, was not the best. My mouth was hanging open as I was talking, yikes, I HAVE to get that gap in my teeth fixed and my little fangs...ugh...and my neck, oh well...at least I'm changing the body for the better. The face we will work on later. The only downside to doing loads of interviews is the time element. It eats it up. We knew with our morning with the press that if we wanted a chance to see anything in Boston, we would have to work on a room for the evening. The word *budget* springs to mind, followed by *time*. Both things that we are always short of. Rather than trying to call and beg for hotels, we figured we would try a HOSTEL. Same letters, different place all together. There is a hostel in Boston that I spoke with earlier in the day. They had told us they could offer us a better rate, but we just can't do it. I try calling some churches with no joy. Yikes, nothing to do but go on with the morning. Just then a miracle happens. The girl I spoke with at the hostel calls me back. They can give us each a bed in a co-ed dormitory tonight! JOY...we are over the moon happy and spend the next few hours celebrating by riding around the city, talking to people, having lunch on a bench and doing phone interviews. There are people who keep doing updates on us. We LOVE this! There are also a few other people doing on-going stories about our journey. It all requires a bit of time but is worth it. I like to think that you never know WHO is going to be watching a tv news report, reading a paper or magazine, discover the journey and start making their very own little changes. That is the exciting part. We wish we could show you all the wonderful emails we have gotten, thousands now, from people saying our trip is motivating them to take control of their own health. *THAT is what we are after!* Plus, we know that many of you just like to read, not write to us...but are still making little changes.

On our way to the hostel as we are walking along a lovely street, a city worker recognizes me from the *Boston Globe*. We chat about how important it is to take care of our own health. He is fit, but has a friend who was over 500 pounds. The man was young and at the end of his rope. He had surgery, complications and died. Tragic. I'm so sad for this person who felt so desperate he would try anything. The man then points to a really heavy woman in her twenties walking in front of us. He gives me a shove on the arm and urges me to go talk to her. He is convinced I can save her. I try to explain that isn't how it works. If I walked up to this obese young lady and told her the benefits of diet and exercise, she would be mortified. Men don't understand this, especially ones that aren't overweight.

Morton and I go to the hostel, get our bikes stored and make our way to our room. It's large, clean and reminds me a bit of summer camp. Anyone that knows me will know my infamous story of wetting the sleeping bag (too shy to use the bathroom in the middle of the night) and how I tried to cover the horrible "accident" by stuffing all my clean clothes in the bag to help dry it out. When that failed, I dumped an entire bottle of *Jean Nate* powder my sister had given me, in the damp and smelly bag. Jeesh, I think I won't drink anything tonight, lest history repeat itself. There are bunk beds and Morton and I each have bottom ones. That is a good thing, but it will be a bit odd sleeping in a room full of strangers. What am I talking about??? It will be great! The first "stranger" we meet has just arrived in Boston today from India. He is going to Harvard. How exciting is that? A new country and starting his life here. We both think it's fate that has us meeting.

I head off towards the large private shower, again...so very clean and take a million dollar shower. We haven't ridden FAR today, but we have ridden hard. The sun was good but very warm. When I come back there are more people as Morton heads towards the showers. Two girls from France, three more guys from somewhere else. Who knows, maybe all 12 beds in here will be full tonight. Morton heads off to wash our dirty clothes. The hostel has wireless, laundry, kitchen and is a great deal if you are on a budget. This is not to be missed. Tonight will be an early one. I MIGHT see 10 pm, maybe 11, but I will not be burning the midnight oil. Tomorrow will be an early morning and heading NORTH on 1A towards Salem.

This journey is just doing the most incredible things, not because of us, but because of the message we are spreading. It brings out the very best in people and each little bit of pleasure we get, is shared, passed on and *THAT* is what is making the world go around...or at least the tires on our bikes!

Day 151 May 31, 2007 - Thursday - *HI Boston*, Boston to *The Salem Inn*, Salem, Massachusetts

Depending on how you look at it, last night might have been one of our oddest so far. We went to sleep with about 4 or 5 of the bunks occupied and we woke up with all 12 beds full. Even the girl that was sleeping in the bunk above me came in after I was sleeping and I never even heard her. Since I have been known to snore so loud I have even woke myself up, I was nervous about that. What if a stranger would have to shake me awake to get some shut-eye? But this didn't happen. The bunk was comfy, I was tired and sleepy and I had no problem becoming best friends with my bunk for the evening.

Waking up at 6 am, without an alarm, I was surprised to see all the people and all the activity already going on. Two people were getting ready to leave, putting their backpacks on, making hand motions to each other to keep the noise down for those of us still in our bunks. There was another person that had just came back in from getting a shower. A few more rolling over and pulling the blankets over their heads and then there was me. Trying to figure out how to get out of the bunk without breaking my neck. Morton had shoved the trailers tight in beside my bunk, so no one else would trip on them. He didn't think however, that I would be up before him, or what about a bathroom call? I worked down to the bottom of the bed and somehow (it looked like a really weird yoga move) got out in slow motion, without having to crush a trailer. I whispered to Morton that I was going to go check my email. Almost 2 hours later he walked out to the computer area to meet me. He didn't have his glasses on, had just woken up and made the mistake of asking me what I was doing! Hmmmm, I don't ever really talk about it on here, but we do have our moments where not all is bliss. This was one of them. He actually seemed to be a bit upset that I was out here cracking on, while he was sleeping. Oh Morton, when will you learn that sometimes *HOW* you say things is as important as *WHAT* you are saying. We both took the comment the wrong way when I answered back, "Working, unlike sleeping for the last 2 hours!" as I said, poor Morton.

He pulled our trailers out, we grabbed a bagel and muffin each to go (I know you think we shouldn't eat them...but they are *FREE* and we do need energy!) Just as we headed out, making our way through Chinatown down to the water, it started to rain. Hard. Again, for the second time today, I was biting Morton's head off. You think that with the weather being forecast for showers that he would have had our jackets on top, but they're buried. Our trailers need *serious* work. They are crammed full of who knows what *(only Morton knows and he's not even sure)* and we want to lighten our load. We have big mountains coming up before we know it and they have to weigh over 100 pounds.

Pulling my orange jacket on, I tried to get in a good mood. It's a size XL after all and the very first piece of clothing I have ever been able to wear from *Old Navy*. Thank you Stella. I remember happy things and Morton gets worried when my mood changes at super-speed from angry to nice. Always something to worry about even if you aren't on a massive bicycle trip for two. We got near the water and there were benches that had managed to stay dry during the rain. Pulling in, we sat and ate our bagel and muffin, washed down with a luke warm water and strawberry protein powder shake. I can't say that I enjoyed it and that had nothing to do with my mood. It was just not nice. This is not a breakfast of champions, but it will do for us. The water ferry took us across the water to the airport side. We couldn't take the bikes on the tunnel, so the ferry was a good alternative. It was cloudy and looked like it could start raining at any moment. The sky looked as moody as I felt. Poor Morton.

We rode without being really sure of how to get to 1A. There were a few wrong turns, a few dead ends, but other than that, it was good. All the people shouting out *HELLO* and giving us thumbs up made my mood change to really happy. The television has a way of making people feel really happy about what we are doing and when they see us out here doing it live and in person, it is even better. My mood also greatly improved because we had a wonderful call from Melinda at *The Salem Inn*, telling us they would give us a room for the night! BRILLIANT! I thought about the room, seeing Salem and my grumpy morning. It seems that can happen sometimes, one thing, one little thing, goes wrong and it snowballs into a bad day that turns out perfect. The big difference with today was, my bad mood only lasted for a few hours, not several days. Being fat doesn't go hand-in-hand with being jolly, at least not for me. Exercise is a big part of it too. The more I was riding the bike, the better I felt. It does all of these great things for us and it dawns on me that I might not have been so moody for most of my adult life if there would have been some exercise in it.

We have to ask a few people for directions to 1A. They tell us that they don't see a lot of bikes on there, but then, we ride a lot of times where someone out for a ride would never go. Busy roads that are reserved for the commuters, delivery trucks and heavy traffic, they don't make the best bike paths. There is a grocery store and I stop in to get some things for us. It is not a dollar store however, so our tuna will have to wait to be replaced. Think BUDGET! With no close calls and only a sprinkle or two, we have done two interviews today and are still arriving in Salem in great time. It wasn't that far away and we were both making good time. I ride faster when I'm angry. Riding down Summer Street we both spotted *The Salem Inn* at the same time. It is impressive, huge and very beautiful. Inside, with Morton waiting with the gear outside, Melinda and I chatted for a bit. She is so kind and had put us in a house two doors down that has a kitchen and jacuzzi. Any traces of *ANY* bad mood that I was ever in, melted away with the words, "kitchen & jacuzzi" could it be any better than this? Actually, yes. As I walked into the yellow house, Morton again, waiting outside, it just kept getting better and better. This is the kind of house that you would have to pay a fee to just go in and look at! Historic, beautiful, the staircase is just stunning and then I turn the key on the brass ring to enter this room, this suite, that just blows me away. The biggest king-size bed I have ever seen, hugged by four posters, hardwood floors that shine with the light streaming through the windows, no trace of rain here, an Oriental carpet, fireplace, period furniture, arched window that you can sit in on two chairs with a table in between, ceilings that seem to never end, wooden carved paneling, then on to the kitchen. It is lovely with a floor that is wood as well, but has been painted with a wonderful effect. The light again pours in from the tall windows, overlooking a balcony. The bathroom is where I just burst in to tears. It is divine. Simply divine.

Little Changes   **205**   *Priscilla Houliston*

Huge corner jacuzzi, lovely tables, windows, tall ceilings and I know I am going to have a million dollar shower there followed by a long soak. My back has been sore all day and it starts to feel better just looking at it! Morton kept saying, in a rather hushed tone for Morton, "This is amazing!" We both agreed that we should have a bike ride, without trailers around the town. Then come back to enjoy this room (Morton was going to LOVE cooking in the kitchen) when we lost the light of day. Everything is close to this inn. You can walk anywhere, which we did in a pedestrian mall, pushing our bikes. A few people said they had saw us on television, asked some questions about the trip and wished us well.

The people in Boston had given us a pass that would actually take us in to the *Witch Museum*. It was in a huge old building that I'm guessing had been a church. The story inside told you about the history of the hysteria, the witch hunt and the tragic fate of those accused. It was heart-breaking. I hadn't really known what to expect, but I came away feeling sad about the fate of those poor people. It is good to remember the bad history, so we can keep from repeating it again, but sadly, even today, there are still witch hunts happening. They just have different names now. Morton and I hop on our bikes and pedal past a lovely green park towards the water and the *House of Seven Gables*. I confess that I have not read the book. Sometime I hope to. The house is lovely, but we don't go inside. We just take a few pictures from outside and I am anxious to get out of the chilly air and back to our lovely room.

Laying on my stomach I work away at the computer as Morton cooks dinner. Sarah calls and we have a little chat, she puts me on speaker phone and I get to talk with her and Graeme at the same time. I really miss them both so much. My intentions are to call my son and his wife too, but the computer has sucked me in for the night. I eat dinner as I'm working on email, then Morton gets to do our tallying up for the month to see how we did on expenses. There are a few things that stand out, like getting the replacement camera in NYC when ours quit working, plus, we discovered that our budget didn't take in to account the $100. a month that it costs for our 2 phones and internet connection. They really have to be a part of the budget. Seeing an email about renewing our domain, *LittleChanges.com*, it means we will have to come up with another $200. before the end of June for hosting fees and renewal of the website. I can't believe it has been a year since I set it up. Wrapping up a month is a good feeling, but sad too. When I think of everything that happened this month, it just makes my head spin. We are going to write a book when this is all over, but there are going to be so many things in it that it will be a *very* big book.

The people, more than the places, are what stand out to both of us. The people, yes YOU, are making this trip so wonderful. I walk away from the computer about 10 pm. This is VERY early for me. I have a shower and spend a bit of time in the jacuzzi (pure bliss) but not a lot, about 10 minutes or so. The big huge bed is calling me and as I climb in and fall asleep, I feel a million miles away from my bad mood of the morning.

Day 152 June 1, 2007 - Friday - *The Salem Inn*, Salem, Massachusetts

Breakfast: *Compliments of The Salem Inn* : delicious quiche, watermelon, cantalope, bagel, orange & cranberry juice We are having a CLEAR OUT today! The day started with a fantastic breakfast in the beautiful dining room at The Salem Inn. Incredible edibles and Morton ate some extra things too, he has no will power! :) We have an interview this morning, it is great on the front porch of the wonderful place we are staying. Then we set off to explore a bit of Salem, find boxes to lighten the TRAILERS (yippee!) and we do something *very* strange and unusual. There is a movie house in town, we spy *Pirates of the Caribbean 3* on the matinee and head in for the film. It was really good, but I felt very guilty. There were so many things to be done today, but it did feel good to have a treat. Morton and I both needed some normal things, our life is very much non-normal right now. We finish watching, head back to the room and we both set at our tasks. I am uploading two months worth of pictures, then burning them on to DVD and then *deleting* them all off my computer. This is a scary thing to do. I also have to find a secure way to ship one set of the DVD's back to Sarah for safekeeping.

Morton has *everything* out of the trailers and is going over the entire load. We want to get every ounce of weight we don't need out of the heavy trailers. Tomorrow we will hit the road, rested, refreshed, a lot lighter in the trailers and on a steady pace that will hopefully take us to New Hampshire. This might be our very last night we spend in Massachusetts. It has been wonderful and we have been so spoiled by the incredible hospitality and new friends we made here.

Day 153 June 2, 2007 - Saturday - *The Salem Inn*, Salem, MA to *Sise Inn*, Portsmouth, New Hampshire

After our second morning of a delicious breakfast at *The Salem Inn*, we pushed our bikes and trailers to the post office around the corner. We had finally loaded up two boxes (still not enough) with *stuff* that we were sending home. Everything from clothing to special things that people have given us along the way. The boxes didn't feel that heavy, but they have stopped our trailers from bulging at the seams. They will arrive to

Sarah on Tuesday or Wednesday and there they will stay for many months until we return home, to create a home. Morton didn't budge on his heavy tool bag, but *he* is carrying it, so I don't mind. That is, until he told me that he has *some* of the tools (all of which he's found by the road) in my trailer in the tent bag. Now I want to camp so I can make sure they exit my trailer. Our route today was 1A and it is a lovely road to ride a bike on. For the most part it was wide enough for us to feel safe. There were some dodgy areas on the edge with pot-holes and breaking bits here and there, but mostly nice. Not too many hills, but to tell you the truth, I think my trailer is still just as heavy. Morton and I had a great break for lunch on a bench in a park, with Canadian geese and their big babies. I shared a few pretzels with them. There was also a softball game going on and I recall a day when my James played ball. My son was not really bothered about the game. He was there for the uni-form, which he did look so cute in. He was just 8 or 9 when this moment happened, but it was one of those things that always make me smile.

The day was really hot out, he was playing *WAY* outfield. I'm sure he would agree with me that he wasn't going to go into a Hall of Fame for his skills, but he did show up to the games. The coach had been clever enough to know that most of the boys couldn't hit the ball anywhere near my son, so he stuck him out on the distant horizon. This time though, a boy on the other team got lucky. Wood hit ball, ball sailed, my heart jumped as I saw it heading right for my son. Now is his big chance to show that he can catch a ball. But James had other things on his mind. James was flat on his back, looking up at the sky, most likely playing the cloud shape game. The people were all screaming, but he heard nothing. In very slow motion, the pop fly ball was sailing against the blue sky, heading right for my baby.

Although it has been nearly 20 years ago, I still smile as I watch these young players hitting the ball and running the bases. It is fun to see the parents and grown ups that are watching too. You see the cringes, the flinches and the sheer joy when a job is well done. Back on that fateful day though, I would hate to think of someone snapping my picture. The ball was sailing, I joined in the yells, trying in vain to get my little day-dreamers attention. I just hoped it wouldn't hurt him when it hit him. Anyone would have given odds on that it was going to hurt though. But miracles happen. The ball landed right beside him. So close that it actually star-tled him into action. He sprung to his feet as if shot out of a cannon. Grabbed the ball and threw it as hard as he could to second base. He didn't catch the fly, but he did stop a home run. He grinned back in at us. After-wards his sister and I gave him a pep talk about the importance of staying on your feet when you are playing ball. So long ago and yet the memory seems like it was just yesterday. Time people, flies as fast as a pop-fly ball, once it starts its descend to the deep outfield. It's never too late to jump to your feet and catch hold of it though. We got back on our bikes and headed up the road. The smell of rain was in the air, but it didn't do any-thing. We rode past mansions that were from the 17th and 18th century. The street looked like it was right out of a page in history. You half expected to see horse and buggies instead of the cars. When we spotted the New Hampshire sign ahead, we were both happy to see another state coming. It is a real sense of accomplish-ment riding your bicycle the whole way through a state, no matter what size it is. We knew that we would most likely just be in New Hampshire for one night, until we go across the top of the state.

Craig, someone who watches the website, had contacted us to tell us he was going to be riding south to meet up with us. Ahead, beside the ocean, I spotted a bicyclist cutting over onto our side and I knew it must be Craig. It was and he was just fantastic. So enthusiastic and in great spirits for our ride. It was approaching 5 pm when I started the daily trek of seeking shelter. The sky was getting more like a storm was going to happen any second. But place after place, I was hearing "NO!" Sigh...so much wasted time each day going in and beg-ging for shelter. Craig kept Morton company and I lost track to how many places I had tried. The weather was starting to rain now. We heard thunder rumbling and there was lightning here and there. I knew it was time to bug Sarah & Graeme for help. Graeme looked up places in Portsmouth and called me back with numbers. The very first one I called, *Sise Inn*, I was lucky enough to get through to Loretta. She kindly listened and said she would call the owner, then call us back. I don't know how I know this, but I could just tell they were going to help us. I rode in the rain feeling a lot better and before long, the phone was playing the *Smurf* tune. I an-swered and was overjoyed. Shelter from the rain. Not far ahead and Craig had to turn back and pedal south like mad to get home before dark. Morton and I said goodbye and made a dash for Portsmouth.

When we came into town, we were on Middle Street. We were heading towards Court Street and were both over the moon when we pulled up to this incredible mansion, that had once been a family home to the Sise family. Morton waited in the rain sprinkles with the bikes and I went inside. The interior is lovely and authentic. They just don't build them like this anymore. It is the type of place that the word, "GRAND" just doesn't say enough for. Even nicer, was Loretta. We chatted for a bit and she had kindly put us in a room that we could just wheel the bikes right in to. No steps, no elevators, just pure sanctuary. Under the cover of the overhang outside, Morton rubbed all the rain off the trailers and bikes. We are ALWAYS so fussy about bringing them inside. They are cleaner then most people's shoes. Just as I started working with the help of free wireless and I heard a noise outside. I thought I heard thunder. When Morton looked out the window, we both thanked our lucky stars that we were inside. It was a full-fledged storm. Water, thunder, lightning and here we were, warm and dry. Life is good. The day however, had really taken it out of me. I got a hot shower and died on the bed. I really wanted to make the new page for the website, but I was falling asleep at the keyboard. It had been a long day and a tough one too. I think the thrill of getting inside after a day like that is so emotional, it just wears you right out. By 10 pm I was sleeping, the storm may or may not have still been going. I was dreaming of fly balls, rain storms and the feeling of home, even if it only is for one night.

Day 154 June 3, 2007 - Sun - *Sise Inn*, Portsmouth, NH to *Dixon's Campground*, Camp Neddick, Maine

I smell like smoke and wet sleeping bag. Our day has been damp all day, now soaking. We are in a tent in the woods in Maine and as I type this, the rain is pounding like mad on the tarp which is hopefully going to hold to protect our tent from the severe weather. It could give way at anytime though, as it keeps getting gallon-sized puddles caught in it that Morton has to step outside and tip. It just might be the best day of my life. True, we didn't get as far as we wanted today, but boy have we came a long way. Making it to Maine is making my heart sail. Tomorrow can downpour all day, I will still smile. My dream of being a fit, normal and healthy person is coming true and I can actually *FEEL* it now. When we had breakfast this morning in the lovely *Sise Inn*, I regretted only being in New Hampshire for one evening. There just isn't enough time though to stop and look around at every amazing place we are going through. The bridge that took us over to Maine was just a few blocks from where we had stayed. I should have known we were this close, but I didn't. It caught me by surprise when I looked at a map online.

The day was dotted with drizzle and the most amazing people who stopped and chatted. We felt a little like we were out for a Sunday drive, minus the car of course. It was wet, chilly and when we crossed into Maine, you could really feel like you were in another state altogether. The thrill of adventure took hold of my thoughts and I started watching the woods. How exciting it would be to spot a bear, moose, deer, wolf or wildlife of any kind on our first day in the state. I did see a very fat little chipmunk running along the stones that were jutting out of the side of the road. We weren't making the best of time, when in the early afternoon, a van passing told us there was a campground up ahead on the left and if we made it there, they would let us stay the night free. Great I thought! We can make camp before the heavy rains come, I can email all the press that we made it to Maine and it would be a great way to spend our first night in Maine. The trouble with that plan, wasn't really trouble at all. It would have been great if I would have gotten straight to work on the computer, but as we rode away from the highway, down the paved road heading to the campsite, I got camping fever. Even though Morton offered to get my laptop out so I could start straight away, I refused. I told him I wanted to help set up camp. Which was partially true. I wanted to build a campfire. This was going to be a challenge with all wet wood, twigs and leaves. My first real trip anywhere was when I was just a few weeks old. My family went from Pennsylvania to Canada, camping and fishing. I spent years going camping with my dad and little brother north of the border. It really is in my blood. I hoped that I could coax a fire to flourish on this damp day. Finding lots of little twigs, leaves dug out from under a log (everything else was soaking wet) and getting Morton to drag a tree branch from the woods into the campsite, I began. With the lighter that Morton found in a campground in Florida, I used the dry leaves to set the little twigs on fire. It was almost like setting a fire for a doll's house. As the little twigs caught, I put on thicker ones. Finally, when they were all flaming, I started to stack like a triangle pointing up, larger damp branches. The fire took a while to get going, but when it did it took away all the cold and damp from the day. Morton had made our tent into our little house for the night. We stretched the tarp over the picnic table and power box so I can work on the computer, but we still weren't ready to head for the tent. It was after 5 pm at this point and something was missing...food. We hadn't had a chance to get any more cans of tuna. The only thing we really have is protein powder, pretzels and a few pop tarts. Oh for a nice warm bowl of Judy or Margie's fish chowder now.

Morton and I walked up to the camp store. There were some bits and pieces, but without cooking gear, we were stuck. The only hot food that we could manage would be toasting marshmallows. The trees that we were under kept us dry as we both worked on getting the fire blazing. We pulled a picnic table close to sit on and soaked up the heat of the fire. We each had about 10 marshmallows and it was just wonderful. Morton said he could eat the whole bag they were that good! But we didn't get the chance to find out if we could. It started to rain heavy and we took care of the fire with the help of the rain and made our way into the tent.

Now here I lay, on my belly, with the smell of smoke from the fire clinging to my damp hair. My nose is already cold but thankfully, Morton feels like a furnace. He's asleep, with his glasses still on. The last thing he said was, "I really cannae be bothered with camping" as the rain pounded so loud it woke him up. This translates to "I really can't be bothered with camping" for those who don't speak Scottish slang. The weatherman says it is going to rain all night. What a way to spend our first night in Maine. Hopefully come morning we will still be here and not washed down the pine tree covered slope behind the tent. Perfection is a dry tent.

Day 155 June 4, 2007 - Monday - *Dixon's Campground*, Camp Neddick to *Captain Lord Mansion*, Kennebunkport, Maine

You must be thinking that I'm crazy, I keep telling you that we have just had the best day of our lives...and it keeps happening over and over. Today was no exception. It only goes to help prove my theory that *every* day can and should be the best day of your life. Even though it rained all night and everything was soaking, it was still dry in the tent. Always a good thing. Morton woke up in a really grumpy mood. He is not a happy kinda camper. Me, I think *ANY* day that you wake up is a great day. I put on my shoes, got out of the tent to head towards the bathrooms and left out a shriek. The water coming from out of the sky was like ice as it hit my semi-warm body. This is what if must be like to jump in an icy lake. I think actually, my yelling put Morton in a better mood. He seemed happier when I came back anyway.

We made the decision to pack it up and head north. There are a lot of miles to cover in Maine and we knew that we weren't going to get anywhere sitting out the rain. The forecast for the next couple of days has rain in it, so we had pretty much agreed on heading out when I got a phone call that sealed the deal.

Morton was still hiding under the sleeping bag, but I was soaking wet from going to the bathroom. It was a short trip, but the rain was just pouring like an open faucet. It felt like it was saving me the trouble of a shower. Sitting cross-legged, I spoke to Rick at the *Captain Lord Mansion* in Kennebunkport. He said they would be happy to have us as their guests in a room with a fireplace. These were the words of encouragement I needed to ride in this weather. We broke camp, Morton doing most of the packing, me trying to get to some email, then relenting and helping him. We had everything double-bagged but I still was worrying about the rain. It was so heavy I knew it was going to be a difficult ride. Condensation from the damp can be a real killer to our laptop, phones and camera. All things we can't afford to lose. After we came out of the shelter of the tall trees in the woods we were staying in, the wind took hold of us. Usually I have been happy to have the wind in my face as I ride fast down the other side of a steep hill. Today though, the wind smacked our wet faces and my eyes stung so bad. I couldn't see with or without my glasses on. I kept them on though, because at least my eyes weren't stinging from the rain as they acted like safety goggles. Morton must have thought I was being sarcastic when I left out a shout for joy. I wasn't though. This is the sort of weather that reminds us that we are alive. It is the kind of weather that invigorates you. It is the kind of weather that when you get through a day of being in it, you appreciate the shelter and warmth like never before. This is the weather that it is alright to scream in.

The woods around us were so many different shades of green, Ireland would have been jealous. The lush ferns curling, tucked under the tall pines, leaves so fresh and new for this year, just starting their life. For just a second, my eye caught a bright yellow leaf on the side of the road and I was reminded how fast time goes by. Another season is always lurking right around the corner. There is a lot to be said for the landscape in the rain, but the trouble is, I can't pull out the camera to take pictures when it is pouring down rain. We would love to have something waterproof, but for today, my camera is tucked in my pouch, under my poncho, beside my phone. In the shelter of my bulk. At times like these, I don't know why, but sometimes I daydream about a pickup truck stopping and asking us if we want a lift. I wonder what my answer would be. It would be tempting, but if it wasn't an emergency, I think I would have to decline. Today however, no one stops. Mine is a mute fantasy. We only talk to people when we pull under an overhang by a dollar store to stock up on tuna. I actually went in and did a BIG shop. I spent $42. but it should be enough food for the next 8 to 10 days. Lots of tuna, whole wheat crackers, things that won't spoil and things that hopefully won't bring the bears in. We have been warned and I know from personal experience that if a bear can smell your food, they will come and try to eat your food. Sort of like Morton and I. The map of Maine is ENORMOUS! We are heading to Quoddy Head, then to west, before getting into some real remote areas, working our way back south and west to New Hampshire. But today I just think about this piece of road we are on. There are plenty of hotels and motels along the way. I'm so thankful I don't have to go in and beg for a room anywhere. It feels just great knowing that tonight we will get showers, be warm, have our dinner inside and a bed. Though my body is really changing, it is still big. Getting in and out of the tent are so much easier, but last night, I was sleeping on a few stones.

I could feel them, but there was nothing I could do about them. We also had the lumpy hard pillows, not the most comfortable way to sleep.

Our REAL pillows got put out for garbage in Provincetown, Massachusetts. We decided they were taking up too much room. Plus, they had been damp and were growing mould...never a good thing to bury your face into at night. The first night of using our pillows had proved frustrating. The clothes are in big plastic bags, but mine all felt like logs. Not sure why, perhaps because they were all rolled. It was frustrating too because the pillow case kept sliding off of the bag and I'd wake up with my face glued to the plastic bag. But tonight..a bed! We need to enjoy these while we can. Soon we will be in a part of the country where the tent will be an every night thing. When you come to Maine, and you *have* to, you have to come to Kennebunkport. Even in the pouring down rain, it is so beautiful. Morton said at least a dozen times, "If only we could take a picture of *THAT*!" about various things we spotted on the way here. Turning down the street that leads to our home for the night, there was a little river running on the edge of the road. At the top of the street, there sat this stunning house. On closer approach and through squinting wet eyes, the sign that said it was indeed going to be where we were staying the night, made my heart leap with joy. Forget mansion, this place is a palace! Wow, if you only ever look at one website from our journey, look at the one for *Captain Lord Mansion*. You also should treat yourself right and come here.

Morton waited with the bikes while I went inside. I didn't want to go in, being soaked to the bone and looking like something the cat had just dragged in. But the kind lady assured me that it was fine, so I walked in the grand entrance very gingerly. The carpets, the decor, the people, all just amazing. I know without a doubt I am dreaming and will wake up at any second in the freezing tent, belly button deep in water. But it isn't a dream. We were thrilled that there is a carriage house that we can stow the bikes in and in just a few moments, we are pushing them inside for the evening. I want to burst into songs of joy and swing from the beautiful rafters. Just to be inside on a day like this is a real treat. I would love to just sleep beside the bikes in the lovely carriage house from a grand time gone by. Morton and I go inside and get a full tour around this huge mansion that was once a private home. We are shown to our suite, *Ship Oriental*. My hands are still shaking a bit from the cold, but in just a second, my whole body starts to shake. I try to hold back tears. The joy of seeing this room, this stunning room, is overwhelming. The lady leaves us and I look at Morton and cry through my smile. This can't be real. It has to be a dream. Without missing a beat, our phone rings and it is a newspaper reporter. We do the story and I am hanging my wet things near the fire to get them dried out. My shoes are soaking, everything I had on is just soaked. Tonight the fire won't be a thing of romance, but a thing of practicality. Beds are something that we are getting to be real experts at. We have slept in over 100 since January. This bed might be in the top 5 in the whole world. It is huge, stunning, canopy on top (not at all like the dome of our wet tent) and hugged with four twisting posts. A carved wooden head board is stacked with lush pillows. It is a bed that we will never forget and I will always want to come back to. The bathroom is something to write home about, so I will! It is perfect in every way, plus it has a huge jacuzzi in it. I imagine that after my million-dollar shower, I will wash it down with a two-million-dollar jacuzzi! That is what they will feel like to me and my sore body anyway. There is a photographer coming out and I try to get my hair dried out and sorted. It is in a mad frizz and tangle. I need to just cut it all off and be done with it, but the ponytail is easy enough to care for. As I brush it, I see strands turning blonde from being in the sun. There are also a few gray popping up. Must be all the close calls. I'll have to watch it or the top part of my head that the helmet covers will stay brown while the rest of it goes lighter. After a really fun photo shoot in the suite, one of the first without the helmets and bikes, I turn to the computer. Lo and behold, my first 3 emails are from people in Maine, inviting us to stay! Yes! This is what we want. It is so much fun to interact with people who know what we are up to out here. We also have an invitation to go to Augusta to the State House. Hopefully we will be there on Thursday. There is a law being signed by the governor making it a crime to come within three feet of a bicycle. Great idea. But tonight, I'm going to work very hard, get all my work done, then go soak away the sore from the night before.

Morton is already snoring...he just can't take the wild pace we are at and needs his sleep. Me, I have more energy then I have in my entire life. Exercise is the key and living in the moment. This is the fountain of youth you have heard of. But then there are miracles that are dancing all around us, constantly. Rarely does a day go so perfect, for a Monday, a rainy Monday. It must be the magic of Maine.

Day 156 June 5, 2007 - Tuesday - *Captain Lord Mansion*, Kennebunkport to *Maine Motel*, South Portland, Maine

One of the best things about getting to stay in a B&B is that in the morning, you get to chat to the most incredible people. Our table had three other couples that we could have talked with all day, but we needed to get our bikes out of the carriage house and head off for Portland. The weather forecast was calling for afternoon showers, so we wanted to get a good early start on the day to make some miles. We met up with the people from *WCSH, Channel 6, NBC* at the *Captain Lord Mansion* as we were getting out the still wet bikes. They handle grips were filled with water, the seats were soaking, but we squeezed the first and put plastic bags over the second. The friendly dogs (who were just lovely!) were roaming around as the camera was rolling and we were talking about the ride, the weather and how we are just having the experience of a lifetime. It was fantastic and soon came the part where we say goodbye and head off.

Today I actually was prepared with directions that would lead us back to US 1. I had put my orange jacket on, but it soon got to be too warm for that. To think yesterday that we were both freezing and in the rain. You wouldn't even think that we were on the same planet today. You have to be prepared for this weather though, it can mean the difference between a great day with bad weather and a bad day with bad weather. The phrase, "All fours seasons in one day" which I had learned while living in Scotland, seemed to fit today's weather. It started out at 6 this morning being foggy and chilly, we'll call that autumn. Then at the start of the ride, smelling the lilacs and feeling the temperature warm up, you would swear it was spring. As the sun really came out, the jacket came off and the sweat on my face screamed, summer. Then, just after we got in a place for the evening, the temperature dropped, very cold and you could feel the chill of winter in the air. All four seasons. Riding along US 1 is really good. We hope the rest of the road stays like this. A wide enough edge that we feel very happy about. There is traffic, but I think most of the cars must be using the big highway to the west of us.

When we stop for lunch beside the road we take advantage of a sunny bank to pull our tent out on. We stake it out, hoping that it will dry a bit. If we have to use it tonight, we will be stuck. It is so soaking wet, I don't think it will ever dry. The big white tarps is still dripping wet as well. Morton stuck a stake in the ground to keep the tent and tarp from blowing away, then joined me in the grass for our lunch. It was sunny and warm when we sat down, but then the sky started to really change. We still had a few peanuts to eat, but I closed the bag and jumped up. You could feel the chill in the air and just knew that the black clouds were not going to be good. We could still see blue skies in the direction that we were riding, so we went as fast as we could to try to outrun the weather. The signs for Portland were getting closer and closer. We weren't sure where we were going to stay tonight and soon we started spotting motels. I thought about stopping in and asking a few of them, but didn't. Morton asked me if there were motels in Portland. I explained that just like him, I had no idea of what was on the road ahead of us. It made me think though, with the sky getting cloudy, the temperature falling and the thunder starting to rumble, I turned into the cute *Maine Motel* that sets beside US 1. Inside I spoke with Jarina, explaining what we were doing and asking for their help. After a phone call, she was able to say yes and Morton and I headed to the room. Not long after we were in, the sky let loose. It felt so good to be watching the storm from the inside, through a window. It lets you see the beauty of nature without having to experience it on your face and body. Right now the sun is back out and bright, so it leaves me with the hopes that summer is going to be back for us for tomorrow. Of course we already know, like today, it will be the very best day of our life.

Day 157 June 6, 2007 - Wednesday - *Maine Motel*, South Portland To *Comfort Inn*, Brunswick, Maine

What a day! Lovely weather, great things to look at, but MOST wonderful...the PEOPLE that we met along the way! There are so many of you now that come up and say you have been on the website, or you watch it every day...we LOVE this! We also love to hear about what you are doing. Today we heard from someone out walking that the paper they read with the story of our journey in it, motivated them to take a walk. This is what we want to happen people! With our trip to Augusta on the horizon, we knew we had to make at least 30-ish miles today. There are a lot of little hills in this area that feel like Mt. Everest with the still heavy trailers. I swear Morton's is considerably lighter than mine. The backs of my legs are really feeling it. Just when I thought my leg muscles were getting good and strong, we have a full day's workout of climbing the hills. Now between my knees and my hips, my upper thigh muscles are just aching. At one point today I get a leg cramp, nearly at the top of a hill and have to just jump off the bike. It felt good to walk, pushing the bike with me. I am reminded of something that happened a few days ago that I forgot to tell you about. It was the day we had left Kennebunkport. We were on US 1, in a town, heading north of course. There were two cars heading south that wanted to turn east, right in front of us. We were coming down a hill at some rate of speed and *WE* had the right-of-way, without one shadow of a doubt.

The trouble is, a lot of car drivers see bikes as things for play, not vehicles of transport. The first car, with an older man behind the wheel, just floored it and went right in front of me. The next car, with a female driver in it, gunned the engine and pulled halfway into our lane, then jammed on her brakes. This was such a close call. Her car bumped me, but miraculously my bike stays up. I can't even tell you how scared I was. Morton and I had just had lunch and I talked on the phone briefly to my son, who was at his home in Pennsylvania, having his own lunch, before heading back to his work. Our conversation had to do with our safety out here. He had heard something on the news, a bad accident and was worrying about me. Promising him I wouldn't get killed out here was the first thing that popped into my head when this woman didn't want to wait for two or three seconds. This is one promise that I don't want to break, but sadly it is not in my control. The woman had looked right into my eyes, which were very wide with horror. I hoped she realized how bad this scared me. I tensed very hard and I'm not sure how, but I pulled a muscle in my stomach. As it was happening, I gave the oddest cry out of, "Jeeeezzz-zookie!" very loud and not what I would expect my last words on earth to be. Morton and I both talked for a few minutes about what a close one that was. What would have happened if we had collided. But I tried to get it out of my head as quick as I could. I don't like to dwell on bad things or even think of them.

Today, while pushing the bike up the hill while my leg was cramping, my stomach still ached from clenching my muscles so tight during my close call. For just a moment, I'm scared again. Then I think..."Hey, I MUST have stomach muscles!" sort of like discovering that I have BONES in my body after decades of them being buried in my fat. I'm the ever optimist. Always have been and it will take more than one driver who thinks they have the right to cut us off, simply because they are in a car, to shake my optimistic outlook. We leave the city of Portland and at once the air changes. It is cool, not cold.

The smells from the trees are like the best perfume you could ever imagine. Pine needles, warmed in the sun. The smell of the sunshine is steaming away all the traces of the heavy rains we had earlier in the week. Paradise found. Morton is wanting to stop and take pictures everywhere. He has never been to Maine before and is shouting out all the Scottish names. I'm reminded of a joke I heard once, but I keep it to myself. Morton can't really hear me on the bike and usually asks me to repeat things over and over. The joke goes like this. There is a man from Scotland, visiting his cousin in Maine. The cousin is flying him around, showing him the beauty of the state from a small plane. They go over the lakes, the cousin says how lovely they are and the Scotsman pipes up, "Ach, aye...but we have brilliant lochs in Scotland too!" Then the cousin shows off a lovely rolling bit of land, to which the Scotsman adds, "It isn't a patch next to the Great Glen in the Highlands, laddie!" The cousin finally spies something that he is sure will impress his Scottish relative. He flies the plane over to the water's edge and says, "Do they have any MOOSE in Scotland?" as the Scotsman spies the large bull moose drinking from the lake. The stunned Scot is speechless for a moment. Then he replies, "Aye, we have MOOSE, and in our country, we have cats big enough to catch them as well!" To really understand that joke, ask Morton to say MOUSE for you!

Since today is a "nothing planned" day for our lodging tonight, I start going into places once we are north of Freeport. I hear several no's, but leave our cards. Hopefully the people will be kind enough to have a look at the website. I'm learning to not take the no's as a person thing and hopefully turn it into a positive by getting them to look at the website and make some little changes in their lives. The air is getting colder and I remember hearing the weather forecast saying that it was going to go to almost FREEZING tonight. At least the tent is dry if we need to pitch it. There is a *Comfort Inn* ahead and we pull in. I had almost gone by it, because it was later in the day and I knew the manager would most likely be gone for the day. The lovely lady Rebecca, at the front desk, listened to my plea for a room. She was kind enough to call the manager, who was kind enough to sponsor us for a room for the night!

Once inside, my laptop warmed my lap up. I had a shower that was worth at least a million dollars, had just enough strength in my to do the photos and the front page of the website before falling fast asleep.

Day 158 June 7, 2007 - Thursday - *Comfort Inn*, **Brunswick to** *Comfort Inn*, **Augusta, Maine**

Lunch : BRIGHT RED 69 cent hot dog, crackers, protein shake with water

Today we bicycled for 36 miles. We woke up early, 5 am, to find two flat tires on the trailers. Still, I have a feeling that TODAY is going to be our best day ever!

Did I mention the hills? We are really hitting them now. I'm not going to spend any time complaining about them because they are incredibly beautiful. It does get tough though and I had to push the bike & trailer UP about 4 or 5 times in the day. I know they won't be the only hills (mountains) that I have to push over. The point is, that somehow, I do manage to get OVER them! The thrill of riding down is worth all the sweat on the uphill climb. Talk about feeling like you are ten again! You really just need to find an activity that will count as your exercise you enjoy. Think back to what you loved in childhood. This morning we started at the hotel in

Brunswick with an interview and some pictures. It was great and I have to admit, we are both getting a LOT better at acting natural. It seems almost "normal" now, to act natural. :) We road across this amazing bridge that had a wild river below it, a brewery on it and Morton was really wanting to stop and get photos.

Today we had an appointment to meet a few people at the State House in Augusta, which meant a 30 plus mile ride over hill and dale. Morton did manage to get lots of photos though. We have discovered that since he is left-handed, the camera doesn't really fit his hand. That is why he is forever covering the light sensor on the camera, the flash and other important things to lead to a picture that he doesn't have to take over. I'm not sure how we can work around this. The curse of the lefty strikes again!

There are not a lot of bathrooms on the road today. There are some homes, but it is pretty sparse in population, heavy on views. Morton and I make a left to a little store beside the road, right after I told him I was getting desperate. When I went inside, I hoped that I wouldn't hear "sorry, no bathroom" that we do hear a lot. My lucky stars were shining though, well, maybe I should say my lucky moon. I was sent back a brick path to a proper toilet that was set in the cutest little outhouse. Complete, of course, with the moon cut in the door. It was a great bathroom, clean and toilet paper (always important) and very appreciated. These are things that people don't really think about when we say we are spending two years on this journey. For the next 19 months, my life is a public bathroom. Morton goes inside the shop for a look to see if they have these huge cans of *Arizona* green tea. They do. He also buys us each a bright red hot dog. I don't want to seem ungrateful, but I'm not a big hot dog eater any time. He has his covered in mustard, ketchup (or red sauce, as he calls it) and relish. He loves it. Me, not so much. They were only 69 cents, but I was worried about WHAT they were and *WHY* they were red. Someone tells me later that it is a Maine thing. Maybe they are moose dogs. We know that today we just have to keep going. There is really no time to stop and smell the honeysuckle, which are everywhere. In my mind I think about all the things I'm seeing, feeling, smelling. I feel like I let you down each and every day but not having the time or talent to tell you about this incredible day.

We have a lot of time to think while we are riding along and most of the time, we spend silent. Lost in our thoughts while looking out on the road for glass, nails, holes and other problems. Morton has a hard time hearing what I say, but sometimes he will rattle on for ages to me. I just turn my head a bit sideways, cutting the wind, then his voice comes through loud and clear. It never fails to amaze me that he really thinks that because I have read the map, have the route written down, I can pinpoint where we are at all times. It is also odd that he thinks I have been down *EVERY* road in America! I suppose it is sort of like people asking him if he knows their grandparents that live in Scotland. There is a trail that looks like it would be great for bikes beside the lovely river that should run us right to the State House. I give a fright to a lady on a bench, who is watching the water. Sorry said, I ask if the path will take us to the State House. She tells us it will run out, but then start again. We decide to leave traffic and noise and go for the path less traveled. All is well until it runs out. It ends with a huge pile of dirt on the path, a rock ledge beside us that we can't get down and a bank on the other side, that we can't get up and over. We have to decide to turn around and backtrack, or manhandle the bikes and trailers through a rather dodgy area that might lead to bad things. Morton steadies the trailers and I pull on the bike. Our feet are slipping out from under us on the loose stones and dirt. I can see an accident coming and call out to Morton to be careful. Somehow we manage to get them coaxed through this. I think about our forefathers going west where there really weren't roads to speak of. Their wagon wheels would have given them a headache or two. Today though, we get lucky and have a clear shot then down the next section of the path. It will be brilliant when it is all fixed. A man tells us to turn up the hill towards the dome we see at the top of a large building. This is one steep hill and we have to push the very top bit of it. I'm not sure what the grade would be, 20% I guess. It is worth it at the top when we can spy the State House, peeking through the trees.

This is our second invitation to a State House and we are thrilled to just be here, even if it is way off our path. Even though I think that it is a personal choice to get yourself fit, laws like these are needed. I'm living proof that a car or truck shouldn't come within three feet of a bicycle.

We make our way into the parking lot, where we meet a lovely State Representative who is just leaving. He chats with us about what we are doing, shares some stories, then gives me a lovely badge that says "Maine - Secretary of State" I forgot to ask him if I have any special duties while wearing this. While we are waiting to meet Jo Dill and some other State Reps, we start talking with another one of Maine's State Representatives. He tells us about the bill for bicycle laws that was in the House today. Morton and I are becoming quite the experts at various bicycle, handicapped accessibility and other parts of highway safety as we are on our journey. It is always interesting to hear about bills being passed to give bicycles certain rights on the road. Again, there shouldn't have to be laws in place for this, but there are people who ignore bicyclists and I have met them and been hit by them. A lot of people (the *FORMER* me, included) feel that just cars should be on the roads. After all, we are a country that is so big, it is built for the car. Did you know there are bridges that you can't cross on foot or on bicycle? How then, could a person take their bike to work if that bridge in on their path? People need to realize that bikes and walking IS an option. Think of all the money you would save if you rode your bike to work. Think of all the health you would have if you did this. The thing we hear out here on a very regular basis is that a person *WOULD* consider walking or bicycling to work, if it was safe. They are shocked at the roads we ride on. Quite frankly, so are we sometimes. The roads can be so shocking for pedestrians and bicyclists. We often comment that if you were in a wheelchair, covering this stretch would be impossible. Take a look at things like gas prices, insurance costs and at least CONSIDER another way to get from point A to B! Enough of my lecture to save the world...here we are, in Augusta Maine, at this lovely State House, meeting all these lovely people. It was a real treat and pleasure, that ended way too soon.

Morton and I went to the library to try to research somewhere to stay for the evening. With not much work at all, the *Comfort Inn*, Larry, to be precise, said they would be happy to sponsor us with a room for the evening. Now we just had to ride there. It was almost 6 pm and we had been going strong all day. My right knee was aching, my back was sore and there was the biggest hill (perhaps it IS a mountain) that we have came across so far. We got our extra energy boost by a lovely lady who pulled over to say hello. She had seen us on the news, thought what we are doing is great and wanted to tell us. We chatted for a few moments. She told us the *Comfort Inn* was not too far ahead on the right. That was just what we needed to hear. Talking to people out here really does perk us right up. It is the reason we are out here. We want to connect with the entire world about how important it is to take care of your own health. Personal responsibility people. Not your doctors, not the governments...YOUR job is to take care of YOU!

As we go inside, I get to meet Larry. He is even nicer in person than he was on the phone! We are so happy when people understand what we are trying to do.

As we go into our lovely room, I think about the fact that Morton and I have really become so nomadic. We rarely stay in a place longer than one night. We have no home, except the tent. It is so odd and suddenly, I become so tired. Exhausted. The shower does the trick and I am human again. I can squeeze about 3 or 4 more hours out of my day to work on the computer. This life is really tiring and as I'm brushing my teeth before bed, I look at my own face in the mirror. It is a person that I know, yet have never seen before. I have wrinkles under my chin where it had been plumped full with fat. I have smile wrinkles around the corners of my eyes, again, where fat had helped fill it out.

Trying to decide if I'm looking older, or if I'm just that tired, I decide that it doesn't really matter what I see in the mirror. What matters is the things I can't see. My heart, beating healthier inside my chest than it has done for decades. My circulation improving in my legs and feet, keeping them warmer at night. My bones that are starting to appear again after being hidden for many moons by my blubber. It is true, getting OLDER is always better than *NOT*. Putting my toothbrush back in the bag, I think about the lady who gave it to me. Stella! Our friend from Cape Cod. If all goes right, tomorrow we will get to see her and her husband Bruce, who are vacationing in Maine. It is a small world. It is a beautiful world. It is a world that I feel like I'm finally, after 44 years, happy to be living in.

Day 159 June 8, 2007 - Friday - *Comfort Inn*, Augusta to South China, Maine

This is the day that almost beat me. Almost. It was the hills really. They started early on and just were one after another. Maybe they were mountains, I have no idea what the elevation is on them. I just know that I'm pushing the bike up them. With sweat pouring in my eyes, heart pounding in my head, I thought I was a goner for the better part of the day. Morton kept coming up with suggestions of WHY I might be feeling so tired! I love him, but at times like that I feel like shouting, "SHUT UP, I'm FAT!" Simple and the real reason why my body was struggling.

When I planned this trip out, I KNEW that I would need two years to get the weight off. Why oh why didn't I think about the hills and mountains in Maine? Everything else before this have been mere ant hills. Not even worth mentioning or complaining about (although I did when I thought I was going to die getting to Mystic!) I try to just focus on getting to the top. One foot after the other. Easy. It was a lot of sitting on the edge of the road today. A pair of steps outside a church were like a slice of heaven for us. It would have been a place that I could have sat for at least a week, trying to catch my breath and figure out just where my body had gone so wrong. The views from the top of the hills were all getting blurry to me. I was so tired that I was really getting upset with myself, with Morton and drank so much water I thought I would surely finish our supply of it. Resting beside the road, I had no appetite whatsoever. I just wanted to stretch my legs out and sleep.

I knew it was the only thing that would help me. My body was exhausted. I hadn't just hit my wall, I was laying in front of it with it on top of me. Above all, I was letting doubts creep into my mind. What was I thinking? I'm way too fat to be riding a bicycle up hills and mountains like this. These are for people who are in shape, on bicycles that *AREN'T* pulling big, heavy trailers. Not for me. I needed to just go home. Being out here is crazy. I miss my family, a nice quiet evening in with them, waking up in familiar surroundings. So what if I'm fat and dying from it, I am happy aren't I? These sort of thoughts sailed through my mind as I kept pushing on. Keeping my opinions to myself, Morton kept telling me why he thought I was so tired. My favorite was that I wasn't eating enough food. Poor Morton, he really does deserve a medal for putting up with the likes of me. Spreading our tarp out, I said I just needed to stretch my legs out. We ate a little food. I couldn't manage a lot all at once. My stomach was sick with all the things I had bouncing around in my head. I was wallowing in my bad mental images.Even though it was Friday, a notoriously GREAT day of the week, I just felt in a funk. I was too old, tired and out of shape for this. Wanting to just go to sleep, the bugs and mosquitoes made me think otherwise. Morton offered to put up the inside shell of our tent so I could sleep, but I said we needed to just keep moving. I knew we were not going to make great mileage today and it was really bothering me. As I put my leg over my bike and was waiting for Morton to get his backpack on, someone went past us in a pick up truck. Two guys. One leaned out the window and threw a penny at me. He also called me a couple of choice, yet unoriginal fat names. The penny hit my leg and bounced off against the bike.

Morton asked if I was alright and then came and picked it up off the ground. It was shiny and new and had no character like the ones that he finds on the edge of the road. Plus, this penny was thrown in anger. What did I do to that guy??? Another reason that I shouldn't be out here. I have had glasses of ice tossed at me, a hand full of nuts and bolts and numerous insults thrown my way. I started thinking about how I was going to explain to my kids that I had to stop. They love me and will support whatever I decide. Then I started to think about all the people watching, the people we have met, the people that email us, the people that just silently read our accounts of our journey. How could I let them down? Surely explaining that I will die if I keep going up these mountains, or hit by a raging penny tossed by a looney, these are GOOD reasons to quit. But there was the word, QUIT. How many times have I said that *FOLLOW THROUGH* is the secret to making exercise work for you.

Thinking back over my toughest day so far, I tried to focus on that one thing that kept me going on. I needed a miracle here and thank goodness, since January, we have seen more than our fair share of miracles. As I started thinking about all the good things, the negative ones got pushed out of my head. I remembered that I just need to listen to my body. This isn't a race or a contest. It is a journey to fitness. Quitting isn't an option. At once I knew what we had to do. We had just gotten almost to the tip top of a big hill that we were pushing up. There was a store on the north side of the road and I asked Morton to go ask where the closest church, motel or campground was. I was too tired to cross the road and stood there rubbing my knee that had started throbbing. Morton went from one building to another. I hoped for the good news that there was something just around the next bend. He hadn't told me that on his way up this hill, he stooped to pick up a rustic lucky penny. He came back saying that the man said we could camp in his back yard. Wow! This was a brilliant result and I almost skipped across the road. The man, Joel, was so kind. He told us to get settled in, chill out in a camper if we wished and even gave us a radio to listen to while we were there. I was really embarrassed that it was so early in the day, about 2 pm I think. But I was just shattered. Morton set the shell up to the tent and I got inside to get the gear we would need in. Foam mats, sleeping bags, pillow cases that were stuffed with our clothes. I laid everything out while Morton was tarping the bikes and trailers. As soon as the sleeping bags were zipped together, I stretched out. My knee was feeling like someone had lit a fire inside it. This wasn't good, but my frame of mind was so much better getting a rest. So what if it took us a little longer to get around Maine because of the hills. I only had to go up one at a time and if I needed to rest a dozen times before I make it to the top, so be it. Morton was saying, "Are you asleep?" as I blinked my eyes awake. It had become dark. But it wasn't because the sun. He had put the fly sheet up on the tent and had even drove stakes into the ground, just inches from my head, without me hearing a peep. I had 5 solid minutes of sleep. That was enough to recoup a bit. I tried to work on the laptop a little. Joel said we could sit on his porch to plug in. His daughter, Bethany, was working in the store and Morton and I went down to say hello and get a few things. She was so lovely and said her dad mentioned my sore knee. I felt like a big cry baby. Bethany is going to college to be a massage therapist and she said she'd be happy to work on my knee later. JOY!!!! This was fantastic. We chatted for a bit and then Morton and I went back to the tent. I was thinking about a power nap, a bit longer than five minutes. But when I opened up the laptop, I suddenly had all my energy back. The emails.

Reading them really gave me this inner strength and joy from hearing what you are doing, what you think of the journey and I got lost in them. My phone rang and I thought for sure it would be the newspaper we were suppose to hook up with. It was a number that I didn't recognize but then I usually don't. The voice on the other end was one that I did recognize. It was our friend Stella. They were just about 45 minutes away. Morton and I popped into the store to let Bethany know that we would be back in a bit. It all happened so quick, it really did feel like a dream. Bruce and Stella pulled in and we all had big hugs. Stella had packed a picnic and we all went and sat by a lake and did a bit of catching up. The food was delicious, but the people, as usual, the people are making this adventure something that is so very special. Stella had brought me a pair of size XL grey short from *Old Navy*, because I can wear that size...finally! She also had baked Morton some of her healthy banana bread. We have to get her to give us her recipes...they are healthy and delicious. It was over though before we knew it. We were saying goodbye, they were heading off for their holiday and Morton and I were at our tent. A wave of sadness came over me and I felt like having a good cry. How can I be homesick for someone we have only met twice now?

Thank goodness, things happens so fast out here. It was coming home time for Bethany and we had this delightful evening together. She is just a treasure and really reminds me of my niece, Katie. We talked about everything under the sun, she thought she saw a bear at our tent and Morton was scared to go out. I had to tease him a bit later about waiting for Bethany to go out the door first. "You're too right!" he said. He added that he wouldn't know what to do if he saw a bear in the wild. Bethany put this great stuff on my knee that made it start to feel better instantly. She said she would work on it in the morning, then we all said good night and headed off to our tent, snugged up in their lovely back yard paradise. Sometime in the middle of the night, I woke wide awake. I had heard something. Listening, I almost jumped out of the sleeping bag. Something was walking in the woods behind us. I listened close. Shaking Morton, who wouldn't really be of any use if it *WAS* a bear, he grunted a bit and said "oh yeah" then fell right back to sleep. Keeping calm, I just listened to the night. There was something there, but you could tell it was an animal. I think it was perhaps deer or maybe even a moose. Whatever it was, it walked right beside our tent, then headed off towards Augusta. Hopefully it will have an easier time with the hills than I did.

Day 160 June 9, 2007 - Saturday - East China to *Comfort Inn*, Belfast, Maine

Everything seems better in the morning. The day started early, with early morning goodbyes after a great knee rubbing by Bethany. I asked her what she was doing for the next year and a half. She said that she just MIGHT come out after she graduates in December and ride with us for a bit. That would be so fun. Who knows, I have learned that *ANYTHING* really is possible! The morning was cool and we started off with our jackets on. The first hill took care of that though. We stripped them off and Morton was joining me as we huffed and puffed up the hills. I knew though, that yesterday was just a thing that will happen sometimes.   These hills won't stop me.

This is tough out here. There is so much I'm asking of my body physically that it is no wonder it gets sore once in a while. I just have to listen to it and be a bit patient. After all, I still have three-quarters of the way to go. We are almost at our first quarter, a brilliant place to be. Since I wasn't all caught up in feeling angry at myself, I was able to really enjoy the day, the views and the sheer pleasure of sweating. The hills seemed a bit tougher, but when we are on the top of them, there is nothing better than letting the bike just roll coming off these giants. There are lots of pictures taken today. In fairness, we could have used up our whole memory card, which holds nearly 600. But we were not that overboard with them. Morton is getting a real talent at getting pictures. Now if he could only quit telling me to say "CHEESE" when I'm sitting there dying.

Something about these hills are reminding me of the Highlands in Scotland. I usually don't think about another place, but even though I'm not a born & raised Scots, it is my adopted home. Living there for five years has embedded it firmly in my soul. The song, *Caladonia*, runs through my mind all day. Caladonia in an early Roman word for Scotland and one of the prettiest songs on the planet.

There is something about all the lakes we are passing, the fishing boats we see and the smell of flowers everywhere that just makes you feel great. Morton is chatting away and we are taking lots of breaks, drinking lots of water and eating small snacks throughout our day. Lots of little meals is a great first thing to do when you want to make little changes in the way you eat.

Being resolved that we might not get 30 miles, we decide to call it a day at Belfast. There is a television station in Bangor that is doing a story on us, so this would be a great place to do it from. Plus, the map shows that there is a *Comfort Inn* there. They have been excellent with sponsoring us for rooms. Fingers crossed, I pedal. There is a bridge, that runs across the bay that will take your breath away, and not from the amount of exercise you will get on it. A sharp breeze is coming off the water and it's the first time in ages today that I feel cool. The sky is now all blue and sunny and I just feel so healthy and alive. My knee has been fine all day, *thank you Bethany.*

When we pull into the *Comfort Inn*, Morton waits with the bikes as I go inside. I tell our story, but there is a slight problem. This is a busy night. Very busy. As in *no rooms available* busy. My heart sort of jumps because I felt sure we would be sleeping here, don't ask me how or why I felt that way, I just did. The assistant manager, Gisele, told me to hold on a second and disappeared. She came back in just a few minutes and asked me to come with her. She took me into a room, a massive room, right beside the lobby. It is marked "Hospitality Suite" and is it ever! There is a lovely bed, a huge massive amount of space, television, tables and chairs, bathroom and a balcony that looks out over this lovely body of water. She asked if this would suit us. WOW! This is fantastic, so much space and bed. Always a treat after a night in the tent, no matter how soft the grass is.

Morton and I get the gear in, I make a few phone calls then a mad dash for the shower. I celebrate by putting on my *NEW* shorts, thanks to Stella and the size XL fits. I am *OVER THE MOON!!!* Wow, I just can't believe my backside got into a size XL! You will be seeing a lot of these shorts in the pictures. They are perfect and I can't wait until they are as saggy and baggy as my size XXXL are now. In the room, I work. Morton tends to the Morton things, is going to do the laundry and my Zen player comes out. With the headphones on, I switch it on. The voice of Dougie comes out and sings, *Caladonia* in my ears. I smile and think about Scotland, but just for a second.

Living in the moment, I'm wildly happy to be in Maine. We have been up almost the entire coast of America on bicycle or foot, over bridges, hills, through cities that scared our families, been hit by a couple cars...what a journey. Thrilled at our wonderful luck, even thrilled at the guy that tossed the penny at us...true, it could have been a twenty dollar bill and wouldn't have stung, but at least he noticed us. Maybe he even knew how we love to find the lucky pennies and was just trying to help us out. You never know what is in the mind of another person and I'm really learning to not judge things by what you *think* they are! The next song that comes on my Zen is Robbie Williams, singing *Angels*. You might have heard this song before by Jessica Simpson, but you have to hear the original by Robbie. It is brilliant. It is going to be a great night and I'm going to try to remember this magical moment for the rest of my life. Thank you for coming along..

Day 161   June 10, 2007 - Sunday - *Comfort Inn*, Belfast to *Bucksport Motor Inn*, Bucksport, Maine

Waking up early, I always feel like I can get a lot done before the day even begins. This was one of those mornings. As Morton shuffled about with the gear and getting breakfast sorted, I got the lovely job of working with the laptop on a deck overlooking the water. It was pleasant as far as the temperature went and I was out of the way of the morning rush of people getting breakfast. Morton made us waffles, which he loves doing. Then he started *PLAYING* with the food. He arranged the fruit and a mini muffin and bagel in a shape like a face. Knowing Morton the way I do, when he came over to take the camera I asked him if his hands were sticky. After all, he was just peeling oranges. They were...so he solved the problem by licking his fingers and rubbing them on his shorts. It feels like I have young children again sometimes with Morton and I try not to mother him, but sometimes it is tough. His answer, without me even asking about the cleanliness of his shorts was that they were going to need washed anyway! Fair enough.

We got an early start, another advantage to waking up early and I was really optimistic about how far we would get today. Surely being this close to the water on the coast we wouldn't have so many hills to slow us down. This was kind of right. There were hills, but not as steep and tall as we had already met, so there wasn't really a problem there. Today our time stealer was going to be bicycle failure. We were going along US 1 and saw signs announcing a bike race. Today. I was interested in seeing some real bicyclists and maybe getting some good pictures of bikes whizzing by us. As we passed their starting point, where they still had a half hour or so to go before their race kicked off, I let my mind imagine if I were in the race. Take away the trailer, put me on a real bicycle designed for speed and I was thinking that I could probably surprise myself. I know I would at least finish, probably not win...but just crossing that line is the important part. I know this now. We were just coming up a big hill that I was thinking about pushing, when I heard Morton screaming out behind me. He usually isn't this loud if he is just finding a lucky penny or spotting a turtle. He shouted for me to hold up and was carrying the back of his bike, pulling the trailer up this hill. I pushed on to a wide spot, just beyond an overpass and he called ahead to tell me to stop, he had a major problem. The derailier had sheared a tooth in one of the cogs, buckled and bent the frame and got jammed in his spokes. It was really bad. I hoped that he might be able to pull off a repair job and left him get on with it. Morton does love fixing things, but he was really worried about this. He kept saying, "I dinnae think it can be repaired." He would go back and forth, studying my bike then his. I sat on the road, leaning against the guard rail and watched all the people that were out for a Sunday race, whiz past us. They were all carefree, on their 16 mile joy ride. The sun was shining, perfect weather and I looked at a few of the guys that were about Morton's shape and size and thought..."I wonder if they have a spare bike?"

It was still early in the day, wasn't raining and we weren't in the remote wilderness. I wasn't panicking about the problem, but I decided to call Sarah and James and let them both know we were sort of stuck for the moment. Sarah offered to find a bike shop for us on the internet, but I told her to hold up. I do have this incredible faith in Morton's mechanical skills, even though he does wipe his sticky orange hands on his shorts. Just four miles ago, we had passed a bike shop, but I couldn't remember the name. Oh well, maybe he would be able to work a miracle, bend the frame back out and we would pedal happily after all the racers. But that wasn't going to be our miracle for the day. No luck with his dooberizing! A man who was working as a flagger for the race came over and asked if we had it fixed yet. He made a phone call and got the man who actually owns the bike shop to come out. It was quickly decided that the repair was too big to happen beside the road. We needed to go back four miles, so we got loaded into his pickup and trailer and went back over the road we had already cycled. Morton was inside while the bike was being worked on and I sat on the front steps trying to chase down numbers that I needed to call. Time slips away as I call on. A television crew that was going to come out to us is called off to cover a fatality on the highways. I thank my lucky stars that we are safely off the road right now, hopefully on our way to being on the road again. The man had been able to repair the bike. It required a new derailer shifter, a new cable and with labor added our bill was just short of $50.00. I put it on plastic, cringing that it was over a tenth of our monthly budget. It meant that we could keep going though, which we did as soon as Morton got the trailers hooked back up to the bicycles.

Retracing our four or so miles, back to the spot where the problem happened, Morton and I had a seat in the shade and had lunch out of our food bag. We said that it could have been worse with the cost of the repair and things would work out, they always do. Soon we were to the split in the road, where 1A and US 1 form a "Y" in the road. We kept on US 1 and were in the blazing noon day sun. The heat was making me tired and there wasn't a spot of shade to be seen. I had drank about 3 bottles of water and really just wanted to rest for a moment. We hadn't done a lot of miles, but we had an early morning and then the mental worry of the bike being knackered and spending money that we didn't really have. There was a little pull off, not big enough for a car, but our bikes tucked right up in it. We spread the tarp down and chased the small patch of shade for nearly an hour. I had more phone interviews with reporters not just up and down the east coast where we have traveled, but from all over the states and the world. We got the word that we needed to go no further please, than Bucksport. There was a news crew that was going to catch up with us and it was just ten or so miles in front of us. It would mean an early sort of evening for us, which suited me just fine.

First, we crossed this amazing bridge that actually has an observation tower in it. It has a bike lane, stunning views and was really fun to ride across. Little did I know as we were crossing it, I would be over it again today. When we came into town, US 1 continued to the right, which I decided to follow. There was a grocery store coming up the hill and then a motel. I told Morton that if we got a room there, he could get some groceries. Crossing US 1, I entered the lobby of *Bucksport Inn*. There are lovely flowers every where, a very friendly dog and Eddie, who listened to my story and said they would be happy to help us. This is the sort of help that we need out here and are getting with great regularity. It amazes me when people are so kind and I hope that I never lose that sense of amazement and wonder. People are, for the majority, exceptionally kind and good. Never forget this and ignore the negatives. As we were pushing the bikes towards our room, we started chatting with the guy in the room next to us. The conversation then started with the couple in the room beside him, who were enjoying the perfect weather and sitting outside while their little daughter was taking a nap. Again the magic of this trip just happened and we became like old friends very quickly. Time passed way too quick and Mike offered to take us to the bridge to have a look up the observation tower. Morton and I were thrilled and the other Mike came along too. Although the tower was closed for the day, they shut at 5, the trip was delightful. We all enjoyed the wonder of this marvel of engineering. Set in one of the prettiest places on the planet, you feel like it belongs there. Nature and progress working like a work of art. The wind was coming off the water cool now, it felt so refreshing after our hot day. The smell in the air was a scent that they should try to bottle. Sea air. Nothing like it! Mixed with the smells from all the pine trees and the approaching cool evening coming, it was pure perfume. This is the air that makes us sleep like babies, the same air that had tuckered Mike's little daughter out.

We got back to the motel and I realized that I hadn't even been inside the room yet. Morton had put all of our things in while I was chatting to the people outside. It was like visiting with friends on a front porch somewhere. You all know how fast *that* time goes by. We had some pictures taken, Mike gave Morton two cold beers to take along and I needed to call Sarah and James to let them know we were in for the evening. I realized as I went inside the lovely room, my phone was still in the carrier on my handlebars. It was the first time in the whole trip that it wasn't by my side. It was like realizing that I had been standing out there naked and talking. I had a bit of a panic, grabbed it like it was life-support and looked at it. Three missed calls. Two from Sarah and one from a reporter who left a message that they would talk to me on Monday morning. Sarah had said she was starting to worry when I hadn't answered and she scolded me for not having the phone with me. She is going to make a great little mommy! I smile as I listen to her tell me about their day that happened so far away from me. Come to think of it, it is pretty rare now to find me not smiling. Life is so very good and I finally understand so many simple things that were out of my grasp before. Maybe there is a relation to gaining brain cells from losing weight. My computer has patiently waited for me. There is wireless internet here and as I switch it on I notice that I have actually worn off a few letters on my keyboard. The letter "N" is almost gone, as well as "M". The space bar is worn smooth and shiny on the right hand side. This little workhorse is really getting a workout. Checking my email, I see someone has sent us money. It is from one of the State Representatives we had met at the State House in Augusta. She had written a lovely email, which I had read just a few emails ago and was thrilled to get. The donation she made was for $50. I was stunned and got chills up and down my arms. Morton was out doing the shopping so I couldn't tell him, so I had to call Sarah to tell her. Earlier on the phone when I had told her about the bike repair, she offered to help if I needed it. Sarah, Graeme and my son and his wife have all been helping us make ends meet when the budget just isn't matching up. I had told her to not worry, things would work out. This was a miracle, plain and simple. I didn't even have to *ASK* anyone for their help. A kind and generous stranger that we had met had solved our budget problem without us even knowing it. Wow! The evening just kept getting better as I read email after email of people from all around the world who are watching our journey and BEST OF ALL, making their own little changes.

I was starting to wonder if Morton had gotten lost, then I remembered how he is in the grocery store. He just had $20 to spend, so he would be shopping for the very best bargains. He came back with four heavy bags, lots of canned goods. We have to stock up while we can and the price is right to make our food budget stretch as far as it can. Telling him the brilliant news about the donation, he was amazed too that the amount was nearly spot on for what we had just spent out-of-the-blue on the bike! We had a very late dinner, almost 10 pm and I got a shower. That was me out for the count. Full belly, clean and the bed was calling. Morton had already fallen asleep and I wasn't far behind him. What a wonderful perfect day!

Day 162 June 11, 2007 - Monday - *Bucksport Morton Inn*, Bucksport To *Primrose Inn*, Bar Harbor, ME

My internal alarm clock was really messed up this morning. I usually wake up at 6 am, but this morning I was wide awake at 4 am. I had a lot of email interviews to do, choosing the high resolution images to send over the internet to papers that will run stories that I will never get to read. Telling myself I would work for a few hours, then catch a quick nap, it never happened. Before I knew it, it was time to ride, almost 10 am with a lot of ground to cover if we wanted to make it to Bar Harbor.

Sending out several emails to places in Bar Harbor, asking for help with a room, we were overwhelmed by the number of people who called us. Memories of all the help from the people of Cape Cod came back to me. These people that live by the water are a special sort, extremely kind and generous. Jeff from the *Primrose Inn* telephoned me almost as soon as I had sent out the emails. It was wonderful to ride with knowing where we were going to stay. It always takes a giant question mark out of our day. We were actually going to stay with them for two evenings, a real treat.

I am embarrassed to say that I just discovered that Bar Harbor, Acadia National Park and some of the most amazing things in the whole wide world are located on this one incredible island that is Mount Desert Island, or MDI as the locals call it. Places like Cadillac Mountain, Seal Harbor and miles of trails, lakes, wildlife and nature all live here! The bicycle ride today, 40 miles, seemed like it was never going to end. Endless hills, views that went on forever and covering a lot of distance all went without a hitch. There was a flat tire near the end of the ride and a swarm of mad bugs that decided my arm looked delicious, almost causing me to crash, but other than that, the ride was excellent. Pure brilliant. Everything that I appreciate each day now came sharply into focus for me.

We chanced upon another person on a bicycle. The young man passed us and said hello, riding off in front. We caught up with him at an approaching store and gas station, where we had pulled in to. This man would really change my whole day. He came over to us and we fell into the conversation of the road. He had came from Texas, on his own. He was telling us about the things that had happened to him along the way. His first bike was crushed by a dump truck in Pennsylvania, leaving him very shaken after his very close call. He also had a horrible attack of road rage in Arkansas that chilled me to the bone. He was riding along, alone, off the edge of the road. Someone came up behind him and laid on the horn. I know this feeling. We jump. It scares us, or at least startles us. Maybe that is the reaction the driver wants to see, who knows? The young man didn't react, but just kept going. The person laid on the horn and stayed right on his tail. When he pulled up beside him, our new friend knew that he needed to just ignore what was happening. The next part is really scary. This person, who first needs to have their drivers license taken away *FOREVER* and then go to jail for this...takes his car, swerves it, with the horn still blaring, into this young man. The man, as any man or woman is, is no match for a car. He goes into the ditch, but has the presence of mind to get the license plate number. The police are called and hopefully they will be able to take the looney off the streets forever, but who knows. Telling us this, I can see he is still really rattled by all of this. Who wouldn't be? Plus, he is out here all on his own. At least I have Morton to cry to and people from the internet to listen to my complaints and fears from wild drivers. Shifting gears, I tell him about some of the wonderful people we have been meeting. People that really should have wings sticking out of their backs. I share a couple of our close calls, nothing compared to his. We both realize that even though we are passed by thousands and thousands of cars, only a few make it a scary place. The odds are not that bad. Thinking of the man who threw a penny at me, the man who threw a hand full of nuts and bolts at me, the man who threw a cup of ice at me and the lady who hung out her window and screamed horrible things in my face, I realize they are a tiny, small, insignificant slice of life. They are not normal. Thank goodness. We both feel a lot better. We hug like we are long lost friends, my heart breaks. He tells me that he sleeps under bridges, in graveyards, anywhere he can. He has stayed with friends a few times, but mostly he is alone. It is a scary thought. I ask him to please email when he can, to keep in touch. He's not far away from his finishing point and will be going home to Texas soon.

Morton and I talk about his journey as we are riding. The man is out of sight in just a few minutes and Morton and I are just amazed. What is motivating him to get back on the bike after having one crushed by a truck? That is really brave, but something that we do hear out here. My thoughts are lost on this young man who will sleep who knows where tonight. We are heading to a destination each night, even if we don't know where it is. We try to take shelter inside. He doesn't even have a tent with him! I am still in awe of it all.

Riding on to MDI was like riding in to another world. There are lakes, islands, birds of every description and very friendly people. The traffic isn't bad and we have avoided by sheer luck, the thunderstorms the day has brought. We could have taken thousands of pictures and still not done the place justice.

As we turn down the street that *Primrose Inn* sets on, we see a group of people on the left, jumping, shouting and waving. It is the most welcomed welcome after a long ride, with evening fast approaching. The entire family, their lovely Corgi and some other people are all saying hello! We are overwhelmed and my thoughts turn inside to our new friend from Texas. What will his evening hold? *Sigh*. This house is amazing. One of the only survivors from a massive fire, built in the days when they knew how to build them. Covered with details, inside and out, surrounded by endless and private porches that hold swings with soft cushion seats, lovely furniture that says, "Sit and unwind" and best of all is the family that own it. They are so kind, friendly and make us feel like we just came home. There is a sign that is beside their front door that I just have to share with you. It reads, *Do not neglect to show hospitality to strangers, for by doing that some have entertained angels without knowing it.* Hebrews 13: 1-2 Words to make you think no matter what religion you believe in.

After I have had my shower with wonderful oatmeal soap, dried with soft, thick, snow white towels and crawled into the most welcomed and comfortable bed, my last thought of the evening was that sign. I hoped that our friend from Texas all alone on his bike was finding some hospitality by strangers. I hoped he had a bed, instead of the ground. I hope that he emails me to tell me he is safely home and I hope that some day, our paths will cross again. It would be a real honor and treat to bicycle with him, if I could keep up.

Day 163 June 12, 2007 - Tuesday - *Primrose Inn*, Bar Harbor, Maine

My first thoughts this morning were that we didn't have to pack everything up and leave...it was brilliant! As much as we love seeing new places and faces each day, it can be very tiring always moving. Today was going to be a bit different. After this lovely homemade breakfast, we met up with Susan from News 5 in Bangor. We could have talked to her all day and nearly did! The camera woman was great and it was a really fun way to spend what felt like the first day of a holiday. The *Chamber of Commerce* had arranged for us to have an *Oli's Trolley* tour, so we took the short walk from the *Primrose Inn* to the spot where you catch it. There we were completely impressed with the next two and a half hours of our journey.

Acadia National Park is beautiful beyond words, or even beyond photos. As I snapped over 300 shots, I later discovered none of them had captured what your naked eye will see when you visit this paradise. In sheer size, beauty and just stunning scenery, I have never seen anything like this before in my life. Even though Morton took his 5 minute nap on the trolley (he ALWAYS does this!) he managed to stay awake for this enchanted trip up mountains, past lakes with beaver dams in them, fields of flowers and stunning rocks that fall away to the chilly blue waters below. There were too many highlights on the journey to tell you all about. A few of our favorites were the Thunder Rock beside the sea where the water would come in, build up force and then *BLAST* out, creating this loud sound that reminded your of rumbling thunder. There was also the view from Cadillac Mountain. The only down side to it was, as always, time. Never enough, is there? I fancied sitting up on the tall mountain and watching the sun peak up over the sea at 4 am, then spending a day on the rocks, painting, snapping pictures, eating grapes, smiling, until the sun was going to set on the other side. Maybe someday. Morton stood by some of these huge ferns that I have been telling Sarah about. There are some that are actually taller than us! They are just like they have been for thousands of years. He looks like a wee hobbit beside it. Beautiful!

There is a wild garden, all native plants and I get a rare picture of Lady Slippers, almost done blooming but still so lovely. There are Jack-in-the-Pulpits that remind me of a summer long ago when my kids were still teenagers. We were remodeling an old farm house. It was surrounded by wild woods and there were the most amazing things to be seen in it. I got a tree that had been twisted by vines that I turned into a handrail on our staircase and I also found Jack-in-the-Pulpits that I coaxed to grow just outside our front door, under a pear tree that was over 60 feet tall and still produced fruit. For a moment I'm back there, with my kids still at school. I smile and Morton doesn't have a clue why I am taking so many pictures of these plants. I think about how quick time passes, good or bad, it all goes too fast. It has absolutely nothing to do with whether you are having fun or not. It flies. Back in the moment, we are heading to reboard our trolley. The tour guide is excellent and loves his calling. He really did a great job and we got quite the education along with the tour.

Morton and I went back to the *Primrose Inn*, to connect with a reporter for a paper. There are so many email interviews and telephone interviews that we are doing as we approach the end of our first leg of the journey. When I go to download my 300 plus pictures from the day, I am shocked to find that my 40 GB hard drive hasn't enough room on it. The only thing I can do is take the time to make the DVD's of the photos and then delete them from the computer (a terrifying job and rather time consuming) but first...I had another shock waiting. When I go to open the program to make the DVD's...I get an error message. There is a part of the software missing, it won't open. This means uninstalling and reinstalling, but it doesn't work. After three hours of frustration, with Morton's help, I am able to move on to the photos. *Whewwww....* Then comes the timely process of making duplicate DVD's of each batch of photos and videos. We have to do this so I have one I can send back to Sarah's and one I can keep to use while we are on the journey. I also upload them to two different free storage places. My pictures are my memories of this adventure, I can't take any chances with them. It is nearly two am before I get to find sleep. I just barely update the site.

In the morning, just a few short hours away, we will leave this amazing place, these incredible people and ride off towards Quoddy Head and finishing the very first leg of this incredible journey. Tomorrow we will stop somewhere and I will answer emails, update the site and all the other things that make our wheels spin.

Day 164 June 13, 2007 - Wednesday - *Primrose Inn*, Bar Harbor to *Mt. Desert Narrows*, MDI, Maine

Before breakfast I always try to check my email. I might not have time to answer it, but it is good to at least download it. I get happy at the view of one from the government saying that Morton's immigration case had been updated. I opened it and it was even better than just updated, it had finally been approved and his paperwork is being sent out. Just shy of one full year and several thousand dollars later. I told him he should have just became one of the illegal immigrants but he found no humour in this whatsoever. He was in the shower and I was on the phone with Sarah. She wanted me to tell him, so she could hear his reaction. I did and instead of the loud cheer I thought he would send up, he just said, "That's brilliant" and went back in to dry off and get dressed. Sarah and I were way more excited about it, but Morton is very low-key. He was shouting for joy on the *INSIDE*, I'm sure.

The day went quick and smooth. We did an interview after an amazing breakfast, then said our goodbyes and started pedaling back over the road that had brought us in to this amazing place, that we didn't get to properly see. TIME! The phone is busy with calls and before we know it, it is past lunch time.

Little Changes   **221**   *Priscilla Houliston*

We sit beside the road, literally and as I'm talking on the phone to a reporter from out west, I start playing with this little stick beside me. There are thousands of them. They are white with a little bit of black on the tip. The tip is pointy. These aren't sticks, they are quills. I almost jump up but then realize they are all up and down the edge of the road. With the exception of one that has poked my leg, they seem to be fine. A lady stops and is talking to Morton to see if we need help. He mentions the quills and she points to a porcupine that is dead in the middle of the road ahead of us a bit. I know what Morton is thinking, *"POOR THING!"* He tells the lady that he fancies seeing a live one and she warns that they can shoot their quills at you when they are afraid. This little one didn't have a choice. It's quills were thrown all along the edge of the road, disappearing into the sand and weeds.

Morton called his parents to tell them the good news of his immigration. He was disappointed to hear that his mom still hasn't looked at the website. He is quiet about his parents, he's not as open at showing his love and affection like my family is, but I can tell that it hurts him a bit. We have family and friends all over the planet and there are so many strangers watching our journey and he is a bit bothered that his mom has never looked at their computer to see it. In fairness, she isn't in to the computer at all and I tell him this. He agrees. When we go back to Scotland, I tell him, we will have to bore her to tears by showing her the entire journey of pictures, in the longest evening EVER. We hope that she has a peek, I think she would be surprised to see her son weighing 165 pounds and looking so fit. :) They won't even recognize me when I'm finished. I doubt if I will. We head up the road and decide that we must get caught up on all the things we have to get caught up on. There is the computer, above and beyond of what I do each day. I have to create some new pages for the end of our first leg, which is approaching so fast. I also have to send out press releases, updates, post HUGE pictures for the media on a special page...all time consuming stuff.

While being inside is ideal, camping is going to be dry, according the the forecast, for the next few days. We stop at *Mt. Desert Narrows* and get two nights sponsored by the people there. *BRILLIANT!* Morton and I ride our bikes to the tenting area and choose a spot. He sets up the tent and I get cracking on the computer in the laundry room. They have a few desks and power plugs, the perfect combination for me. Working away, I start chatting to a lady who is in doing her laundry. I'm just editing pictures, no real thought process required, so we have a chat. I really should say, a wee blether! She is from Glasgow. It is good to hear the accent. So is her husband, who is in their motorhome. They are getting ready to do a 45 day tour of Nova Scotia, Newfoundland and the other outer areas of the great north east. She invites us to stop in when we are done, for a little visit. Just as the sun is thinking about peeking out for the first time, it is almost time for it to be setting. We walk down by the water and I get a few pictures. Then we pop in to the lovely RV for a wonderful time of just talking about everything. Again, hearing the accents are lovely. I could listen to them and Morton for ages, but since I got up this morning at 4 am, I knew I would have to go to sleep soon. They needed to get ready for their big adventure as well, so we said our goodbyes outside and Morton and I walked back to our tent, holding hands and carrying the laptop and discs.

The sky was so pretty, there were people here and there, glowing lights on in the RV's and I thought for a moment, just a brief moment, how much different our trip would have been if it would have been eight of us instead of two. Things didn't work out that way though. The shelter of the motorhome was wonderful, just not meant to be. Tonight it is just the two of us, in our little tent for two, warm enough, full enough and we have a midnight snack at 9 pm (because we couldn't stay up until midnight!) of pop tarts. I fall asleep by listening to Morton reading out loud to me from a book he picked up in the laundry room. It is not a classic of sorts, it is a book of adventure about Conan, the barbarian variety. His voice feels like home and I fall asleep listening. Another perfect ending to another perfect day.

Day 165 June 14, 2007 - Thursday - Mt. Desert Narrows, MDI, Maine
Stats for the day: Breakfast: cold pop tart, peanut butter
Lunch : 1 bag of tuna mixed with 1 can of sweet corn (we split this) with 12 wheat crackers, 1/2 bag of m&m with peanuts (little bag), pretzels
Dinner : hideous cold canned spaghetti with meatballs, Morton made this even worse by putting 1/2 a can of sweet potatoes on top of it (don't ask me why!) this was without one doubt the WORST thing he has ever dished up to me. I was hungry though, so I ate it, soy nuts, animal crackers

You know the jobs that we *have* to do, but we really don't want to? I have had this big one hanging over my head for a while now. You see, each time we do an interview, I promise the person to update them as we approach milestones. It would be a simple task, if I had been keeping a database of email addresses for doing so. But I haven't. Remember, I'm not a PR person. As we get close to our first MEGA milestone, bicycling up the entire east coast of America, I need to tell them about it, before we get there. This means spending a bit of time on the computer, compiling a list that is bigger than I imagined it would be. I also needed to fine-tune the site with some additional things that have sprung to mind since starting our journey. Today was going to be the day that I tried to make it all happen. Morton and I parted ways early in the day. It was 7:30 in the morning when I first logged on to the laptop in the laundry room here at the campground. Little did I know that it would be almost 11 pm before I would shut it off for the day. As I sat and worked, it was noon before I knew it. I kept my headphones on, listening to music, so I wouldn't really have to chat with people coming and going. I did a bit, but I was really good at giving the "short version" of what we are doing. Morton came and went a couple times, I only got up and walked outside to go use the bathroom. Other than that, on my back-side, in front of the little screen ALL DAY and most of the night. About 11 pm I realized how horrible I felt. My eyes were aching, I had a headache, I'm sure I was dehydrated, my joints were all aching (even though I did some stretching during the course of the day) and as I went to go back to the tent, ahead of Morton, I thought I was going blind. It was so dark outside that I couldn't really see or focus right in front of my own face. I had went into the restrooms and came back out and just stood there. It looked like the little lane that led to our tent just faded into nothing. I was going to turn around and try to find my way back up the hill to Morton, when he came walking along. He was fine and could see, nae probs, so it had to have been my eyes were just so tired from working on the computer all day. He got into the tent but I decided to go for a shower. We wanted to get an early start the next morning, so getting it out of the way would be a smart thing to do. It also might make my muscles stop aching. My left knee was killing me.

Another problem that I was facing was a medical one that no bicyclist wants to get. For the first time in my life, I had hemorrhoids. A bicycle seat does not make for a happy trip. I was in agony and had spent the day shifting from side to side, using my pillow to prop one half of my butt on to try to get a bit of comfort. Morton offered to bicycle the distance back into the town where a pharmacy would have something that would help shrink them away, but it wasn't a good idea to go backwards and alone. Too many "what ifs" popped into my mind. I could have stayed in the shower all night. I was finally warm. My hands and feet had been like ice all day long. It was tough getting out of there and walking back to the tent. I was hoping I would wake up with no more hemorrhoids and be ready to ride like the wind instead of whining like the wind. I want to call my daughter-in-law to ask her what to do, but it is late.

The sky was so very black, inky black, with the brightest stars I think I have ever seen, just floating in it. There is a little pond on the left and I hear the frogs singing their night tunes. So tired, exhausted really, I get the worst wave of homesickness that has hit me so far. Will it ever go away? Climbing into the tent, or actually, falling into the tent, I pulled my shoes off. Morton had fallen asleep, but my mind was wide awake. I couldn't even think about sleeping. The tent was freezing, my hair was wet, my "pillow" that is really just a big *Ziploc*, filled with my clothes, covered with a pillow case, and was as hard as a rock. The sounds of the frogs came through the paper thin wall of the tent and I remembered all those nights that my little brother, my father and I would be camping. It was another lifetime a go. A place that I can never go back to, only in memories. They were the happy, simple times that we never realize are perfect, as we are going through them. I was too young to know, how could I, or anyone, know this? But tonight I knew. I knew that this moment, this tired, golden moment, is all I have. I might not ever see my family again. I might never have a home again. Who knows and who can say. Tonight though, I have a tent. A sore body that is alive, hemorrhoids and all, frogs singing and Morton snoring. It is my home in the outdoors, under an inky black sky that is dotted with a million bright stars.

Day 166 June 15, 2007 - Fri - *Mt. Desert Narrows*, MDI to *Faith Bible Fellowship Church*, Millbridge, Maine

This morning as Morton tore down camp, I tore up the computer keyboard. There were still a lot of things I needed to do, but I was fairly pleased with the things I got done on the computer. I am only one person and am only human. The real important thing was that my backside was feeling a lot better this morning. The day break off of it was a great thing. I wished it could be longer, but I have to keep going. I did try to ride standing up as much as possible and considered trying to ride side-saddle.

We headed off the island in the sunshine and had a bit of back-tracking to do. We kept seeing the sights and smells of lobster dinners everywhere. There were loads of little places, all steaming pots outside and I couldn't be certain, but I think I saw Morton's tongue hanging out of his mouth. I know mine was. The thought that we would soon be turning inland and this would be our only shot at getting fresh Maine lobsters, got the better of me. Scott, the guy in New Hampshire that we had bicycled with, had given us a $20 bill to treat us to dinner. Morton had this tucked this paper money in his wallet as an emergency fund. I know what you are thinking, having a lobster wasn't an emergency, but I'm only human. We saw a sign saying $16.00 for a dinner and there were picnic tables *with* umbrellas to shade us sitting there. We *HAD* to do it. Morton was shocked as I stopped. He really wanted to have one but didn't have the courage to tell me. The first time Morton ever ate lobster (there have only been two times in his whole life) was just after I met him in Scotland. There was a local supermarket that had a special on them and I got two of them to have at his house. He didn't know what to do with it, so I showed him. The second time Morton ate lobster was at a place in Florida, back in 2002. It was an *ALL-YOU-CAN-EAT* lobster feast, or as Morton likes to call buffets, "eat 'til you burst!" He had three small lobsters there and loved them. Today was the third time. He talked to the man at the pots and asked, "Is this where they meet their fate?" The man had to ask Morton to repeat the question, but got it the second time and laughed as he nodded.

There is no denying that today's lobster was the best Morton ever had. It was also all the better knowing that our lunch of a can of tuna would still keep for later. The only trouble was, this splitting of the meal was just a tease. It was actually worse than just smelling all the food cooking. It made me want to sign Morton up as a lobster man and see if I could ever get tired of eating this.

My mind, even though we are really living in the moment, keeps floating back to old memories. Sweet, wonderful memories that carry me through my homesick spells. This one was a real golden moment. The family, mine, were all packed up and loaded in a motorhome and headed north from Pennsylvania to Newfoundland. A whole other world away. My dad knew a family that lived in a small town called, Daniels Harbor. We were going to camp in their front yard for two weeks that would stay with me for the rest of my life. The people we stayed with were just so kind and wonderful. Much like the people Morton and I are meeting out here. Our family was like the circus coming to town and I think all the people in the town came through our old motorhome to have a look. Again, sort of like the looks we get with our bikes and trailers. Same concept really, the grass is always greener, even if it is lobster red. These people in this small town were all lobster people. They lived beside the sea and from the sea. Our host, my dads' friend, even took us out in his small boat to pull up the traps. This was a real treat for us. My mom had packed a lot of hot dogs on ice to feed her five kids that were along on the trip. These became barter for swapping hot dogs for lobster. The people of the town wanted the hot dogs, we loved the lobster, everyone was happy. I suppose you can get tired of eating anything if you have it all the time. But lobster is something I would like to try with. But not today on our budget. If there are any people out there with traps and want help pulling them, Morton will gladly volunteer...me too!

In Newport with all the beautiful mansions, the servants of long ago had it in their contracts that they wouldn't be fed lobster more than so many days a week. It was cheap and plentiful and they got sick of it. Oh to be a maid to the rich in the olden days! After our treat, we got back on the road, then made our way on back roads, with lots of hills, heading to our destination EAST! It was a lovely ride, not much of a road's edge, but we made it to US 1 with no trouble. The sun was really hot and right after a rather big hill that I had to push up, there was a lady up in front of us on the side of the road, waving us in to a parking lot. She had seen us on the news, then stopped us to give us the best gift ever. Ice-cold watermelon! Talk about a miracle. We sat in the shade, ate this delicious food and thanked our lucky stars that this earth angel was kind enough to stop us and share. It was a great break and we got back on the bikes 100% refreshed and ready to ride. We kept pushing on, finding no rooms along the way. There were a few churches here and there, but we couldn't get in touch with anyone to get permission to camp. Before long though, as the sun was now set and we weren't making long shadows anymore, we came to the town of Millbridge. Someone earlier had told us that we would find a motel there. We did, but it was full. It was now dark. Sigh....we have been here before. There is one thing that we are learning...it will all work out. There was a church in front of the motel, but the pastor when we spoke to him, lived 30 miles away. He had no way to get us inside. I felt bad because I kept calling Sarah to bug her for phone numbers. She had a long day, was really tired and I could hear a combination of worry and weariness in her little voice when we spoke. She found me the number for the police department and from that moment on, I didn't need to bug her again. We talked to a great officer who made some calls. There was a church, about a mile away and the pastor drove out to us. The officer had stopped by where we were and was chatting as Rev. Rolfe pulled up. These two gentleman gave us the best escort we have had to the church in the country. One was in front guiding the way and lighting the road, while the other was behind protecting us from being hit by a passing car or truck. It was a very welcomed sight as we pulled in, then went inside. Talk about sanctuary! It was nothing short of a miracle. We had a safe place to make our bed for the night, power to charge our phone, bathroom with nice hot water and even a kitchen! JOY!!! Once I ate my warm noodles, I was out for the count though. I wanted to do the page and photos that night, but it wasn't meant to be. I fell asleep at home.

Day 167 June 16, 2007 - Saturday - *Faith Bible Fellowship Church*, **Millbridge To East Machias, Maine**

I'm not sure about Morton, but I needed a day like today. It started out with me working on the computer, him loading the gear after our bed on the floor of the church. There were several wonderful ladies who came and went, cleaning, brining food in for a funeral that was going to be happening and just talking to us. The somber occasion of a funeral, which is in all of our futures, is a reminder of how fast our lives go. Sadly, we only all have so much time and each and every day I see reminders of this. Today was a tough one. I know that it is a short ride, this little thing called life. I also know that my dad's 82 years just weren't long enough. As we ride today, he is all I'm thinking about. My heart is breaking as I remember his voice and then think that I will never hear it again. It is really hard and has been, each and every day since he's left this world. My emotions are really out of control today. Each white birch tree I see, each glimpse of blue water I see, each garden getting ready to grow is reminding me of dad.

Morton and I have our normal bike riding conversation. Shouts from me warning of *"HOLES, GLASS, BUMP"* may or may not find their way to Morton in time. It is quite often he's looking off to the side, trusting me to sing out about dangers on the road, only for me to hear the crunching of the glass as he runs over it. When he stops to put his trailer back on the bike after it's been knocked loose, I know that he didn't see the bump he was about to hit. Today these shout outs take me back to riding in the front of the little boats we would use while we were fishing with dad. My little brother and I would climb into the front, keeping our eyes trained on the water and call out, *"Deadhead, 1 o'clock!"* Dad would make the need adjustments on the boat to take us away from the danger. A deadhead was a floating log, not a fan dressed in tie-dye. A few times, when there were loads of rocks all around, dad would keep the motor pulled up, just dipping the prop into the water enough to keep us going. He didn't want to damage it by hitting a rock when we were so far away from civilization. We did have paddles and sometimes Paul and I would get to push away from rocks and dangers. Oh the sheer power we felt in our child-arms as we saved the boat from a horrible crash on the rocks! All these thoughts are coming to me, thinking about my long lost days of carefree youth. It's not my youth I'm missing though, it's my dad.

Morton and I stop at a gas station for the bathrooms and to split a sub for lunch. I eat mine and call my sister Cindy as Morton goes back inside because he "fancies an iced-lolly" that we call ice cream sandwiches. When he comes out, I'm in tears, sobbing memories with my sister in Hannibal, Missouri as we remember our dad. Funny stories, sad stories and we say almost at the same time, that through our whole lives with dad, we always felt loved. For that we are so thankful. Not sure what to do for me, Morton just handed me the ice cream and I ate this comfort food, while sitting on the ground crying like a baby. People must have thought I was a bit mad, but it really is that I was just missing my dad. The cry made me feel a bit better. We both agreed that he will always be missed and still always be with us. Life is short, very short, even when it lasts for 82 years, it is never long enough. *Sigh.* Dad would be proud that I am really following through with this journey. I know he would. He would shake his head in disbelief and ask me what the fish were biting on, but he would be proud.

The only thing biting today though are giant horse flies. There is a spot on my arm that they seem to love. It is hot and swollen now and there is this one fly that has been following us for days (at least I THINK it's the same fly) that keeps trying to eat my arm. After all, the size I am I must look like a real feast to him. Bugs, bugs and more bugs. I'm glad though that they are all little problems. Not only are my legs getting a workout on the hills, the way I'm waving my arms around, people must think that I'm doing bicycle aerobics. The trick is to not fall off as you are trying to shake a fly out of your helmet that is sinking it's teeth (or whatever they have) into your scalp.

We stop beside the road in a patch of shade and watch a baby squirrel. It has no fear of us, as it sits just a few feet away. I'm reminded of how bad I want my Samsung camera back, as this one is just not cutting it. I have to figure out a place for Sarah to ship it to. I have been wishing though, that they would just say that they are coming to see us. But I have to start thinking a bit more realistically and know that they can't. We are far from our family now. The next time I see my children is when I become a gramma. Sarah is going to call her doctor and then call me. At that point, Morton and I have to SPRING into action. Depending on where we are, we are going to rent a car and head to Pennsylvania as fast as we can. We might try hitching a ride if we are in the right area...you never know. Even though the baby is due to be here at the end of July, which isn't far away, it feels like years, whole lifetimes away. I have to shake this homesick feeling so I turn to the beauty of the state we are riding in. I tell myself, *LIVE in the present.*

Maine has whole seas of trees that seem to just keep rolling as far as your eye can see. There are hills that are a real challenge, but they also give you the most amazing views when you get to the top. For one brief moment, that hill is all yours. Blueberry bushes are everywhere, but we are a tad too early to enjoy the fruit. It would be lovely to be here when they are ripe. I'd even share with the bears! There is sandy soil that starts to remind me of childhoods spent fishing in Canada on so many summers, so I try to change my thoughts. I stop for a moment to have a drink and try to call my mom, but my phone has lost it's signal. That reminds me...I might not be able to get computer signal or phone signal if we get a bit remote or on the wrong side of the mountain. I remember in the Outer Banks of North Carolina how I scared over 4,700 of you to email *"ARE YOU OKAY?"* when I wasn't able to update for two days. PLEASE check the tag board. If I can't get connected or get a signal, I will phone Sarah or James, who will update that we are alive and kicking. That is, if we ARE alive and kicking! Fingers crossed and bicycle firmly planted with the shiny side up and the greasy side down.

Tonight we are heading for a family that we are going to be staying with. A kind lady had seen our story on the news and emailed us the offer of a place to stay. We love it when this happens. It is our favorite way to stay out here. As evening was coming, we were almost there. It had been a long emotional day and this brief moment of feeling like we were part of a family was really what I needed. When we arrived, we all just started talking as if we were old friends. They are just wonderful people, who we will treasure forever. They also have a delightful shower which we got to use. After a shower, feeling human, we all ate this delicious home-cooked meal. The evening went way too fast, they always do and Morton and I were getting ready for bed. I felt for the first time today, NOT homesick. It was wonderful to go to sleep feeling content, clean, fed and ready to face our end of our first leg in the morning. *Life is better than good...life is BRILLIANT!*

Day 168 June 17, 2007 - Sunday - East Machias To *Quoddy Head Station*, ME
Today we bicycled 24 miles Weather: Temperature was in the 70's, with nothing but sun until we got to Quoddy Head. The fog set in, it got cold and then rained

Capturing today is going to be a tough one. I won't be able to really get this across to you, but I will try. Work with me on this and use your imagination a bit. We had a beautiful breakfast with this beautiful family. It is really tough to set off after being made feel so very welcome, but we leave, hoping as we always do, that we will get to meet these people again someday. Morton and I head down a lovely side road to join up to US1. He tries to catch a bullfrog and doesn't manage it. I videotape him. We laugh easy and smile always. It is a carefree ride dotted with memories.

Even though it is Father's Day and I'm missing my dad so much, I'm more concerned that my phone isn't getting a signal. I am really needing to speak to my daughter and my son. Just hearing their voices is such good medicine for me. Here and there I will get a bar or two on the phone, but no joy. It has me thinking, "What if they needed to call me?" then I think about the hundreds of miles of wilderness that we are going to be in, where a phone signal will not happen. Come to think of it, electricity might not even happen at that point. There are a lot of kind people we meet today. One will always stick out in my mind. This lovely lady was coming out her drive, waving at us from the left side of the road. I crossed over where they offered us cold water with ice. She has been watching our journey on line and it was a real treat to meet her, her son and her grandson. The ice water was just the frosting on the cake, she was the real treat. As we left this family, we met a man who had passed us jogging. I know what you are thinking...*"Priscilla, HOW SLOW are you guys going?!"* But trust me, he was REALLY fit. He had bicycled 100 miles, a century, just the day before. This man is amazing and inspiring. My mind thinks a moment that someday, I'm not sure when, but someday on this journey, Morton and I will crack 100 miles in one day. He gives us his card and tells us if we need anything in the state of Maine to call him. Morton files it in his wallet and we head off, up another hill, pushing the bikes and pulling the trailers.

The sun is out and the weather is just right for riding. When my shirt gets wet on my back from going up the hill, it dries out while it's flapping against my back coming down the hill. Morton and I are a bit stunned and dazed with just how incredible the views are here. Morton is getting just like me and saying, "Would you just LOOK at that!!!" about every five minutes. As we get closer to our first *huge* milestone, the weather turns. It happens fast, the fog pushing in off the water and the air feeling wet and cold. We put on our jackets and keep going. Only four miles left in this first part of our incredible adventure. Will we hold out an more importantly, will the weather? The road is a bit winding, with hills, but again, it looks out over some of the prettiest sights on the planet. My big worry is not getting back to Quoddy Head, it is getting out of there. The fog has our clothes wet now, visibility is really low and even with our bright jackets, I worry about cars being able to see us. Morton has the blinking light given to him by Stella hanging off his back like a beacon. Traffic is quiet today. It is nearly 4:30 and I imagine lots of people are at home now, celebrating Father's Day with a meal around a table.

I try to get my blue thoughts out of my head. This is a day for a great celebration. This is a day that I thought would never get here. My dad wouldn't want me to be sad and missing him. He'd want me to find out about the fishing. The weather is turning so fast that I know we have to think about staying put. It is a road out to the lighthouse, not a lot on it, then back in to civilization. All in fog. There is a place that I had seen on the internet, *Quoddy Head Station*, a refurbished former Coast Guard station. Suddenly we were in front of it, just a bit away from the lighthouse. I headed in and Morton followed. We were lucky to just get there minutes before the office closed. We were also lucky they had a spot...and not just a spot. This is an apartment so big, roomy, comfortable and well-equipped, I wanted to just move in. The red and white tile flooring, lovely wooden ceilings that are so tall and a real, life-sized refrigerator and stove. The girl made our night when she told us there was a free washer and dryer we could use too! Morton and I wasted no time in getting our gear in, then heading off with just the bikes to the lighthouse. The fog had firmly took hold of this enchanted place I had been thinking about for the last 168 days of my life.

A fog horn was keeping sailors safe and Morton just loved it. It was damp, wet, cold, we were ex-hausted, but we had made it. The noise from the horn sunk through my damp coat all the way to my bones. Melancholy melody.   At first he put the camera on a post and we did a few pictures together. We were the only people there, so we couldn't ask a stranger to snap a picture please. He also made a little video, of the two of us, then put the camera just on me. I had told myself that I wouldn't cry. Even though along these last 3,013 miles I have shed my fair share of tears, I am not a real cry-baby. There have been times, some very tough times, that I couldn't help myself. Today, right here and now, all my emotions were swirling around with this damp fog and I just couldn't help it. I was so happy, sad, exhausted, homesick, in awe that I had not only lived to do this, but the journey seems to be taking other people along on their very own journey...it was a bit too much for me. I broke down while the camera was rolling and even though I tried to be happy about this mas-sive achievement in my life, I just couldn't find it. Morton didn't know what to say. He wanted to walk down to the lighthouse and I was just too tired to. I felt like I might never be able to move off that rock I was sitting on. He asked if I was going to be alright, then walked down the path to lighthouse without me being able to answer him. As soon as he was out of ear-shot, my tears turned into sobs. I searched the woods with my eyes, looking for a reason to all of this. Why am I on this journey? Why am I so far from my family, feeling my heart breaking with homesickness that can only cured by going home? I am going to be a grand-mother and here I am riding my heart out and my butt off, so cold, so tired and so alive. In the woods I could see no answer and no rea-son. The trees told me nothing. Trying to see if I could feel the presence of those around me, I couldn't. I felt all alone sitting on that cold rock. Morton was down trying to take a video of the fog moving and the horn blast-ing. I could see him walking back up the hill to me. Poor Morton. I held my head in my hands and tried to wipe my tears with my sleeves of my raincoat. He stood in front of me and pulled me up to give me a bear hug. This is just what I needed. We didn't talk, we didn't need to. We had both experienced so much in these last few months. Terror of living on the road, fears of things that might never even happen, feeling so very isolated from our families and the world. But we have each other. Who could really ask for anything more?

We headed back to our lovely sanctuary. We both know our evening routine now. He does all the do-mestic side of our day and I do all the computer side of it. The wireless internet here is brilliant and in no time I'm looking at the smiles on the faces of all these people who are making this dream come true for us. I even get to chat with my daughter on the computer for a little while, without feeling homesick. The joy of the day is sinking into my bones. Morton makes a meal out of nothing, he is very good at that. We are safe, warm, dry, with the sad cry of the fog horn in the distance. 3,013 miles is a long way, but when you think that we still have another 13,000 miles to go, we are really just getting warmed up. Literally.

Day 169 June 18, 2007 - Monday - *Quoddy Head Station*, Quoddy Head, Maine

This is one of those days that was filled with interviews, computer and a lot of bicycling to nowhere. It was important because the press is really helping us get the word out there. Without them we would still be doing this, just as many people wouldn't get a dose of getting their own lives changed with little changes. We decided today that we are going to make a dash for the west coast now. It is going to be a long and lovely ride and if we are lucky, we will escape winter. This evening, after a really long day of acting natural, we had thought about riding into town. The trouble was, if we did it to have something to eat, we would most likely be in the dark for the ride home. Not safe or clever.

One of our visitors to the website had made a donation and told us to get ANOTHER lobster. We were thrilled when we called a local restaurant in the town of Lubec, that would deliver to our private sanctuary for the evening. Before we knew it, we were having the most delicious dinner (we both decided Morton *will* get a job as a lobster man when we are finished with the journey) followed by a sweet surprise of dessert. We didn't order the dessert, they had just put it in the bag. Today was filled with work, well-wishes, planning for what happens next and endless phone calls. Having two nights here is not just a great idea, it is almost a requirement for where we are at this wonderful point of our journey. Tomorrow we ride WEST, for the next several thousand miles.

Day 170 June 19, 2007 - Tuesday - *Quoddy Head Station*, Quoddy Head To East Machias, Maine

Morton and I are very excited about getting to see Cindy and her family again as we turn our bicycles around and head back west. This is something that hasn't happened to us yet, getting to retrace our path for a short while before heading WEST to the state of Washington. As Morton is packing he takes the bikes out the front door. He tells me that I'm not going to believe what is out there. I get worried, because he's so excited. I'm thinking bear, moose, maybe a snake or wolf. But whatever it is, it has Morton almost squealing. Sitting cross-legged, balancing the computer, I make the needed movements to shuffle up. Morton sees that I'm actually in the middle of working and stops me before I get up. Someone has left a gift bag on the doorstep! It is actually the lady that works at *Quoddy Head Station*. She brought the most amazing things for us and just popped it on the step and left. There is also a wonderful note and Morton and I are just blown away. The kindness of strangers....amazing! We have the fresh yogurt and keep the other goodies for later. Morton is thrilled that there is more bug spray. It seems the biting things *LOVE* him. He has been wanting to get more and we have been using our current spray very sparingly. The bugs have left us alone here at Quoddy Head though. It is a bit windy and we heard that they don't like that. We know that there are others waiting in the deep wooded parts we are going to be going through.

As we head back the same road we came in the other evening in the fog, you wouldn't even know we were in the same place. The fog had been so thick, we didn't realize we had been riding beside the water at some points. The lilacs are also in *full bloom* here, so the 4 miles were heavily scented with the purple and white blossoms. One of my favorite smells. When we got back to the road that takes you to Lubec, we headed west. It is going to be odd now, looking for the west bound road signs. This one looked familiar, since we had ridden the other way on it, yet everything was different. It actually felt like we were riding home today. Getting to spend another night at Cindy's is a treat. It is the closest feeling we will have out here of getting to see family. Morton and I both just keep pedaling today and make very good time. Before 4 pm, we are pulling in, parking the bikes in their garage and heading in the house to say *HELLO AGAIN!* It is a great day, a great evening of wonderful food and conversation and it all feels like something we have done a million times before. Morton and I actually go to sleep before 11 pm tonight, with the invitation to stay for another night if the weather proves true and is rainy in the morning. My computer has to wait for me, it was a night of not a lot of sleep on Monday night and I just can't keep my eyes open. With emails to answer, pictures and videos to upload, interviews to do....another day might be just what the doctor ordered!

Day 171 June 20, 2007 - Wednesday - East Machias, Maine

Morton and I had an amazing day. *BIG, HUGE, GIANT NEWS COMING!!!* A phone changed all our plans. We are sorry to be secretive about it, but we have been asked to not discuss it yet.
I can say that Cindy & Malcolm and their family have just been wonderful to us, we will be sad to leave but we know that we will all get together again. Today Malcolm gave us a fantastic tour around on some wild roads that our bikes would have never gotten over. It was like being on a safari ride, only no lions in sight! We spent another perfect day with these great people & I felt horrible for being stuck on the computer for most of the day. With only so many hours in the day, it doesn't seem to end...this lovely thing called "laptop" I also think of it as good therapy for my knee, it's nice and warm.

Day 172 June 21, 2007 - Thursday - East Machias, Maine to Central Pennsylvania

Someday we will fill you in on all the WHO, WHAT, WHERE & WHEN questions about the last day or two. Right now, we have so many things that we HAVE to do, that it is impossible to catch you up with it all. James & Mari drove up from Pennsylvania to Maine to pick us up, then I was able to drive back, since James had driven all night on Wednesday. When you are having things happen so fast in your life, they can seem like a bit of a blur. That is how this trip was. Though my mind was racing about all the "What ifs.." I tried to stay in the moment. I would look over at Morton, who looked about as shocked and stunned as I did. The funny thing was, my daughter hadn't even really told my son why he was having to drive over 700 miles to pick us up. He just did it. As I filled him in on what might be happening, he seemed to be a bit more interested in sleeping. The miles raced by at a frightening speed, though I wasn't speeding. After spending the last six plus months either walking or on a bicycle, this was all happening so quick. The car breezed by as we chattered away inside.

I drove past Boston, Cape Cod exit, saw signs leading us to places we had just made a turtles-pace past, then felt like I was nearly back to Pennsylvania when I saw the bright lights of New York City. I knew it was only three hours or so from there. About 11 pm I got worn out. Today was tougher than being on a bike. It was one of those heavy mental days, with so many images and thoughts dancing about my head. I had to just give up, pull over and my son got back behind the wheel. Since Morton has been in America longer than a year now, his International Driver's License isn't valid any longer. James does a fine job and I sleep sitting up in the back seat. At 1 am, we pulled into his driveway and I rushed to his spare floor. He wanted to get the air mattress out, but I was so tired I just wanted to fall asleep standing. He insisted on the mattress, so I leaned against the door frame as he danced on the pump that blew the mattress up. Morton and I fell right off to sleep, me dreaming about what was going to happen on Friday. After all, now I really do know that ANYTHING is possible.

Day 173 June 22, 2007 - Friday - Central Pennsylvania

With butterflies the size of Brazil in my belly, I woke up feeling like I was having a dream. The surroundings were familiar, the day was just coming in the windows and my alarm hadn't gone off yet. It was 5 am. Not good when you only went to bed at 1 am.

There were so many things to do today, I had a hard time getting everything done that needed to happen before 8 am. Maybe tonight there will be more than 4 hours of sleep for me. The day really just flew by in a blur. Bits and pieces were actually sticking with me. Images of seeing my daughter Sarah, with her 8-month pregnant belly coming towards me, smile on her lovely face. Giving the furry dog Max his first cuddle. He has lost weight and so have I and we both sort of had to look each other up and down. Since he is a dog, I couldn't ask him how he has been. He did tell me though with a wag of his tail. He has been fine. Before I knew it, the day was almost over. We had all met back up at my son's place, for a cook out. The weather was perfect for it. Not too hot, not too cool. It was a reflection of the day...everything was just right! As the day had been one of those ones that dreams are made of, I just enjoyed sitting in a folding camp chair that I would have NEVER dreamed of getting into a year ago. Max came up on my lap and I thought that is just couldn't get any better than this. Then I tasted the dinner. It was so simple and so lovely. We all spent the evening catching up on what all has been going on in each others lives, how the next few weeks would be fantastic, being here. The schedule we are going to be filming at is pretty hectic, but after a 3,013 mile bike ride, it will be a breeze!

Day 174 June 23, 2007 - Saturday - Central Pennsylvania

Today was a great one. It began with Morton & James DOOBERIZING the neighbor's lawnmower. They managed to get it going. Since it was Saturday, it was a semi-relaxed day, but I have so much stuff to do on the computer and with film & photos...I could use about 2 months for for that. Morton had made blueberry pancakes. He is looking forward to the thought of cooking indoors for the next few weeks, but he better not get use to it. I have a feeling we are going to be camping out, cooking out, riding around and doing a LOT of things that surprise us all. The urge to just sit back and suck up the time with visiting and catching up, has to be curbed as much as my appetite. I'm worried about eating too much, not moving enough and actually putting weight on over the next six weeks of filming. Now that I know this though, I can prevent it.

We are going to be filming right now to work on a documentary being made about this massive journey. It was all accidental, fast and perfect timing. We have been given the chance to work with a company who are going to help us get LittleChanges out to the world. We will be filming in Pennsylvania for the next few weeks, then driving out to the West Coast to beat the seasons. It all happened with a flurry of phone calls, snap decisions being made and lots of following our gut instincts.

This being the weekend, getting up early as usual, I fall in to the WORK thing. Remember, our days have all ran into each other. We can't tell a weekend day from a Monday morning anymore. It is a bit like bringing a wild animal inside right now. I'm still in shell-shock over what is happening and it makes me a bit nervous, ordinary things. The access to a clean indoor bathroom, cold water, ice cubes...all luxuries that I'm not use to anymore, now wait at my disposal. We are going to get together later on today with Sarah & Graeme for a bit of mini golf, but for now I have to work on the computer. Staying focused is tough. My bike is calling to me from the shed and it feels very wrong to not be on it, heading thirty miles somewhere. I have to get an early morning REAL ride in...from 6 to 8 each morning, I'm going to try to make that happen. Now I know what all of you who are writing me mean! It is tough to find the time, even 30 minutes, but I have to just do this. Feeling horribly guilty, I stretch, clench, twirl my arms and try to raise my heartbeat as my computer is uploading things. Sigh...the grass is always greener on the other side of the tent, isn't it?

Nothing has changed with the journey EXCEPT there are going to be cameras working with us for the rest of it. This is fantastic, because we will really get to get the message out to everyone that we all NEED these precious 30 minutes a day. (Clenching my leg muscles as I'm typing this...and release) We are NOT going to be living in the lap of luxury in some 80 foot long motorhome that drives itself. It is still going to be a very pure journey, with Morton and I on the bikes, riding everywhere and still begging for places to sleep. This ISN'T going to become *The Simple Life*, or reality television. I'm not sure who would play Paris and who would play Nicole...I can NEVER picture Morton with blonde hair. We are really going to be just as we were, plus a cameraman. A lone cameraman that might be met up with OTHER cameras from time to time. No reality TELEVISION here folks...just the ride. We are also NOT going to have any scripts or set-ups.

It is going to be the same ride, acting natural and I hope in time we forget that there is a camera. It won't film us every single second and we will hopefully have helmet cameras that will allow you to see what we are seeing, including each other, when they are on. Exciting stuff really, because there is so much we miss with our cameras. Plus, now that we are back in the area where my daughter is, we have joined up with our LOVELY *SAMSUNG* camera that was sent out to us as a replacement for ours that died right before NYC. I love it so much and the pictures it takes are just amazing. Morton is going to keep the "spare" camera of inferior quality (NOT a Samsung!) but it does all right in a pinch. This way we will both have still cameras on our bikes, video cameras on our helmets and a REAL video camera trailing us all during the day. I hear what you are thinking...YIKES for the people that we visit! Don't worry, Morton and I will *never* film or even take a picture in your home or business if you don't want us to. Actually, from this point on we need to get signed releases for any filming that we are going to do that might end up on the television or in the movie. Today though, we are HERE. With the family for a weekend of getting together, doing some press, doing some computer work and a lot of being thankful we are living in the moment.

Change in Plans

When the calls and emails came in to get to Pennsylvania as quick as we could to meet with and talk to producers who were interested in getting our ride captured on film, I didn't hesitate. Morton wanted to go more cautiously, but I never really listen to the logic of my husband. This was one of those mistakes that turn into a beautiful blessing and would have me saying, *"you were right"* to Morton. The reasons we came back to Pennsylvania were all just and over the next several days I did a mad dash to jump through every hoop I could on the hope that our project would take wings. Morton kept reminding me we were already doing it, but I just tuned him out.

With my only experience of television and Hollywood being several screenplays that I wrote years ago that did actually get a phone call from Hollywood, I felt that I knew so much more than my husband. Did I already mention I had to say "you were right?"

So with the ups and downs of things that weren't meant to be, we found ourselves in Pennsylvania with my daughter ready to give birth, me wanting to hang around for that and a production company interested in having me film for the next couple weeks to get footage of my body at this weight. It was going to be alright, just a bit out of the ordinary.

We wouldn't have a cameraman with us for all the time, a relief really, just for certain parts. Now we needed to keep the journey moving even though our wheels were just going to be turning in Pennsylvania until baby Alexander was born. This is my only daughter having her first baby, nothing, not even my wonderful journey was going to take me away. Remember, there is always a plan B and good things are waiting to happen if you just look around you.

Back to the journal and back to the journey Day 183 July 2, 2007 - Monday - Central Pennsylvania
Dinner : Courtesy of *Market Cross Pub*, Carlisle : cup of shrimp bisque, 1/2 salad, 1/2 piece of fish, 10 french fries (chips), 1/2 beef & ale, 1/2 fresh green beans, 1/2 mashed potato, 1/2 piece white chocolate cheesecake, 1/2 piece Snickers cheesecake
This was a long, but pleasant day. It is a day that I discovered a lot of things I never knew before. Morton and I found a family of three groundhogs living in Sunken Garden, beside the river in Harrisburg. We discovered that the State Museum is closed on Mondays (why???) and we, well I, discovered that I'm still FAT! How do I keep forgetting this fact?

The trouble with having to lose almost 300 pounds is that it is a LONG process. I now know why I have failed so many times. You do start to feel better as you lose weight, but then you get to a point where you feel (me anyway) like you just can't be bothered any more. I still have over a year to go on getting rid of all this. THAT is a long time! One whole year. But it isn't. A year flies by. I have to keep practicing patience.

Little by little...one meal at a time, as a very wise Stella said. Today though, I was on display in my size XL shorts, doing exercises for the camera on FULL display in this lovely setting in Harrisburg. I have driven past here hundreds of times, but never actually went in it before, or even noticed it. How many other incredible things have I driven past and never noticed? But things slow down when you are on foot. My knee is sore and I blame lack of movement. I have been riding an indoor bike at Sarah's, but it just isn't the same. I don't like the sitting in a chair to pedal. Give me the seat of a bike as long as it doesn't feel like a brick wrapped in a hankie. As we walk today, it feels better. But when I sit down in a lovely gazebo to do an interview, it starts to cramp up. I start doing some stretches, then it turns into a full blown work out session...of sorts. There is a lot of re-peating a move. It is a bit odd because people are walking by and looking. They have looks on their faces that show they are puzzled. What is the idea of this fat lady out here exercising for a film camera, still cameras and why on earth is she smiling? Everything is alright, a bit uncomfortable being on display, but I am getting use to being a circus...but then a group of three guys walk by. They are in suits, on their lunch hour I imagine. They start laughing and one says after seeing me, "Whatever happened to that fat girl you use to date?" I feel my face turn red and my heart started to pound in my ears. Talk about feeling embarrassed. I wasn't even the FAT girl in question. This cooth-less trio stopped, stood, watched and discussed with loud voices, the FAT girl. They acted like I was in a sound-proof booth, rather than a gazebo. I wanted to shout...*"I CAN HEAR YOU!"* But I didn't. Instead I kept doing my pretend exercises for the cameras. Why oh why did these guys have to come along and rain on my sunny day? Thinking that they couldn't have the whole afternoon to just stand there and watch this train-wreck of me doing leg lifts, was the only thought that kept me going. Just when I thought it couldn't get any worse, one turns to the other (the guy who actually DATED the fat girl) and says, "But she wasn't THAT fat!" With that, they were off. Tears came up in my eyes but I didn't cry. What was the point. They were just three unkind people, who all took a bit of pleasure in taking cheap shots. Wasn't I someone who was actually TRYING to change? These are the times that the words "Comfort Food" come in to play. Attitudes like that had always gotten to me in the past, but not today. Not now. Now that I know things are changing with time and lots of little changes.

Before I knew it, Morton and I actually had a little time to ourselves. Not long though. We were going to pop inside the State Museum to use their bathroom, suck up their air conditioning and fill our empty water bottles at their water fountain. This wasn't to happen though. They are closed on a Monday. When we were all done with the filming, we headed back to Sarah's to get showers. We were going out for a meal tonight and getting to meet up with *Tim Pratt*, from the *Hanover Evening Sun*. They have been fantastic on following our story and Tim is the very first newspaper reporter who covered us.

We arrive early (I love being early) and get some outside shots. I am so use to doing all the photos myself, it is hard to let go of that. I do hand over our camera to get some that I can use on the website. The evening goes WAY too quick, it is ten o'clock and time to go, for a very early start the next day. Tomorrow we actually *ROAD TRIP* with filming happening, but feeling a lot more like we are back on the journey. As I go to sleep I remem-ber the guys that were slagging me, in a very off-handed way at the park. I thought that even with their mean comments, my day was still the best day of my life.

Day 184 July 3, 2007 - Tuesday - Dillsburg to *Churchtown Inn*, Churchtown, PA

The bikes get stowed in the trunk. Everything is broken down, packed up, pushed in and we set off. Today we hit the road, cameras in tow, to cover some mileage in a car, then get some footage as we pedal in Lancaster county. It feels like we are forgetting something, because one of the trailers stay behind at the home of my son. Our goal is to get some award-winning film shot. Film that will make people weep with joy, soar with inspiration, laugh until their sides hurt, or perhaps, just keep them entertained for two hours while the movie is playing. The important thing is to have fun with it...at least that is what we are being told. Have fun and act natural. My only real direction given for filming LittleChanges. The weather was good for filming. The sun was out, but not glaring as we unloaded the bikes and headed out for the *Churchtown Inn*. It was a few miles, not our biggest day, but we were getting to ride straight through. The bike felt strange and naked without my trailer. It threw me off my ride.

Things like my mirror seemed impossible to adjust. My legs stretched too far when I pushed the pedal down. My seat felt like Morton's seat. I had ALMOST forgot how to change my gears. What was happening? By shooting this part of the film, am I losing focus on the journey? I started to worry. Then, a pothole bumped me back into real life.

Scrambling to keep my balance, my natural bicycling instincts switched to high gear. I suddenly felt like it was alright. We were on the road and even without my trailer and the next leg of our journey to long for, we were in our element. Then I remembered something very scary. The hills. The gentle rolling hills of Lancaster. How beautiful they are, one almost rolls right after another. Looking like a soft Amish quilt of greens, they are lovely to look at. A real thing of beauty. They are also tough to ride up, with or without a trailer. Today I was lucky though. I only had to walk once. Just once.

When we arrived at Churchtown, the *Churchtown Inn* was very easy to spot. Large, lovely (kind of like me...just kidding!) and sitting right across from a historic church. The front door was opened straight away by Jim, the innkeeper. His wife Chris, was out at the shops and would be right back. He took us on the grand tour of the grand home, filling us in on the history. Showing us to our room, a former dance hall, Morton and I felt like trying a tango. It was incredible. Canopy lace bed, fitted with a quilt across a never-ending mattress that made me miss my grandmother, Grace. She was a great quilter. Pennsylvania Dutch, lovely and my dad's mother. Suddenly I'm a million miles away, remembering how her house smelled, seeing her quilts, some stretched out on the frame she was creating them on. So very long ago, yet just yesterday. We got settled in, then had a lovely chat with Chris, then needed to head out to get something to eat. It is really different for us, this special filming time. It is like the journey, but not quite. We also have the sheer, deluxe, luxury of knowing where we will be for the next few nights. No scary feelings at 10 pm when it is too late out and we are still pushing the bikes around looking for a place to spend the night. There is also a car involved. As long as we have our phone charged, help will only be a push button away. How on earth did this all happen to a fat lady who couldn't even tie her own shoes a year ago? Miracles and movement, the two go hand in hand.

Day 185 July 4, 2007 - Wednesday - *Churchtown Inn*, Churchtown To *B F Hiestand House*, Marietta, PA

"I'm a Yankee Doodle Dandy".... I woke up with this song running through my head. It was the *FOURTH of JULY!* The best part about this holiday is when you are in America to celebrate it. The very first summer I lived in Scotland, 2002 and I had called my parents in Pennsylvania on the Fourth. My dad asked me if they celebrated the 4th in Scotland. I reminded him just what happened so long ago, where the British really didn't have a heck of a lot to celebrate about that day and he said, "Won't you at least be having a cook-out?" To that I told him that it was a little chilly that day.

Today though, we woke up in the lovely *Churchtown Inn*. There were so many things to do today, but first there was breakfast. The second "B" in bed and breakfast. Chris made this amazing breakfast that was going to set us up and carry us for the day. What a long day it was going to be. We chatted with a lovely couple at the breakfast table, in the lovely dining room that really feels like you are sitting outside. The huge windows look out over the Welsh Mountains. It is a terrific view. As we say our goodbyes and cycle off towards Marietta, my phone rings. Oh the phone. I am always just getting going when I get to pull over for a break of talking. People are surprised to find that I answer the phone and can do a number of multi-tasking when it comes to the phone. I eat lunch while chatting sometimes, careful to not chew in anyone's' ear.

We keep getting filmed, our photo snapped and in general, lots of "acting natural" for the day. As we ride into Marietta I realize how little I know about Lancaster County. This town is a brilliant. So many historic homes and buildings you aren't quite sure if the year is 1707 or 2007. We could have rode around all day just looking at things.

We did get distracted by baby toads, stopping to photograph them. We could have just filmed all day on everything but out journey, but we did keep focused and did the job at hand. It is easy to get pulled away by beauty and the simple little things that I'm seeing that I somehow never noticed before. My life has already changed with my journey. It now just keeps getting better.

When we went along to *B F Hiestand B&B* and met Dallas and Mr. Biggs, a lovely yellow lab. We were charmed instantly and also felt right at home. The B&B is a mansion that isn't like a museum. You feel like you could live here. Dallas showed us to our room and I claimed the study in it for my workspace. It is really tough right now, as you can tell from my lack of writing on here, to focus on the website. I don't want to neglect it, but we are so busy living in the moment right now, it's tough to do. The cameras get set up and we get to do a bit of "acting natural" and talking about the week to come. The first time it was terrible, then we did it again. This was MAGIC! Morton and I had one of our funniest and best bits ever of "acting natural" that even made us laugh. It was great and I was thinking that was really what we want to capture in the movie. Then, as any great crew does, we check back over the days film. The part that was brilliant movie magic, was there, but soundless. The mics hadn't been turned on. We tried to do this over, but since we aren't trained actors, we failed miserably. I told Morton that we needed to always check, re-check and then check again. We are learning as we go, we will make mistakes and you know what? That is fine and dandy. We are TRYING! If you never try, you will never know what all you can do.

The afternoon and evening just fly by. We chat with Pam, our lovely hostess who I could have spent ages talking with. We talk about the trip, kids, grandkids (come on Sarah and have our grandson already!) and like too many other people we have met, we just don't have enough time to talk as long as I'd like to. Morton and I head for our suite, as fireworks sound off reminding me that we are independent of Britain, I smile thinking of my Scotsman, who I'm very much dependent on. The house here will forever feel like a special place for me. It is something that has a wonderful feeling of family, from the moment you step on to the huge porch. You aren't overwhelmed, just charmed, invited to come inside and stay a while. We never get to stay as long as we'd like but we have the hopes of returning someday to all our special places. I work into the wee hours, I let my mind drift to what the post-production process of our film will be like. It will consist of someone being in one spot, pouring over tens of thousands of images, watching endless hours of film. They will be looking for that one special clip. Our project on the front porch of this home will hopefully find it's way in to the story. Perhaps someone that does lip reading could tell Morton and I just what we were saying and we could Milli-Vanillie it.

Day 186 July 5, 2007 - Thurs - *B F Hiestand House*, Marietta to *The Artist's Inn & Gallery,* Terre Hill, PA

Bed and BREAKFAST...as in DELICIOUS FOOD that isn't coming out of our food bag, is what Morton and I got treated to this morning. We were in a rush and as soon as we walked down the grand staircase, the world seemed to stop. The smell of food took over the urge to race at a breakneck pace to the pretzel factory we were going to be visiting and filming in. Pam is a brilliant cook. The food was so good I wished we could stay for a week, a month....forever? Who knows, maybe we will have to take a room here when it is all over for a while. I could quite happily see myself working away upstairs as Morton helped Dallas paint, do projects or even polish up his cooking skills in the kitchen with Pam. We have a great chat, but then it is time to head out. This part ALWAYS comes way too quick. Always.

There are pretzels waiting though and since I'm such a lover of the pretzel, it is enough of a draw to pull me away. We have been kindly been given permission to film and to make it even GREATER...we were going to be doing a newspaper interview there.

When we arrived at the *Intercourse Pretzel Factory*, we got taken in on our own, soon to be joined by the reporter. Morton and I can never, and I do mean never, count on twisting pretzels to make a living. Mine was pretty good, but I was shockingly slow. Morton produced a *MONSTER* pretzel with two or three twists in it. It's odd shape looked like it might be tasty though. Who knows, maybe he will start a trend..."How many twists would you like in your pretzel sir?" It would taste good I'm sure, but it did look rather odd. The tour was very interesting, fun and we loved getting our hands on the dough. What a great idea for anyone to do. The place is just one of those things that you HAVE to do, whether you are a tourist or a local. We highly recommend it. We finished the interview on the porch, then were invited to come inside and get some pretzels to take away with us. Talk about PERKS!!! Pretzels...hard and crunchy with just a dab of salt to replace what we are sweating away each day. Delicious and eaten in moderation. As we were leaving, we saw a place across the way that was having heart tests happening. We went in, spur of the moment, to make some shocking discoveries. Morton went after my test and discovered that he is a candidate for a stroke. His age on his veins and arteries log in at 48 years old. He is only 40 so he is worried. Me, I am mortified! My age checks in at 69 and I am just 44! How did this happen? I will tell you. Decades of abusing my body with food is showing in my heart and veins. I am a candidate for a heart attack. Just hearing those words and my heart starts racing. How is it possible? I bicycle EVERY DAY. But then I think about it a bit more logically. For the decades I abused the food, didn't take any exercise and pretty much stuck my nose up in the air about my health, my body had no choice BUT to get in this condition. I ate away committing a slow form of suicide, happy with the thought that my weight was only hurting me. I wasn't puffing second-hand smoke into anyone's face, I wasn't using drugs, I wasn't drinking and driving, but I was committing suicide by food. Combine it with no exercise and it is lethal. My weight also does have a real bearing on the lives of those around me. Do my children want to bury a forty-four year old fat mother? I wonder how high it would have placed my age a year ago, when I weighed in at over 400. The man giving the test assures me that as my weight comes down, so will my age. Next year I will do this again. I will have shed another 100 pounds and hopefully a decade or two from my age. Exercise will turn back these vicious little hands of time.

People, do NOT stick your head in the sand. Morton and I had a conversation about "knowing or not knowing" and we decided it is *ALWAYS* better to know...always. When it comes to your health, how can you fix it if you don't know!? We had a lot of figures thrown at us with this test, but the man giving it explained what they all meant. The big thing he said, was to get our weight right and keep exercising. The next time we get together, hopefully we will all get a pleasant surprise.

From here we went to Terre Hill. We had seen signs for this place before. As we are driven up it, I thank my very lucky stars that the bikes are in the back. We are not having to struggle as I'm sure that we would be doing. The *HILL* is more like a mountain, the sky is clouding up and the rain is getting ready to soak the lovely rolling hills that fall off on the smoky looking horizon. I jump out to go to the porch. The house is lovely. There have been so many wonderful places in Lancaster County that it would be tough to decide where to stay. We recommend staying a week or two and bouncing around. Try several and then you can always pick out a favorite. We couldn't though...too many choices.

When I rang the bell, I was too busy looking around me to actually listen to hear if it made noise. Waiting just a minute, I rang it again, then saw people coming towards me through the curtains. I apologized to Jan for "double buzzing" and hoped she wouldn't think I am an impatient person. Even when I'm frantic, I really try hard to practice patience. It costs nothing and saves millions in stress.

Once I am in their home, the word "Gallery" takes on a whole new meaning. I have been in many galleries, even had a try at having our own gallery in Scotland (it was a failure...but hey, we did try!) Morton and I have explored galleries in Scotland, England, France, Holland, Italy and many other exotic locations. But this gallery, this has to be the best we have ever been in. To call Bruce an artist is an understatement. To say he is good, talented and creative again fall way short of the mark. He is this *UBER-TALENT* that is contained in a person who is so charming, witty and genuine, that it takes a while to realize that you might have just met one of the greatest artists in the world. His style is just...BRILLIANT! You must see his art, buy his art, buy his book, visit them and fall in love with this gallery. We went from drawing to drawing, artwork to artwork and tried to take it all in. We tried to choose a favorite, but couldn't. I am very partial to a pair of pigs, one smiling and one not, titled *"Sweet & Sour Pork"* but there are just too many to choose from. The other fantastic thing about his art is that when you see the prints, you *KNOW* someone who would love it. Someone that would fall in love with that piece. It is the art that has spoken the loudest to me and made me laugh and enjoy it more than anything else we have encountered. Jan had been an angel and arranged for *Channel 11* to come out and interview us there. The skies were really cracking now with a storm and clouds. Water left loose from above and we had to forget the idea of filming on the porch for a while anyway. Instead I floated between the Kris Kringle room and the Garden Suite, looking at pictures, oohing and aahing and wishing I had a home to hang some art in. But it wouldn't work well on the bikes. Maybe at the end of all of this I will have to come back and get some incredible prints for the sheer joy of art!

When the news crew arrive, the church bells are playing and the rain has eased off a bit. It is decided that while we have a break in the weather, we will film. Morton and I don't mind riding in the rain at all and this is just a drizzle. Even though there are small streams running down the road beside us, we ride. The joy of riding really comes to me at times like this. I am trailer-free, going around in circles with the rain splashing on my nose and nothing else really matters. Of course I do have to think about not running over the cameraman. But today there are no mishaps. After a short time we all head on to the huge side porch for the interview part. Slipping the microphone up my t-shirt and clipping it on my neckline is something I'm getting really good at. We have lost track as to how many times we have done this now...not enough though. It is always a thrill and a privilege to get to talk to people on such a wide scale about how important their health is. If we get through to just one person with each interview...that is all that matters.

We had a city editor with a newspaper once tell us that he wasn't interested in covering our story. He had ran stories before about obesity. He couldn't be persuaded that our story was unique or different. *Already covered that.* I think about the funny side of that. Would he limit how many stories he would run about the weather, politics, accidents? Hmmmm...I also don't remember the obesity problem being cured. We DO need to talk about it, try to beat it, before it claims more lives. Being fat is killing people daily but for some reason you never hear about *that* on the news. Plain and simple. People die, as in being dead, breathing no more...because they are too FAT. Why don't we talk about this? Why isn't it making headlines? We are eating ourselves to death America, while other people are starving to death. HOW did this happen? More importantly, HOW can we solve it? The answer is easy. One person at a time. One story at a time. One set of little changes at a time. This all takes time and if we need to do a million interviews to get the message out and motivate people, bring on the cameras.

As the interview goes on I'm thinking about the things I dare not say. I want to shout and scream for people to wake up to the fact that being FAT is deadly. Your doctor can't help you. Only you can help you and the sad thing is, we don't listen. The doctor can tell you things, give you tests and ideas, even medication, but when it comes down to it, at the end of the day...only YOU can help you. We pay the medical people for their advice and then don't take it. Why don't I ever say this? I don't want people to think I'm preaching to them about FAT...dangerous fat. Forget all the stereotypical reasons people have for not wanting to be fat. The one that should shoot straight to the number one reason isn't how you look in a pair of jeans, or in my case, sweat pants...the number one reason should be *BECAUSE IT IS DEADLY!* Look at me. Just lost 150 pounds and *STILL* at age 69, rather then my real age of 44...all down to my lack of a bad diet and no exercise for decades. I have to pick up the slack I suppose, get braver, step outside my comfort zone on camera. There are lives to be saved, including my own.

When I finish talking (sorry that I run on and on, but I am so passionate about our journey, I get lost in it) they put the mic on Jan. She is *WONDERFUL*. Her personality is so bubbly and she is very photogenic. A great smile, witty and I am really enjoying watching this. She is the reason, along with so many others who are helping, that our journey is working. Will she even know just how much she has helped us? Hopefully some-day, but I don't think that is why people help us like they do. I think that people, most people anyway, are very kind and good. We forget this because we only hear the bad things a lot of times. But tonight's news will be filled with hope and good things, at least our little part of it. When the crew is leaving, there is a couple arriving with their bikes, who are staying for the evening. We don't really get a chance to do more than say hello, then we head for a little meeting about today's shooting and what is on the schedule for tomorrow.

Did I mention that we are the luckiest people in the world? Even if my heart attack that I am a candi-date for would happen tonight and I wouldn't wake up in the morning, my life has been so full and blessed. I fall asleep in another magnificent place, amongst strangers & family, counting my blessings. This of course came after we had watched Bruce star in his delightful DVD. He is working on the second one and I can't wait to see it. He told us that he always wanted to be a stand-up comedian and he really is. His humor is almost a motivational type of comedy that makes you laugh and think.

Even though I'm up too late, didn't eat lunch and found out my veins are more than 20 years older than my birth certificate says they should be, this my friends, was a perfect day.

Day 187 July 6, 2007 - Friday - *The Artist's Inn & Gallery*, Terre Hill to *Zook's Motel*, Leola, PA
***Ode to a BREAKFAST* at The Artist's Inn & Gallery**

Up late, smells great
Down stairs, in pairs
Plates down, glasses crown
Food to swoon, use your spoon
Blueberries for all, art on wall
Laughs abound, hospitality astounds
We will meet again, new friends
Terre Hill or Scotland

Breakfast that inspires poetry...even *IF* it is bad poetry, has to be special and this was. It just kept coming, we are very spoiled now, maybe even ruined forever. *Lancaster County....we love you.* Our table is filled with this great feeling of conversation, food to ride for and laughs. Lots of laughs. It makes us feel fuller than all the delicious food. Again, the *CLOCK THIEF* comes and just steals time. Today we need to stay on schedule as we are having a dream come true, so we need to leave faster than we would have liked to. It is my hope and dream that we WILL get together again. We have to get together again. I am in awe of this dy-namic couple...they could have put Batman & Robin to shame as the REAL dynamic duo. They are a perfect couple, if ever I saw one.

This is just like Christmas morning when all the presents are *JUST* what you wanted. The doll that you have to feed and change (and NOT have to share with your little brother), the lipstick flower tree (that was really for your big sister) and of course, every little girl or boys dream...a pony! Today I get to ride a horse. I was lucky enough to get one once, many moons ago, for my birthday. She was a lovely pony, but too little. I hit a growing spurt so I only had one golden summer of riding on her swayed back. Today I was eleven again. Today I rode a horse.

When we got to *Allimax Farm* we met Joe and the rest of the wonderful people there. My mind flew back to all the brilliant smells from a barn. Instant memory. They reminded me of sitting in the hayloft, above my precious little pony. It could have been the summer of 1974 today, but it wasn't. Today was the day that I would face a fear and follow a dream. I had been worried that my weight was too much for a horse. I have seen stables that have riding limits posted of 250 pounds. My weight hasn't been that for over a decade, plus I was worried about getting on and off the horse. Lets face it, I didn't even like to go through narrow doorways.

When I first asked Joe if we could have a carriage ride, he was kind enough to say yes. I told him via email that my dream was to someday ride a horse again. Joe wrote back, *"Priscilla, Your trip is an inspiration to all of us, you just jumped in and did it. Never put off til tomorrow what you can do today. So, why put off your horse riding? We have several horses that can carry weight. So, weight is not an issue here. Why not just cross that hurdle when you are here!"* Thank goodness he wrote that. Who knows how long I would have waited, but today, thanks to Joe, was the day.

Now Morton growing up on a hearty diet of John Wayne films in Scotland, dreaming of the wild west, had only ever been led around a paved parking lot on a horse when he was a teenager. He has always wanted to ride, though I think he probably was hoping for a pair of cowboy boots, a big black cowboy hat and a six-shooter or two. Today, for one brief moment, Morton would be the Duke, at least in his mind.

We saw the horses we were going to be on and I fell in love at first sight. I remembered when I got my pony and my parents couldn't drag me away from the barn. I wanted to sleep in it too. That lovely barn smell all around us, I even jumped in today and moved a pile of fertilizer that had fallen. Fresh country air!

There was a CBS news team coming along to do a story on us. Just as we were heading out to the riding ring, their van came pulling in. I had *Starr's* leather reins in my hand, holding on to her and hoping that she liked me. There was also the thought of her legs just buckling when I got on her. I had whispered in her ear earlier that I was sorry for what I was about to do to her, which was climb onto her back. As Joe steadied the ladder I was about to climb, everything happened so fast I didn't have time to be nervous. Morton was already up on *Brian's* wide back and riding around barrels like he WAS a cowboy. Now there was no chance to back out, the cameras were rolling as I lifted my leg, while holding on to the horn and pushed up and over. Just the leg lift alone would have been impossible a year ago, never mind climbing the little ladder to mount the horse. Sitting in the saddle, for the first few seconds, I was terrified. Just terrified. But Joe, who must have sensed this, said that he would walk with me until I felt comfortable. *Whew!*

The cameraman was running backwards, sticking very close to me as I hit the trail. I was worried about running over him. I worry about doing that on the bike too, but somehow I think a 1,200 pound horse would be worse. He was a real pro though and knew just where to stay. In a few minutes, I forgot he was even there. Suddenly I was a child again. My face was smiling, the sun was shining and all was right with the world. How happy I am that Joe reminded me of my own philosophy.

Today was really just red letter beyond words. Morton and I both felt it was over in sheer seconds. Before we knew it, we were saying goodbye and riding the bikes off to meet up with Reynaldo at *Zook's Motel*. One dream over, now another on the horizon, it is always a life in movement.

The miles just flew by. My leg muscles could tell the difference between a horse and the bike. It was a really different kind of workout. There are the inner leg muscles that get used when you ride a horse. A horse, a lovely horse, my lovely horse. I recall a song that was sang by *Father Ted*, a British comedy about Irish priests, called, *"My Lovely Horse"* all the more funny now. I could sing a song about a lovely horse quite easily. Maybe even win the *Eurovision* song contest.

It was quite warm as we pulled into the pretty white and yellow motel. There is a lovely house that sits beside the road, then the motel rooms are nestled in the shade behind. Reynaldo was cutting the grass and met us with a very warm welcome. Chatting a little, he sent us off to our room. First though, we had to get some pictures. We were going to build a website for *Zook's Motel* and we needed the goods! It was a snap though...lots of nice things to photograph. The evening was spent with me working away, getting lots of input in from Morton. I was finally happy with it. The internet is an amazing place. It was yet again an incredible day. So very diverse, so very wonderful and all made possible by little changes. Reading back over my journal I decide that even though this is something I repeat a lot, I mean it each and every time. I hope it doesn't bore you but rather that it inspires you to take the world by the hand and make today the best day of your life. Follow your dreams, especially the impossible ones.

Day 188 July 7, 2007 - Saturday - *Zook's Motel*, Leola to *Lititz House B&B*, Lititz, Pennsylvania

Today, if there was ever a day I COULD have slept in, should have been that day. My BAD body clock had me up and at 'em by six am though. Oh well, I had a lot to do for the new website, wanting to make it as good as I could. Reynaldo kindly offered to take us out to breakfast, but we had to say no. There was too much for me still to do on the computer. He is so very kind though, really a one-of-a-kind of man. Easy to smile, incredible personality and this kindness that just seems to go forever. When we got his website *LIVE* on the web, it was time to pack up and head off. We had about 11 miles to ride, a little day really, but the sun and heat were really tough.

It is a bit of a heat wave right now and we are riding right in it. Earlier in the day we had met a lovely older gentleman, Paul, at *Zook's Motel*. He wasn't able to speak, but he had so much to say. He used a pen and paper, which Reynaldo had saved for him, to tell us a bit about his life. It was really staying with me, our conversation with the written word and the hopes that this person would hopefully write down his thoughts, stories and someone would be able to get them out to the whole world. If we would have had a bigger trailer, I would have invited Paul to hop in and ride behind us, seeing this wonderful country, then maybe the world. But I couldn't. Chances are very good that I'll never even see him again. It makes me sad and I think that someday, when we have finished, I want to go back and try to talk to him again.

At a red light in a small town, Morton is adjusting my brakes and I am talking to my mom. I'm only 90 minutes away from her in a car right now, or a three days bike ride, but we have to film. The phone might be the next best thing to being there, but I can't help but feel like I'm the worst daughter on the planet. :(It is a good conversation, part of her on-going therapy is to have as many conversations as she can. I wish I was twins. Morton has given me the nod and hand signals that the bike is ready and hands me the hot bottle of water. Solar power really works and just earlier in the day he was talking about being able to cook with a sun-cooker. Morton thinks about inventions a lot on the bike. How to get power is a big one, since we always need energy for recharging our things. This heat is draining me and I drink the water, hot from the sun, until the bottle is empty. It is wet and that is all that matters. With winter on his mind, Morton is also thinking about how to make *HOT* things when we are stuck in the snow. I draw the line at eating road kill, but you never know what we might have to do to survive out there. I've already done so many things I never thought I would, just because we had to.

Mom and I say goodbye and I get back on the bike gloomy, guilty. Riding lifts my spirits a little and thinking about what is still ahead of us for the day helps me to focus on the "right now" part. Hills, mountains, lots of buggies loaded with passengers. That would solve the problem of how to take my mom along, but I wouldn't want to see how the horse would handle the long stretches with no water. Horses couldn't just sleep anywhere and as you all know, sometimes we don't even get offered a stable to sleep in. But not tonight. Tonight, as all our nights thus far in Lancaster have been, we are going to be hosted. Pat, the owner of the *Lititz House Bed & Breakfast* is the person that greets me at their lovely front door. Again, I am ashamed to confess that I grew up around this area, sort of, an easy day-trip, and have never been to Lititz before today. The town is really pretty...I mean REALLY pretty. I am not sure on the history of it, why it is here, what it has done, but I know NOW it is meant for strolling in. Even a bike is too fast to enjoy this town properly. After Pat shows us to our lovely room, with a sitting room just outside our door, I set about working. The house is very impressive. So much lovely dark wood on the tall doors with windows above some of them, letting the light pour into the halls. From attic to basement, this huge home is stunning. Pat surprises us with a gift certificate to a local restaurant. This is a real treat! I was setting my tastebuds up for a can of tuna, instead...the luxury of dining out. The best part about it wasn't just the delicious food, it was the stroll to the place, through a park, then the stroll back to find the house just glowing for the evening.

Little lights twinkled on the house, peeking through windows with curtains framing them. The stairs on the rear decks were lit with soft glowing light. It was an enchanted evening and I didn't feel stuffed, just comfortable. I also felt like I might have enough energy in me to get caught up on everything that needed catching up. Inside our room I stretched out on my belly (another sign that I wasn't too full) and began working on the computer. I promised myself that I'd stop at 11 pm. There are so many things that I need to be writing down, recording to remember, but I don't have enough talent or time. Headless chicken syndrome overtakes me most of the time, with the overwhelming things we are seeing and experiencing. We end our evening with Morton falling asleep while using a MASSAGE & HEAT machine on my back. It is wonderful, but I know that he is sleeping when it just stays in one place for ages. I nudge him and he starts moving his hand around a little, but the snores are coming and he is gone. Putting the laptop away for the night I wonder as I fall asleep if I will see Paul again. The man who communicates with his written word, writing down in neat handwriting that he had been to college for four years, various things he has done with his life, that he now walks everywhere, the reason he looks so fit. It is hard to meet these people and NOT interact with them. Human connections. When this is finished, we have no idea where we will end up. We don't know which country or state we will end up living in. For a moment I let my mind wander and toy with the idea of a large lovely home, like the one I'm sleeping in. Shared with strangers, all who have stories to tell. Maybe someday it will happen, after all, dreams do come true if you help them along their way. Morton and I both agree that the worst advise our mothers ever gave us was "Don't talk to strangers!"

Day 189 July 8, 2007 - Sunday - *Lititz House B&B*, Lititz to *Lovelace Manor B&B*, Lancaster, PA

To put it mildly, today was HOT...very hot. The morning started off great with a fantastic breakfast that Morton had seconds and thirds on, then a nice shady moment in the garden at the lovely *Lititz House B&B* with Pat & Jim. We are meeting so many wonderful owners of the lovely B&B's of Lancaster County that Morton and I might have to end up putting a whole chapter in the book about just that! Fantastic place to see and again, come for a few weeks and dot about the place. It got hot as soon as we pulled out of the shade from the parking area, in the backseat of a black car. The thermometer was pushing 90 as we pulled into the *Lost Treasure Golf* on Route 30 in Lancaster. We were going to be filming and frolicking AND sweating today for the cameras. A lot of sweating. The course, actually two different ones, is lovely. There are huge trees, including one that is over 300 years of age, that provide you with lots of natural shade. There are also waterfalls you go behind, caves to play inside and even a pirate ship that you board to play a hole. It is a really fun course, maybe the funniest that I have ever played on. I do love to play regular golf too, but mini golf is all my body has managed for the last decade or so. We did both courses, but since we weren't technically REALLY playing, more just getting photos and film, it was too much like work. Mini golf is a FANTASTIC way to get your 30 minutes a day. There is lots of bending, stretching, walking, laughing when a wild thing happens and wouldn't you know it...the time we AREN'T keeping score is when I get a hole-in-one! After the golf we did a maze that is there. It is timed, very fun, frantic and Morton and I were running around looking for things in it. I use the word "running" loosely. I was more like speed-walking and trying NOT to have a heat stroke. The whole thing was filmed from above and looks VERY funny on film. Think two lab rats, one fat, looking for the items in the maze and then the exit. We are going to speed up the 14 minutes it took us to about one minute, the miracle of film.

We needed water, had lots of it and then did some more filming before heading off to the lovely *Lovelace Manor*. It turns out that a few days before we had actually PASSED this large brick mansion. Now we were going to get to go in and explore, with the owners Lark and Michael as our wonderful hosts. Michael and Lark have a real passion for the house, with good reason. The history, the name and the whole story are fascinating. You can see the house in the television show, *"If Walls Could Talk"* where they tell the story about all the treasures they discovered when they bought the house.

Once we get settled into our room, we only have a few minutes before we head out to *Dutch Apple Dinner Theater* to see *Peter Pan*. This is going to be a real treat! We are going to be able to do some photos, a bit of filming before and after and best of all, get to spend some precious moments with family. Sarah and Graeme join us, where we are shocked to learn that Graeme has never seen Peter Pan. He doesn't even know the story! It is just a fantastic evening where we all feel like we are flying, full of food, fun, laughs and the best thing of all, spending time together. There are families there, children of all ages and everyone is smiling. It was perfect, bliss and an evening of great joy.

When we come back to *Lovelace Manor*, we are all feeling very lively and set off for the basement. There is a pool table, loads of games and a karaoke machine. Oh, the possibilities! Morton gives us a few tunes on the guitar, then grabs the microphone and belts out his own version of standard songs. His rendition of *"A Boy Named Sue"* defies explanation. He loves this song and has heard it loads of times...but tonight he howls through it with a tune that sounds nothing like it. It was a bit, ummm, how do I say this nicely, diabolical! Since Morton was properly microphoned, you SHOULDN'T be able to hear me snickering as it was happening. Somewhere in the house though, another guest thought they heard singing. We found this out a bit later and thankfully we stopped before the police needed calling and the cats started howling outside.

The bed in our room is huge, soft, sheets that make me hate our sleeping bags and sleep and I soon find each other. When I first looked at this grand room with it's lovely desk, I had visions of sitting at it and writing the great American novel. I think if there is any place that I could squeeze out some great writing, it would be here. But alas, the time thief is on the prowl again and I run out of steam just approaching midnight. For now, fragments of my memory will be planted on these pages, to be harvested at a later date. Tonight I sleep.

Day 190 July 9, 2007 - Monday - *Lovelace Manor B&B* to *King's Cottage B&B*, Lancaster, Pennsylvania

Today we filmed LOTS of long shots, action shots and spent way too much time in the sun. It was a really hot day, VERY hot indeed. By the time we had finished our breakfast at *Lovelace Manor* (you need to VISIT them and hear the incredible story of how they got to be in the house and the treasure they discovered there!) we said our goodbyes.

After several hours in the scorching sun, so HOT that our bicycle helmets actually melted, we headed to *The King's Cottage Bed & Breakfast*, where we met Ann, Janis and Sampson...the cutest little white fluffy dog we have ever seen. He was so friendly, again we are dog-struck.

Today I'm going to be getting a real treat. Ann is giving me a massage. The only catch is, it is going to be filmed. Massage is something that I long for, dream of and relish. This is a recent love affair. Not too many years ago, just the thought of getting a massage would make me cringe. Why on earth would I let anyone see me, let alone touch me, with just a towel on! But then one night in Scotland, something wonderful happened. We were at a "race night" in a little town called Carrington. It is a great way to spend an evening with friends, where you bet on pre-recorded horse races. You can buy a horse, bet on it and all sorts of other things I didn't have a clue about. Morton and I were just there for the laughs and accidentally won £80. Someone at our table won a coupon for a free massage and I was given it. The massage was one where the lady came to your home. In this case, our little place in Scotland, while Morton was at work. It was safe. The person giving the massage was wonderful, Geraldine from Ireland. It made me want to have them all the time. My fears were all gone and I wondered why I waited almost 40 years to do this. After that first massage, friends in Scotland gave me a massage for my 40th birthday. They didn't give it to me personally, rather a voucher for a massage at a castle. Dalhousie Castle. It was another incredible experience. It leaves you feeling so relaxed, so renewed and just wonderful. Today was just as wonderful. If I had it my way, we would have a massage therapist with us. If only I could talk Morton into taking lessons, but I don't think there is any hope of that. It was a bit embarrassing though at the Dalhousie Castle. You see, my husband being a local always pronounced it Dalhoosie, so I did the same to the amusement of the staff there. They were use to Americans calling it Dalhousie, remember the joke about the mouse and the moose?

The massage today in Lancaster, Pennsylvania was wonderful, though I couldn't fully relax with the cameras. Massage is best with just you and the therapist. It did make me feel so much better though, it always does.

We have a special treat and get to go to *Miller's Smorgasborg*, a Lancaster tradition. My dad had lived and worked on a farm owned by the owner in the 1960's and early 70's. We grew all sorts of fruit and veg for this place and today, we were going to get to eat there. The dishes are all like memories come to life in the form of food. My grandmother could have been in the kitchen herself cooking. It was a trip down memory lane for my tastebuds and I wished that my dad could be here.

When we went back to our rooms, the food, which I didn't over indulge in, had settled and I was ready for sleep. Emotional, tasty and full of filming, my legs and body was relaxed. The air conditioner hummed as I drifted off, hoping the weather would ease off for the rest of our time here.

Day 191 July 10, 2007 - Tuesday - *King's Cottage B&B* to *Walnut Lawn B&B*, Lancaster, Pennsylvania

You have heard of the Bridges of Madison County? Well this is the Bed & Breakfasts of Lancaster County. Much tastier! Breakfast tastes so much better when you have it at a Bed & Breakfast. If you have never done this, you have no excuse. Make it happen. Janis is as good of a cook as Ann is at massage...both perfection. The heat hadn't eased up. It was going to be hot and my big fear of riding through the desert comes to haunt me today. If I can't make it through a day of filming in Central Pennsylvania, how am I going to survive hundreds of desert miles?

Today we visit *Dutch Wonderland*. It's this family amusement park in Lancaster that I had always begged my parents to go to. I really didn't have any memories of it, except the monorail. Today, we met the lovely Bethany who showed us around and helped look for good shots. Oh the heat! It was just a really tough day, but I did have my bathing suit on under my t-shirt and shorts. There is also a water area that I was looking forward to, but first we did some other "FIRSTS" for me and my new body. Climbing into a log boat ride, flying over head of people in sky chairs and even riding a little roller coaster is something I would have never done last year. My weight stopped me from living. I would have also NEVER climbed the three-plus flights of steps to ride down the giant slide in a burlap sack. Today, I did it. My heart was in my mouth when I got to the top, but not from being out of shape. It was tall and I know that I'm still about 250-ish. I pictured SHOOTING down the slide so fast that I would knock down the cameras, the people watching and not stop until I hit the water. But sometimes your fears DON'T come true...most of the time actually. Today though, the big slide was just a big blast. It was fantastic. Morton and I were side by side, laughing and playing like kids. This is what I had been cheating him out of for the first part of our life together. I can make it all up to him though. Now I have him on the adventure of a lifetime, our lifetime, our *healthy* lifetime. The heat gets to us and we all head towards the water part of the park. This morning I made the wonderfully terrible discovery that my bathing suit has become too big for me. It is so loose on the bottom, it hangs down about 4 inches. It is not suitable to wear in public, without some serious taking in. Since I didn't have time to stitch it up, I had to just leave my shorts on. My legs aren't my problem anymore, thanks to the bike. My trouble is my big, rolly-polly arms. There is just so much of them that I worry about the skin not going back. I have to keep doing my arm exercises and hope for the best. As my shirt comes off, I see some looks. I don't worry about them anymore...I'm changing! This is a tough moment as the cameras are snapping and I know that this isn't going to be pretty. But, the water is calling. The weather is so hot, I am wishing my suit fit so I could take off the shorts. Soon Morton and I were splashing, playing, again I think about all the times I said no to him about swimming. Poor Morton...but not anymore. I won't hide away and not be active anymore. The day zips by, we still have more filming to do so we have to say goodbye to Bethany and head out. The heat hits us as soon as we leave the lovely cool gift shop at the entrance to *Dutch Wonderland*. The car is roasting. We have to do some more outside filming and I just want to get inside. I'm melting.

There are times when you need to listen to your body, but today I wasn't. My head had gotten sunburnt, I wasn't drinking enough water and I was really tired. We should have headed right for our room then and there, but we didn't. I insisted I was fine and kept going. We went finally, to the *Walnut Lawn B&B*. It was lovely, great setting and again, very friendly people. After a chat, we headed upstairs to our room and I got an ice cold shower, by choice. I was so warm from the day, even the rain that happened didn't work to cool me down, but the shower did. After getting cooled down and clean, we headed out for dinner at the *Historic Revere Tavern*. Now you *KNOW* we love food. We have also been lucky enough to eat in some amazing places along our journey. We can say that tonight we were impressed beyond expectation. It was brilliant. This might be the best food and atmosphere in Lancaster, that isn't a smorgasbord! I didn't overeat. It feels great to enjoy food and not abuse it. That night when we were getting ready to sleep in the lovely Quilt Room at *Walnut Lawn Bed & Breakfast*, I felt so very blessed. Well fed, lovely bed and great filming to share our journey. It is a fantastic end to what is again, the best day of my life.

Day 192 July 11, 2007 - Wednesday - *Walnut Lawn B&B*, Lancaster to Harrisburg, Pennsylvania

The day started with a wonderful breakfast, conversation and too fast with the good-byes at the lovely *Walnut Lawn B&B*. Sarah made a great breakfast, Tom kept the conversation lively and we wished our big wish of this trip. More time. We had to see a man about a horse. I always wanted to say that. We were back to Leola to *Allimax Farm* to visit Joe & Valerie and get an education with a buggy ride through the lovely countryside. Going back the lane that the barn is on, I was thinking about the great time we had there riding the horses. Today was going to be another great one. The buggy ride is something that everyone needs to go on. We learned more in those two hours than I had the whole time we had been in Lancaster. Joe drove the team of two lovely horses with an expert hand, over the little roads, past the Amish farms, even through two covered bridges. We pulled into the Amish blacksmith that Joe uses for his horses and we got to get out and have a chat with the man who was actually putting new shoes on a horse. It was a real highlight of our trip. Winding back to the farm, we said our good-byes as the rain began. It was really a downpour and I jumped in the car that was still blazing hot by the sun. I can't be sure, but I think my pants actually sizzled on the seat.

My stomach started going in the to flips and my heart was pounding in my head. I was spinning and I just wanted to lay down. I had been drinking water, but not enough.

The day before I got too much sun on my head. My hair is not thick on top, very thin in spots and those spots had all turned red. Someone had told me that they put sunscreen on their head and without my bicycle helmet on, I need to start doing that. The part that was the worst was the part. My scalp was raw feeling there and my heart was beating the hardest there. After group decisions, long roads and lots of turns, the diagnosis was *"EXHAUSTION"* (like I didn't know that!) so it was off to Sarah's house to occupy her spare room. Without a second thought, as soon as my head hit the pillow, I was out. Exhausted, with no bicycling in sight, I think that the filming is harder than any mountain I have had to climb so far.

Day 193 July 12, 2007 - Thursday - Harrisburg, Pennsylvania

Resting in bed, curtains pulled and air conditioner humming, I try to beat exhaustion. How do you do it other than just rest? I did manage to convince Morton that FRESH AIR is what I was really needing and we went for a tiny bike ride in Harrisburg. We did a bit of veggie shopping at a market, took a wee walk and then back into the air conditioning. The trouble with being sick (or exhausted) is boredom. I just can't stay in bed and felt like a big baby for even being there. My head was dizzy and woozy though, so I suppose I do need to rest...just not now please!

Day 194 July 13, 2007 - Friday - Harrisburg to *Massage Therapy*, Camp Hill to *Kromer's Bed & Breakfast,* Ephrata, Pennsylvania

Still feeling a bit shaky and tired, we headed towards Camp Hill to meet with Beth & Karen. Today was going to be sheer joy...we were both getting a massage at *Massage Therapy Associates*.

When we arrived Morton needed to fill out his paperwork, just a few questions about his health and background. I was happy to see Karen again and she was going to be giving Morton his massage, while Beth and I were brainstorming. With Morton tucked under his sheet, he relaxed so much, he even fell asleep. After Morton had his massage, it was time for mine. Beth gave me this incredible massage that took all the stress and strain out of my neck and shoulders. My body is really missing the daily grind of the bike. I think I'm going to pay for it when we ride off in a few short weeks. Saying goodbye, Morton and I got a very special treat. Beth sent us with some creme for our muscles, some flavor packets with vitamins for our water and a few bagels and orange juice, which became our lunch! Delicious!!!

We had a big treat then, it was sort of a private treat...but as a FUTURE gramma, I have to share it with you! Sarah, who everyone knows, is having a baby boy, Alexander. Today I was invited to the hospital to see an ultrasound to check his size. This was perhaps the most incredible thing I have seen in my life, which is a big statement to make, because I have been around the block a time or twelve. As the person rubbed the wand covered in jelly over Sarah's tummy, we could see this black and white image on a screen on the wall. Morton has waited in the car, not wanting to crowd the room...but what came next, I wish he could have seen. This is where science fiction comes to life with what I saw in front of me. There on the screen came the 4-D ultra-sound image that I had seen in the many baby magazines that now dot Sarah's home. We didn't think she was getting one...but here it was! I had promised to leave the cameras outside and now I regretted it. I was looking at the face of my grandson. Smiling and crying, I tried to not become too overwhelmed, but it was tough. He is the most beautiful baby, as every baby is. But today, looking at this little man in her tummy, it really hit me that my baby is having a baby. His eyes were closed, sleeping just like a baby, with his little arm tucked under his chin. He has Sarah's lips and nose, but when you look at the shape of his eyes and his forehead, it's Graeme! There is hair on his head and we think, a dimple, like Sarah's, in his chin. Did I mention he is BEAUTIFUL? The kind lady doing the scan gave us a range of photos, all lovely. These pictures and seeing him, made me wish Sarah would just go right in to labor! After all, the estimated his weight at 8 lbs, 2 oz...he's ready and so is Sarah. But not today, we will wait and he will come in his own time.

From there we headed to Ephrata, filmed our little hearts out and headed to Elmer & Linda at Kromer's B&B. They put us in the lovely "Hannah" room, named after their grand-daughter and all decorated in soft shades of purple. Talk about relaxing! It was all done in lilacs, lavenders and just the best place to unwind. We all know though, relaxing in the room is something that I don't get to do. So I set about working and managed to get some things done that really needed it. Where oh where does the time go? It had been a wonderful day, not too shabby for a Friday the 13th!

Day 195 July 14, 2007 - Saturday - *Kromer's Bed & Breakfast* to *Tree Top Bed & Breakfast*, Ephrata, PA

Do you know the story of the *Ephrata Cloisters*? It was founded by a man, half-hermit, half-teacher, half-composer...an incredible person and the whole story makes me want to read all about him.

My legs loved the stretching and even with some filming beforehand, Morton and I had a few hours to ourselves, to stroll about this place. It reminded me of a place I had been before, but I really couldn't put my fingers on it. Maybe I was here on a field trip I've forgotten or with family ages ago. Before we got a guided tour in the Cloisters, we got to walk about on our own. There is a museum with these incredible artifacts in them. A cloth shoe from the times that had been found in a closet. There was also something that has caught my imagination. It is a huge trumpet made from glass, laying in a case. This was really odd seeing it there, then they had little signs putting questions forward to you about *HOW* did it get there, who put it there and that was pretty much all my mind needed. It was off and running on a story, as Morton walked about the incredible museum, reading signs. I stood and pondered. *WHO?* That was the question which led to *WHY?* Then, just in a wink, a story popped into my head. I took a few pictures, made a little audio tape on the outline of the story, promising myself that when I got a few months to sit down, there will be a novel come out of this mystery that I have solved, in a fictional sense of course.

Morton didn't have a clue as to why I was lingering. He really never does, he just leaves me to it. When we had a good look around the grounds, it was time to gather for a film about the place. Now, I can't watch anything without thinking of all the technical behind-the-scenes thing that go to making a film. I wonder if I will ever be able to watch a show or film again without thinking of lighting, sound, what is and isn't *IN FRAME*? The subject was interesting but I just wanted to head out to the very old buildings, built with a German-style, that can't be found anywhere else, at this age, in America. There is something about the unique and different feel that fascinates me. Our guide was a lovely lady dressed in clothes of the day of the Cloister. She was very good, knew her history and gave a great tour. We were in the kitchen of the Sister's House, when a man came up and asked if I was Priscilla. This happens to us now, but it always does seem a bit odd. This was a real surprise though, because this man was Max from *Dutch Apple Theater*, who had arranged for us to see *Peter Pan*. We finished the tour, then met up outside to have a chat about the journey, life and this amazing place we were standing in. Always good, like today, sometimes great! It was too short though, never enough time for visiting. Morton and I spent the rest of our time just strolling around in history. My mind kept walking back to to the trumpet in the case. Before we left, I needed to have just one more look and a few more photos. The Sister's House, which one held 36 celibate woman who all believed that Christ was going to come back to earth between midnight and two a.m., which led them to be awake each night, was locked when I wanted to get a couple of more photos from there. I suppose it is better to lock up something like this...after all, you can't really replace it.

We headed off to our very last stop in Lancaster county for the night, *Tree Top B&B*. After this marathon location, we feel like we might have a career in B&B keepers, advisors or at least, the people who enjoy it! We had a chat with Bonnie & Paul, loved all the views from each window and then went to bed somewhat early. My body is still not getting the rest it needs and I want to be able to film each and every day that we have it scheduled for. Rest is what the doctor orders to fight exhaustion. With our last night in front of us, we did the very exciting thing of falling asleep before midnight and thankful to be inside, in a bed, with our cans of tuna in our bellies, that made us homesick for our beloved road.

Day 196 July 15, 2007 - Sunday - *Tree Top Bed & Breakfast*, Ephrata to Harrisburg, Pennsylvania

The best thing about B&B's is the company, the food and the company. Did I mention the company? Today at breakfast, Morton and I were talking to a lovely couple who are over visiting from France. They live in Paris, were delightful and it made me homesick for Europe. Why oh why are we never happy and content where we are? Why don't I take my own advice and embrace the now? The food was great, we said our goodbyes and then were off! It was our last big car ride together, hopefully for some time. We want to GET BACK ON THE BIKES...we need to ride!

Our bikes were waiting for us, with the cameras, in Harrisburg. It was going to be a VERY short day, filming wise, with the promise of a big bike ride, just on our own. Hey, we can dream can't we??? The day just slid by, so very fast, finding us back in Sarah's and Graeme cooking us dinner. It was so nice being here, all together, just like so many of my daydreams I had while I was far away from them. Sometimes words just won't come, or they are too special to record. This was just a day, another very special day.

It feels a million miles away, our life on the road. I am homesick for the road.

Day 197 July 16, 2007 to July 17. 2007 - Harrisburg, Pennsylvania

Filming, riding for cameras and general moving about the streets of Harrisburg. Trying to rest a bit and get ready for the next bit in this big adventure. Pure family bliss.

Day 199 July 18, 2007 - Wednesday - Harrisburg to *The Keystone Inn Bed & Breakfast,* Gettysburg, PA

"Four score and seven years ago..." we all know THAT part, but do we know the rest of it? Being that I'm American and Morton is from Scotland, he's shocked that I don't know it. "Don't they make you say that in your schools?" he asks. I tell him that he is confused with pledging allegiance to the flag of the United States of America.

Whipping out a little blast from the past, I give him the preamble to the constitution, thanks to Schoolhouse Rock! Ahhh, the things that you DO learn on tv.

Filming in Gettysburg is really tough. It is humid and worse yet, filled with so many memories. How many can my poor heart hold before it just breaks? This is where I come from. This is the road I drove my mother over for her rehab after her stroke. These are the roads that my dad would ask about stopping for ice cream on. It was just a million yesterdays ago. I'm finding it extremely difficult to smile for the camera. The gravity of what happened here is pulling on me. This is sacred ground where this anything but CIVIL war happened. This doesn't seem right and I have to just talk about what we are doing for the next two days. It's not going to be happy and carefree riding. It is serious here. You can't walk about these battlefields without feeling something, whether you were from the North or South or even Scotland. Morton is feeling this too. There is a monument here. Really there are hundreds of them. They depict all the different people that came here to fight. So many people died, just one civilian, Jenny Wade. Killed by a bullet that came through the kitchen door while she was baking. When you think the townspeople all just stayed here, that was a miracle that only one "innocent" died. But then they were all innocent, weren't they? The monument I'm talking about is a rather huge one, covered in the names of the dead. Somewhere on there I will find my maiden name, from a great uncle of my dad's (maybe even a great-great) who had walked here to fight. He was a farmer, this relative of mine.

Taking his gun and putting his walking boots on, he just walked in to Gettysburg, fought the good fight, then was lucky enough to be alive after the three day battle and headed back west to the hills. The family was near Altoona. I often wish I knew more about him. I couldn't even tell you what side he fought for, the north I suppose. That isn't important though. Neither is finding his name. Just looking at all of them I want to cry. They were all sons. Sons who died way too soon and without a real good reason.

Today has been long. Very long. We got up early and it was after dark when we finally made it to *The Keystone Inn*, where we will be staying tonight. The house should be the SECOND most famous Gettysburg address...it is beautiful! The location is perfect, in town but OFF the touristy bit. You can walk to Lincoln Square, but you don't have loads of people or cars making noise outside. This house is really like coming home. The large house, wrapped in an inviting porch, reminds me of my Gramma's house. My dad's mother. It was always her house, even though loads of people lived there. You couldn't step on the porch without smelling bread baking. You would also see her with her apron on over her housedress with the straight sleeves that came just above her elbows, stepping out to meet you. A million memories join me as we approach the front door. Why can't we go home? Why can't there be a way to get back to a place in our lives that was so easy, so simple?

Wilmer shows us up to the top floor, over a spectacular wooden staircase. The door tells us that this is *"Grampa's Room"* and I'm glad it didn't say *"Gramma's Room"* that would have been too hard to take. This room is so lovely. A big round mirror on a vanity that is just like one I had. Mine was rough though, bought at an auction in a horrible state, I worked a shabby-chic bit of magic on it. With special paints, I first dissected it, turning each side into a night stand. Then the big round mirror became the floating headboard over my bed. You had to see it, trust me, it was lovely. Sarah is still using the night stands. But this vanity is lovely. Perfect condition, with a silver brush and mirror resting. There is just the right amount of furniture in the room and a lovely rocking chair. I set my eyes on the chest that is at the end of the bed. This is going to be the perfect place to lay on my stomach and write. Tonight I can write.

The million dollar shower feels refreshing and I eye up the huge claw foot tub and dream about having a nice long soak, but just for a moment. There are so many things I need to do on the computer. It calls to me and I have to answer. Even though I should be exhausted, I'm not. My mind has been racing all day. I wanted to pull out the laptop so many times and just lose myself in writing. There are so many stories to be told from here, it can just never be done. I won't live long enough to tell all there is to be told.

The heat is really a humid variety today. It has me drenched, with hair plastered to my face for the majority of the day. When you think that the battle was fought at the first few days of July, you realize just how horrible this had to be for the men here. Today I slather myself with sunscreen and my bare legs stick out the bottoms of my clam diggers.

Back in the day, or days, that Gettysburg became world-famous for all the wrong reasons, there was no sunscreen. These brave men baked in their wool clothing. What a horrible battle it must have been, I can't even begin to imagine. There is a painting I think about that is in the State Museum in Harrisburg. Today makes me want to go look at it, stand in front of it and try to make sense out of what happened here. I'm not sure of the title, or who painted it, but it is enormous. Massive, covering a huge wall and depicting the scene here. Horses looking like they are almost as brave as the men on their backs, soldiers dying, mass destruction on this painting that freezes this moment in time.

We see children running and playing on fields that had been the spot for the fiercest battle our country has ever had on it's soil. This soil, under the heavy amount of traffic, has nothing special about it. You look at it and it looks the same as many other parks, fields and rolling landscape all around the world. But this soil is different. It was the bed for all these soldiers, fighting for their reasons. For the first time in the many dozens of times that I have visited Gettysburg as a tourist and not just a resident on their way somewhere and passing through one of these hallowed fields, it dawned on me. This was the temporary home for these soldiers. The soil was where they fought, slept, ate, went to the bathroom and the very unlucky ones even died on it. This is indeed sacred ground.

Most of the place is very well preserved. There are the fast food joints, loads of things built up to cater to all who visit here, but it holds the ancient feel as well. This battle happened so very long ago now, but here, today, it feels like it could just have happened yesterday.

Curiosity has gotten the better of me, reflecting on the day, as I write my thoughts down. What IS the rest of the Gettysburg Address? I try to remember. Does it hold some important meaning that we should all know? So I found it in a matter of seconds on the internet...lets read it together, shall we?

"Four score and seven years ago our fathers brought forth on this continent, a new nation, conceived in Liberty, and dedicated to the proposition that all men are created equal. Now we are engaged in a great civil war, testing whether that nation, or any nation so conceived and so dedicated, can long endure. We are met on a great battle-field of that war. We have come to dedicate a portion of that field, as a final resting place for those who here gave their lives that that nation might live. It is altogether fitting and proper that we should do this. But, in a larger sense, we can not dedicate -- we can not consecrate -- we can not hallow -- this ground. The brave men, living and dead, who struggled here, have consecrated it, far above our poor power to add or detract. The world will little note, nor long remember what we say here, but it can never forget what they did here. It is for us the living, rather, to be dedicated here to the unfinished work which they who fought here have thus far so nobly advanced. It is rather for us to be here dedicated to the great task remaining before us -- that from these honored dead we take increased devotion to that cause for which they gave the last full measure of devotion -- that we here highly resolve that these dead shall not have died in vain -- that this nation, under God, shall have a new birth of freedom -- and that government of the people, by the people, for the people, shall not perish from the earth."

President Abraham Lincoln - Gettysburg, Pennsylvania

As I said friends, today we were walking on sacred ground, somber, sacred ground. We all need to remember those people, this place and never, ever take our living & breathing for granted. They fought for our nation and now as a nation we are eating ourselves to death while others starve. The day turns in to tomorrow as I listen to my Zen and *Bob Marley* is singing and strumming *Redemption Songs* in my ears. It has been a reflective day, a hard day, a day full of memories with big hopes for tomorrow. "None but ourselves can free our minds."

Day 200 July 19, 2007 - Thursday - *The Keystone Inn,* Gettysburg to Middletown, Pennsylvania to *Caesars* , Atlantic City, New Jersey

If you blink a day or miss a day on LittleChanges.com everything can change! As much as I say to people that you NEVER know what is right around the corner, I still get caught off guard by it. Today was one of those days that I just couldn't seem to catch up with, physically or emotionally. It was a tough one, but I spoil the ending and tell you there was NO better way we could have spent our 200th day on this brilliant trip. It began way too early. Since I had been up until after 3am, working on the computer, the alarm going off at 6am was just too soon. My head started to hurt at once and even though I was in the beautiful *Keystone Inn*, I felt very unsettled. I should have gotten more sleep. I'm running on nearly-empty and as long as the filming is going on, I see no other way around it.

The lovely people at *The Keystone Inn B&B* were kind enough to get us a bit of breakfast, even though it was shockingly early. Again I feel like there is not enough time for what all we are getting done. It makes my head hurt just thinking about it. I know exactly why I passed out with exhaustion and can do nothing about it. We have to go our separate ways today, Morton and I. Thinking of an excuse to tell you of why I couldn't be in Gettysburg, I decided to face my demons and just tell you. It is so emotional for me, it really is something that I just can't do right now. There are shots that have to done, but thank goodness Morton is willing to do them.

The day takes me to Harrisburg area on my own, doing a telephone interview that lasts for 2 hours for a newspaper in California. It amazes me of how the world really is learning about our journey. The lady doing the interview, Patty, promised to send me a link to it. As she's saying the words I'm thinking of my neglected press page. There is so much that I haven't kept up with, but I am only one person and there are only 24 hours in a day. Google me already! As I'm waiting in a park for Sarah, who is kind enough and BRAVE enough, to take me into her doctor's with her, I finally have a moment that I'm on my own. It feels odd. No one to talk to, no Morton, nada...just me. I am going to nip into the library to work on the laptop and try to stay awake for an hour and a half, until it is time for the appointment. But for now, I have about 30 minutes to waste on a picnic table in the muggy shade of a big green treen. Since I was so tired and my head was already spinning, I decided to NOT use the 30 minutes for exercise. I knew I was going to be doing a lot of walking today anyway. Because boredom is something that never seems to get to me. I looked down at my feet and this idea popped into my head. Gathering a hand full of pine bark on the table, I laid out the pieces to form the name, *Little Changes*. It was my attempt at stop photography and I think it worked. We won't know for certain until I edit the pictures, turn them into an animation and see if it paid off or I wasted 40 minutes! It was fun, even though the workers who were mowing the grass, thought I had a screw loose.

As I went into the library in Middletown, Pennsylvania and settled into a newly upholstered wing-back chair, my laptop on my lap, I remembered how much I really love libraries. When I was in college, I worked in the library. It was fantastic and it was always my fantasy to start at one end and read my way right through to the other.

Sitting amongst all those words, inspiration kicked in. I started working on a story that I'm doing an outline on. But then, tempted by the lure of my email, I just had to check it. The story stayed open, sitting nice and patient at the back of my email screen. The words that people write to me are far better than anything I could do. Reading, enchanted and inspired, I wish that you all were putting these incredible emails on the blog. Share it with the world! Even if you are shy about people recognizing who you are, make up a name! Think of it as your writing alias! There was a man and woman who came in and were looking at the furniture I was sitting on. It was very comfy and they were telling me it had just been reupholstered. We started chatting and the lady had seen our story on the news and the talk turned to the journey. The man she was with, her brother, disappeared and her and I kept chatting. I figured, in my mind, that he was bored listening to woman compare notes on *WHY* diets don't work! In a few minutes, the man returned and said he had called the local newspaper and they were sending someone right out to talk to me. This was the first experience today of anything can happen! The man arrived and it was a really in-depth interview. One of the best, I can just tell. The reporter really understood what we are doing and why. Brilliant!

The time slid by, as usual and I found myself walking to Sarah. It had rained a bit and you could smell that hot rain smell that only happens on a thundery summer day. The leaves on the trees were showing the underside of their leaves and I could hear my dad saying that meant a storm was coming. It's nice to think that a storm won't bother me today, no bicycle around.

Memories of my father are very bittersweet. 82 years was not enough, though some people will argue that 82 years is a long time. When will I quit missing him so bad that it hurts my heart? Missing Morton, feeling very down and like a baby for not being able to do the filming that they want in Gettysburg, Sarah turns my day around. Sharing this experience with my daughter is a blessing that can erase any amount of heartache. Especially when it includes listening to her little son's heartbeat in her tummy. While we are in the examination room, I feel like I'm going to swoon. Not over love, over exhaustion. I need to sleep more. What is wrong with me, pushing so hard and not able to just take one simple day off? The room is really hot and my forehead beads up with sweat, even though I'm not walking or bicycling. I go to the bathroom and feel like I'm going to be sick, but I'm not. There is the room with the scale and I'm tempted to get on it. The way we haven't been riding lately scares me. Combine that with real food and I walk back to the room and step on. Smiling, I'm very happy with it and head back to Sarah's room where little Alexander's heartbeat is playing through a machine. He is fine, not ready to come out yet and we head off. Sarah has to go back to work and I'm meeting some people from the filming. Things change fast for us and our plans are now taking us, me anyway, on a very unexpected road trip.

I need to be in Atlantic City for 6 am. It is 3 hours away. I have no car, but have to get there. There is also no way for me to get in touch with Morton to let him know this. Panic sets in a bit, then I remember that I do have a cell phone number for the one person he is working with. After a lot of rushing, setting things up and with the brilliant help of Chris from *Caesars Atlantic City*, there is a room arranged for me. Now I just have the lovely task of sleeping in the backseat, while being driven to Atlantic City. I sort of felt guilty about that, but I needed those 3 hours more than any other sleep of my life. So here I sit, 12:30 am now, in a lovely room on the 47th floor at Bally's, arranged by Chris and ready to jump into the lovely bed, with my name all over it. The pillows are singing and tonight I won't even have Morton putting covers on me when I'm already hot! The ONLY thing wrong with this picture is that I have to wake up at 5 am, be ready for filming at 6 am on the boardwalk. *Did I mention the fact that they want me on the beach in a bikini?*

Right after I got here, even though I had slept the whole way and was still exhausted, I had to just get on the boardwalk and smell the ocean. The Atlantic has been our friend and companion since January and it was going to be good to see the grand lady again. The waves were snow white against the black sky and the seagulls that flew high overhead looked like some sort of wild snow storm. The only thing missing was Morton, but they didn't need him for the filming that was happening and it meant I would get here about 4 hours sooner. He also has things that he has to do tomorrow in Harrisburg. While walking on the boardwalk, I got an ice cream cone. It was not huge, delicious but the girl who gave it to me, wrapped a napkin around the cone that was more like a tissue. It glued itself to the cone and I couldn't get it off. I had to squeeze the gooey cone like a tube of toothpaste, to get the last of the ice cream out. Not wanting to just throw this away, I went to the very edge of the boardwalk. Even though I knew better, I was going to feed the seagulls.

Little Changes   **245**   *Priscilla Houliston*

Just as I was throwing it away, a man came up to me and said, "Don't give that to the seagulls..." at which point I thought I was going to get a seagull-feeding-fine. But no. "I'm starving" he finished. It was only a cone, stuck to a napkin, I explained to him. He said that was alright and kept walking, looking in garbage cans for food. My heart was breaking as I went back to the table where one of the people I'm filming with was eating a huge ham sub. I explained what just happened and the cameraman said I could have the one half of the sub for the guy. Thrilled and sorry that I didn't have my very own food bag here, or enough money to take this guy out for a meal, I found him as he was just ready to started eating a pizza crust he had pulled out of the garbage. The sandwich, which was on a plate, did look good. He was really happy to have it and as I walked away, I wished that I had the time to just talk to this guy and hear his story. Never, ever, judging books by their covers, he really peaked my curiosity. The people that I was with had a little discussion about the homeless. They are both from NYC and a little jaded I think. After about 20 minutes, we decided that the solution to the problem is for everyone to get involved. Everyone. This means you too! Ask questions, listen and then see if there is anything you can do to make a personal difference in someone's life. I bet you can. But for now, I couldn't save the world. I had to just try to save myself and head for the bed. In just a few minutes I'm going to be sleeping, thankfully NOT starving, without Morton, but in a room that is as cool as I like with no humidity...life is very good.

Day 201 July 20, 2007 - Friday - *Caesars Atlantic City* and *Bally's,* Atlantic City, New Jersey to Harrisburg, Pennsylvania

Lunch : Chris at *Phillips Seafood in Atlantic City*, provided me with the most incredible lunch. I had crab chowder and a chopped salad, mixed VERY fresh at tableside by the great waiter Joe, with the largest, tastiest shrimp I have ever had the joy of meeting and eating.

How do I get this emotion to come out on this computer? Today is one that I'm going to have the hardest time relating to you. It was great, don't get me wrong. No matter how stressed I sound, I wouldn't have traded it for anything in the world. Starting weird, waking up on my own, I tried to remember the last time Morton and I had been apart for an evening. It was ages ago, when we lived in Scotland and I went to France for business, without him. It was really sad, being in a lovely castle with lovely people in this picture-postcard place and not having Morton. I remember the pangs of homesickness for him that made my stomach twist and turn, that even the French countryside, charming markets and incredible company couldn't replace. Today I had that same feeling, only I shoved two breakfast sandwiches in my gut to try to override it. It was early, too early to be homesick. I had a tankini (bikini that is sort of like a one piece, only easier to go to the bathroom with) that was looking up at me, waiting to be worn. Knowing it would fit from my quick try-on the night before, I waited until the last possible moment to put it on. There is a wooden ring that is on the bottoms, placed to lay flat on your stomach, if you have a flat stomach. Mine was more at a 45 degree angle. It also revealed a BARE spot of belly. Looking closely in the mirror I breathed a sigh of relief that this wooden circle did indeed land on the ONLY place on my stomach that there isn't a scar or a stretch marks. I felt better instantly! Covering up my new outfit with my baggy gray pants and t-shirt, I went to face the morning. Stepping out on to the boardwalk, smelling the salt air, seeing there wasn't huge crowds of people, all helped ease me in to today. The moment of truth came faster than I thought. I was to remove my "hiding clothes" while still on the boardwalk, then walk, *"ACTING NATURAL"* of course, to the beach. Now if they had any idea how a 250 pound woman works, they would know that I would keep bundled up in my cocoon of clothes until I was at water's edge. I've even been known to dive in fully clothed. Then, after looking around to make sure no one was looking, I would have made a made 15-second dash into the water, no matter HOW cold it was. I would have ducked down as low as I could get, with just my fat face bobbing on the waves. There I would have remained until the people I was with wanted to leave, then I would dash out, bundle up in the clothing, even if it was inside out, heading home feeling a great amount of self-loathing. But not today. Today was so different. It was a really freeing experience. Like watching in slow motion, the whole experience as surreal as it was, has helped me like my body a lot more. There were no laughs, pointing, nudging a friend to get a load of the beached whale. I was working. Even though it was walking in a very unrealistic way, doing something I would never even considered a year ago, this was perhaps, the most liberating day of my life. A few people would talk to the people around me about what was going on. They would give patches of the details and a few tourist snapped photos. The cameras were not as terrifying as they have been before. It was all for a purpose.

Don't ask me how, but I just know there are people out there who feel just like I do. Trapped in a body and world we have created for ourselves, not having any clue on how to get to normal from here. Now I know. I also know it is my mission to share this with everyone who wants to listen. Not being super-human, you will see and have seen, I might add, all my weaknesses, joys, fears, pains, warts and all. There is nothing special about me, I just finally get the big picture of a few simple facts.

Fact One : Diets don't work. They have a beginning and end. When it ends, you have to mentally go through the struggle of doing this for the rest of your life. Think about this. The diet industry makes BILLIONS, yes *BILLIONS* of dollars a year. If it worked, if *ANY* of it worked, it would only be in business for one year. After that, we'd all be fit and fine.

Fact Two : Eat what you like with *MODERATION* followed by a big serving of *MOVEMENT!* Think small when it comes to food and *BIG* when it comes to moving!

Fact Three : Exercise can be what YOU make it! My big lie that I always told myself was that I didn't have TIME to exercise. This is just 30 minutes a day people...think about it, we WASTE more time than that! Sarah told me, and I love this, that she *WASTES* more than 30 minutes a day *THINKING* about if she should exercise or not! We have to just get it in our heads that we need this 30 minutes a day. It has to come as regular for us as breathing.

Fact Four : Make some human connections. Network for your exercise, find what you enjoy doing and get a friend involved. Talk to strangers, get out of your comfort zone, don't worry about what anyone thinks and most of all....love yourself enough to do this right.

Fact Five : The **BIGGEST** and last fact. Don't take this as an insult, it's not meant to be (the last time someone said that to me they REALLY did insult me, but I promise that ISN'T what I'm doing here!)....**HUMANS LIE**! This is a fact, no matter how good and noble we might think we are, we all lie. We delude ourselves sometimes so much, we start to believe it. There have been so many times I have said, *"I tried that diet and it doesn't work"* when the truth was, that I just didn't stick to it. We all make excuses, (little white lies) as to *why* we can't beat our weight problem. ***WE ARE OUR OWN WORST ENEMY*** when we do this.

Today, stripping off from my *COMFORT CLOTHES*, walking across a beach and then getting loads of film and photos done in front of ANYONE who happened to be there, was a real moment of truth. This is the bare honesty that makes my heart beat faster and lets me know I'm alive. My body is far from being where I want it to be, but that is fine. I'm working on it, putting a very honest effort forth to make it happen and being CRAZY enough to put it all out there for anyone to see. This I do for a reason. For the first time in my life certain things have become crystal clear. Life isn't worth living if we can't help our fellow man. Period and simple. I want to help. No matter what shape you are in, we all need motivation, inspiration, positive encouragement and FRIENDS. That is what this journey is about people. You give to me just what I need in a very big way and I hope, on some level, you are all getting something from this.

But here I am on the beach. Not cracking a single joke about being a beached whale. For decades I would crack the fat joke before someone else could. It was easier that way and I knew then that I was in control of it a bit. But I think my days of putting myself down are going to get less and less. Leaving Atlantic City I felt that I was the biggest winner that ever visited. No one knew this but me. This feeling of facing my fears, living through them, even without Morton by my side to give me a little word of encouragement, showed me that I'm going to be fine. After all, the tankini fit and my confidence went a few notches higher. Priscilla - Atlantic City, NJ to Harrisburg, Pa *THANK YOU* to Chris at Caesars Atlantic City for helping me with a room for this whirlwind defining moment in my life, again.

Day 202 July 21, 2007 - Saturday - Harrisburg to Dillsburg, Pennsylvania

It was late for me this morning when I woke up at 7 am. This was luxury sleeping until this strange hour. Morton and I were going to go by bicycle over to the radio studio, just 4.5 miles away, but there were delays. So many things to do, a meeting that was going to happen to decide just where our next leg is going to start from and time, who I am still working on mastering, slipped through my fingers. We had to use a car to get there, since we always like to be early for these things. My head is not set for lateness and it just gets me too flustered. I always like to get there early and waiting gives me time to reflect on what is about to happen. A good time to pull my thoughts together, rather than just winging it.

Today, even though I am a bit early, so is Kelly, the lady who is doing the interview. She is fantastic and we have a great chat about every sort of topic, before heading back to the studio. I fight back the urge to crack a joke about me having the perfect body to work in radio. I tell myself to stop being my own worst enemy. Giving myself a big mental hug instead, I smile and sit in the chair with arms. Ahhhh....the chair with arms. A year ago you were out of my league. If, perhaps, your seat was wide enough, I might give you a try. But too many times have I been wedged into a chair with arms that left big welts on my legs from my fat pushing into the arms. It wasn't the chairs fault, trust me. I knew to sit on the floor (even though it was hard to get up,

I always had the excuse the my leg had fallen asleep, therefore needing a hand from Morton) sit on the couch, even sit on a cement block...anything but a chair with arms. Today though, I sat in it, with room to spare. It was divine! The studio was exciting, but you have to just think about it being a room with some people chatting in it. Still learning, with a long way to go before I can safely say that I know a thing or two, about a thing or two. I like to learn. The best way to learn is to listen and watch, but today I needed to speak up too.

The show started and in a matter of seconds all my butterflies had flown away. The chat was great, fast and the hour sailed by with me not getting out a lot of the things I wanted to say. This journey is *BIG*, very big and I think the whole idea of it sometimes is too big for just an article, story or even an hour segment. When we are driving away to get Morton's passport photos done for his British passport which needs renewed, we listen to the radio. The doctor who was on, says something about how we afford to do this. I think a lot of people must think we are fabulously rich....not true! We are getting by on the kindness of strangers, a very limited budget, t-shirt sales, sea glass sales and banner advertising. The doctor also says something that makes me wish I was back in the studio. He says about gastric by-pass surgery working for some people. That some people can't lose weight (or words very similar) and he has seen good results from this. *YIKES....*where is that time machine that will get me back there!? Surgery, under any circumstance, is risky. I know this. I have had surgery, several times in my life. This surgery however, is a life-long commitment to on-going medical care and is *VERY* risky. Since we have started our journey, Morton and I have lost count over how many people we have actually met who have had a loved one die from this surgery! *DIE* people, as in cease to breath! Being fat is horrible. This I know. It is so unhealthy, but the point with the surgery is that it is *NOT* magic. Some people gain weight, some people have horrible eating problems, all bad things...but the thing that really scares me is some people die. Dying is what I want to avoid. The other thing that people fail to see is, this isn't a quick fix. You still have to do all the work. It takes time, unless you are like a man we met in South Carolina who couldn't eat more than a few spoons of soup before becoming sick. He had to stay in the hospital for over six months, lost his job and lost weight so fast that his skin is just hanging. The doctors wanted him to have surgery to get it removed, all the extra skin, but he told us he is so scared of surgery now, after having it four times to correct problems with his initial surgery, that he just can't face it. Some people feel that the surgery is their only hope. *PLEASE* just give yourself an honest try at doing this with moderation and movement first people. Just think, the money you save on the surgery, you will be able to buy a new wardrobe when you get to your healthy new size. Best of all, you will have made the *LIFESTYLE* changes that are vital for being healthy and keeping the weight off. I see the surgery as the medical professions way of trying to help a situation they feel is hopeless...but *YOU ARE NOT WITHOUT HOPE!!! YOU*, yes you, can do this. If I can, so can you. There will be tough days, I'm not telling you it's all peaches and creme. There will be days that you don't WANT to move for 30 minutes. But then there will be the days, like days I'm experiencing now, that you KNOW, without one little doubt, that YOU really do control your own body. *HELP YOURSELF PEOPLE!!!* I did make a call back in to the radio station, maybe while I'm still in the area I could pop back in for an update on finances and gastric bypass but our schedule is rather full. Did I mention I'm getting a grand-child? What a great reason to stay alive.

Sarah & Graeme have a lovely image of our little guy, still waiting to see when his birthday is going to be, but her doctors are thinking next week. Isn't that exciting? Alexander will soon be here and all will be right with their world, except for the sleeping at night part. My mind lets go of the things I didn't say in the interview, I think of Alexander. Even though I won't get to be around him for the first part of his life, I will be alive (hopefully) to be there when he is learning to walk, run and then ride a bike. I will play with my grandson in the park. There was a time when this was a far out of touch dream for me. I never thought I would be able to ride a bike, now I am thinking about all the things that I will be able to do. Run, swim and not just splash about in the pool, rock climb, ski, who knows, I might even try snowboarding and skateboarding....anything is possible.

Day 203 July 22, 2007 - Sunday - Dillsburg, Pennsylvania

For those of you that have never been, Hanover Pennsylvania is a great town to shop in. There are a lot of stores, great variety and best of all, incredible bargains. If we are going to outfit ourselves for the next leg of the journey, we need a wee budget to do that.

We are taking the money from the sea glass sales, not a penny more, to make this happen. Morton and I have to really pinch all our pennies to get the needed gear and this is the place to do it. Flipping back the pages of my memory, James is now 8 instead of 24. We are doing back-to-school clothes shopping. On a budget. There was the bargain of the century, name brand jeans in his size, an 8, for only $2.00 a pair. Not only did I get 4 pairs for that size, I decided to go ahead and get the 10's, 12's and 14's as well. After all, jeans never go out of fashion and they were only $2.00 a pair. This future shopping in Hanover happened at a very good time. James hit a growing streak and actually grew into the size 14's over the next two years. It happened just right, much like life does and we never seem to notice. Today we left James at home. He was reading a book and Mari, Morton and I were going to shop until we dropped. And we nearly did.

Store after store, bargain racks were piled through. I still find it really hard to not go for the largest size in the store. It is weird being able to actually shop in the regular ladies department, rather than just the plus size. It has opened up a whole new world of choice for me...and bargains. Turns out though, the mens department held some great treasures. Morton and I really need bright colored day-to-day shirts that aren't 100% cotton. We have learned that not only does white look bad fast out there, when it is cotton is stays wet all day if you get caught in the rain. We also need rain jackets that breath. Again, after hours of combing the shops, we really strike gold and get pretty much all our clothing for under $100.00. There are a few bargains that really thrill us. The 50-50 cotton/poly BRIGHT green t-shirts, name brand, that are 2 for $5.00. My packs of three undies for $1.00 (that is just 33.3 cents a pair!) and our breathable weather-proof jackets for $29.00 each. How we needed those! The trip finished with a visit to the grocery store. Since we have been back here, we have been ruined by the kindness of our family feeding us. I know they don't think twice about it. But we do. We really can't just say, "No, we don't want to eat *your* food, we will sit in this corner and eat our canned tuna and green beans combo!" yet it feels like a horrible bit of sponging we are doing right now. Not for long though, soon we will be back out there and Morton will will be opening cans for our dinner. Hopefully though he has learned the hard way that I don't want my cold canned sweet potatoes dumped on top of my cold canned spaghetti, juice and all. Ugh...the worst meal of my life, but still PERFECT because I had food to eat.

Day 204, 205 & 206 July 23, 24, 25, 2007 - Monday, Tuesday, Wednesday - Harrisburg, Pennsylvania
Route : The doctors visit turned to a three day waiting game for the wee one to arrive! It was SO worth it!

For all the people reading and waiting for the details...here is a BRIEF account of the long story I'm working on for here. Right now I'll just let you know he was 20.5 inches long, weighed 9.4 lbs., has lovely skin, is the most beautiful little love and is my *FIRST GRANDSON EVER*! His birthday is July 25th and he came into the world, after not wanting to leave his mommy, at 8:44 am.

The details of these last three days are so full of emotion. From watching my child go through the pains and joys of childbirth to holding my grandson, it has been a real rollercoaster of feelings. Many are very private and going into my offline journal, but I will try to explain how the days went. Sarah and I were finally going to get some time together on Monday morning at her doctor's office. On the way in though, she said that she wasn't feeling right. She called her boss and said she thought she might be going in to labor and might not be in today. She was half right. The doctor sent her to the hospital, where we spent the next 48 hours and more waiting. Sarah, poor Sarah, did all the work.

But then, after all the waiting, he was born and nothing else mattered. It is odd how it felt that time not only stood still for a moment, but time also felt eternal. Seeing my child holding her child made me finally understand the word "eternal" and appreciate it. All those worries, fears and doubts about what my future holds, her future holds or his future meant nothing anymore. All that matters is this moment. This precious, baby-scented moment that will be forever embedded in my mind. Alexander has completed my life. Even though Sarah had been through over 24 hours of labor, 3 hours of pushing and then a c-section anyway, she remained like a peaceful mother on a mission. No crying, no screaming, but the look of pain did cross her beautiful face. This was a look that broke my heart and made me love her even more...it that is possible. As her mom, I wanted to take her pain from her, but that isn't how this thing works. She had no choice, but remained calm and even managed to keep a sense of humor about her. Since Sarah and Graeme had been kind enough to share this experience with me, I got to be with her right until they rolled her away for the longest hour of my life. My job was simple then, just sit with the gear that Sarah & Graeme had brought with them to the hospital, waiting in the waiting room and trying to think *HAPPY* thoughts. There was another new gramma to be and we shared a bit of chit chat and then that moment I have been waiting for my whole life happened. Graeme and the lovely nurse who had been helping Sarah for the last few days, casually pushed up in front of the glass windows that I had taken my eyes off of. There he was. With a little cap on his head, wrapped snug in his blanket and looking as peaceful as his beautiful mother. Leaning close to him, I whispered that he had been a naughty boy, making his mommy wait so long to see him. But it was worth it. My heart felt like it would burst with love, daisies, butterflies and all things BABY! This is what true love is. Graeme let me know that Sarah was resting now. We were both worried about her, but the worst was far behind us now. Happy days were here and will be as long as the little man is with us.

Seeing my grandson for just a moment was all I needed to fall hopelessly in love with him.

Little Changes   **249**   *Priscilla Houliston*

NOW I understand how doting grandparents carry thousands of pictures and never stop telling you how fantastic *THEIR* grandchild is...and *THEY ARE RIGHT*! Never again will I be in a hurry or listen half-heartedly. I get it.

The time slipped by, evasive, fast, forever. Morton was at Sarah and Graeme's house giving our bikes a new paint job. The world I'm sure, ticked on, but I was counting the moments to get to actually hold him. Really though, as much as I wanted to hold him, I wanted to see Sarah with him in her arms. When this moment arrived, I thought I had prepared myself for it. I knew it would be heaven. Little did I know it would be like what it must be to see an angel holding a baby angel. Not one for being a cry-baby (unless the road is giving me a *REAL* hard time!) my face was soaked with tears. This sight, this pure vision, is what all of my dreams have ever been made of. Perfection, peace and this joy that was going to make my heart burst!

So many people have been emailing your congratulations and he even shares the same birthday as several of you, but one question that keeps going through is, *"Will you still continue your journey?"* To that I say, without hesitation, "YES!" As tempting as it is to lose the rest of my 100 pounds on taking Alexander for walks, the whole purpose of this mission we are on is to wake people up! We all need the 30 minutes a day and as long as I'm breathing, I'm going to be spreading that word. Now more than ever.

My mind goes back to one of the most special moments that we have had since starting the journey. It was the gramma we met who was out with her grandson, age 6, for their first walk together. She explained that seeing our story on the news got her to think that she had little changes to make and the first was going to be going to the park each day with her grandson. This story, which had already touched my heart, now makes me want to go back and follow up with her, let her know that now I understand how important it is to her to be healthy for her grandson. Finding that THING that makes us smile, makes us want to get up in the morning, is the real key to happiness. Seeing our little Alexander is the one special thing, combined with thousands of others, that is going to make me ride harder, faster and further than I have ever ridden before. He will be with me, as you all are, along the way. Life, I'm happy to report, is beautiful. So is my grandson, but then, aren't they all?

Day 207 July 26, 2007 - Thursday - Harrisburg, Pennsylvania

Today we were suppose to be in York, Pennsylvania, for our last full day of non-stop filming. But little Alexander changed that. We were also suppose to go and see Cindy and her mom in York...again, they were kind enough to let us reschedule for next week. Today I got to go spend the entire day, while Graeme was at work, with Sarah and son. Don't worry, I'm not going to rattle on with my non-stop love fest of words trying to describe him or how I feel. Just put this down and the best day of my life, as they all are! While we are still here, I'm going to be walking this very tight rope of making sure everything is getting set for our trip to resume, while squeezing every single second of family time in. It is going to be tough, but hey, I work well under pressure. Since I have learned to live in, and love, the moment...everything seems to be easier.

The day was full of special, tender times and I kept crying...pretty much all day. This feeling of love is just overwhelming. Since Sarah and Graeme have let me share in so much of it, I actually know more about his birth than the birth of my own kids! I can also watch from a distance, savoring each second I see the three of them together...family. While Alexander lays on his mother's shoulder and sleeps, I realize that is what they mean when they say, "Home is where the heart is" he is home, so near to his mommy. It makes me start to cry again, not sobs, just tears rolling down my cheeks. Sarah smiles and gently teases me about it. Sarah and Graeme are lucky enough to not only have this child, this miracle, this blessing, but they are lucky enough to understand just what that means. They will be the best parents on the planet. This baby is so loved.

When I leave the hospital in the evening, Morton and I run a mad-dash series of errands for things we have to do. We still have to focus on how we are going to get to the north-west and if we can even go to Alaska right now. Even though Morton has gotten his immigration resident card now, he still has to get his British passport renewed. It is always something. We have both learned to be so flexible. Rolling with the punches is the only way to be happy. Plans change always and being open to changes has become our credo.

Day 208, 209, 210 July 27, 28, 29, 2007 - Friday, Saturday, Sunday - Harrisburg, PA

These were busy, beautiful family days. We were lost in the glow of a new baby and all that goes with that. From bringing baby home to listening at night for a cry that I was needed, I relished every second of it.

Day 211 July 30, 2007 - Monday - Harrisburg, Pennsylvania

This morning I woke up with a sore throat and fever. I started getting sick yesterday afternoon and I put a distance between everyone and me. Thinking about just being in the hospital, where it is *FULL* of sick people, I remembered each and every person that hacked my way while we were in the crowded elevator. I can't be sick right now, but almost hacking my lungs up, I decided I mostly likely am. There is no money for a doctor to confirm this, I just have to wait and see what happens. Taking my laptop to a corner of the house without people in it, I try to work. My face sweats as though I just rode my bicycle up Mt. Everest. The keys seems to wiggle out from under my shaking fingers. Trying to focus on work, I make some phone calls that need made and edit some photos. Seeing the ones of Alexander (I have taken over 1,000 now and still not enough!) I miss him, though he is right upstairs. I know I need to keep away. It would be the worst thing ever to pass this on to that dear little soul.

Since the clock is ticking on our departure for the west coast, I start putting the feelers out for a lift WEST. We are going to stay in this area for another two weeks to help Sarah. She has to recover from her surgery and as her mom, I have to be here for her right now. This means that we will start in the state of Washington, bicycle south and not be in the tight wrath of winter. Loading up with vitamin C and other drugs, I wonder WHY we don't have sore throat lozenges like the ones in Britain. They have antiseptic in them and just one or two kills anything that is growing in your throat. We are all out of them though and I suck on one from America that really doesn't do anything my make my throat numb for about five minutes. My eyes start to get hot and swollen and I'm so glad I have been staying away from Sarah and the baby. I wonder where Michael Jackson gets his wacky masks and wonder if I can get a hold of one of them. For now though, I work on the computer, trying to get caught up on things that I haven't been able to get going.

Cheap airfares show us that we can get out west for about $200 each. Right now that might as well be $200,000 each. The sea glass sales haven't been as good as we were hoping for. Something will turn up...it always does, so I'm not going to fret or sweat about it. I'm too busy right now sweating from this fever. Morton and I spend the day in isolation, then decide to go to my son's house to be away from the baby. As sick as I feel I'm not sure when I'll be back in his little world. Tomorrow we have loads lined up, but I'm not sure what I'm going to be able to do. As it is right now I can't really swallow, have a temperature of 103 to 104 and think I will try to upload all our files that I have been working on. Maybe I'll take two aspirin and call you in the morning.

Day 212 July 31, 2007 - Tuesday - Dillsburg, Pennsylvania

Several months ago when we were in Myrtle Beach, South Carolina at the *Court Capri,* we were being interviewed by a lady in lovely shoes. They were more like a little boot, tall heels and way to petite for my feet. We started talking about weight and shoes because she mentioned something she had seen on *Desperate Housewives.* The reporter told me that there was a line about one of the ladies gaining weight and saying something about at least her shoes would still fit her, but that isn't how it works. When I explained to her that it wasn't true, she said she had never thought about it. But as long as I can remember, I have had fat, wide feet. Today I got a pleasant surprise.

Since the filming of us on the bicycles was off today due to my sickness, we decided to go to York to get our shoe size taken. MBT, who are providing us with shoes for the entire journey have a shop that is a dealer. I had been in there last August, for the first time ever and fell in love with the shoes. The people in the shop had fitted me, when I had been in the last time and even had a file on my feet! This was fantastic. A photographer from the *York Daily Record* had came out to photograph the fitting and it was a real thrill to have gone from a size 45 to a size 43. These sizes are in EU sizing...I think it was 12, then 10 in the US sizes.

Today I feel bad, breathing on everyone. It is tough to be out, head spinning and trying to smile through it all...but I have to keep moving. The ride is going to be starting again soon and there are still so many things to do. After the shoe fitting, we stopped for a brief moment in the *Harley Davidson* factory. We were going to speak to someone about doing a trip around the shadow of our journey, right after we finish. It would be great for going back and getting some footage for the film...but we have to wait and see. Today I'm way too sick to do any flogging of our ideas. I just needed to get home and put my head down.

The car was about 1,000 degrees inside. My shorts were stupid to wear, as I burnt my legs when I sat in it. We got the windows down and were heading back to Dillsburg. Not long in the car, Morton asked to pull over. He thought he was going to be sick. It seems that I had given him my BUG. Sorry Morton...but you *DO* say that I never give you anything! Morton takes a walk beside the car, looking back at us every once in a while. He stops to bend over slightly, but isn't sick. Instead he gets back in the car and leans his head back until we are home to James & Mari's house.

The cool air conditioning is a blessing. The water that comes out of the sink is a blessing. I don't even sit on the sofa, instead I lay right on the floor. Not as far to fall if I pass out. There are so many things that need done on the computer, I try to focus and pretend I'm not sick. My eyes are sore though. There are spots in front of them. If feels like my chest is so tight. Being healthy people, is priceless. After several hours, reading LOADS of emails (you are all getting very creative on how to get us out to Seattle) and somehow I even managed to get some new T-Shirt designs uploads, I switch off. Stay tuned for tomorrow is the FIRST of August, a day closer to the journey starting again and a day closer to leaving the comfort of a home and a place to lay my fevered head.

Day 213 August 1, 2007, Wednesday Harrisburg, Pennsylvania

It is always a joy when a new month rolls around. Today was no exception. We woke up early to catch a ride back to Sarah's. I figure that if I keep my distance and just admire him from afar, I won't make Alexander sick. Plus, I think I'm on the upswing of this throat thing. The website has been growing so much, there have been a lot of changes I have been wanting to make with it, just haven't had the time. Today is going to be my day to pull it all together. I have to make all the pages load faster, the images more efficient and get our banners and advertising under control. It has been a good six months now and we can see what is working and what isn't working.

Ahhh, the baby! He has his first check up today, a call from Sarah tells me he has gained a pound plus. The only time it is alright to be fat, is when you are a baby. Maybe that was my problem, I grew up too quick and didn't lose my puppy fat.

I'm not sure if anyone else had ever had this happen, but at my school, we would have several lessons in *"why it ISN'T good to be fat"* all through the year. First, the lunch aid, a volunteer mom, would stand guard over your eating. Our hard plastic molded plates would have to be cleaned up before you could leave. If you were a little pudgy, you would hear, "A big girl like you should be able to finish your lunch!" True, but hurtful. The other cringe time for me at school was when we would get weighed in. *WHO* on earth came up with this system? The school nurse would push the big scale with proper weights on it in the room. We would line up, along the edge of the classroom by the big windows, facing the chalkboard and the scale. I would take my time lining up so I would be near the back, but not the last person. I learned very young how to keep my humiliation factor to a minimum. The school nurse would push the weights around, clanking the big bulky one up to the next highest level if you were over a certain weight. She would then tap and fiddle with the little weight until she could determine just how much you were weighing in at. It always seemed to take hours when I was the person on the scale.

Stepping on it, with my shoes on, I would hope for the best but expect the worst. The nurse, always a female in my day, would tap, adjust, force the little one to TRY to get up to the very end and get my bulk weighed, but then she would always have to reach for the heavy weight. Pushing it over, she would then have to tap the little one back, one click at a time, until it rested in the dead center. By this time I would be sweating, dizzy and wishing I could be like an uncle of mine who jumped out a window in the sixth grade, never to return to school. The room would always go silent. The rustling of papers, passing of notes, whispering of playground antics, would screech to a halt. The only sound that could be heard would be the teacher's pencil, tapping on the desk, waiting for the figure to be called out across the room and recorded. This, was the worst part of my school days. All eyes would fall on me. I was the fattest girl in the class and everyone would want to know just how fat that was. The little buggers who couldn't pay attention at any other time, were now all ears, waiting to hear the number and then tell it to me when they would ask how much I weighed. Kids are cruel, but so are the nurses and teachers that put us through this. This was more than 30 years ago, when childhood obesity wasn't really a problem. Looking back, I wasn't even THAT fat. But in the day, I was huge.

When the nurse called out the number, the teacher would call it back to her. Though they were only standing four feet apart, loud, outside voices were used. Once in sixth grade, which was my biggest year in elementary, the nurse had to repeat my weight TWICE, since my teacher had his pencil in his ear, using the eraser like a q-tip. It was the worst. The boy I had a crush on and just might have liked me, was right at the front. The angle that he was at, I knew he had to hear what was said. If not the first time, surely the second or third. But this year, I had something that was on my side. I was putting on weight ABOVE the belt. A classmate with the nickname, Greaser, shouted from the back of the room..."*AND it's all on top!*" when they made the third call out of my weight. That was alright. As long as I wasn't going to get picked on about the weight, I could handle the teasing of my body changing. This was really the start of my upscale struggle with weight. The next two years my parents put me in a private school with no exercise and the weight just piled on. Eighty pounds in two years and I can assure you, it wasn't *ALL* on the top! By the time I went into high school, I wanted to just die. I was so much bigger than everyone. I didn't fit in. I didn't want to put my gym clothes on, it was easier to take an "F" in that subject. The battle with the bulge had began and would grip me for over 30 years.

Today, eating ice cream at lunch, I think about these things. The ice cream is to help my throat, hmmm. That sounds good, but I know me. I have to just control what I eat, or more importantly,

HOW MUCH I eat. With all my fat ghosts from the past to remind me and my fat legs still sticking out the bottom of the shorts that I'm wearing, I make a new pledge to myself that I *will* go for a bike ride tomorrow. A long one. Early, to beat the heat of the day. My baby fat is finally coming off and I want to keep it that way.

Day 21| August 2, 2007, Thursday Harrisburg, Pennsylvania

This warm-glow feeling that comes from being around family you love should be captured. All the warm-fuzzy moments are just too sweet to load the page up with, but trust me, this is the medicine that will carry me down the long and winding road that is waiting for us. Morton and I are on our own for a bit today and that is when it really sets in that it will soon be like this again. Just the two of us. No camera crew, except when we are meeting somewhere to film or doing interviews. No "acting natural" and worst of all, no family around. I have talked with Sarah about how I'm going to cope being away from her little new family. The changes that will happen to all of them during the next 18 months are going to be lost forever, unless I can *stress* to them of the importance of keeping a journal, in pictures, words, videos or all of them! I hope I get through. Drifting back, as I like to do, I see a brown leather covered book. A big book with a lot of faces on the cover. The shape of a tree is embossed on it and the words at the top, printed in gold letter, announce that it is my family tree. The last name is the name of my first husband, Sarah & James' father. This book was a gift from my sister, the start of what should have been something beautiful. When my Sarah first arrived, I was as good as gold about writing in it a lot. I even toted it to my new relatives and asked for missing links to solving this puzzle. Sarah was my first-born, arriving just 10 months and one day after her father and I had eloped to Florida. My family was in shock, my whole world had changed and I was just 18. Looking back now, I wonder how it all worked out. I was just a child when I had her, but I wanted to do everything right for her. My whole world has never been the same since that day in September almost 26 years ago now. The first couple days I was home from the hospital with her I wrote in the book often. Things were different then, pre-digital, with photos. I tried to take a lot, but on my 110 camera, which was horrible, I knew I would have to get the film developed and we were on a budget then that is almost as tight as the budget we are on right now with the journey. As my days got busier, I'm ashamed to admit, the book got stuck away and barely written in. By the time Sarah was three I really never wrote in it again. Little reflections on her changing face, the appearance of her golden curls, the way her twinkley blue eyes would light up at the mention of going to see Neen, all observations that would have taken mere minutes, passed without notice. Blinking my eyes, twenty-six years have gone quicker than the time it takes to type this paragraph. Perhaps one of the reasons my grandson feels so very special to me is that I get to be part of this chain now. Telling Sarah the words my mom told me, trying to get her to savor every second, without scaring her that she will never be able to record it all, I decide that I have to just get back in the moment. Twenty-six years behind and twenty-six years ahead don't really matter at this moment. Now is the time.

Day 215 August 3, 2007, Friday Harrisburg, Pennsylvania

It seems odd to be bicycling without our trailers, but that is just what we did today. After loads of real work, hours on the computer and phone, Morton and I pushed the bicycles off for a nice ride. Eight miles is nothing to me anymore, but still feeling a bit under the weather and with the real weather being so hot and muggy, eight miles seemed to be just right. We couldn't find my glasses before we set out. I searched all over and Morton peeked in the places that I might have missed. I even called my sister to see if she had grabbed my glasses by mistake, but touching her head, she confirmed the pair holding her hair back were indeed her own. Thinking that my vision is a lot better than it actually is, I soon discovered that I really need to get an eye examine. Even when I have my glasses on for distance now, my short sight is coming up...well...short! There is this sweet spot, about the length that I work away from my computer at, that I can actually see in. Closer or further and I'm left squinting.

Morton has put a little jingling bell on my handlebars, which will come in handy on the miles ahead and as soon as we get beside the river, I waste no time in testing it out. It is old-fashioned sounding and reminds me of a bike from childhood. It had been a hand-me-down bike, made for a boy I think, but it had the same, tingle-ling-ling bell on it. I liked it then and I like it now! There are people that chat with us when we stop to take some pictures of sculpture beside the Susquehanna River. We stick out like bright orange fluorescent thumbs and that is what we want. We hear peoples stories about what stage of health they are in, tales of relatives who they are sure can get some inspiration from our trip and even ideas are exchanged, on topics that DON'T include exercise or health.

As we ride and I look across this river I remember growing up thinking of it as a great divider. We would go in to the "big city" for renewing car registrations, anything to do business-wise, but NEVER, ever, for pleasure. Since my dad grew up on a farm in western Pennsylvania, the city was his idea of a nightmare.

Traffic, crime, red lights, cramped quarters, no privacy, no nature, no need to visit. Last summer I tried, to no avail, to talk my mom and dad on a trip in to the State Museum in Harrisburg. I told them how I could drop them off on the corner, we could have a wheelchair for my mom and then go in and spend a few hours in this incredible time machine. Neither one of them wanted to. The city was still a place they would only go if they were forced. For a long time, I had felt the same way about cities. Cramped, crowded, loud, nice places to visit, but I wouldn't want to live there. Then I moved to Scotland. You could hardly say we lived in a city. It was a little market town, with only one or two stop lights. But this was city to a country girl. My husband's house sat right on the main road where the bus, truck and car population was heavy. Double-deckers would start rattling by as early as 5 am. Morton was always closing the curtains, as soon as I would push them open. The neighbors could indeed see in, but I wanted to see the sun. I learned really quick though how right he was, as a whole top-deck of bus passengers heading to work one morning looked right in our second-story window, as I was shoving the curtains open in my pajamas. This would be the lack of privacy that my dad had been on about. Today though, riding the bike beside the river, I saw this city for the first time. It was quiet by the river, even though there was a steady stream of traffic moving beside us on Front Street, the soft green five foot sweep of grass that separated us was enough. There were lots of people out walking, roller blading, jogging, bicycling and just strolling. The benches held people who were chatting, reading and just looking out over the wide brown river. It was a peaceful scene. Not scary, not crowded and even though there were many people around, it didn't feel like there was a loss of privacy. Morton and I could have sat down on the grass, discussed the meaning of life and no one would have looked twice. People were going about their own way, even though we were bright orange. It felt nice and easy. The view across the river is lovely. Little islands come and go, depending on how high the river is. There is a couple in the water, wading out towards one of the islands. There are Canadian geese walking beside us in front of the governors mansion. Two little boys throw their bikes down and the peaceful scene gets shattered.

We had stopped to get some pictures of the geese, one of my favorite creatures, when these two boys decide to interact with nature. Morton and I are both on our bikes, at the edge of the path, just watching. I quickly look around to see that there are no parents with them, then I guess them to be about six and eight years old, brothers I would also guess. They set about chasing the geese, but in a very scary fashion. They are trying to drive them out into the traffic that is just a few feet away, shouting, swearing and even trying to hit and kick them. Morton and I stand as helpless observers while I wonder what has gone wrong with my peaceful, easy moment. The boys are bad. Of course you could get into the discussion of who, what, where and why they ended up wanting to do bodily harm to geese at such a young age, but my computer would die a natural death long before we could finish that. These boys are just bad. Simple. The geese are running, flapping and trying to get away from these bad boys. The boys, very street wise, stop short of running into traffic themselves, but they do manage to chase one of the geese on to the road. Cars and trucks line the three-lanes of pavement and behind us is the stately home the governor lives in. What should we do? What are we allowed to do? Is it acceptable for me to yell at them to knock it off? How about stepping out to stop traffic? Instead, I do what a lot of us do in life, nothing. I watch in horror and hope for the best, the true sign of a person in a non-active role in life. This can't be good. There are brakes squealing, horns blowing and a few near misses, but I'm glad to report the goose made it back to the sanctuary of the grass. One of the boys headed down a ramp that led him to the river's edge. The other, younger brother, followed him. The geese by this time were all down there, trying to get away, yet not seeming to want to get out on the water. Things were being thrown at the geese and the older boy kept both his middle fingers in the air, shouting curse words, as he tried to get the goose who had been in the traffic. Kicking and running, it all happened in about three minutes. The geese were then all in the water, with the boys standing at the edge, picking things up and throwing them at the lovely creatures. Bored, they got back on their bicycles and headed off. Morton, who hadn't said a word as we watched this terrible show unfold, looked at me and raised his eyebrows so high I thought they would meet his hairline, which is at the BACK of his head. "Wonder where the parents are?" he asked me. We sadly both knew the answer. The parents were missing their children growing up. Instead of being out here with them, they had sent them out to play. There isn't anything wrong with that, but they should have first taught their children to respect other living things.

Our ride had taken on a new feeling now. The sunset bike beside the river now had these images of innocent people being caught in a wreck by geese being chased out on the road. We always imagine the worst, or at least I do. This is a habit that I have to break. I don't like it and have been doing it way too long. If the phone rings late at night, I'm thinking of only bad things. If a loved one is late arriving, again, I think the worst. This is something that I will change. It will take lots of time and effort on my part, after all, I've been doing it most of my adult life. Children never imagine the worst. They are incapable of that I think. They live only in the moment, not thinking even three seconds ahead. That is why these boys could chase a goose out into traffic. They never stopped, for one little second, to think of who would have or could have been killed. A goose, an innocent stranger in a car or even themselves, could have all been killed. But not today. Maybe the boys aren't bad boys. Maybe they are just living so hard in the moment, they can't even imagine what the next 60 seconds will hold. What if all the energy I wasted on thinking of the worst happening, I could just let go of? It would lighten my heart. Of that I'm certain. It will be a challenge, but then, since discovering that I really can do anything in life that I put my mind to, I'm up for a challenge. *Always look on the bright side of life....da, dum, da, dum, da, da, da, da, da-dum!*

Day 216 August 4, 2007, Saturday Harrisburg to Dillsburg, Pennsylvania

Saying goodbye and seeing people go out of your life that you love is tough. This morning, I'm reminded of this as my sister and niece head off to Florida. Where did our little seconds together go? Blinking the tears from my eyes, I actually manage to not cry. We will all get together soon, but then thinking realistically, the next time will probably be in 18 months at least. Sarah and Graeme have been so kind and gracious to us, letting us invade their space, block their kitchen with our bright orange bikes, eat their food and get in on the very first moments of them becoming a family. Graeme is a very special guy that I feel safe to say, is perfect for Sarah. I don't want to ever become a monster-in-law, so I decide to go spend a night or two with my son and his wife. Morton and I have been working hard to get our things in order, last-minute everythings taken care of and gearing up for life on the road again. How fast it will be here! The thought of not having a clean shower to step in to each day is at the front of my mind. So is drinking out of a glass that has water and ice in it and not just a re-filled, luke warm or hot, plastic bottle of water that has been filled under the tap of a bathroom at a gas station.

We want to step up our game of who we are coming in contact with while we are out there. There are so many people that we want to help, meet with, speak with, motivate and get this message out that we ALL need 30 minutes a day. From press, politicians, groups, public schools and all the others that we want to reach while we are going by, is very important.

It shouldn't be an issue at all, but someone actually had emailed me when we were in New England to ask if I was Democrat or Republican. They had seen a photo of me with a State Representative and wondered. Health should never be based on politics. It is something that we all should strive for and who knows, it might even build a bridge or two of communication. Common healthy ground!

The short answer is, I have been living in Scotland for the last 5 years, then living on the road for the last six month. I am as far away from politics as you can imagine. There is no statement I'm trying to make, other than, *MOVE 30 MINUTES A DAY!!!*

Today though, I have some email from a number of Pennsylvania politicians who are wishing us well. It makes me really want to outline a challenge that people can hold close to their hearts. I don't want it to cost a cent, not to the person hearing it, not to the taxpayer, nothing. A free message, as free as the freedom of speech.

We are trying to do that with this website and journey. Putting forth a strong and positive message that, like our newest t-shirt design states, *"Anything IS Possible"* and we all have to take personal control of our own health and well-being. Morton and I know the feeling of just having 57 cents in our pocket. People might think we are joking about this, but we aren't. We know that we always get by, people are kind to us. We get fed by strangers, allowed to sleep In strangers spare rooms, backyards, motel room, church floors, even some incredible B&B's...but this feeling of funding is really getting to us. It is tough out there when you are down to your last 57 cents. These fears, even though you don't want them, take your mind away from things you should be thinking about. Like traffic and riding your bicycle in it. The sea glass is working, it is selling, but we still have MORE of it. We have sold almost 20 pieces so far. Nearly $400. but then, almost as if life knows this, Morton's fees for renewing his British passport are $300. Money isn't the root of all evil, not when you have it anyway. Things will happen, whether we worry about them or not. It is good to TRY to be prepared though. We don't want a fortune, just enough to get by.

A very wise man in North Carolina told me something that I will never forget. He said, "Everyone knows the word "more" but it's rare when someone knows the word "enough" --- very well put! This is something that I will hold with me, in lots of practices.

There was a time when I did think that if only I had loads of money, anything would be possible. But look around you at people that do have loads of money. Are they happier than I am? Nope! Happiness has no price tag. Remembering my grandmother, with her twinkling blue eyes, in her housedress, always smiling, I picture happiness. Real happiness. If she had her garden to putter about in, she was happy. When she held her grandchildren on her lap, she was happy. Simple pleasures in a world that is too often measured by wealth to equal success, is where we can all find happiness.

Sarah is catching a nap with her son sleeping on her chest and I'm watching, looking over the laptop with a map of the USA on the screen. So much distance, so many miles, so far away from them. Moments are frozen as I see them breathing up and down together. His little pink arm is tucked under his sweet face. His hand is just a shadow away from her wedding ring, held by a chain that she wears around her neck now. Her swelling at the end of her pregnancy is still with her, but any day now that ring will be able to go right back on her lovely hand, where it will stay. Sigh...what else in life is needed.

My eyes fall back to the laptop. I wonder for a second how much longer I'll be on this earth. We are all just here for moments. Just a few moments. The time for action is always now, since there is no other time. I still have a good 18 months of bicycle life, then after that, there is going to be at least six months of interviews, film releases, bicycling the shores of Britain and everything else that will keep me away from my two sleeping babies. The route is planned, the journey is in motion and I know it is possible. It won't be easy, it won't be fun all of the time, but it is written inside my very soul now that I have to do this. Not even a pull as strong as my very first grand-son can divert my attention from this. As my weight comes down and I feel more alive than I ever have in my life, I have to keep moving. People have to be shown that the weight issue can be beaten and we want to show then that. Not with things you have to buy, devices, tools, contraptions for losing weight. The answer is right inside all of us. How bad do you want it? No, really. How bad do you want it? If your mind is made up that it is what you need to do, you will get there. One foot in front of the other, one moment at a time, one reason after another...we can do this together. Of that, I'm 100% certain.

When Graeme comes home from work, Morton and I head out to stay with Mari and James for a night. I miss seeing them. I feel my "baby fever" has taken over my life. I also wonder just how many precious moments that I have changed for Sarah, Graeme and Alexander. Instead of just being the three of them, they have been "plus two" for the first 10 days of becoming family.

Exactly how this whole journey happened isn't as important as the fact that it IS happening. Just a few more days and I'll be thousands of miles from my family and Morton will be even further away from his. For tonight, I stay up late, until 1 am, working on the never-ending computer. Trying to have everything in order before setting out on our next leg, I smile as I remember all the hundreds of golden moments that today has held.

Day 217 August 5, 2007, Sunday Dillsburg, Pennsylvania

Since we are back on the road in just a wee while, Morton and I are getting TOUGHENED UP by sleeping on the floor in our sleeping bags. Believe it or not, it is actually comfortable. Today we are having a bit of last minute purchases for some items we still need. We get bright orange jackets that will be our only long sleeve attire. I'm delighted that I can fit in an XL. We also bought 97 cent bright orange ski hats to pull on over our bike helmets to keep the wind out and make them more visible. While I'm in the plus size section, looking for one pair of shorts that come above my knee, the only thing I find is $7.00. A bit more than I wanted to spend and Morton SHOCKS me by telling me that I should try the regular ladies department. Hmmm...perhaps I should. His little tip paid off. I found a pair of XL shorts that fit me and were only $5.00. It is so weird to be able to shop in this part of a store now. People must think it's odd when they see me squealing over wearing XL...let them wonder though. XL beats the heck out of XXXXXL.

Before we head for bed, we watch a DVD from Scotland, "Chewin' the Fat" and I get a twinge of homesickness for Scotland. The accents and the banter! Oh the banter! It is class. Pure class! You have to watch it to understand. We stay up late for having to get up at 5am, but we will have time to sleep later. Right now, we are squeezing ever last second out of our short time here.

Day 218 August 6, 2007, Monday Dillsburg to Harrisburg, Pennsylvania

There are way too many phone calls today. Morton lends a hand with helping me, but trying to arrange everything ourselves is a mind-boggling day. We keep at it though and then I get to head off for a doctor's appointment with Sarah. She is fine, baby is fine and I even SNUCK on the scale to see that I had lost another 3 pounds since I was there the last time. I'm shocked! My big fear while we are here and not riding for 30 miles each day, is that I would put on weight. But since I was just in there and snuck on their scales just two weeks before, seeing the scales show three pounds lighter was a thrill. This shows that my 30 minutes a day and moderation with food does indeed work! Who would have thought that the professionals that told us to watch our diet & exercise are right?

Little Changes   **256**   *Priscilla Houliston*

Day 219 August 7, 2007, Tuesday Harrisburg, Pennsylvania

We got a MEGA THRILL today. Our emails were stuffed with people saying they had seen the story in the *York Daily Record*. While I was working on the website, Morton rode to a newsstand and bought a paper. We were both over-the-moon that our story was on the front page! It also showed two photos on the front page of me trying on MBT's in York. I lost two shoe sizes in the last year.

The weather has us pinned inside today. I wanted a nice bike ride, but the humidity calls for some indoor exercise. It is going to hit 100 degrees today. A lot of you are emailing me that as this heat wave grips the country, you are getting your 30 minutes inside in the air conditioning. *GREAT IDEAS* people! From walking in the mall, to doing laps around your living room, jogging in the basement and using your exercise equipment that has been doubling as a clothes basket...you are really doing it.

Today, holding my grandson, we had a long chat about the journey. Actually, he just listened, adding a little grunt and wiggle here and there. He does understand that gramma just has to do this. Not just for him but all the other little babies out there that want to *KNOW & LOVE* their gramma's for a long time! Morton has hooked up a web cam for Sarah, who has promised to let us see him a lot out there. We also have a web cam now, so expect to see us a lot more. There is a way to capture it as video, so we just might come to you from some very exotic locations and some, not so exotic locations...like the tent.

Tomorrow we build up each trailer and load it with all the things Morton has assembled. We are then going to go for a ride over to City Island, where there is a big scale that is going to weigh the trailers. If mine is over 60 pounds, I will have to come up with a plan for a lighter load. Tick, tick, tick. The clock teases me, lures me and lulls me in to a false sense of security that there will always be more time. I know this isn't true, as the road calls.

Day 220 August 8, 2007, Wednesday Harrisburg, Pennsylvania

When it seems like panic was just really setting in with me, everything just clicked and worked out. I know this happens and I tell people all the time not to get flustered, worried, upset, etc...but when you are faced with the dilemma of getting yourself, your husband, your bikes, your trailers and your gear transported 3,000 miles to start riding and with so many people from all around the world watching, the pressure can set it. The car rental agencies weren't able to help. There are many reasons for this...too far, out of certain zones, too many people that have to review and decide. I don't blame any of them, it is how they do their business. It is just one of those things that should have worked but didn't. I know this is how life happens.

We had posted pleas on the internet for anything going west that we might be able to hop a ride on. I was actually considering hitching a ride from a truck stop...not a joke, but I didn't voice this to Morton, who would have not gone for it. It is a different story if you are asking a stranger to drive you over a bridge your bikes aren't allowed on, then to asking a stranger for a 3,000 mile ride that will last several days.

When my phone rang with a number I don't know, I was ever hopeful. The voice on the other end took all my worries away when she explained her situation. She is moving west, needs someone to driver her car and the dates work out great for both of us! We chatted for 20 minutes and are working out all the final details, but this, my friends, is how we are going to get out west! It is a giant load off my mind. Funny how our minds work though. As soon as that problem was solved and my phone was still warm from my conversation on it, a new set of panic problems set in...there is still so much to be done.

Morton has been doing his VERY best to make sure all our gear is in order. But he also knows that this time I'm going to be really hard-line on making sure the stuff doesn't weigh more than 60 pounds... total! This is a hard mark for him to reach. It might sound odd, but trust me, I know how heavy these trailers are when we are pulling them behind our bikes uphill. Any hill. They weigh a ton then. Just think of how heavy they will be with real mountains that are waiting ahead of us! Things like my hairbrush are getting replaced with a hair pick that I found from a bad perm I had back in the 80's. Who knows why I saved it or how I found it, but there it was in a box Morton had been going through. We are also looking through old camping gear that I had, also vintage 80's and are going to use a light that straps around your head to put on the front of my bike for night time emergencies. Even though we don't want to get caught out after dark, we all know that it happens to us.

Filming this journey out and the next 18 months are going to be just Morton and I. We will meet up with various film crews along the way, but we are going to be 100% on our own. We won't have a vehicle that can come and rescue us. We have to make our way, just as we did up the east coast of America...just the two of us. We don't want our journey to change and become an unrealistic reality show. People are different when you have a camera stuck in their face. We have better gear for filming, plus we are going to start doing live web cam chats. There is going to be a lot more filming, photographing and getting the feel of the trip captured.

Don't worry though, we will never film or photograph anyone we meet unless they agree to it.

Today we get a surprise delivered to us from Melissa at *Little Capistrano Bike Shop* in Cape Cod. She has sent us an incredible bike tool kit. It is so small, compact, light and perfect for what we need. Morton knows that this means his big, heavy, thirty-plus pound bag of "tools" he has found along the roadside will have to stay here in Pennsylvania now. He is going to be not too thrilled with giving up all his treasures, but I will allow him to hang on to the lightest of the two hatchets he has, for hammering down tent pegs and splitting wood for campfires. Besides that, the tool bag is history! Melissa has also sent us a computer for my bike that tells all sorts of things that will be incredibly useful for here. It will save me time at the end of each day as we can record our mileage from off of there rather than relying on a web mapping program. It will also be nice to be able to look down and see how fast we are going. It might make me cry going up the hills when I'm topping out at 3 to 4 mph and it might terrify me when I'm coming down the hills and hitting 30 plus. Either way though, it will be nice to know.

At a dollar store we found these packs that are for back-to-school lunches. They have a bit of padding on them and are bright green and orange! They look like they would just hold a sandwich, few treats and aren't huge, but what we want them for, isn't food. Morton is going to put all his tools, thanks to Melissa and his tire changing & patching kit in his. Mine is going to hold sunscreen and the first aid kit, which is also going on a serious diet before we leave here. Morton has it crammed with every medicine known to man and woman. Things that we never needed are riding along and taking up precious space and adding weight. Our bottles of drinking water are now going to sit neatly in the front of one of the trailers, where the huge tool kit and giant medicine bag had been. Our bottles had been crammed in here and there. We are also going to just switch to having 3 gallon jugs, with twist on caps, that we can fill our water bottle that is on our bike with. Again, we have Melissa at *Little Capistrano* to thank for these. This way, it will be easier for Morton to fill our fresh water each day and we will always start off with 3 gallons, plus our two bottles. We will splurge every few weeks to replace these gallon jugs, so they don't get nasty. Planning is something that this time we are a lot more prepared to do. When we first set off in January, we didn't have a clue. It was through a lot of kind people, dumb luck and not having any other choice that we managed to do the first 3,013 miles. We learned lessons that no school, college or even just every day ordinary life can teach you. We learned *road rules* the hard way. Now we want to be ready for the next part, wiser, healthier, more on top of things. I know though, that no matter how much planning we do, the first day out there we will both remember something we forgot. Let's just call this "life" and instead of panic, just solve the problem!

Day 221 August 9, 2007, Thursday Harrisburg, Pennsylvania

Tonight, during one of the biggest rain storms I have ever been caught in, we were all going to go visit my mom. Sarah, Graeme, Alexander, Morton and me...piled in the car during the crashing, the raining and the downpours. It was a night that we should have had better sense than to go out in, but we wanted to get a picture of our four generations. My mom, myself, my daughter and her son. The kind of thing that is WORTH going out on a night like this for. But alas, it wasn't meant to be.

We had just left Sarah and Graemes house and my lovely girl was just on the phone to her gramma to see what she wanted us to bring her to eat. But before Sarah could make the call, in the pour rain, with me behind the wheel, there was a loud, "CRACK" on the windshield. I thought for a split second that lightning had hit a tree, that broke a branch, then smacked in to the windshield. What had actually happened was the wipers, both of them, had flown off the car.

Turning around, we headed back to Sarah's to come up with a more sensible, PLAN B. It was stay in, safe and dry and wait until the rain was gone to fix the wipers. The rain, even though I was only in it for a total of 4 to 5 minutes, had soaked me. Memories of being on the bike in the rain grabbed me and I thought about how incredible it is to have a house to come in to and get dry. Morton scolded me about why I didn't use my new rainproof jacket that breathes and I tried to explain how the things for the trip couldn't be used right now.

Our white t-shirts, that we had made ourselves last November, are getting packed in boxes to be saved as mementos of the journey. They are well-worn, stained, torn here and there, but they have served us well. My size 3XL are baggy now, with the v-necks on them being way too loose. The new t-shirts are a 50/50 poly blend that are in bright green and orange. We also have 2 bright green tops that are 100% polyester, to help with the sweat problem. They dry faster than the cotton and although I have never been a fan of polyester, I'm hoping they will do the job.

Tonight though, we have a roof, towels a spare shirt and some amazing conversation with family. Plus, I get to end the night with giving my grandson a bath. Perfection.

Day 222   August 10, 2007, Friday Harrisburg, York Springs, York, Dillsburg, PA

We had arranged to visit a new friend from the website, while we were filming in York. I had gotten a really bad sore throat though and didn't want to contaminate anyone at the retirement center that she stays at. Our postponed trip happened today and was just BRILLIANT. Morton, my mother and I all drove down to York to catch up with Cindy (you know her as Cindyrella, from the BLOG) and finally get to meet her lovely mom, Gene. We pulled into the pretty place she lives and my mom got her work out walking down the long, lilac-bordered, halls. The staff and the residents we met were just so nice.

The best thing came when I knocked on the door and the ladies told me to come in. Cindy and her mom were all smiles and hugs and at once, I felt like I had known her mother my entire life. You could see kindness, fun and this lovely twinkle in Gene's spirit that spoke volumes to me about how I want to live my life. SMILING! Sure there are always things around that we can complain about, but why not try this...*SMILE* and *CHANGE* them. I hear you saying, "What about the things that can't be changed?" But look about you...*EVERYTHING* always changes. Why not for the better? Positive thoughts and actions active positive changes.

We had a few short hours chatting away, munching some of the goodies the ladies had out for us and I regretted leaving. This was a feeling that again stirred memories of childhood. It turns out, we had all lived in the same sort of areas for many years. We were just all great friends that had never met. The computer is a wonderful thing that bridges miles, ages, distances of all lengths and has the real power to do as much good as we want to do on it. This was a friendship that had started that I hope continues for the rest of my life. When we left to go back to my mom's house, instead of taking the faster, quicker, newer road, we decided to take the old trail that we had gone down almost every Friday night of my childhood. Mom would drive then, but not today. Today it was me behind the wheel, as mom and I drove literally down Memory Lane. Morton saw the first mile or two, then quickly started napping in the back seat.

In the days of my childhood, we would have been in a long, big, fake-wooden sided station wagon. There would be different colors of them along the way, but always a long station wagon. The mini-van of the 70's for us. They all had a front seat that held three, a middle seat that held three and a rear-facing third seat that held three children. If I was in the front, I would lean forward and bite the dashboard. It was a horrible habit I had that would get me scolded. I have no idea WHY I did it, I wasn't teething at 10, but it was just habit. As we rode along today, there were a lot of new and different houses at the first part of our familiar ride. Then we turned left, on to a really old back road. It is the kind of road that Morton says they got a snake drunk and then followed him to make the road. This one had stop signs in places that I hadn't seen for thirty years, hidden around corners that I remembered. Mom would panic a bit, thinking I wouldn't remember, telling me about the stop ahead...but I did. It seems that you can go home, at least drive past it.

We turned on to the road that my mom and dad had named. My dad built a lot of homes, developments and we moved around a good bit when I was growing up. This home that we were about to drive by though, would sum up most of my childhood. At least the best and worst times of it. The evergreen trees in the front that were now about fifty feet high, flashed back to little green wisps in pots that I helped my dad stomp the dirt around. The giant pony barn in my mind, turned in to the old large shed that sat down a path. It was all there. Including the *GOLD* colored metal siding on the house. The high-tech stuff of the times that looked tired and dated today. We stopped in front on the road, mom talking about the people that had bought it and wondering if they still lived there, me wondering how many life times ago I was there. The place was so familiar, yet completely different. My mind had the front yard being at least 10 good acres. In reality, it was perhaps 1/3 of an acre. The trees, so many trees, that we had planted were now all big and mature. I would like to say the same had happened to me, well, the BIG part had, mature...never!

At this moment, I would have traded anything I have or ever will have, for just one day back here. 11 years old, the summer everything in my life was still right. Still young enough to play *"Sassy Weasel"* in the front yard with my dad when he was cutting the lawn, with my little brother running, laughing and so much time still in front of me. I could have looked at the yard forever, but a car pulled up behind us and one was coming the other way. I had to keep moving on.

This road led us past houses of the people of my childhood. We would sing out names, mom and I, as we rode down a dirt road to what my dad called, "The Project" - which was an understatement. It was about 100 acres that he had bought with the idea of building a house at the top of it, amongst the giant rocks where mountain lions were said to live and roam. *The Cat Rocks.* We never made it to the top of that mountain though. Instead, my oldest brother and my father, started putting in lots for mobile homes to rent. Please don't think *TRAILER PARK,* this wasn't. Not in our day anyway.

Little Changes   **259**   *Priscilla Houliston*

This was a landscaped development, with incredible views, up the side of a mountain that we were never meant to live on. Instead, dad and my brother kept building "pads" for people to park their homes on. There were streams, giant fields of grass that we kept mowed for people to play and picnic on and best of all, it had *PRIVACY.* They designed it this way. It was laid out on large lots, some of them are over 1/2 an acre, beside streams, but all private with nice views. Today I saw the process of aging in my face. Talk about a wake up call for how fast time goes by. The sales lot, where dad had a collection of the latest mobile homes for people to purchase, was now a lot for a house. I remember the day when they used dynamite to move a rock face to make this lot happen. It was great watching from a distance. I wished I would have taken some pictures of it. If there would have only been digital cameras then, my library of images I have would be over 3 million, instead of just 300,000.

When we entered the park, it was bittersweet. Many of the very same trailers that my dad had sold, were still there. The trailer that I had *"SOLD"* when I was just 12, was setting on it's lot. The lot number had changed, the weeds were growing, but it was still there. My dad had given me a commission of $200. for taking the people through the homes, riding around in their car with them, showing them lots to sit the home on, that were available, then heading back to the office, I even pulled out the agreement I had seen my dad use before, had them sign it, took a deposit check from them and really impressed my parents. This was the first real money I had ever earned and I liked it. I also liked the fact that when I would walk past this home, with a family inside, there was this little satisfaction that I had helped put this together. I was a grown up now, at least in my head.

While we were driving through, remembering the people that made up this community, we were both laughing, smiling and remembering the past. One of my very best friends in my entire life, had lived there. Her mom still does and we were going to pop in and say hello. She was not home though, but it really was a treat just walking up on to the porch that I had sat on for ages, talking and laughing with Karen and her mom. Sweet memories that push me into dialing Karen's number. I hadn't talked to her since I have been in the area. Her mom is out she tells me, with a flat tire and we make arrangements to get together for a brief visit on Monday night. Karen is one of those friends that when you see each other, it feels like it was just yesterday that we were together. Time melts and smiles run rampant.

There were so many good things and bad things that happened here. Now the thought that just seemed to haunt me was, "I'm glad dad isn't seeing this." It would break his heart. Pot holes, weeds overgrown, the pavilion where so many picnics would happen is long gone and the shape of the homes themselves is shocking. This place isn't cared for anymore. Dad never went back after selling it to retire. Now I know why.

The road we came to next had an ice cream stand on it, that sold sandwiches too. This was only open in the summer and we were regulars. We would go in a few times a week for their home-made ice cream and beef b-b-q sandwiches. Today we stopped and found that the 30 years that have passed, haven't changed this place. The lady that was working in the kitchen, was the lady that owned the place. She cares, which is what makes a difference.

Now, we finally wound our way back home, driving past the graveyard where my dad is. My sister had just had my mom there and I asked if she wanted to stop. She said no and I was glad. My dad is buried there, but he's not there. He didn't believe in graveyards. He believed in Heaven, so much so, that no matter what your belief is, you would be certain that my dad is now in Heaven. That is how strong his faith was.

As we pass the graveyard, not stopping, my mood gets a lot lighter. I think I had been worrying that my mom would want to stop in. It is the feeling that there are at least 10 people in there that have been immediate family members or very close relatives, that I don't like. It reminds me too well that we are here for so short of a time. I take a deep breath, feeling so grateful to be alive. Life really is our most precious gift and tool, that we seem to fritter it away without much of a real thought to it. Me, I want to look closer, laugh longer, be kinder and really be alive.

Saying goodbye to mom back at her house, it breaks my heart driving away. She is on her own. She has people that look in on her, but really does love the company. I know my mom isn't a special case. There are so many people out there like this. Lonesome and wanting things to be as they have been in the past. That can never happen because the past is just that, past.

Day 223 August 11, 2007, Saturday Middletown, Dillsburg, Pennsylvania
We are off to sell stuff to raise funds for our gas going west. While it was still dark this morning, we pulled in to the old parking lot of a big former department store, that is now used to sell produce, this and that

and just about everything you can think of. This is where people came to sell their things they were tired of owning. In Scotland, this would be called a "Car Boot Sale", the "boot" being the trunk of the car. Here it is a flea market, though I have never actually seen anyone selling fleas. Call it what you will, it brings out a certain kind of people. On both sides of the pond, early morning shoppers are out with flashlights poking in the boxes, asking if you have any tools, movies or cd's. Standard stuff really. When we pulled in, there was a man putting up a tent. I pulled alongside him and Morton, with his window down said, "Excuse me, can you tell me who you see about setting up?" The man, coming closer, said, "WHAT?", to which Morton repeated his question. Speaking slow with his Scottish accent. The man, sticking his face almost in Morton's said, *"SPEAK ENGLISH!"* in a very loud and angry voice, at which point I stepped in to ask the same question. The man then said, just set up anywhere you don't see "reserved" on the ground.

Pulling away, I apologize to Morton for my fellow American. I wanted to go back and tell him that manners go a long way and remind him that it was indeed the British who taught *US* how to speak English. If France would have been the people we were fighting, instead of helping us fight the British, we might be speaking French. I also wanted to tell him that statements like his gave Americans bad reputations. Instead, we just tried to laugh it off and get on with the day. It does make you feel odd though, when someone, just because they can't understand your accent, gets angry at you. The day was a wash. We headed back, disappointed but not disillusioned. We are all different, different ideas, different natures....different. We were be able to laugh about the statement of speaking English. I joked with Morton about being a fuzzy little foreigner. He isn't amused.

Day 224 August 12, 2007, Sunday Dillsburg, Mechanicsburg, York Springs, PA

If I have said it before, I have said it a million times..."What a difference time makes." Just 24 hours and everything seems so much more in focus.

Our day of selling things to raise funds turned out to be a great day. We were setting under the trees in Williams Grove and talking to the people that strolled by. We did manage to make enough to pay for the gas out, hopefully.

Today we had our big bright green banner hanging out. I didn't think about it, but since the banner reads, "LittleChanges.com" on the top line, then "Bicycling 16,000 miles to battle obesity" on the second line, it might have been a bad thing to hang up.

There were people that would read it, keep walking and not even make eye contact. I think the word "obesity" freaks people out. Especially if they think they are obese. Not now, but a year ago I would have never stopped and talked to me. Even in the store, on a magazine, I would feel my face becoming hot if I saw the words, *"FAT, OBESE, DIET, EXERCISE"* or things like that. They felt like they were screaming at me and I wanted to ignore them. Why is it that we can't just come to terms with our own bodies? We should know them, love them and appreciate them better than anyone else, yet I chose to ignore mine for decades. Pretending that one day a miracle cure for fat would be discovered and I would wake up a size 8 any day now....it took ages to figure out that only *ME* can fix *ME*! Quit complaining and start changing!

People have commented that I'm shockingly honest with this journal. I say things they don't expect a person to say. The thing is though, I'm *not* an honest person. For decades I was the biggest liar on the planet. There was always a *reason* for why I couldn't lose weight. It was always anything else than the truth. This honesty thing is great though, it really frees you up. Today I think though, the world, or at least the shoppers at this market, might not be ready for the word *"OBESITY"* as the truth really can hurt.

Several people stop by who have came out to say HELLO! Thanks to all of you that did. Several others ask us questions, say they have seen us on television and talk about any given subject. Many people ask if I have had surgery to lose weight. The answer is 1000% NO...never, nada. You don't need it. *HONEST!!!* YOU can do this. Take the money you were going to spend on your surgery and use it to buy a new wardrobe at the end of this battle. There is an image on my desktop of an old ad for *TAPEWORMS*. It promises to make us free from fat. It is something that medical people had even recommended. The thing is people, you have to want this. Really want it. You also have to be prepared to work. It isn't easy always, but it is worth it. Letting the banner up, after seeing the hundredth person cringe, I thought it needed to stay there. A moment of truth. Nothing wrong with that.

My eyes looks around this old park. This was a delight to bring my kids to when they were little. Easy, affordable, fun, picnic area...but things change. Today the rides all sit in ruin, covered in spider webs. Weeds grow through the rollercoaster track. The big rig trucks that my son loved were sitting to go to rust and ruin. I took pictures and the new found film person in me thought it would be an excellent place to make a movie at.

The movie, though you would think might be a fright fest, would be a trip down memory lane with these stunning visuals. Death of a rollercoaster.

We get the exercise of loading and unloading and after paying for the space and the gas for my dad's truck that I had borrowed, we net $150.00 This will help get us out west. Stopping at the store to pick up things for on the grill, we bump in to my son and his wife. It makes me feel so domestic, yet so totally homeless. Morton tells me to "not go mad" as I look at a pack of pork chops to take to my mothers. Instead I go for the "buy one, get one free" pack of hot dogs and a watermelon. Mom has said that she made pasta, so I don't go mad on the money. Cheap and cheerful.

At my mom's, it reminds me of the amusement park that has closed and the mobile home park that is overgrown. There are weeds that have taken over my dad's garden. I wonder if it will ever see a caring hand plant it again. There are signs everywhere that the person who has cared for this is gone. Mom would, but her stroke doesn't allow it. She tries, but it is a lot to take care of.

We laugh, visit and I let my laptop in it's case. I had fully intended to work on it, but not right now. This time is too precious. I'll stay up late and do it, even after waking up at 5 am-ish the last two nights. There is going to be a meteor shower tonight. We talk about watching it, but I know I can't stay awake from 1 am to 3 am. It won't happen. The evening gets cooler and we say our goodbyes to mom and leave her on the front porch. My heart breaks as we drive off. We need more caring. There has to be someone within a few miles of my mother who would love the company and sharing the house. I think about how it would work, if it could work. Morton and I had a dish of mom's pasta with tomato sauce. The sauce she told us, was stuff that she had made herself. I didn't think about it, even when my stomach was cramping so bad I was crying as I tried to sleep. Morton kept telling me that I just needed to go to the bathroom, but I knew that it was something more. Morton couldn't feel what I was feeling, then the phone rang. My mom was going to the hospital in an ambulance. She was suffering from severe stomach cramps. She is fine, at home now, brought home by Morton and I at 5:30 am on Monday morning, but the stomach cramps are still there. For both of us. Morton tells me that as he was cleaning up the counter, the bag that had the frozen homemade sauce in it said that mom had made it the summer of 2004. It had meat in it and we reckon that it was the culprit. Morton escaped because he had put his in the microwave and technology killed whatever bug had crept in to our bellies. What a rollercoaster of a day! From seeing the death of the rollercoaster to the shocked expressions and sideway glances at the word *"OBESITY"* on my bright green banner, to our medical trauma from sauce from long ago, it was a day of memories. Old mixing with new, nostalgia mixing with the moment. Fantastic to be alive.

Day 225 August 13, 2007, Monday Camp Hill, York Springs, Harrisburg, PA

One of the emails this morning is from a place in Jackson Hole, Wyoming that is going to have us for a night. It is breathtaking. I get that feeling again of when you are packing to go on a vacation or holiday that you have been looking forward to. Joy!

The homesickness is only going to get worse. I just have to admit this and deal with it. Each day that passes, my grandson will change. I'm leaving a little baby wrapped in a blanket to come back to a little man who will be walking. Those moments I will never be able to get back and they break my heart. My heart. Which only has so many beats in it, that no one really knows how many, but I need to keep it going. All the things that are in store for him, I want to be around to see them.

Then I get to my turning point of how I feel for the day. The pain in my stomach is gone, almost. It's still a bit tender, but I know the worst of it is gone. We go in to my daughters and she asks me if I would like to give him a bath. They have been very kind in sharing their first-born son with me and these special moments. The evening melts away and I get to spend moments that I will replay in my head a million times while I'm riding and missing my special guy. Sarah takes him off my lap at 9 pm to head up to bed. I have just spent 3 golden hours with him. Smiling, I look at the display that tells me who is calling as my phone is ringing. It says "Karen" and then it hits me. I just stood up one of my dearest friends. Telling her what happened, how I got swept away with the baby and the pleasure of taking care of him, we both laugh. Morton and I were going to go for a visit, but we rearrange for Thursday. Now that we aren't leaving until Saturday, it isn't a problem. She will fully understand when she has one of these treasures called "grandchild."

Morton and I head for bed about 11. There is a very full day ahead of us tomorrow and I need a real night's sleep. As I'm getting ready to drift off, I smile thinking about my little guy on the floor below us. He's already asleep and dreaming and if I listen really hard, I might get to hear his soft breathing and commit it to memory. This very special night.

The love I feel for him is the perfect thing to fall asleep thinking about.

Day 226 August 14, 2007, Tuesday Harrisburg, Pennsylvania

We have been so lucky on this trip to get to meet a lot of famous and important people. Names that ring bells like, Toby McGuire, Kirstin Dunst (actually the entire Spiderman cast) people at the Today Show & the David Letterman show, Ray Ramano, many state representatives & senators. This part is always thrilling for us. Today we were getting another thrill. Heading to the lovely capital building in Harrisburg, we got to meet Senator Mike Folmer. He met with us in his office and we talked about many things, including Scotland. People like to talk to Morton, when they can understand him, about his native home. We had left our bright orange bikes parked outside a security booth, climbed the stairs and then played tourist inside. It brought back memories of field trips long ago and recent stops at other state houses and capital buildings up and down the east coast of America. The building is stunning, free to tour and I highly recommend it.

If you set on the steps outside, looking at the carvings, you might for a moment, feel as if you are in some far away European country. There is a certain feel to the exterior of this building that follows through inside.

On this same day, we got an email message that the governor of Pennsylvania wouldn't be able to meet with us this time, he was out of town. Maybe when we come back. As we bicycle away from our meeting, I wish I had time to get a real movement going. This journey though, is very time consuming. It sucks the very hours off of the clock and makes time race away. Plus, the real message of the journey isn't one that needs to involve the government. After all, our health isn't political.

Taking charge and personal responsibility for our health is the message we want to share, which we do right here. I guess I don't have to beat myself up for something I *SHOULD* be doing...I already am in a way. Morton and I have so much on our plates over the next few days. We have things to pack, things to sneak in the trailer without the other one seeing and most of all, we have to spend as much time as we can with our family. It's going to be ages before we are back, but then, no...it will just be the blink of an eye.

Day 227 August 15, 2007, Wednesday Harrisburg, Pennsylvania

Smiling is something that comes easy for me, but not for Morton. He was telling us that he always got in trouble when he was young for looking so grumpy on photos. Today we were having photos done for an up-coming story on our journey in a magazine and poor Morton was really annoyed. He tried to explain that his look on his face *DOESN'T* mean he is in a bad mood...it is his relaxed expression. Me, on the other hand, always seem to have a stupid grin on my face. When I smile though, I can't help thinking about the gap in my teeth. UGH! It really looks silly in pictures and I'm getting more self-aware of it. I suppose it is all of those make-over shows and advertisements on television showing us how our teeth should look. They are not yellow and not white. I have never drank coffee, tea or smoked, so they aren't stained or crooked. They are, however, gapped. I think of the slogan in London for the tube..."Mind the gap" and smile. With my lips closed of course...since there are cameras going, I do want to "mind the gap" and not show it off. Sure there are glamour shots of women who can pull off the GAP in the teeth. I'm not one of them.

Fat arms. It is the thought that pops in to my head to take my mind off the gap. My fat and flabby arms that HAVE to get more work done on them. They don't have as many rolls on them as they did when I was over 400 pounds, but they still are scary. I worry about them flopping out of my t-shirt and injuring someone. Who designs these clothes for heavy people? What are they thinking? I remember spending hours searching for tops that hid my fat arms and not even considering shirts where the sleeves didn't come past the elbow. Give me a three-quarters sleeve shirt, no matter what time of year it is. One that doesn't have horizontal stripes. Again designers, it is not rocket science. Just think about who is going to be buying a size 5x shirt. Today my arms wiggle and as I'm told to lift my arm and push on a pole, I have to just quit thinking about it. At least I have arms and I can change them after all. I think about all the exercises people have told me to do on them. Once in a while, in the shower, I will. But I'm NOT doing it on a regular basis.

Right then and there, while we are working with three strangers, I call out to Morton who is trying to SMILE. "Remind me to work on my fat arms when we get back on the road!" He nods and understands. Thankfully he doesn't go in to telling how he does tell me to do arm exercises, I just don't listen to him. He also tells me to do crunches. Perhaps I'm going to incorporate a 30 minute training exercise into each day, along with the 6 to 8 hours on the bicycle. After all, I already have a gappy smile, I don't want to have flappy arms as well.

Day 228 August 16, 2007, Thursday Harrisburg, Pennsylvania

This day is a tough one. It is the birthday of my brother who left this world in 1975. It brings back the reminder of just how short our life is. He was in his very early twenties and had so much more living to do.

I call my mom, as I do most days. I know she will know what day it is, but I don't bring it up. Instead we talk about when I'm leaving. It would be so much easier if I didn't. I could stay and help my mother, spend my time split between changing diapers, or nappies, as the British call them, on young Alexander and cooking healthy stuff for my mom...but I can't. As the clock ticks away and the time to leave comes closer, I know I'm making the hardest choice of my life. To leave, I follow my dream, hopefully help others and finally become free from fat. My health is greatly improved and it is the best thing for me. To stay, I take care of duty. Helping my mom, getting to enjoy Alexander while he is so little and being drenched in this wonderful thing called family. I have to think about this leaving like strapping on my own oxygen mask on a plane that is falling. I have to save myself before I can try to help anyone else. Either way, staying or going, leaves me with the feeling that my choice is something I'll regret forever. But there isn't really a choice. Of course I'm going. This journey has to be completed. I know there are still so many people out there that have to get the message that everyone needs 30 minutes a day.

Day 229 August 17, 2007, Friday Harrisburg, Pennsylvania

Burning the midnight oil, Morton is sitting on the floor going over our gear for one final time. I did manage to get him to part with some of his tools, but he still has some that he insists are vital to the journey. He has promised they will ride in his trailer.

For one final time I get to give my grandson his bath. He is extra sweet and cuddly tonight and I snuggle him afterwards in a rocker and sing to him as he is going to sleep. This moment is sealed in my mind and will replayed often over the next 18 months. It all starts again tomorrow. We ride in a car out to the west coast, stopping at some amazing places along the way. We have so far to go, but then, we have already came so far we know we can do it. Bring on the homesickness...I'm ready to ride!

Day 230 August 18, 2007, Saturday Harrisburg, Pennsylvania to Washington DC & back to Dillsburg

Washington DC is really a great place and I have been there a lot in my life. Today though, I seemed unable to find it. How is it that our nation's capital could be so tough for me to find? That was the case though as my son and his wife gave us a ride to pick up the car we are taking to Portland, Oregon. Driving in the traffic, even though the nine to fivers should have been off the road, we kept getting held up. It was a trip that should have taken two hours and ended up feeling like years. Just as it was getting dark, we pulled on the lovely street that the car was at. Nadine met us with her beautiful little short haired wiener dog. She introduced us to the car, we went over all the details, insurance, where what lever is to pop what item on the car, then almost as fast as we arrived, we left. We will have a proper visit and chat when we get to the west coast. We are dropping the car off on September 6, which leaves us time to really see some things, do some press and meet people as we go west. Now James was following me, as we set off in the lovely little car. We just had to go out Pennsylvania Avenue, pick up the parkway and that would be us out of the city. But not tonight. Nope, today was my *GETTING LOST OVER AND OVER* day. It was a great tour of the city though. The weather was mild and there were people all dressed up for a fabby Saturday night as we made our way past monuments, buildings and sights that we have all seen on television dozens of times. I was more worried about seeing the right road sign. After my horrible mix up getting us here, the least I could do was to make the going home trip painless. After all, my son needed to get to work eventually...if we ever get out of DC. There were so many familiar sights to me. We walked past there, we bicycled past here, but where do I turn? Streets that surely would have taken us out were pointing the wrong direction and my bearing were all messed up. This is really unusual for me. I am a natural navigator. My dad started me young by handing me a map and saying, "What roads do I need to take to get there?" Which might not sound odd until I add that I was just 6 or 7 and we would be heading to Florida. Dad knew how to get there, he just wanted to make sure I could navigate the 1000 mile trip.

Tonight though, I was missing the map and relying on memory. This isn't good, when my mind is so full of other things. I thought I had us going the right way until I hooked a left over a bridge that led to 50. It was signed that it would get us to the belt way and I knew that once I was on that, I could get us up the road to Dillsburg. Or so it would seem. This road was dotted with red lights, seemingly every block or two. It was also very congested. My driving had to be slow, since my son was following. I was glad I couldn't hear what he must be saying behind the wheel of his car. My phone did ring to ask me if I had any clue as to where we were going. He didn't buy it when I told him I was giving him the ten cent tour of DC. Eventually, with what seemed like years later, we found our way back. It was then just a matter of driving up the familiar roads that landed us at his house when it was approaching 11 pm. He had to be at work at a shocking time, maybe 2 am. I *AM* a bad mother!!! We decided to spend the night at his house, wake up early and go in to Sarah's to see if we could get the bikes to fit.

It felt great to lay down and spend one last night with my son just sleeping several rooms away. Max, the wiener dog with long fur, decided to spend the night in our room and I rolled to my stomach to let my backside have a break from being sat on all day. Plus, I had to give it a rest for the long ride west.

Day 231 August 19, 2007, Sunday Harrisburg, Pennsylvania to Hannibal, Missouri

Bright and early, we did get up and get moving. Morton had to do a bit of maintenance on the car and then came the task of packing. Nadine had half the car neatly packed with her items. She was kind enough to have a selection of tapes for us to listen to and even had flashlights (torches, for my UK friends and family) inside. This was the hard thing. Leaving Alexander.

With my grown children, I know I miss them fiercely when I'm gone. But they don't really change that much. Sarah might have her hair a bit different and James may or may not have a beard, but they are pretty much done surprising me with growing spurts. They should at almost 26 and 25! But Alexander has changed every day that I have been with him. He will be a little man the next time I see him. We all knew this wasn't going to be easy.

Morton was focused on the car and packing and I got the job of putting everything in order in the room we had taken over. It had looked like a tip, even Graeme had commented on the state of it, but out of chaos comes order...sometimes. As I went up and down the stairs, I fought the temptation of peeking in the room at Alexander & Sarah. I knew once I saw them I would want to just stop and stare. Instead I got my big workout on the steps. One the last trip down the stairs, I peeked in. There he was, in the crook of his mommy's arm, sleeping. So was Sarah. What a picture the two of them are together. This is what pure love looks like. Graeme was standing up, going to the the side of the bed, so I popped in for a moment. My little guy was fast asleep and didn't really want bothered. I had to have one last cuddle, diaper change and kisses.

Someone needs to hurry up and invent a human transporter that is Star-Trek-like. This is a place that I need to pop in to at the end of a long day of riding. Just seeing this little family would fix any day, no matter how many hills I climbed or cars that had bumped me. *BLISS.*

Morton and I headed off. I promised myself that I wouldn't cry and I didn't. Instead we plugged a tape in and sat in the lovely car, flying over miles that it would have taken us weeks to cross with out butts on the bikes. Speaking of butts, mine was killing me. It was one long car ride. The weather was stormy, humid and when it got dark we got treated to a great lightning show. Morton sat snoring, filming or feeding me. We both ate way too much. Graeme had given us a bag of drinks, bottles of water and sports drink. It was like a non-stop food fest and I got that old horrible feeling of being out of control. Telling myself that I was munching this to stay awake, my old eating habits were right there in my face. *WHAT WAS I DOING?*

Thank goodness we were running out of road. Just 60 miles to go and we would be at my sister's house in Hannibal. I hadn't ever visited her here. She bought it while I was living in Scotland and the way my life goes is that the only idea I had over it had came from the images I saw on the computer. But the last miles were just too tough. It was so late "our time" and my body had just 5 hours sleep the night before. I'm getting too old for this kind of living. It seemed like the state of Missouri was just an oasis on the horizon. I knew the Mississippi River was somewhere ahead of me in the black night. The pink-grey glow on the horizon just might be Hannibal. There had been lots of little glows we had seen and passed, never knowing just what was lighting up the sky.

At a last ditch effort to keep awake I got a diet cola and a special peanut butter cup from an all-night gas station. The sugar and soda would do it. I ate and was waiting for the rush to kick in, but it just never happoned. Instead, my head was starting to nod and I know the first rule of night driving is to pull over as soon as you get sleepy. We just had to pull over and sleep. There was an off ramp that had a semi-truck pulled off and sleeping on it. Closer to the stop sign and under a light, I parked and used my new bright orange jacket as a pillow. This worked enough to let me sleep in sweat for about two hours. I kept waking up to see Morton standing outside the car or sitting on the seat with his legs out the open door. He would look at me and say, "It's too sweltering to sleep" and I would be off again. Poor Morton. His knee was locking up on him too. It would crack like a gun when he stretched his leg. Me, I was just so worn out I could have slept on the edge of a brick wall. But it was hot and humid. It was bad sleep. I gave it up as a bad job about three a.m. and jumped out of the car. I took a walk, jog and run (well, maybe a BRISK walk) around the car. Anyone driving by would have thought I was quite mad. I also took a bottle of water and washed my face and hands with it, drying them both on my t-shirt. Starting the car, we kept going west and talking about what was coming up ahead of us. The only time I had cried today, was just for a moment when a sad song came on the radio. It was "I would give everything I own, just to see you once again" from the 70's or 80's. Lovely and one that I had heard before, but now it just got to me. At the end of the music, the DJ said the singer (he had been the lead singer for BREAD) had written it when his dad died. It's too much to take and the tears come, but just for a few seconds. This is the future, this is the moment, this is what I have been waiting for my entire adult life. No time for tears while life is right here waiting on me.

We pull in to my sister's house, after I phoned her and woke her from her own dreams. It is more of a mansion than a house. Giant. Huge. Stunning. As we park the car and head inside for late night hugs, she gives us the tour. It feels like this could be one of the delicious B&B's we have stayed at. Tall ceilings, delicate touches that only historic homes see to have from staircases to glass door knobs, I drink it all in. Seeing her pictures, books and belongings in this mansion in her dream home in her favorite town in America, it is a familiar scene. It feels like we have been here before.

My sister is one of those people who can do anything she puts her mind to. She is a doctor, knows how to fly a plane, is a published author and is now following another dream in Hannibal, Missouri. I'm not big on idols, but if I ever said I had one, it might just have to be my lovely sister. Really a hero of mine and others. She is very special indeed and we are going to have a fantastic two or three nights here.

Tonight I get the "Becky Thatcher Room" in pinks, but very soft and gentle. Sitting on the dresser with the big round mirror, is a stuffed teddy bear that was a toy from my sister's children's childhood. On a chair is a quilt my grandmother had stitched by hand. Little girls with big sun bonnets on their heads. There are so many memories in this new old house. Morton is snoring as I switch off the present to dream of the future. Books, adventures and endless possibilities are all on offer. Hannibal, Missouri on the street where Mark Twain lived!

Day 232 August 20, 2007, Monday Hannibal, Missouri

"Be good and you will be lonesome" is a famous Twain quote, that Jimmy Buffett echoed in a song a century or so later. Today, Morton and I were on our own, but not lonesome. I guess we aren't that good!

My computer is screaming at me to work on it. So many things to do, but what my heart wants to do is sit here in my sister's lovely living room, looking out the big window with the lovely little panes of glass in it, writing for pleasure. Sigh...if I only had the luxury of time. Like so many incredible places we have stayed at, this one is shouting at me to sit a while and write. Maybe take a sketchpad on to the big front porch and try to capture some slices of time and place. But not today.

There is the email, the updating, the phone calls, things that make the morning leap forward further than any bullfrog that Mark might have ever jumped. I wonder for a moment what sort of things this great writer could have gotten up to on the computer. Would he be distracted with emails, web sites and things that keep us from our work? I doubt it. He was focused. He was dedicated. He really was one of the best writers this country, and even this world for that matter, has ever seen. On the stand beside our bed there is a copy of *Tom Sawyer*. This is a book that I have read several times, but always find something new and fresh about it. Perhaps that is the way a timeless book should be. You can never fully put your finger on what makes it so special, because you always take away something different when reading it.

Today though, my stab at the great American novel would have to wait. I do get an idea for a good story as we are walking about town and I mentally remind myself to write it down when we get back to the house. The town is different than I pictured. There is a vibrant main street with lots of period shops that if you peeked in the window, you might expect to see a young lad in bib overalls ordering a stick of penny candy, while wearing a straw hat. There are also a lot of artists here. Galleries abound. There is a glass blowing place that I make a mental note of wanting to check out. I have always fancied having a shot at that.

In 2006, Morton and I were in a little town in Germany, where a glass blower had a fantastic shop that had been there for 300 years. They did demonstrations and even offered lessons, but I wasn't able to try. It came down to the fact that I spoke no German and Morton, though willing to translate (since he CAN speak German) wasn't allowed to. The man was afraid that I might catch myself on fire or something. Perhaps here in Hannibal, I just might convince the nice glass blower to let me have a try. They also make marbles and paperweights. Interesting indeed. The banks of the Mississippi River was streaming with life. People out taking walks in a park, holding hands in the humidity, watching the river roll by. It is a lovely sight that would surely be worth sitting on a bench and watching, or even better, joining in on the walking. Morton is overjoyed to see a barge passing and we talk just briefly about how this river provided industry to towns like Hannibal, the whole way down to New Orleans. There are many businesses that echo the Mark Twain theme, but they don't seem to be big neon, jumping and glaring "tourist traps" that my dad always avoided. This town seems to be keeping it in good taste, the memory of it's most famous son. There are lots of things we are going to explore tomorrow, with my sister, but today Morton and I just have a walk around.

There is a lighthouse on a hill, something I wasn't expecting to see inland. I thought when we left the coast of Maine we wouldn't see another lighthouse until we got out to the Pacific. Hmmmm, interesting. We will climb the hill that it sits on tomorrow. My sister is an expert in everything Twain. I don't type those words lightly, she is. She has been one of his biggest fans since first falling in love with his writing in the fourth grade. Being here in this place, is her dream come true. I think if Morton and I tried to look around without her, I would be letting Morton down. After all, he always asks a million questions and I would have to just fake my knowledge of Twain. I do know a bit, but everything I know really was gleaned from listening to my sister.

The rain is coming and we can both feel it. The humidity is so high it feels like we are walking through a solid hot mist. There isn't a breeze and I'm thankful that we aren't going to have to sleep outside in a tent with this heat. Memories of walking through the Florida Keys pop into my head, I think it might have even be hotter there, but the humidity wasn't this tough. Bring on the DRY heat!

Back at the house, after our two-hour foot tour of the town, self-guided, Morton and I settle into our grooves. Me, on the lovely blue chaise lounge that looks out into the trees and Morton tinkering with the car. He is setting about trying to make sure the transmission fluid level is *JUST* right and the fluid is clean, not smelling and able to take us across the mountains. He knows cars, but I haven't got a clue. We are good like that, certain things we both click on and like to do together, others, we are as different as the sun and the moon. My eyes keep going to the staircase in this house. It has two landings on it, lovely windows, again, with odd panes of glass and is the real focal point from the living room and the library room. Since this house is over 100 years old, I like to think about the people that have gone up and down those stairs. Did they realize that they were getting their exercise on them? Lives were so much different then, it was rare to see someone fat enough to be called obese. There was physical exercise in everyone's lives in 1907. From doing the daily housework to walking to your work, we moved then. Really moved. Even if we never even left our little town, we moved. People also ate very differently in 1907. We didn't have a corner store to buy frozen meals to pop in the microwave. We had to peel the carrots (burning calories) then we had to carry in the wood to build a fire to cook the carrots on, then we had to carry the bucket of water in to wash the dishes with. When you consider that you would burn off 800 calories to prepare a meal of 400 calories, it was no wonder there wasn't an epidemic of fat people.

Today though, we use our fingers more and our legs and arms less. There have been times that I have actually been to tired or lazy (or a combination of both) to even open the freezer door to get a meal out to tear the cardboard lid from and put it in the microwave. I couldn't be bothered. Instead I would open the cupboard door and get a bag of something that was meant to snack on and eat that for my meal. People don't believe me when I tell them that I could eat whole bags of chips, cookies, half gallons of ice cream and other really bad food from the year 2007. Convenient and deadly.

Tonight Morton nukes a cardboard box of the worst of the worst. Beef and noodles. People should never eat food like this. The sodium content is so high, the chemicals they put in this stuff will keep my body alive for at least a decade after I quit breathing. Morton and I both complain and agree that we should have just eaten peaches from our big bag from Pennsylvania. *Diet and exercise.* The words would have been way out of place in this town a hundred years ago. *Food and work.* That was a time when people ate food that would stick to their ribs and carry them through the day. Now we eat food that sticks to our hearts and carries us to an early grave. Why are we killing ourselves with poisonous food and it isn't making the headlines every day? Past the window walks a boy and his mom. They both could lose weight, at least fifty pounds each or a bit more. Hopefully they are on their way down to a healthy life. Leaving the frozen death in the freezer, peeling the carrots and cooking a meal. Morton and I agree that we won't do this kind of eating any more. Even a can of tuna mixed with a cold can of green beans would have tasted better.

Within an hour, Morton is passing out the peanut butter cups to me. They are mini ones, not bad if you eat two or three. Over the evening though, with being lost on the computer working, he worked his way through half the bag. This isn't how you lose weight. This isn't even close to how you lose weight. Morton says he won't buy them anymore like that. He is as bad as I am, when it comes to eating the stuff if it is around. Of course after several hours of munching on these sweet treats, I want salty food. He opens a bag of pub mix snacks and I start eating them. Pretzels, odd shaped things that cut the roof of my mouth but taste great and my favorite, the hard little circles of brown crunchies, sort of like melba toast, only coated in flavor. Chemicals can be delicious. Why oh why did he buy these? We had the talk about only getting the things that won't pile the weight on. Morton gets on the scale in my sister's bathroom to discover his is 10 pounds heavier than when we stopped in Pennsylvania. Those 10 pounds don't show, but they are there. After a night of eating, he really thinks I'm going to go get on the scale too. I can't. I know what it will say. I will have at least the 10 pounds and more likely, 20. I haven't told him, but my bra is tighter. The scale can just sit there, I won't get on it and feel like a failure. Even if I do have an extra 20 pounds that came about with the filming in Pennsylvania and the days of me not getting my 30 minutes of movement in, I don't need the scale to tell me that. My body has been screaming for the last few weeks to *MOVE*. That, we are about to do.

This dilemma of diet and exercise, as recent as it is, has to be conquered by each of us in our own way. Try to find what works for you and don't quit, even if the scales move in the wrong direction. Keep trying.

If I wake up tomorrow, it will be a whole new day where anything can happen. One of the things that I will work on changing is saying *no* to the food that kills. Even if it does taste delicious (or not) I have to break this horrible food addiction I have.

When my sister comes home, Morton tries to push the peanut butter cups her way. She just says no, doesn't want to eat all that sugar. Morton is going to be forced to either finish the bag himself over the next few days or toss it out. Either way, they won't cross my lips again. Back to the computer I come across a page that is talking about obesity perhaps being caused by a cold-type virus. What sort of thing would that be to discover? Why didn't people "catch" obesity to the epidemic state a hundred years ago? Too many questions and distractions. Right now I'll disconnect from the internet, write a bit about the story that popped in to my head on the streets of Hannibal and try to think about things that will not just make me a better and healthier person, but ways that I can share them with others.

Day 233 August 21, 2007, Tuesday Hannibal, Missouri to Quincy University, Quincy, IL "The love of literature has no age boundaries" is a quote on one of the many pictures I was unpacking in my sister's office in Quincy University. I was surprised to read this was a quote from her, under a picture of Mark Twain sitting in black and white. I wondered as I set it on her bookcase, just where this came from and why my sister would have a quote from herself on something like this. She is not one to blow her own horn, even though she could if she wanted to.

Morton and I got lost in the boxes of my sister's treasures, unpacking, unwrapping, stacking, sorting, dusting and arranging. Morton hooked up external hard drives, ran cords to reach far away wall plugs and we just made ourselves at home, while my sister was off teaching a class. It felt odd doing this, a bit like we were on one of those room decorating shows where neighbors swop houses and do terrible things to them. Then at the end of the show, they pretend they like the new shiny green slime wall color and the way they sawed the legs off their antique dining room table, made throw pillows out of toilet rugs and now eat while sitting on the floor. I hoped that my sister wouldn't scream when she came back in her office.

Being at this incredible campus I feel a strong desire to go enroll. There is something about this time of the year that always puts me in the mood to go back to school. We should never stop learning, the term "continuing education" is a brilliant one. Now my mind wanders to the day when our journey is over and I picture Morton and I going from school to school, with a life-sized fiberglass statue of me at 440 pounds, telling the young minds that they have to remember and always consider the physical side of their education. After all, what good is it a great education if you aren't alive to use it.

Walking down a hallway of doors to get to the ladies room, I hear my polyester pants rubbing. It is a loud noise. A very loud, "swish, swish" that seems like it should have heads sticking out of doors to see what all the commotion is about. This noise, unsettling as it was to me, is one that I enjoy hearing. It reminds me that I'm wearing *TIGHT* polyester pants, not to make a fashion statement, but to bicycle in. It reminds me that once my road education is finished, it is a noise I won't hear anymore. The next time I walk these halls, to visit my sister when our journey is finished, the noise will be forever gone. Enjoy it while it's here.

Inside the bathroom, the mirrors are set on an angle where you can actually see yourself from behind. I'm still getting use to clothes that fit, having left all of my three and four XL sizes of clothes back in Pennsylvania. The size XL t-shirt I have on is tight, for now. Too tight for my liking. After all, I have been trying to disguise my rolls of fat with layers of loose clothes for the last 30 years. The pants I have on, 100% polyester, are hot, (not hot as in sexy, hot as in high temperature) tight and something that I would have never been seen in, at home or out. They fit like leggings, with an orange and white stripe up the side. I chose them to be easier on the bikes. Cotton gets wet and stays wet, which isn't good. So here I am, in my skin tight polyester pants, tight fitting bright orange shirt and feeling very, very fat and conspicuous. I have to walk back the long hall, having just gave myself a good once-over in the mirror. It felt like I was worse than naked, with clothes that look almost spray painted on. This is embarrassing and I get very red in the face. At this point in my life I'm not sure if it is the change of life or just blushing from my shame of fatness. On the walk back, smiling faces say hello.

No one points and stares, not a gasp to be heard. Just the swishing of my polyester thighs.

In the office I close my sister's door behind me. Morton knows nothing about my secret shame. He doesn't even notice my red face. His head pops up from behind her desk, where he had been getting her external hard drive sorted. Going back to the boxes, I keep pulling out her treasures and tools to make her work space her own. Books, so many books, great books that make me want to sit down and read them. A complete set of *Childcraft Encyclopedias*, just like the ones we had growing up. I wanted to organize these here so they will be easy for her to access. My days of working in the library when I went to college come back to me. I want to organize them the way they *SHOULD* be, if they were in a real library...but I know that the way her work goes, it would be easier if these books were grouped. Trying my best, I lose myself on the shelves and my cheeks are red now from work, not shame.

When I pull a picture out of a box that is a poster of animals getting on to the ark, it all sort of hits me. I know this poster. I know the story behind it. There is just one single nail sticking out of one of the walls that begs to have it hang there. Morton, who has been in on the discussion that we aren't going to put up anything on the walls today, asks why that is going up. Trying to do the story justice I tell him of how that poster is the reason my sister went back to school. She was on a field trip in Florida to a zoo with one of her children. Her lifelong dream of being a teacher had fallen by the wayside. We had both gotten married young, had our children young and hadn't gone to college in the traditional order. Since childhood my sister knew she wanted to teach, it just hadn't happened. But on that sunny day inside the gift shop of the zoo, that poster jumped out at her. The thought that it would look great hanging in a classroom of her very own students was so strong that she bought the poster went home and enrolled in the community college. She worked so hard over the next several years, earning degree after degree, holding down full-time jobs, beating the odds and making all her dreams happen with a lot of hard work and studying. Now, a few decades later, she is a doctor, a professor, an author and her degrees, awards and certificates all started with this humble poster. It is fitting that it is the one that goes on the lonely nail.

Just like the television shows, as I'm putting the last finishing touches on her newly set up office, her door swings open and in she comes. I worry if she likes it. Again, this moment is just like the television shows. She is looking around, just sort of saying, "Oh my" and I can't tell if she is loving it or wondering why I just didn't sit quietly and work on my laptop. She starts saying she loves it and being her sister, I can tell that she really does. My heart swells with this feeling of joy that comes from doing a good thing for someone else. I do love this feeling. Forget fame and money, just give me a bit of praise for a job well done and I'm a happy. polyester clad, fit person in training.

Making a mental note to ask her about the picture with the quote on it, from her, slips to the side as she is busy with the telephone and taking care of business. Morton and I keep on task and take boxes of bubble wrap out to the car and head back towards Missouri. On the ride home, I fall asleep in the car. I'm exhausted. I think I'm still catching up on our big road trip. My sister is on the phone talking to a friend in Florida and I hear my sister say that she will be sure to tell me. I hear her say this a few times and through my sleepy thoughts and I wonder what she is going to tell me. Right now though, I just enjoy my 15 minute cat nap. These power naps are something that I haven't really gotten in to before, but they work. The conversation ended in about 10 minutes and I was wide awake, refreshed and in another state. Morton was still sleeping in the back seat. His batteries must take a bit longer to recharge.

Cindy started telling me that her friend on the phone had a son in Florida that had been part of a writer's workshop that my sister was running. It turns out, the photo of Twain with a quote from my sister on it was a gift that the lady had given Cindy. Her son was a few years shy of the program, but his love of literature was the reason that he was able to participate in the program. He had read the required reading three times on his own and really wanted to take this creative class. Age should never be a factor in whether or not we find our dreams. If the passion and desire is there, anything is possible. My sister hadn't noticed that the picture was up on her lovely book shelves. Tucked in with the volumes of words waiting to be discovered by new people and revisited by my sister, who like me, will read and re-read what she loves.

Today we did a lot of things we didn't plan on doing. We talked with a lot of people who made me all homesick for the road. Meeting all the new people along the way is a thrill I will never get tired of, or get enough of.

At dinner, in the best spot in Hannibal to eat, *LuluBelles,* we are at a table beside the "official" Becky Thatcher. She is charming, lovely and kind enough to let us get a picture with her. It is a nice way to end an evening beside the big river.

Little Changes   **269**   *Priscilla Houliston*

Today has been one of those that every turn I took I saw proof that anything is possible, with ambition, desire and dreams followed by a strong constitution of work and dedication. Dream and do and never stop learning.

Day 234 August 22, 2007, Wednesday Hannibal, Missouri to Quincy University, Quincy, Illinois We have found a new profession to do AFTER our journey is over, "Office Makeover" as we did yesterday. Today, we can also add "Picture Hangers" to our resume. Morton and I tagged along to Quincy University again with my sister. We took along her ladder, loads of framed artwork and a selection of nails and hangers. We had everything to put up from a poster of a cockpit of an airplane that she flies to a selection of framed Mark Twain stamps, an odd shelf and of course her diplomas.

While I could have done it, Morton chose to be the one climbing the ladder while I stood on the ground saying, "To the left, to the right...just a HAIR" and so on. But as good as my directions might have been I have to admit, he did have to pull out the odd nail or hook and move it another few hairs. Things never look quite the same until you actually get them up there. Then you have to make a few minor adjustments. They were just needing a few little changes to be perfect and we tried to get as close to that as we could.

After doing stunts of ladder climbing and clinging, Morton was pretty well worn out. He's not afraid of heights, or at least he never told me if he is, I just think he was tired of the clinging to the ladder and the huge pictures while we stood below making our minds up.

He and I drove back to my sisters. There were a few interviews to be done and this is where Morton got his own back. While I sat and worked on the computer and interviews, he laid down on the lovely hardwood floor, on a wee four foot rug that ties the room together and snored loudly. One interview was from across many miles, Australia to be exact. The man on the other end of the line even asked what the noise was. He thought it must be a problem with the connection and offered to phone me back. I assured him that the connection was fine, but my husband on the other hand, was knackered.

The weather is a bit muggy and oppressive. We watch the weather channel to see a picture of what is in store for us when we head west. There are floods in Ohio that we had just driven through and there is cold weather back in Pennsylvania. Morton is always amazed with the size of America that there can be floods in one area, droughts in another and bang on winter in still another. Since Scotland sits on the top part of the is-land that is the United Kingdom, with England to the south of it and Wales to the south-west, all sharing the same island real estate in a rather small package, he isn't use to great temperature differences. Scotland is fa-mous for getting all four seasons in one day, but there are times when your roses are still blooming in the gar-den at Christmas if the season has been a mild one. There is even a place on the west coast of Scotland where palm trees grow. Not at all what you would expect, but I can assure you, they are there. I have seen them with my own eyes and touched them to make sure they weren't made out of plastic.

The weather today traps me inside. There is a huge porch here I want to sit on to work, but as soon as you walk outside, your clothes get damp. I can only imagine what it would do to my poor lil' laptop. It is already showing signs of wear with it's dings and bumps that it has gotten along the way. My screen is getting blurry (at first I put this down to spending 12 hours at a time on it and my eyes were playing tricks that made it LOOK blurry) but it really is. It is a thrill each time I turn it on and it actually starts. I worry about the shelf life of this computer with me dragging it all around creation on the back of a bicycle.

Watching the sun go down, sitting on this comfortable chaise lounge chair that I could sleep in, my mind wanders about 100 years ago. How different would the view out this window be? The house is sur-rounded by huge trees, so it would have been close to being the same I imagine, just instead of the odd car going by, it would have been horses. The town holds so much history that the surface is just scratched by most who visit. I would love to spend time here and write, paint, talk to the locals, stroll along the Mississippi and of course, sit on any one of the locations from the book and re-read Tom Sawyer. Maybe someday.

Day 235 August 23, 2007, Thursday Hannibal, Missouri

BUY THIS BOOK...You might be familiar with *Tom Sawyer* & *Huck Finn*, but Mark Twain wrote so much more. *The War Prayer* wasn't printed when it was written. I'm sure it had to do with the message it car-ries. This book is something everyone should read, regardless how you feel about war. Insight of how war never really changes. We have had a fantastic Thursday. There are so many things to see and do in this area, we really are spoiled for choice. Today however, we did the Mark Twain tour, that you must go on when you visit Hannibal. We met people from England, France and heard some German accents. People really do come from all over the world to see this page of history. A few people did a head-turn when they heard Morton rolling his "R's" and the eyebrows went up trying to place his accent. He gets mistaken for Irish, Australian and occa-sionally English. Today was no exception.

My sister had taken us to the starting point of the Mark Twain tour, introducing us to several people along the way. We were going to have a few hours to explore on our own and then meet up with a television news crew for an interview outside of the real and actual boyhood home of young Mr. Twain.

When we were handed the map of all the homes and businesses on the tour, I tried to work out in my mind how long it would take to get through them to end up at the boyhood home come interview time. I seriously underestimated the treasures the places would hold, capturing not just my attention, but Morton's too. We all know Morton loves to read signs, take pictures of signs and really try to learns as much as we can about the areas we are travelling through. When he does this, I can picture him at the end of our journey reading as many books as he can about the places we will have been. Me, I'm more a "live in the moment" kind of person and a fiercely fast reader, which makes us an odd couple to tour places like this. Today though, our pace was almost perfectly matched.

Lingering over facts, quotes strategically places and fascinating memorabilia, we got lost in this slice of Americana as sweet and tempting as a slice of my grandmothers apple pie. It was all I could do to keep looking at the time on my cell phone and keep nudging Morton along. He was so curious, of course reading everything and since we did have a schedule and a place to be, it was up to the mother in me to keep my guy going.

The house that Huck Finn lived in is the only recreated house. The other homes and offices, shops and areas are all from the real time and place. Even in the Huck Finn house though, with it's two rooms, rough wooden floor and location amongst the others, yet on it's own, you feel that this isn't some made up amusement park. This is a living, breathing, historical gem. How many American's have made the journey to see this? If people are willing to fly halfway around the world, surely you can take the flight or drive that will get you to this special place.

We get to the boyhood home with just a few minutes to spare and decide to take a peek inside. Morton looks at the statues they have placed of Twain and asks me how tall he was. I'm stumped. I should know this question and I'm glad my sister isn't there to see me stumble. Since I'm suppose to know a bit more than Morton on all things American and I do well with trivia, he files this question away to ask my sister later. We both decide he must have been close to the size of the statues and then head outside to meet the reporter. You couldn't ask for better weather, sunny, the humidity seemed to have gone on down the river and not a cloud in the brilliant blue sky. The interview is fast, wonderful and Leslie, the lady doing the interview, was really great. It seemed a bit surreal, doing an interview right here in front of such a famous place and not having the focus on the interview be Twain. We did talk about a wonderful story that Twain had written about the bike. I want to share it with you and know this, when he talks about HIS experiences on it, I can easily relate. Especially the bit about dogs. Mark Twain was the greatest American writer, humorist of the mega variety and this piece really illustrates that. Enjoy and then catch up below with with how Morton gets his Twain questions answered.

Taming the Bicycle By Mark Twain

From: *What Is Man? and Other Essays* (New York: Harper and Brothers, 1917)

In the early eighties Mark Twain learned to ride one of the old high-wheel bicycles of that period. He wrote an account of his experience, but did not offer it for publication. The form of bicycle he rode long ago became antiquated, but in the humor of his pleasantry is a quality which does not grow old. A. B. P.

I thought the matter over, and concluded I could do it. So I went down and bought a barrel of Pond's Extract and a bicycle. The Expert came home with me to instruct me. We chose the back yard, for the sake of privacy, and went to work

Mine was not a full-grown bicycle, but only a colt -- a fifty-inch, with the pedals shortened up to fortyeight -- and skittish, like any other colt. The Expert explained the thing's points briefly, then he got on its back and rode around a little, to show me how easy it was to do. He said that the dismounting was perhaps the hardest thing to learn, and so we would leave that to the last. But he was in error there. He found, to his surprise and joy, that all that he needed to do was to get me on to the machine and stand out of the way; I could get off, myself. Although I was wholly inexperienced, I dismounted in the best time on record. He was on that side, shoving up the machine; we all came down with a crash, he at the bottom, I next, and the machine on top.

We examined the machine, but it was not in the least injured. This was hardly believable. Yet the Expert assured me that it was true; in fact, the examination proved it. I was partly to realize, then, how admirably these things are constructed. We applied some Pond's Extract, and resumed. The Expert got on the other side to shove up this time, but I dismounted on that side; so the result was as before.

The machine was not hurt. We oiled ourselves again, and resumed. This time the Expert took up a sheltered position behind, but somehow or other we landed on him again.

He was full of admiration; said it was abnormal. She was all right, not a scratch on her, not a timber started anywhere. I said it was wonderful, while we were greasing up, but he said that when I came to know these steel spider-webs I would realize that nothing but dynamite could cripple them. Then he limped out to position, and we resumed once more. This time the Expert took up the position of short-stop, and got a man to shove up behind. We got up a handsome speed, and presently traversed a brick, and I went out over the top of the tiller and landed, head down, on the instructor's back, and saw the machine fluttering in the air between me and the sun. It was well it came down on us, for that broke the fall, and it was not injured.

Five days later I got out and was carried down to the hospital, and found the Expert doing pretty fairly. In a few more days I was quite sound. I attribute this to my prudence in always dismounting on something soft. Some recommend a feather bed, but I think an Expert is better.

The Expert got out at last, brought four assistants with him. It was a good idea. These four held the graceful cobweb upright while I climbed into the saddle; then they formed in column and marched on either side of me while the Expert pushed behind; all hands assisted at the dismount.

The bicycle had what is called the "wabbles," and had them very badly. In order to keep my position, a good many things were required of me, and in every instance the thing required was against nature. That is to say, that whatever the needed thing might be, my nature, habit, and breeding moved me to attempt it in one way, while some immutable and unsuspected law of physics required that it be done in just the other way. I perceived by this how radically and grotesquely wrong had been the life-long education of my body and members. They were steeped in ignorance; they knew nothing -- nothing which it could profit them to know. For instance, if I found myself falling to the right, I put the tiller hard down the other way, by a quite natural impulse, and so violated a law, and kept on going down. The law required the opposite thing -- the big wheel must be turned in the direction in which you are falling. It is hard to believe this, when you are told it. And not merely hard to believe it, but impossible; it is opposed to all your notions. And it is just as hard to do it, after you do come to believe it. Believing it, and knowing by the most convincing proof that it is true, does not help it: you can't any more do it than you could before; you can neither force nor persuade yourself to do it at first. The intellect has to come to the front, now. It has to teach the limbs to discard their old education and adopt the new.

The steps of one's progress are distinctly marked. At the end of each lesson he knows he has acquired something, and he also knows what that something is, and likewise that it will stay with him. It is not like studying German, where you mull along, in a groping, uncertain way, for thirty years; and at last, just as you think you've got it, they spring the subjunctive on you, and there you are. No -- and I see now, plainly enough, that the great pity about the German language is, that you can't fall off it and hurt yourself. There is nothing like that feature to make you attend strictly to business. But I also see, by what I have learned of bicycling, that the right and only sure way to learn German is by the bicycling method. That is to say, take a grip on one villainy of it at a time, leaving that one half learned.

When you have reached the point in bicycling where you can balance the machine tolerably fairly and propel it and steer it, then comes your next task -- how to mount it. You do it in this way: you hop along behind it on your right foot, resting the other on the mounting-peg, and grasping the tiller with your hands. At the word, you rise on the peg, stiffen your left leg, hang your other one around in the air in a general in indefinite way, lean your stomach against the rear of the saddle, and then fall off, maybe on one side, maybe on the other; but you fall off. You get up and do it again; and once more; and then several times.

By this time you have learned to keep your balance; and also to steer without wrenching the tiller out by the roots (I say tiller because it is a tiller; "handle-bar" is a lamely descriptive phrase). So you steer along, straight ahead, a little while, then you rise forward, with a steady strain, bringing your right leg, and then your body, into the saddle, catch your breath, fetch a violent hitch this way and then that, and down you go again. But you have ceased to mind the going down by this time; you are getting to light on one foot or the other with considerable certainty. Six more attempts and six more falls make you perfect. You land in the saddle comfortably, next time, and stay there -- that is, if you can be content to let your legs dangle, and leave the pedals alone a while; but if you grab at once for the pedals, you are gone again. You soon learn to wait a little and perfect your balance before reaching for the pedals; then the mounting-art is acquired, is complete, and a little practice will make it simple and easy to you, though spectators ought to keep off a rod or two to one side, along at first, if you have nothing against them.

And now you come to the voluntary dismount; you learned the other kind first of all. It is quite easy to tell one how to do the voluntary dismount; the words are few, the requirement simple, and apparently undiffi-cult; let your left pedal go down till your left leg is nearly straight, turn your wheel to the left, and get off as you would from a horse. It certainly does sound exceedingly easy; but it isn't. I don't know why it isn't but it isn't. Try as you may, you don't get down as you would from a horse, you get down as you would from a house afire. You make a spectacle of yourself every time.

During the eight days I took a daily lesson an hour and a half. At the end of this twelve working-hours' apprenticeship I was graduated -- in the rough. I was pronounced competent to paddle my own bicycle without outside help. It seems incredible, this celerity of acquirement. It takes considerably longer than that to learn horseback-riding in the rough.

Now it is true that I could have learned without a teacher, but it would have been risky for me, be-cause of my natural clumsiness. The self-taught man seldom knows anything accurately, and he does not know a tenth as much as he could have known if he had worked under teachers; and, besides, he brags, and is the means of fooling other thoughtless people into going and doing as he himself has done. There are those who imagine that the unlucky accidents of life -- life's "experiences" -- are in some way useful to us. I wish I could find out how. I never knew one of them to happen twice. They always change off and swap around and catch you on your inexperienced side. If personal experience can be worth anything as an education, it would-n't seem likely that you could trip Methuselah; and yet if that old person could come back here it is more that likely that one of the first things he would do would be to take hold of one of these electric wires and tie himself all up in a knot. Now the surer thing and the wiser thing would be for him to ask somebody whether it was a good thing to take hold of. But that would not suit him; he would be one of the self-taught kind that go by expe-rience; he would want to examine for himself. And he would find, for his instruction, that the coiled patriarch shuns the electric wire; and it would be useful to him, too, and would leave his education in quite a complete and rounded-out condition, till he should come again, some day, and go to bouncing a dynamite-can around to find out what was in it.

But we wander from the point. However, get a teacher; it saves much time and Pond's Extract.

Before taking final leave of me, my instructor inquired concerning my physical strength, and I was able to inform him that I hadn't any. He said that that was a defect which would make up-hill wheeling pretty difficult for me at first; but he also said the bicycle would soon remove it. The contrast between his muscles and mine was quite marked. He wanted to test mine, so I offered my biceps -- which was my best. It almost made him smile. He said, "It is pulpy, and soft, and yielding, and rounded; it evades pressure, and glides from under the fingers; in the dark a body might think it was an oyster in a rag." Perhaps this made me look grieved, for he added, briskly: "Oh, that's all right, you needn't worry about that; in a little while you can't tell it from a petrified kidney. Just go right along with your practice; you're all right."

Then he left me, and I started out alone to seek adventures. You don't really have to seek them -- that is nothing but a phrase -- they come to you.

I chose a reposeful Sabbath-day sort of a back street which was about thirty yards wide between the curbstones. I knew it was not wide enough; still, I thought that by keeping strict watch and wasting no space unnecessarily I could crowd through.

Of course I had trouble mounting the machine, entirely on my own responsibility, with no encouraging moral support from the outside, no sympathetic instructor to say, "Good! now you're doing well -- good again -- don't hurry -- there, now, you're all right -- brace up, go ahead." In place of this I had some other support. This was a boy, who was perched on a gate-post munching a hunk of maple sugar.

He was full of interest and comment. The first time I failed and went down he said that if he was me he would dress up in pillows, that's what he would do. The next time I went down he advised me to go and learn to ride a tricycle first. The third time I collapsed he said he didn't believe I could stay on a horse-car. But the next time I succeeded, and got clumsily under way in a weaving, tottering, uncertain fashion, and occupy-ing pretty much all of the street. My slow and lumbering gait filled the boy to the chin with scorn, and he sung out, "My, but don't he rip along!" Then he got down from his post and loafed along the sidewalk, still observing and occasionally commenting. Presently he dropped into my wake and followed along behind. A little girl passed by, balancing a wash-board on her head, and giggled, and seemed about to make a remark, but the boy said, rebukingly, "Let him alone, he's going to a funeral."

I have been familiar with that street for years, and had always supposed it was a dead level; but it was not, as the bicycle now informed me, to my surprise. The bicycle, in the hands of a novice, is as alert and acute as a spirit-level in the detecting the delicate and vanishing shades of difference in these matters.

Little Changes   **273**   *Priscilla Houliston*

It notices a rise where your untrained eye would not observe that one existed; it notices any decline which water will run down. I was toiling up a slight rise, but was not aware of it. It made me tug and pant and perspire; and still, labor as I might, the machine came almost to a standstill every little while. At such times the boy would say: "That's it! take a rest -- there ain't no hurry. They can't hold the funeral without you."

Stones were a bother to me. Even the smallest ones gave me a panic when I went over them. I could hit any kind of a stone, no matter how small, if I tried to miss it; and of course at first I couldn't help trying to do that. It is but natural. It is part of the ass that is put in us all, for some inscrutable reason.

It was at the end of my course, at last, and it was necessary for me to round to. This is not a pleasant thing, when you undertake it for the first time on your own responsibility, and neither is it likely to succeed. Your confidence oozes away, you fill steadily up with nameless apprehensions, every fiber of you is tense with a watchful strain, you start a cautious and gradual curve, but your squirmy nerves are all full of electric anxieties, so the curve is quickly demoralized into a jerky and perilous zigzag; then suddenly the nickel-clad horse takes the bit in its mouth and goes slanting for the curbstone, defying all prayers and all your powers to change its mind -- your heart stands still, your breath hangs fire, your legs forget to work, straight on you go, and there are but a couple of feet between you and the curb now. And now is the desperate moment, the last chance to save yourself; of course all your instructions fly out of your head, and you whirl your wheel away from the curb instead of toward it, and so you go sprawling on that granite-bound inhospitable shore. That was my luck; that was my experience. I dragged myself out from under the indestructible bicycle and sat down on the curb to examine.

I started on the return trip. It was now that I saw a farmer's wagon poking along down toward me, loaded with cabbages. If I needed anything to perfect the precariousness of my steering, it was just that. The farmer was occupying the middle of the road with his wagon, leaving barely fourteen or fifteen yards of space on either side. I couldn't shout at him -- a beginner can't shout; if he opens his mouth he is gone; he must keep all his attention on his business. But in this grisly emergency, the boy came to the rescue, and for once I had to be grateful to him. He kept a sharp lookout on the swiftly varying impulses and inspirations of my bicycle, and shouted to the man accordingly:
"To the left! Turn to the left, or this jackass 'll run over you!" The man started to do it. "No, to the right, to the right! Hold on! That won't do! -- to the left! -- to the right! -- to the left -- right! left -- ri -- Stay where you are, or you're a goner!"

And just then I caught the off horse in the starboard and went down in a pile. I said, "Hang it! Couldn't you see I was coming?"

"Yes, I see you was coming, but I couldn't tell which way you was coming. Nobody could -- now, could they? You couldn't yourself -- now, could you? So what could I do?"

There was something in that, and so I had the magnanimity to say so. I said I was no doubt as much to blame as he was.

Within the next five days I achieved so much progress that the boy couldn't keep up with me. He had to go back to his gate-post, and content himself with watching me fall at long range.

There was a row of low stepping-stones across one end of the street, a measured yard apart. Even after I got so I could steer pretty fairly I was so afraid of those stones that I always hit them. They gave me the worst falls I ever got in that street, except those which I got from dogs. I have seen it stated that no expert is quick enough to run over a dog; that a dog is always able to skip out of his way. I think that that may be true: but I think that the reason he couldn't run over the dog was because he was trying to. I did not try to run over any dog. But I ran over every dog that came along. I think it makes a great deal of difference. If you try to run over the dog he knows how to calculate, but if you are trying to miss him he does not know how to calculate, and is liable to jump the wrong way every time. It was always so in my experience. Even when I could not hit a wagon I could hit a dog that came to see me practice. They all liked to see me practice, and they all came, for there was very little going on in our neighborhood to entertain a dog. It took time to learn to miss a dog, but I achieved even that.

I can steer as well as I want to, now, and I will catch that boy one of these days and run over him if he doesn't reform.

Get a bicycle. You will not regret it, if you live.

Citation: Twain, Mark. "Taming the Bicycle," What Is Man? and Other Essays (New York: Harper and Brothers, 1917)

Now *THAT* is how you write. As I was reading this out loud to Morton, we were both laughing and picturing this scene in our mind's eye. That is the mark of a real writer, one that can take you there.

Morton and I meet up with my sister at the *Mark Twain Museum*, her most favorite place in the world. She takes us inside and we get a tour that is second to none. She knows all the stories, the behind-the-scene things that there isn't enough room to put on the signs and Morton and I eat it up. This is the best tour and I wish my sister had the time to take everyone through this enchanted place.

We have a stroll through the cemetery where you go at midnight with a dead cat to get rid of warts, we walk through the cave where Huck and Tom explored and even sat in a stagecoach. All in the air conditioned comfort of the museum. There are benches that look like you are on a raft, where you can sit and watch a bit of Huck Finn, stairs that you climb that look just like you are inside a riverboat, with a wheel to steer at the top and a whistle, which we both delighted in blowing. This of course, overlooks the Mississippi River which is right outside of the window in front of you. This place really is hands on. We love it. At the top, you see the original Norman Rockwell paintings for the Mark Twain books, *Tom Sawyer* and *Huck Finn*. These are wonderful, again, Cindy gives us the details and insights that we love to hear and then we move on to see a tall bicycle, like the one Twain tried to master. It is a Penny Farthing and Morton and I can't resist a picture with it. Neither one of us would be brave enough to attempt it, but maybe when we are all finished with the journey and quite fit, we will have to give it a go.

We get to meet Henry Sweets, a true expert of Mark Twain who asks us if we have any questions. I can't think of any, but Morton, who asks more questions than a four year old belts out his of, *"How tall was Mark Twain?"* Henry tells us that he was 5'8", but then disappears in to his office to return just seconds later with a book. This is the mark of a true expert, not only does he know his facts, he can also put his hands right on the spot that backs the facts up. Henry read to us the following passage that left us all standing in the hallway of the museum having a belly laugh.

[In applying for a German passport on May 7, 1878, Mark Twain described himself to the authorities]--My description is as follows: Born 1835; 5 ft. 8 1/2 inches tall; weight about 145 pounds....dark brown hair and red moustache, full face with very high ears and light gray beautiful beaming eyes and a damned good moral character. - letter to Bayard Taylor written May 7, 1878 (in German); reprinted and translated in "New Letters of Mark Twain," American Literature, 3/1936, p. 48.

This is a sense of humour in the highest degree. Subtle, thinking and so quick.

We say our goodbyes and make our way back to my sister's house. I ponder on the way about perfect jobs. Since the people that work in the museum have such a love and passion for Mark Twain, their jobs have to be such a pleasure. Once I heard that working in a flower shop, arranging flowers to be exact, was the perfect job. Today though, I saw otherwise. Working in this town, in this museum, has to rank right up there with astronaut and pirate.

Day 236 August 24, 2007, Friday Hannibal, Missouri

Today Morton and I both got stuck in to working on the computer. I'm trying to train him how to help me with the photo editing, but it reminds me of the saying about old dogs and new tricks! He is so smart about most things, but he seems to be *NOT* learning on purpose, just because then I'll have him do it. We take advantage of my sisters huge porch and the cooler temps and sit out all day. Only once do we have to push the table back to get out of the reach of the rain. My sister made a delicious leaving dinner and we spent a wonderful last night together in the lovely town of Hannibal. We will be back.

Day 237 August 25, 2007, Saturday Hannibal, Missouri to Gothenburg, Nebraska

We drove and drove and then drove some more. My sister had gotten us off to a good start with goodies to eat along the way and the further west I drove, the less I felt like running back to Pennsylvania and Sarah. The Mississippi River is really a great divider. Nebraska is really pretty. There are fields of sunflowers, tall corn and the road is long and straight. Morton sleeps as I drive on. My mind kills time by thinking about what is waiting in front of us. Since it is impossible for me to even know anymore, I turn my thoughts backward. Something pops into my head and I am sitting in my parents room flipping through a copy of *Wild West* magazine that my dad always read. There were articles in about gunslingers, old men panning for gold, stagecoach robbers and the bold riders of the Pony Express. As I was thinking about our trip west, lo and behold there was a sign announcing a real Pony Express station at Gothenburg. I woke Morton up long enough to ask if he wanted to try to find a cheap motel off that exit. Cheap being the word. We are spending money on gas only. We had agreed that we would sleep in the car on our way to Cheyenne, but neither of our seats will go back. After our two to three hours of sleep in the car on the way to my sister's house, we thought it might be more comfortable to sleep on the roof. It was a stroke of good luck that we found a cheap room in a little motel and it was clean and close to the Pony Express station. Morton fell asleep FAST and I tried to stay up and work, but all the driving had me worn out. I would have NEVER made it as a Pony Express rider.

Day 238 August 26, 2007, Sunday Gothenburg, Nebraska to Cheyenne, Wyoming and *Howdy Pardner Bed & Breakfast...*the ONLY place to stay in Cheyenne. *Dinner* | Calamity Jan made us a HOME COOKED meal of delicious salad, stuffed green pepper (DELICIOUS!!!) fresh sweet corn, watermelon, two homemade cookies, a lovely treat in our room of this scrumptious homemade sweet that Calamity Jan makes herself.

We got up early and made for the Pony Express Station. We figured that it would be shut on a Sunday morning, but we were hoping that we could get some pictures. We were thrilled to find it not only opened, but staffed with a wonderful lady who told us all about the history of it.

The road sailed under the tires and Morton and I both felt a little sad that we weren't getting to really see what we were breezing by. Life is slower on a bicycle and better. You really see things. Today we were looking for a sign that said WYOMING.

Morton commented about the way that the corn grew in this country, row after row. We talked about using it for gasoline, eating it, grilling it and all things corn.

We made good time, great time actually. I had forgotten about the clocks slowing down and turning back out here. We passed a sign telling us we were in Mountain Time and I knew we should have had an extra hour of sleeping.

The signs for Cheyenne got closer and before we knew it, I was following Calamity Jan's directions to the lovely bed and breakfast known as *Howdy Pardner*. We arrived early and were met graciously by our host and hostess, such lovely people.

Morton and I got our gear inside with the help of Herb. Morton was blown away by the house, being decorated with a real Western flair and I couldn't get over the views. The best you can imagine. We were doing an interview with *CBS Channel 5* in Cheyenne and they were kind enough to come out to the B&B to do the interview. Sitting on a log, wired up with a microphone I got lost in the journey and rambled on and on. The thing about the interview is, you never really know what parts of it they are going to use. The reporters are usually lucky if they get to ask me three questions. Just one questions starts my wheels rolling and I'm soon talking faster than I should about our journey. I'm passionate about what we are doing and really want to share the journey with the world. It is the best feeling I have ever known, being able to inspire someone to see the light about moderation and movement. To get motivation, we must try to give it.

The interview was great, then over and Morton and I went in to have a chat with with our host and hostess. It was great and we could have talked all night. My computer was calling me and I had to download pictures. Just as I was getting going, Jan brought the most amazing dinner down for us. The stuffed peppers were out of this world. We were both just so impressed with her cooking, her hospitality and again we feel the sting of having just made friends and then having to leave. When we are finished, we are going to be back. Morton and I enjoy the rec room where there is this bar with the best bar stools. They are seats from tractors, so fun and comfortable. Our room holds a secret. Our turned down beds have lovely mints on them, with chocolate and there is a window scene that is lit up, like a night light for us. It is so lovely in the big log bed we fall fast asleep, loving our first night in Wyoming. Morton says he could stay here forever, after all, he always wanted to be a cowboy.

Day 239 August 27, 2007, Monday Howdy Pardner B&B Cheyenne, Wyoming
Breakfast | stuffed french toast with peaches & creme cheese, fresh fruit with creme, sherbet, oj, bacon * Lunch | delicious fruit smoothie at *Rubyjuice on 17th St,* with lovely wraps and a bag of chips * Dinner | 1/2 salad of teriyaki chicken, 1/2 wrap at *Synergy Cafe*...BRILLIANT eating in Cheyenne!

We had an entire day to explore Cheyenne and we wished we would have at least two weeks, but sadly we still need to head even further west.

First we had a Trolley Tour of the town that was really good for getting our bearings. Then we saw the *Cheyenne Botanical Gardens*, the museums, the trains and all the charms of this magical city. There are eight foot high boots scattered around the city that have been painted lots of different ways. My favorite I saw was one with a deer and antelope playing cards on it. For those of you that don't get the joke, think, *"Home, home on the range...where the deer and the antelope play..."* It was all good fun.

We had FANTASTIC food today at *Rubyjuice* and *Synergy Cafe* and even met some people who knew what we were up to. It was one of those days that flew by, was gone before we knew it and found us heading to bed after a stunning sunset and what looked to be a full moon.

When you come to visit a place like this, it is impossible to squeeze everything in to a day or two. We could keep busy and occupied in Cheyenne for at least a week or two. Actually, come to think of it, you could find different things to do for the rest of your life here. I have a feeling that the COWBOY FEVER has grabbed Morton. From the way his face lit up when he put a cowboy hat on in the LOST LUGGAGE bit of the train station museum (DO NOT MISS THIS!) and he grabbed a pair of six shooters in a holster, it was all over for him. I didn't have the heart to tell him the hat he had on *and* the six shooters where meant for kids to play with.

Take the time out of your life to GO SOMEWHERE, even if it is just exploring in your own backyard. There is no substitute for travel and adventure. If you are working on weight loss like I am, incorporate a sense of adventure with it. We got an email from a lady who is making her weight loss an adventure and noting it along in a very clever way. She started with a big, white sheet of poster board and took a picture of her at her heaviest. She then takes one whenever she reaches her *"during goal"* of 20 pounds. This way, she can look and see the progress. We think that if FANTASTIC and really recommend doing this. Pictures don't lie and it will give you a clear outlook of where you are.

Today we had a fantastic talk with Liz, from Synergy Cafe in Cheyenne. She and I were talking about this clever way of marking your progress to keep you going when you think there is no point. (Trust me, there are days that I think it *IS* too tough, but thank goodness I won't let myself fall into the old QUITTING ways of the past) Liz said that she had read in this fantastic book that it was a good idea to take pictures and make a collage of lots of images of yourself, including pictures of your face now, on the body you wish you had. I think I would choose a normal sized, toned body...but not SUPER MODEL level. Anyway, the idea is that your subconscience sees this image and accepts it as the normal. You can TRICK your own mind into seeing you normal sized and helping you get there! I am going to do that! To often, when a person has so much weight to lose, it feels like our journey is never going to end. The truth is, it isn't. I know that since I had weighed over 400 pounds, I'm inclined to abuse food and forget exercise. THIS IS WHERE I HAVE TO GET TOUGH! I have to commit to being healthy and do what I need to do FOR THE REST OF MY LIFE to first get there and then stay there. Thinking about the words like "yo-yo diet" and people that have told me they have lost thousands of pounds in their lifetime, I know what is in store for me. The only difference is, my mind has finally figured out that being fit has nothing to do with how I look. This is a matter of staying alive, living longer, being active and actually having a life that is worth living. I want ALL of these things. My diet will never end since I'm not on one. I will practice moderation and quit eating whole bags of chips, whole cakes, huge portions. I will also make sure that my adventure with exercise never ends now. There is nothing I enjoy more than going on a walk, slowing down and seeing this wonderful world we live in. Even on a bicycle, it can be too fast sometimes to stop and smell the roses. If only we had more time we might just stay awake and watch the stars twinkle. We could almost reach up and grab one here. If I wake up in the morning, it will be hard to leave this place and hit the trail, but there are miles to be covered. We aren't leaving big ruts in the land that can still be seen decades and centuries later like the wagon trains, but hopefully we will have gotten through to JUST ONE PERSON in Cheyenne that there *is* hope. It is all inside you waiting to come out. Have a plan and then be prepared to follow through with it. That is the secret to success in anything. Like the cowboys who ride the bucking broncos and wild bulls know, if you hang on tight and give it your best shot, it's one heck of a ride!

Day 240 August 28, 2007, Tuesday Howdy Pardner B&B, Cheyenne to Bentwood Inn B&B in Jackson Hole, Wyoming

Waking up at five am today, I hoped to get writing done. It wasn't meant to happen though. The emails, the photos and the clock that seems to have extra fast hands kept me chasing my tail.

Jan made us our second scrumptious breakfast in the same number of days, then gave us a bag with goodies in it when we said goodbye. Her and her wonderful hubby will get added to our long list of people we hope we get to see again. All of this travel is tough people. This is day 240 of being somewhere different, living out of giant Ziploc bags stuffed with our clothes and a heap of perpetual motion. We hoped our cameras would not fill up before we drove over 400 miles through Wyoming today. One of them did fill up, 480 pictures. The other one ended up having almost 500 pictures on it and you know what, there wasn't one bad one.

We saw pronghorn deer, lots of cows, the prettiest horses, a buffalo and lots of rabbits along the way. Even though the animals were everywhere, the big scene stealer today was the landscape. Morton kept saying over and over that no one will believe just how big this place is. Pictures aren't enough to fit it all in, no matter how large they are. It is just stunning. After gasping all day, we reached the lovely Bentwood Inn and had to start gasping all over again. The logs used for the inn have came from Yellowstone. We strolled around their massive yard taking lots of pictures. Everything from white toadstools in the lush grass to Morton sipping wine.

We debated for about 5 seconds if we should get back in the car and drive around before the sun sets, but after a full day of it, I needed to just get to the computer, downloading almost 1,000 pictures and trying to find sleep before midnight. If you haven't noticed, my time is just getting tighter and tighter. When you think we aren't even spending 7 or 8 hours on a bike right now, I start to worry. Morton has to step up to the plate and kick in with some help on the pictures. They are a vital part in our journey, now we are doing serious filming as well. This trip is either going to kill us or make us able to do anything. I think we'll choose the second.

Tonight we enjoy the sheer luxury of being inside. The temperature is suppose to dip in to the 30's. Tonight is what we have. Tomorrow, it is back on the trail of *NOT KNOWING* where we will stay. Something will turn up, we know this.

Morton and I are both longing for dropping the car off in Portland and just being us and the bicycles again. It is so much easier and cheaper. True, we don't cover as many miles and things are slower on a bicy-cle, but what you miss in a car that you see on a bike you could fill a library with. Then there is the horrible cost of gasoline.

The smells, the breeze on your face (or ice cold rain on your face) and just the wonderful feeling of being alive and outdoors is really something. We are both addicted to it now. It isn't always the easy thing to do, but it is the right thing to do. We know this.

Adventures come in all shapes and sizes, just like people. We want our adventure to inspire you to turn your life into one big journey that is just full of adventure. Open up your mind to the idea that you can do anything, really *ANYTHING* that you put your mind to. Don't be realistic. Take chances. Care enough about your health to put that on a high priority in your life. After all, if you don't have your health, you have no life.

Our email is full of people from around the world in various stages of health. Some are very fit, some are bedfast due to obesity. There is the simple truth that all of us, yes, even *YOU*, needs 30 minutes of exer-cise each and every day. If we don't get it, bad things happen to our bodies.

Even though most of our day was spent sitting in the car, Morton and I went for a lovely stroll when we arrived at the Bentwood Inn. Our legs needed stretching and our bodies are missing all the exercise they are use to. Tomorrow we park the car and hit the park. Walking, walking and then more walking. This all ac-companied of course by a healthy dose of "ooohing and aaaahing" from the sights we are seeing. Tonight though, we have an indoor bed that very well could be the last one we see in a while. So I'm off to dreamland, smiling and thinking about all the sights we got to enjoy out the window. They would have all been a million times nicer if we would have been walking or bicycling through them. I think at the end of our journey we are going to have to spend a summer in Wyoming on the bikes. But then, come to think of it, we could really say the same about all the other states we have bicycled through so far.

Day 241 August 29, 2007, Wednesday *Bentwood Inn B&B* in Jackson Hole, WY

We didn't really have a clue to where we were going to stay tonight. All we knew this morning is that the breakfast and the conversation was lovely and we were off to explore. After all, something always seems to turn up. Using the map to negotiate up the one side of Grand Teton National Park, Morton and I weren't ex-pecting to come to a park entrance booth. It was $25. for a weeks pass or $80. for a year pass that would get us into all the National Parks. Since there are quite a few of them and we haven't been able to get the NPS to become a sponsor, we bite the bullet and shelled out the $80. It really is a bargain if you think about it. It means that we will have to make up that $80. of the budget with food though, which is a good thing. We need to cut back on the grub. Driving into this paradise, we knew in a second it was the best $80. that had ever been spent. Either side of the road were a million "ooohs and aaaahs" just waiting to be photographed.

We had read that the park tenting spaces fill up quick, so we stopped to pitch tent in the only camp-site area that offers showers. We are having two nights here, tucked under pine trees that sway about 70 feet in the air. The ranger tells us that there have been bears in this camping area daily, to know the bear rules and follow them. At the same time, there are two rangers of some sort that are there setting a bear trap in the area. Morton is so excited he squeals and gives up a rare smile.

While we are pitching the tent, something crashes in the woods and Morton and I both jump. It turns out it was a squirrel that thinks our campsite is his. He doesn't have a lot of fear and while Morton is setting the tent up, he almost runs inside at one point. We throw the sleeping bags in and get outta camp to see some more before the sun sets. The wildlife is stunning. Morton has a close encounter with a little herd of buffalo, a deer right at the car window, beautiful horses that I couldn't even thing about riding because they have a weight limit on of 225 pounds per rider (the next time I come here I will be able to do that) and there are birds of every description around.

The day is spent with lots of photographs, one telephone interview with a newspaper far away that I promise to send high resolution photos to and a shopping trip at a dollar store! Morton and I are happy to get stocked up on our cheap eats. We are starting with the normal road eating again, today getting enough food to last us a week or so. $41.00. A bargain.

This area is a bit overwhelming. I think that you would never get bored with looking at the sky, watching the clouds move in shadow across the mountains, seeing the wind push the sage bushes and grass in the breeze...pure paradise. It is brilliant times a gillion. We fill our heads with images we will never forget and we fill the memory cards on the camera. We need power and we have none at the campsite. There is the option of standing in the bathroom, but neither one of us are thrilled with that thought. Not when there is a sky like the one above us to gaze at. When we get our gear sorted for the night, I build a fire with dead wood that Morton has chopped with his hatchet. It starts on the first time and we sit and watch the silvery blue sky turn into a velvet blue with a million little stars, steady glowing.

There is a picnic table that I use to lay back on and watch the process of the stars popping out. There are none at first, when the sky is still a light blue. But then it begins. I see the first one, right above me. It is strong and bright and if almost by magic, another one appears to the left of it, slightly out of line. Why have I waited 44 years to see this show that happens every clear night? I was enchanted. Morton didn't seem bothered, just giving the odd glance upwards as he poked the fire.

His mind was on the bag of marshmallows we had gotten. He had a metal fork he was determined to toast them on. I warned him it would be too hot, but he still made a great effort of it. Soon I was eating toasted goodness that varied from raw to charcoal black, after being set on fire by Morton. He likes them that way, I'm more of a "golden brown" sort of girl. We were like children tonight, eating toasted campfire candy, taking pictures of the flames and me, enchanted by the way the stars all came on. I counted them, while they were still few enough to count. 27. Then, all of a sudden there were thousands. An endless sky of tiny white lights.

Just beyond our tall trees are the mountains, invisible now in the dark sky. We watched the fire burn out and called it a night about 10 pm. We both wanted to get up early to see wildlife. Seeing the sun come up in a place like this should be a requirement. The tent, our NEW, old tent, is smaller, lighter and able to handle lower temperatures. Since the forecast was calling for the 30's, I was glad. I was sorry though about a big mistake that I had made. We left our foam mats at Sarah's house. We did this because they take up so much room, add weight and I figured we are always sleeping on grass or sand. But not tonight. Tonight we were sleeping on pebbles. Thousands of them that felt sharp and cold in our backs. Morton tried to say it was my fault and I told him that if we wanted to play the blame game, I could bring up the fact that we have the cheapest sleeping bags on the market that are tissue thin and offer no real insulation or mattress type quality about them. We laughed as we discovered that our pillows, our jackets shoved into pillow cases, were the best bit of our bed. At least it was a clear night, lots of stars and not a drop of rain to be found.

Day 242 August 30, 2007 Thursday Grand Teton National Park, Wyoming

When we look back on today, we will dot it with animals, birds, stunning views and some very interesting people we met along the way. First I have to tell you that I got up with the sun, which was easy since my back was in agony from our cold stone bed. This is not a beauty therapy I would recommend. It made me feel very tired and old, but thank goodness the weather motivated me to move as soon as I climbed out the hole in the tent. We are now using tent number 2, a tent we had gotten before the walk that is more suited to cold weather. The trouble was, when we tried in on for size in a "practice" scenario in my mother's yard, the tent fit me like a glove. We were squashed in it and Morton and my son both had to give me a hand to pull me out of it. When we were back in Pennsylvania for July & part of August filming, I tried on the tent again. Since I am minus 150 pounds or so, this time it was a much better fit. Still smaller then tent number one (an old one we had bought in Scotland about 4 years ago) but tent number 2 was lighter, wasn't falling apart like tent number 1 due to many nights in service and tent number two was also going to keep us warmer. It might have worked, but somewhere between marshmallows toasting and us climbing in the hole of the tent (it really is a circle about a foot off the ground!) Morton, being the first night we had actually camped in this tent, didn't zip the outside flap. We were freezing come sunrise. During the night I was wishing we had upgraded the sleeping bags. I also wished I would have taken the two minutes to pull my socks out of a bag in the car and put them on my freezing feet.

We were sleeping on a downhill bit, on a bed of rocks with sharp little points and the almost full moon had made for a very cold evening. Morton, human heater that he is, wasn't cold at all. But me, as soon as I popped out of the rabbit's hole on the tent, I sprinted to the bathroom. After throwing ice cold water on my face and drying it with the bottom of my t-shirt, I was off to wake my sleeping bear. Getting Morton to wake up was fairly easy. Since we were camping in a place that has signs about bears everywhere, I took advantage of a feisty chipmunk that was making way too much noise for something so little, just about twenty feet from the tent. Once I had unzipped the circle I paused for a second. I knew Morton had half an eye open and was waiting to see what I was going to do. Get back in the cold sleeping bag or get up to see the sunrise. The chipmunk got loud and I looked back at him, as if I was peering into the woods. "What on earth is that?" I said in a whisper. Morton was up like a shot. After all, the chipmunk could have been a grizzly bear. Morton was pleased to see the chipmunk and when he saw the purple, pink and golden sky with a almost full moon still hanging high in it, he decided waking up this early wasn't bad. Our early morning wake up was well worth it. If you come here, make sure you get up with the sun or even a bit before. By lunch we had seen a mother moose and her calf, elk, a whole herd of buffalo, an eagle, a bull moose and any number of "grizzly" chipmunks. Morton was still waiting to see his real bear though.

We spent the day driving to various points in the park and then getting out of the car and walking. This is the only way to see it. If you come through on a bus and it stops anywhere, make sure you get out the door and walk in this wilderness. There is something about getting away from the crowd, down an empty path, where you don't hear anything but nature. Even though so many people visit here, it never felt crowded once you were off that main road. The history of this area is fascinating and Morton and I both agree that someday we will sit down and read a book or two about it. But right now we are here and want to take in every second of it we can. Morton had spotted with his keen eye, a patch in a field that turned out to be a coyote chasing something. Maybe one of the fierce chipmunks. We watched for a bit, but he never seemed to catch what he was after. We all know that feeling. Morton and I decided that maybe he didn't like an audience and drove one.

Since our sunset at our campsite is hidden by the trees, we agree to go to this bend in the water where a whole moose family seems to live. The Tetons are behind it in the distance and it has to be one of the prettiest sights on the planet. The sun should set right behind us, making this a perfect place to set for a few hours and be amazed by the way the scene changes with the light of the day. We aren't disappointed. A mother and her calf, moose of course, are in the water at the edge. They watch us and the other people there, with little or no interest. They have been seeing this same show for ages. People stopping in their cars, getting out, taking a million and one photographs, we are nothing knew to them. The pair don't even get flustered when a squad of people in kayaks and canoes come down the little river, passing just 10 feet from them. They barely stop eating to turn their heads and acknowledge anyone is there. The bull moose is off in the other part, attracting his own group of onlookers. My interest is with the mother and her calf. Even though the calf is getting really big, I notice the mother always has herself between us and her child. She is protecting her. If anyone of us made any move to get closer to her calf, I know it wouldn't end up pretty. Some of the photographers, men and women, creep down the edge of the bank and approach the water. The mother watches them, but knows there is a river between them. This is her space and we feel lucky to get to peek into their private life. I'm happy to watch from this distance and put the zoom feature on my camera to work.

When the sun sets, the mosquitoes and flies have been out for ages. Stupid as I am, I don't walk the 100 yards back to get the bug spray. After all, the light is fading fast now and I still have a few dozen pictures to get of the mountains, their reflection on the water and of course the mama and baby moose. I slap the bugs and snap the photos. Morton is busy with his own camera doing the same only he does more of a dance to shake the bugs off him. If he had a tail like a moose or a horse, I'm sure he would have been swinging that as he was taking pictures like a man on a mission.

Driving back to our camp, we were both thinking of burning the rest of the wood Morton had gathered from the woods and split. After all, he had gotten a blister in the process, so it only seemed right to burn it all up on our last night there. But when we got back, our big long day caught up with us. We were both so tired that the thought of crawling into our tissue-paper like sleeping bags on the pointy gravel, seemed like heaven to us. We gave the marshmallows a swerve and instead fluffed up our jacket pillows, with the *outside* flap of the tent zipped, we settled down for the evening.

Day 243 August 31, 2007, Friday Grand Teton Natl Park, WY to Big Sky, Montana
This morning was a tough one. I woke up sore, cold again but my toes didn't feel like popsicles today. I had this incredible urge to use the bathroom. Hopping out of the tent hole with surprising spring, I sprinted to the bathroom block. To my shock and horror, they were *CLOSED* for cleaning. I wasn't the only person that was there crossing her legs, there were several people hopping up and down and we were all wondering why they would chose this time to clean the bathroom. After all, when you are in a place like this, it becomes a

ghost-camp after 9 am. Everyone is off to see the sights. Whatever the reason was though, both the mens and the ladies were closed. I walked funny back to our campsite, sat down on the picnic table and whispered my plight to Morton through the tent hole. His idea was to go off in the woods, which I would have done, but there were tents all over. No safe cover. He suggested heading down to another set of bathrooms, but I knew my bladder would not take that. Instead I just kept a hawk eye towards the toilet and waited for the golf cart looking cleaning car to take off. They finished first with the men's bathroom and five guys all went in. Three women, still standing and waiting, looked at the men's room but didn't make their move for it. I held my ground at the picnic table. My bladder isn't the best at the best of times and combine the cold morning and the feeling of not being able to use the facilities and it is the recipe for an accident.

Finally, they were finished and I waited until the ladies line had died down. Making my sprint there, a man stopped me as I was almost at the door. He wanted to chat about the park, where to go, what he and his wife had seen and endless other things that I would have found fascinating if my back teeth hadn't been floating. Finally I got to run in the bathroom, relief, then to the mirrored sink to wash my face and hands. My ponytail during the night had shifted. Instead of being down the back of my head, it was now high on my head, half the hair hanging down, the other half in a big knotted nest hanging out of the ponytail. I looked hideous, far worse than any other morning. I questioned the sanity of the man who had stopped me for a chat outside. I did look quite the sight. Oh well, he'll have a funny story to tell about the dancing woman with the wild hair who was running for the bathroom.

Morton and I were breaking camp this morning, off to Yellowstone with no plans for the evening. Since we had to pay $3.50 each to have a shower here, we decided to wait until morning, then were shocked to find the showers didn't open until 8:00 am. We hoped to be up to Yellowstone by 8, so it was a mad rush to brush our teeth, scrub up in the bathroom with the cold water and head off, eating our cereal bars along the way. The drive was not disappointing. The trees are what really captured my eye today. Morton and I were looking at a map of Yellowstone trying to figure out what campground we would use. When we got into the park, driving up towards Old Faithful, we stopped at every little turn off we would come to. We walked back paths, climbed stairs and Morton hung out the window trying to capture pictures of this place that is impossible to photograph. There isn't a camera or lens large enough to take this all in. You just need to come here.

A friend of mine from Pennsylvania, Lois, had told me about a path we should take. She had told me that her and her husband had been a bit disappointed by Old Faithful but found that getting off the trail and discovering all the little side paths, they had enjoyed the smaller bubbling and steaming holes in Yellowstone far more than the famous one that attracts huge crowds. Lois was spot on! This is just what Morton and I had felt too. Don't get me wrong, Old Faithful is stunning, but when we got off of the main road, did some of the walks that are up on boardwalks so you don't burn your feet, we discovered paradise. Colorful holes filled with boiling water that would spout off, sometimes as we were passing, had us feeling like we were in the land that time forgot. The other people disappeared and Morton and I just tore up the cameras. So much so, I filled up my camera card and needed to download.

We went to one of the visitor centers so I could get power. I was thrilled, overjoyed and smiling beyond belief at an email we had gotten from a lady named Kathryn. She had invited us to come to and spend the night with her in Big Sky, Montana, just 45 minutes from West Yellowstone. This made our whole day. We were sorted for a night to sleep, a SHOWER and best of all, company! Morton and I could really just enjoy our day now. We had the pressure off of us on *where* we were going to sleep. We explored, walked, climbed and even ate our lunch watching the ground bubble in front of us, over a cold mountain stream. It was a brilliant day, perhaps one of the best ever.

When we finally headed west towards Montana, Kathryn and I spoke on the phone for the first time. She asked if we would like to have dinner with her, gave us our directions and we pointed our eyes to the side of the road to keep a look out for beasties along the way! Driving through a beautiful and brief storm, we were thrilled to see a rainbow over the mountain where we would be spending the night. We stayed up past midnight and made a fantastic new friend. Now comes the time of saying goodbye, always hard to do, but we have a long way to go. But what a view!

Day 244   September 1, 2007, Saturday Big Sky, Montana to Yellowstone National Park, Wyoming

This morning we woke up in paradise. A beautiful bed, a bathroom, breakfast, perfect company and just this wonderful feeling that the day that starts this great can only keep getting better. And it did. Kathryn took us on a wonderful walk up the side of a mountain to watch Chris, someone who works with troubled horses, work miracles with a pair of beautiful horses. This was something right out of a movie, but it was happening before our very eyes. We sat on the fence that is put up at angles because the ground is too rocky to sink a post in. I was enchanted and Morton watched with great intent. This backdrop was as amazing as what we were seeing. Against the brilliant blue Montana sky, there was this handsome cowboy working with this horse of a beautiful color, in a ring surrounded by wide open spaces. Just after a few minutes I knew we were witnessing something very special. The way he became so in tune with this horse he had never met before was amazing. He didn't whisper anything in it's ear, but rather used body language and really just got in tune with the horse. Before we knew it, they were leading the horses to the trailer, with the lesson finished. Chris watched as the owner tried to get the horse into a trailer. It had never been properly trained and she had explained it took several hours to make this happen. Sure enough, the horse did just what the owner said. She refused to go up the ramp, standing firm or even backing up. Chris took the rope that was on the halter and as if by magic, led this naughty horse right up the ramp. She actually went up herself, with Chris putting no pressure at all on the rope. The most remarkable thing about this was the owner's face in pure disbelief. She was stunned. So were we. The next few moments Chris led this horse, actually, he let her lead him, up and down the ramp as if they had worked together for the eight years she has been on this earth. It was as natural as anything could be. Afterwards, Chris told us that the horse just went up with him, because that is what he expected to happen. The horse trusted him, sensed no fear or worry that she wouldn't walk up the ramp and just did it. *Natural.*

As he was speaking I was thinking that this lesson can really be applied to humans as well. When we put up our own roadblocks and hurdles, we turn and run before we even get a chance to go up the ramp. We talk ourselves out of, mentally sometimes, many things that we feel are beyond our reach.

Morton looked a bit worried when I asked Chris if he could work with Morton to get him to listen a bit better to me. He said he wouldn't go there, so we headed back down the hill, smiling and walking with Kathryn. Saying goodbye to our new friend was just as tough as all the people we have been blessed to meet along the way. My dad use to always say, "The good Lord willing, we'll meet again!" whenever he would be leaving. As we drove off I hoped that someday we would get to visit with Kathryn again. She is wonderful and someone I would love to call *friend.*

Morton and I drove the way she had told us would be spectacular and it was. Seeing all the men in the river that ran beside the road fishing, up to their hips in water, casting on the breeze, I wished that I would have learned how to fly fish. My dad took care of teaching my little brother and I how to cast a reel, but we never dabbled in fly fishing. It looks like a dance, gentle and easy. It has to go on my list of things to do someday. Heading back to Yellowstone, we were glad we had looped into Montana. It, as the rest of the great west, is stunning. The mountains, the streams, the fields but most of all, like everywhere, the people are making this journey so special for us. Brilliant!

The gates coming into Yellowstone from the north are impressive. Tall, stone, arched and of course, looking at this incredible view behind them. On the way to the camp we were heading to, we passed Mammoth Springs and had to stop. We just had a very quick peek, not wanting to miss the space at the campground. With the holiday weekend on us, we knew there would be lots of campers out.

The campground was better than we hoped for and at $12. a night, it might be the best bargain in America. Our space is wide open, dotted with giant pine and we got to choose it ourselves. We also got to see a mommy deer with twins that still had their spots on them. Paradise! Morton set the tent up, found a big dead log and started chopping it. We wanted to have the wood ready, since we planned to watch the sun set by the mountains and we knew it would be after dark before we made it back in to the camp. He, like me, likes to be prepared for what happens at night, when we can't see anything.

After seeing the sunset, bison, deer, elk and chipmunks galore, we made our way back to the camp. We were both looking forward to a fire, watching the sky and of course, toasting the marshmallows. Morton and I both let out yelps when we looked in our fire ring to find it empty. There were little twigs that was still there to make lighting the fire easy, but the three big pieces that he had chopped with his wee, dull hatchet, were missing! Beside us, there were some younger French men, with a campfire blazing. The logs looked strangely familiar. Morton was upset, but neither of us said or questioned anything. Instead, Morton popped on this headlight flashlight that he had brought out of my old camping box when we were in Pennsylvania. He looked like a miner preparing to go deep in the earth as he took off into the woods, dull hatchet in hand. I got the twigs going as he searched in the dark for more down and dry wood. Just a few minutes later, I saw the bright light bobbing back towards me. There comes Morton dragging a MASSIVE log, at least eight feet long. He didn't say a word as he took the dull hatchet to it. I think he took out his frustration of having his chopped firewood stolen out on the big log. He was like a man on a mission, moving in the dark, piling the wood in a tipi shape in the fire around my little blazing twigs.

The men around the questionable fire were cooking something that smelled delicious and watching Morton. I sat on the edge of the picnic table as Morton chopped just what was needed for a big fire this evening. He took the rest of the log, now about five feet long and pulled it on the ground to lay beside our tent that was glowing from the blazing campfire. Morton stowed his hatchet, came over and sat by me on the picnic table. "Now hopefully they won't pinch that wood!" he said, gesturing towards the tent. "That is just bad camping manners." Morton finished. He was done with his anger. We toasted marshmallows as we smelled the delicious food the Frenchmen were cooking. I told Morton that we should expect a bear to come in with that smell. That did wonders to cheer him up. The smell made me want to go over and pinch some of their stew, while their three logs burnt down to embers. Morton and I tried not to think that people could be cold enough to steal the logs out of your fire ring and after all, maybe it wasn't this group of Frenchmen. There were other fires glowing. Perhaps, Morton reflected, whoever took it didn't have a hatchet or a way to cut it. We heard a baby crying as we were laying on our backs, watching the stars from the front of the open tent. Maybe, I told Morton, the family that had that little baby had pinched the wood and the baby was now sad that the fire was going out. Morton told me to stop talking rubbish and go to sleep.

The ground was soft and the night was still warm. As I looked up in the black sky with at least a billion stars, we both saw a shooting star. Morton didn't make a wish, he said he doesn't believe in that. I did. He turned over to nestle into his jacket shoved in a pillowcase pillow and I saw the biggest shooting star of my life. It looked like it was four or five inches wide and just slowly moved from east to west. The baby was still crying and the beautiful French accents floated into our tent as I fell asleep in Yellowstone. Somewhere in the dark our stolen logs were now just ashes.

Day 245 September 2, 2007, Sunday Yellowstone National Park, Wyoming

Today we went back to Mammoth Springs only to discover, we hadn't seen ANYTHING just driving past it. Once you start walking the trails to discover one perfect view after the next, we felt like we had landed on some strange and magical planet.

Morton kept saying he expected an alien to pop out of this strange landscape, but the closest thing we saw to it was a chipmunk that looked more grey than brown.

We loaded up the cameras, going all over walks, trails, climbs and things that would have been impossible for me to do a year ago. Feeling very fortunate that I had started making my little changes and glad that I was around to be doing this, I spotted a young lady with her parents.

The family was really overweight. They had driven to the edge of a trail that you needed to walk back just 1/4 of a mile to see the most stunning view of a stunning subject. My heart broke as the daughter, in her early twenties, looked at the sign and then told her parents she would just wait in the car. This was me last year. Since there isn't really any point in me trying to change the lives of people this close, without running the risk of insulting someone or hurting their feelings, I say nothing. What I want to do is gently tell her in a quiet way that life shouldn't be lived like this and it can change. Her body can change. Mine has and I'm not even all the way down the scale yet. But I don't say anything.

Once, a long time ago, I went to Mexico. As soon as I crossed the border in Larado, I was approached by so many Mexicans trying to sell me diet pills, abortions and even one that said, "Lady, you want the lipo?" My face was so red as these street hawkers wouldn't leave me alone. A big fat American was an easy target. Surely I had crossed the border to become thin, not to look at the shops. It was really embarrassing and the person I was with kept laughing about it. For me it was a nightmare.

Never will I walk up to a stranger, no matter what their size is, to tell them how they should live. It is a really personal subject. Now on here, it is a different subject. I can preach away about how important it is to get your body right. Nothing to do with how you look in that dress, pair of jeans or the latest fashion, but this is about how we feel people. We want to be able to be alive and able to walk out to see the view, don't we?

There were places today that made me red in the face. Climbs that were steep, paths that seemed to never end. But Yellowstone rewards it's visitors with the most incredible things hidden all over the place. Traffic jams that were caused by bison trotting down the road, people pulling over to take pictures of moose and elk, all at a slow pace. No one seems to be in a big hurry here. This is a place that you need time to see and Morton and I realize this is our day to just explore and suck it all up. How fantastic there aren't bowling alleys, mini malls and gift shops everywhere. This 2.2 million acres is special and I would need at least another few years to write about everything we saw and did today.

After a very full day of it, we headed back to our beautiful camp site. We were happy to see our logs still laying beside our little tent, waiting for Morton to chop them up. We were glad no one had pinched them. He still went in to the woods to drag out a third log, while it was still daylight. We were going to have a great fire this evening, being our last night in the park.

Morton had seen on a survival show on the way to boil water over a campfire. You take a plastic bottle, tie it with a string and dangle it over the fire. In a few minutes, or twenty as we found out, it boils! This really does work and we have video to prove it.

Sometime though, during this procedure of getting the fire going, Morton got a migraine. This is something he hasn't had for about two years and it scared the life out of me. He started slurring his speech and said his arm was tingling. He sat down and I felt helpless. There was nothing that I could do, except get him aspirin and send him off to bed.

Our fire got drowned with water, the extra logs still laying for the next camper to use. Morton's migraines can really knock him off his feet and when he started mixing his words up, it reminded me of my mom's stroke. A stroke can grab any person at any age and the fear of this really got me. I have to take better care of Morton. We talked for a bit about what might have brought this on. We had did a lot of hiking today, at a high altitude. He also had just did a good bit of exercise, chopping the wood we were going to use this evening. We also had a very late dinner. So many things, but no one can really say for sure. When our flashlight was out, I was watching the stars on my own as Morton was sleeping. It was good he was sleeping, hopefully in the morning, his head would feel fine and I would take it easy on him, exercise wise.

Day 246 September 3, 2007, Monday Yellowstone National Park, Wyoming to Boise, Idaho

Today, while driving from Yellowstone to Boise, Idaho, I was speaking to my sister in Hannibal on the telephone (joy of getting a signal!) and we were both talking about the past year, how it had really flown by. Today was the first anniversary of my father's death and being here, in a place that the two of us had talked about, watched television shows about and read about, I was reminded of him everywhere I looked.

My mom had seemed in good spirits when I talked to her on the phone earlier. I wanted to mention the day, but my dad was all about living and being happy. He wouldn't want my mom to be sad that he was gone (though it's impossible not to miss him almost every waking moment) and he would want everyone to smile, not cry, when thinking about him. I know this. Yet I can't help but think, "what if..."

Today when we were almost ready to leave Yellowstone, one of the last pictures I took was an older couple, hand in hand, walking off into the mist of one of the hundreds of geysers. The picture is lovely, thought provoking and made me sad. What if dad and mom were here? What if they were that very couple, enjoying their golden years together? Would I realize how precious my time with them is?

Even though I'm missing my dad so bad, my thoughts turn to my mom. She is in Pennsylvania, on her own and my phone isn't even getting a signal to call her. I hope the others remember to call or stop by if they can. Mom is a tough lady, but it has to be so very hard on her. This is one of those moments that I wish our original plan of eight of us, including my mom and dad, going on this incredible journey, could have happened. But that wasn't what happened. Now I have to forget the "what if's" and deal with the here and now. It is hard to live in the present.

We drive and it gives us lots of time to think. I have no clue as to what is going on in Morton's mind, busy with my own thoughts, until he speaks up. We are in Idaho and he has been busy looking out the window at all the mountains in the distance. The land has opened up and we keep seeing signs for the Oregon Trail that the pioneers used so long ago. "Can you just imagine what they thought?" was the question Morton asked. Of course he was talking about the people who had headed west to settle in this part of the country. His mind had been thinking about the past, just like mine. The difference is, my past I was thinking of was just one sad year ago.

We arrived at Boise to meet Asheley, the lovely person we are staying the night with. We had a great dinner, conversation into the wee hours and found ourselves all settled for the night. Our only night in Idaho was a perfect one and we will see this state again, the top of it anyway, on our bicycles when we are heading east.

Day 247 September 4, 2007, Tuesday Boise, Idaho to Portland, Oregon

Today we did something we NEVER do...we slept in! It must have been all that driving, the late night talking and staying up a bit for the computer. It was 8 am that I woke up! This is really late for me and we had loads to do today.

Our story is good news and with the press, sometimes we have to wait while other things are going on. That is what happened today. There is big news afoot of scandal and intrigue in Idaho and our story is put on the back burner. It's alright, we still do phone interviews with two newspapers and one online interview. It seems a Republican senator was caught in the mens room at an airport doing something he shouldn't, or so they say. The news has to jump on this because after all, we ARE in Idaho.

We get word that we need to head to Portland ASAP for filming in the morning. Our plans seem to be changing at breakneck speed today and I have no time to really get to chat with Asheley. Morton makes up for it though and chatters away while I go at the computer. Before long, we are heading off...on the road again and we have another friend that we want to keep in touch with. I had told Asheley that mom's should grow an extra set of arms, since she has an 18 month old, she can relate to this. I'm thinking that I need to grow another set to be able to work on two computers to keep up with everything. We drive, or I should say, I drive. Morton does the camera and then we find NPR on the radio and I spend the next several hours listening to all sorts of various stories. I recall our visit to the NPR headquarters in Washington DC on bicycles.

Morton is loving the sky and sunset as we travel towards the coast, following the trail of Lewis and Clark. Again, Morton is asking me loads of questions about history and I haven't a clue. We are going to have a few days in Portland and I intend to learn a bit, take a few hundred pictures and "act natural" for the film crew we are hooking up with the first thing in the morning. We are here, ready to assemble the bikes and trailers and ride SOUTH. It seems like a million years since we were in Quoddy Head. We have lost a bit of time filming, but it is important to share this adventure with the world.

Day 248 September 5, 2007, Wednesday *Terwilliger Vista B&B*, Portland, Oregon

This day was golden. We were enjoying a look around these two incredible gardens in Portland when the phone rang with Charlie, the manager at the *Terwilliger Vista B&B*. He invited us to come for the night and has done a huge bicycle trip himself. We had a room that a person who has a B&B was going to let us sleep in for the night (in his own home) but since we had a very early start the next morning with filming, we thought it would be more polite to be in a place where we wouldn't upset the household with early morning filming.

After a few phone calls, things were sorted and Morton and I went on taking loads of pictures in these two magical gardens in Portland. One Japanese, one Chinese, both beautiful.

Day 248 September 6, 2007, Thurs *Terwilliger Vista B&B* to *The Lion & The Rose B&B*, Portland, OR

We were up very early today, packing our gear and heading to the set of a live television interview. I was their first guest, but while waiting in the green room, got the thrill of meeting a man who founded and organizes an international bicycle film festival. We chat a bit, exchange emails and then I head into the set, all wired for sound and ready to go. The video story before mine was a man who was riding a lawnmower a few hundred miles. I only caught a bit of it, but it was a nice ice breaker to talk about leading into our massive bicycle ride. The interview was incredible, but over in the blink of an eye and we were off to see a bit more of Portland. This city is green, filled with trees, friendly to bicycles and oh-so beautiful. Morton said he had no idea that a place like this existed. Then we headed to the beautiful bed and breakfast, *The Lion and The Rose* to spend a wonderful evening.

Day 249 September 7, 2007, Friday *The Lion & The Rose*, Portland, Oregon

It is going to be tough to capture the highs and lows from today, but I will try. The day started out with a brilliant breakfast, conversation and then the packing and loading from *The Lion and The Rose B&B*. Morton and I were giddy and had talked about staying in Portland to check out the bicycle film festival, but the road was not just calling us, it was screaming. We had to ride.

Last evening we had driven the car to the lady who had us bring it west for her. We decided to walk the seven plus miles back to *The Lion & The Rose*, seeing a bit of Portland on foot. It was long walk, but beautiful. It felt great to be moving.

This morning, we packed our trailers, hitched our bikes up, made sure we had all our water bottles filled and with the freedom of NOT having a car along, we headed west to get to the very coast of Oregon. The bicycles felt so familiar under us, we both commented that having the car was really a hardship and expense we could have done without. Now free of it, we wanted to head to the coast, turn south and not stop until we got to Mexico. After all, still being fat I didn't want to get bombarded with people trying to sell me diet pills or the lipo.

As we crossed one of the many bridges that connect Portland east to Portland west, we were stopping for Morton to pump up the tires on my bike. The front and the rear were a bit soft. Morton was doing his thing and I was chatting with a few people in passing. I also had my camera out, snapping away at this lovely city.

Standing beside my bicycle, I had no clue that the whole journey would change with what happened over the next few seconds. Morton was getting something in my trailer, I have no idea what, but my bicycle fell over. Morton's bicycle had moved from the wiggling in his trailer and was knocking them both down like dominoes. I was turned away from it, with my back on an angle beside it. The metal pedal caught my heel, side of my ankle and to make matters worse, I jumped and twisted to try to get away from it all while trying to catch it. It all seemed to be in slow motion and I'm still not sure what I was trying to do, I just know it all ended very badly.

There was a cross between a pop or a snap in my knee. I knew this wasn't good. The first reaction was to the stinging burn in my ankle and heel, with a big amount of pain there. I just needed to take a few steps to see the really bad thing was my knee. Since 1999 my knee, my left knee, has been a problem. It was hurt in an accident, required surgery and I went through two long years of pain with it. The whole time too, my weight increased, making it even tougher for my knee to stand a fighting chance at healing.

This knee, this left knee, has been a source of worry ever since we started. There have been a few days that it has been tender, but I have been respecting my body and listening to it. I've also been shedding the weight which has to be making the knee feel better. Our bodies weren't built to carry an extra 300 pounds on them, or even 50.

Feeling very stupid to get an injury like this, poor Morton thinks it is all his fault. It is an accident I tell him. But I think he would have been much happier if my knee had to pop and snap, it would have done so while I was bicycling up a tall mountain. Not while I was standing there taking pictures and he was digging around the trailer. The thought of denial came into my head. In my gut, in my knee and in my ankle I knew this was a bad injury. But my old friend denial was quick to jump up and tell me to ride it off. So just giving the back of my heel a rub, I climbed on the bike and started going downhill. My leg was really killing me. Burning on either side of the knee cap, the pain really just ran the whole way down, shooting with certain ways my knee moved. Trying to hold my left leg out and just pedal with my right proved impossible. Morton had no clue as to how bad it was until I let out a scream and stopped. Pulling the map out of my pouch on the bike, I consulted it looking for a little red cross on it. There I found one not too far away, or so I though. The tears were stinging in my eyes and I wasn't sure if they were from pain or frustration.

Using my bike like a crutch I leaned over and let the bike take my weight off the bad knee and ankle. We were pushing for what felt like miles and ages, asking here and there about how far the hospital was. This was the kind of thing that makes you realize the importance of one step after another. I knew that we would eventually get to the hospital, it was just a matter of my knee exploding before we arrived.

Seeing the large building was like seeing the line in Key West, Florida that I will see again someday. It felt like we had been walking and pushing for years, but it was only about an hour. There were benches outside where Morton was able to sit with the bicycles and trailers while I headed in.

My big fear wasn't just my knee and ankle. My big fear was the bill. We have no health insurance in this country. I do have a National Insurance card for Britain, but I'm far from there right now. Can't just pop in, be seen to and leave. As I got checked in, my stomach felt empty and sick. Churning with all sorts of bad thoughts I did have to fight to hold my tears back.

There wasn't much of a wait and soon I was taken into a room where some information was being taken. I expressed my payment fears to the man asking the questions and he put my mind at ease by telling me that no payment would be due today. Good thing too. Morton had a whole two cents in his pocket, not counting his lucky pennies. He can't spend those anyway, but has to give them away.

There was one kind person after another. A few had known about what we were doing and the passion of the journey really helped me feel so much better. This wasn't going to be an end to anything. It also wasn't going to be a pity party for me. When they took me down to xray they used a big, oversized wheelchair. I had room to spare in it and could have fit in a normal sized one, but instead, got the perspective of the feeling of having to ride in a chair designed for a fat person. It groaned under me and I felt embarrassed at not being able to walk. Has my weight finally done me in?

On the table in the xray room, my fat leg seemed even fatter than normal. The left ankle is swollen, it has reason to look fat. The trouble is, the fat doesn't stop there. My leg is really still so big. My knee is hard for the girl to see with the fat around it. I feel like it is all my fault these normal sized people are having to feel with their fingers to see where my knee cap is. This is something that still makes me cringe thinking of it.

Bending me knee for one shot is tough. It is crunching and growling. Never a good sign. I am leaning up, holding a film board in one hand while I prop myself up with the other. My mind starts thinking to how hard this position would have been a year ago with an extra 160 pounds on my body. The xrays show no breaks.

The doctor is fantastic, beyond fantastic really and we talk about the journey. The doctor assures me that they will help with the bill, giving me one less thing to worry about. I'm surprisingly upbeat at this moment. Truthfully, I think I'm in a bit of shock about this.

My stomach is sick and my knee feels like it is grinding and sanding itself down with each bit of movement. Riding the bikes is out of the question, but I can use the bike as my crutch. I have to rest the leg, which is in two braces, ice it and keep it elevated. All hard stuff to do while you are living on the road.

Morton and I sit outside the hospital on the shady bench and discuss what to do next. There have been very kind people we have met in Portland who have helped us, but you don't want to bother anyone. We are in a mixed-up sort of panic. We didn't expect or really prepare for something like this. We need to decide just what we are going to do while my leg heals, then see if I need surgery. We are talking months, not weeks and we have no family here in Portland.

Logically we have to head east. We can stay at my son's, daughter's or mother's house. Morton can get a job. We can raise money as my leg recovers and then continue the journey. These words all sounded wrong, but we both convinced ourselves we had no other choice. After all, my leg in braces could do nothing.

There was a train station we passed, not too far away and all down hill. I'm thinking about the upcoming night and I know it is the worst night for finding somewhere to stay. The weekends are great, when you have a roof over your head. Putting our tent up isn't an option, but I figure the train station will be open all night and we could sit safely there. We can stay up all night talking about what we should do.

On the way down, my leg is throbbing. I have people stare, then stare even harder as I try to just coast, with my double brace hanging off the bike, down the hill. This doesn't work and Morton starts getting on my nerves by asking if I want him to film me trying to ride the bike. The answer was no. Not unless he wants to visit the emergency room to have the camera removed from where the sun doesn't shine.

The journey down to the station feels like it will never end. The sidewalk is our new home. At least for now. At every bench I see I stop, sit and put my leg up. It is throbbing and the urge to just sit and cry my head off is overwhelming, but I hold my tears. I also hold my tongue from taking my anger and frustration out on Morton. At the bottom we find the station. To our shock, the station closes at night so waiting in it would not be an option. Along the way I see a *Holiday Inn* van. Instinct takes over and I dial the number that Sarah has gotten for me and get to speak to Tim, who was kind enough to arrange for us for a ride and a free room for the evening. My leg could take no more bicycling, walking, limping and just needed to go up with some ice on it. The van would solve that problem.

When we got all the gear in to the room, it sort of all hit me. This isn't what we expected. After all, for over a year now I have been doing GOOD things for my body. There are a lot of decisions to be made, but this I know. The journey will not end here, not like this. This journey will be completed. This is a very temporary setback and presents us with a chance to catch up on all the things that we never have time for. Writing, speaking, organizing photos and film footage, doing interviews, planning a bit better and serious training to get my knee better than it has ever been. This ride isn't over.

Just as my spirits sink so low, even though I have my laptop out posting on the website for ideas, a knock comes on our door. It is room service delivering a meal from our friend in Big Sky, Montana. She sent a delicious miracle to us that made us both appreciate everything we had. My leg would heal, it has to heal.

Day 250 September 8, 2007, Saturday *Holiday Inn Portland-Downtown*, Oregon

We were rescued by Holiday Inn van at the train station. They were even kind enough to give us a lift back to the station the following day to take the four day train across the country. This was a low moment. It would have been easy to just give up here, go home and call it a day, but that isn't happening! This isn't a set back, this is a chance to experience what it is like to not let an injury stop me from my road to fitness. I am going to practice what I preach, moderation and movement and when we set off again, my body will thank me for it!

Dr. Andy Mones gave me a very personalized set of discharge instructions. Knowing that we were on bicycles and telling him that I had leaned and limped into the emergency room on my bicycle, he said that I could use the bike for substitute crutches. This worked like a charm!

We had four days on a train from Portland, Oregon to Pittsburgh, Pennsylvania. This was one long ride while in pain. No sleeper car (too much $$$) and sitting up in a chair, leg propped, sick to my stomach for most of the ride.

I knew this was going to hit me, the shock of stopping with an injury. I just wasn't expecting it so soon. Depression set in almost as soon as the train took off.

Day 251 September 9, 2007, Sunday Somewhere in Montana & east

It had all the makings of a perfect story. We were living our dream, smiling, ready to ride, when boom, I get injured in the weirdest way possible. I thought surely that it would be a crazy driver that put me in the hospital, *NOT* Morton. But there is always that thing called fate that reminds us from time to time that we need to just be still and listen. Today, spending a full 24 hours on a train, I am reminded of what it feels like to sit on the sidelines and watch the world go by. People that are out and about wave as we glide by. I wave back when I think they might be able to see us. There are not a lot of power sockets on this train and my laptop has been buried high on an overhead luggage, waiting to by clicked on. The first day that we were on here, how long has it been now, was tough. My outlook and actions were equally depressed. My leg hurt, I was faced with the fact that our food bag would be empty before the train pulls into Pittsburgh and pulling my bright orange jacket over my head, I buried myself in a shell of pity and tried to sleep. It didn't really work out well.

At some point in the day I figured that I would just go for it with my laptop battery. It would give me just less than an hour of power and it might be enough to help me snap out of this funk I have worked myself into. I typed and the therapy of releasing all my thoughts to an electronic piece of paper was just what the doctor ordered.

Sitting behind me, a man who I shall forever think of as Mr. Stinky Feet, helped with this process as well. He didn't speak a word to me, but his smelly feet provided the bit of humour that I needed to smile again. Morton and I decided that we were going to eat a hot dinner and I limped to the dining car for an 8:30 pm seating. The trouble is, my leg didn't want to fit under the table that we were first going to be set at and the hostess had to put us somewhere else. This time, we got a lovely older gentleman at the table with us. Up until now, I haven't been doing any real talking to people. Morton has been my voice, assorted people that have a million and one questions, some having known about our story and others just finding out about it. Communication, which is one of my strong suits, seems to have left me. Morton and the older man have a great conversation. The salad comes and even though it is just a small bowl with nothing really exotic in it, it is delicious. Morton chatters away and I crunch the croutons and listen. He has worried me these last few days. Morton feels like it is his fault I'm injured, on paper that it true. But the fact of the matter is that an accident is an accident. He has nothing to feel guilty about. Even though I have told him this, I see him looking at my leg and then starting to bite his nails. It is a nervous habit he developed over the years. His condition of the Darriahs disease makes his nails split at the base and shoot up in odd directions. The twenty years he spent working in the same printing factory in Scotland, hands covered in ink, didn't persuade him not to bite the nails. My nagging over the last six years won't do anything either. He gnaws at them and thinks. But right now, his nails aren't in his mouth, the salad is. More importantly, words are in his mouth. He is relating our journey to our dinner companion. Morton now is showing the zest that I always had. It feels good to see this.

His words encourage me to join in. After all, he is sort of talking about me as if I'm not there. *"She was over 400 pounds last year"* he tells this stranger. The man looks at me and smiles, I imagine he might be thinking about what I weigh now. Our meal goes by fast, with lots of ice water. At the end, Morton and I decide that the two rolls that are left in the basket won't be missed if we take them along. My mind clicks back to a Shirley Temple movie called *Heidi*. She takes some bread for "the grandmother" and keeps it tucked in her pocket to offer up later. Ours will be eaten along with a can of green beans for breakfast.

With full stomachs, we make our way back in the darkened cars to our seats. Morton and I are going to try to sit side by side, legs up. This doesn't work though. My leg can't stretch straight out, it has to be at the side, over towards Morton. He is an odd sleeper and I don't want him to give it a kick or a shove in the middle of the night.

Instead, I ask him to find another seat. He goes forward three spaces and I just catch a glimpse of his feet sticking off the seat. Nestling down for the night I wish that we were in a sleeper. My comfort level is rather low. Depression abounds for just a moment. Then I think about the big picture. We are safe, dry, inside, full stomachs, warmish and most of all...we are breathing. The most important thing in life. Tomorrow, if I wake up, will bring a whole new day, again spent on the train, but ALIVE! This journey is about moving, right now I'm just doing it on a train.

Day 252 September 10, 2007, Monday Somewhere on a train heading east

Waking up from a sitting position, with my leg stretched out flat and propped with pillows, it hits me again. The depression is something that I never thought I would feel about going home, but here it is. Feeling like hopes and dreams have been stolen at the twist of an ankle and the pop of a knee, I want a pity party. It's gloomy, the track goes on forever and *I AM STILL FAT!* Woe is me.

Morton has moved to another seat during the night and I look for him as we are pulling into a station. I like to use the stopped times on the train to head for the bathroom, which is down the stairs. It is less jerky on me and my fear of falling and crushing a fellow passenger is lessened. Morton is not moving, zonked out. I try a few, "psssts" that don't work. I whisper his name loudly, no movement. Ugh, I crawl out of the seat and head towards him as the train is jerking to a stop. He needs to come back to all our gear, laptop, cameras, etc., that need to be sat with. People get on and off on the stops and I haven't had time to download the cameras and don't want them stolen from the train while I'm in the loo. Morton gets back to our seats and I make a dash for the steps. These steps remind me of the double decker bus in the UK. They didn't have carpet lining the wall on them though, so no real brush burns if you have to rely on leaning on the wall a bit to get up and down.

When I get to the handicapped bathroom, the only one on this train, I find it occupied. I lean against the wall, taking all the weight off the dodgy leg. La, te da te da...waiting for the bathroom first thing in the morning can seem like eternity. Finally the door opens, just as the train is lurching and pulling out of the station. A lady with no visible problem comes trotting out of the bathroom. "There's more room in this one" she tells me, holding her beauty bag and looking like a million bucks. I might have growled at her.

Inside, the mirror shows me a sight that I don't want to see again, hair every which way, looking like something the train ran over. The bathroom was full of smells that you get when you put your face on and fix your hair. Spray, powder, perfume and mouthwash. Jealous a bit that I wasn't prepared to have a mini-bath in the handicapped bathroom, I gripped my way back up to my seat happy to have not wet my pants.

Breakfast didn't help put me in a better mental mood. One stale roll from last nights feast left my stomach wanting more. Smells from the train hit me reminding me that we really are hungry in the morning. My most important meal of the day was supplemented with 1/2 can of cold green beans that fell short of the mark as well. Morton was chatting to some people and I forget that this is out here for the world to read. Two ladies stop by the seat and say they are sorry to hear what happened. I wonder when Morton was talking to them, then they say that they have been watching since we were in Maryland. So odd, but incredible. We chat for a few minutes and they walk on. I feel like a fraud because even though I'm telling them that this won't stop me, just slow me down to recover, I'm not sure if I believe it. Depression.

Sitting in the train, my mind turns over so many things. Trying to stay focused and keep the big wolf of doubt away from the door, there is a mental list compiled. Things to do, not counting the what if's, thinking, thinking, thinking. My mind goes back to a bridge in Florida. It was a hot day (weren't they all?) and the sun felt like it was about 5 inches from my back. The bicycle was groaning under my weight as I climbed this bridge. I hear the words in my head, "I think I can, I think I can..." echoing from a childhood story about a little engine that could. Something happened along the way. Somewhere between west and east, my head clicked into place. This isn't a set back. This is just what happened and how good or bad it is, depends on my attitude. Being sore, hungry, tired, smelly and still fat doesn't make it hopeless, after all, I'm still breathing. Life is only beautiful when you are around to appreciate it. Now it all makes sense. This is just where I need to be at the moment. We get to Chicago and I remember my times that I have been to this lovely city before. I never made it into the train station, but I did now. It is busy, very busy. It is big with a long walk with a bum leg to the place we need to be. Morton is worried because the seats are all taken as we wait for the next train and I have to stand. This feels like pure pleasure though. Standing without the fear of being jerked to the ground by a shift in the track. The layover isn't long. Morton and I wonder if our bikes and trailers will be loaded on to the next train that will take us to Pittsburgh. Fingers crossed, we head for the food court. We need to get something for dinner, our last supper on the train, affordable, semi-healthy and hot, would be our choice. We found a Chinese place that had things that sort of fit all those boxes and got it to go. Working our way down to the waiting room, we decided that we should go ahead and eat while we wait. This way it will still be warm. As I'm eating I'm hoping that the lady across from us who is watching, gets curious about our bright orange jackets that say *LittleChanges* on them. There on my sleeve it says, "Bicycling and walking 16,000 miles to battle obesity" as I chow down the Chinese. Talk about mixed signals to send.

We get on a new train being taken on a bit before the other passengers because of the leg, we are told where to sit. We get the top floor right in front of the doors that slide open when you hit the button, to take you to the next car. This is not a spot I recommend sitting in. Ever. With our bellies full, I figured I would fall fast asleep. This train was an express train, which sounded great but felt horrible on the leg. I thought I might be feeling more twists and bumps because of the sore knee, but the yells, screams and laughs of the other passengers in that train car confirmed that is was one wild ride. At one point, this is a true story, I called Sarah to tell her if I didn't call her in the morning at 5:30 am saying we arrived in Pittsburgh, *not* to come pick us up.

That would mean the train jumped the track and we would want our money back. Sarah was laughing about this as she heard the screams and yells from the people on the train. She knew at that point, I wasn't just exercising my sense of humour.

We asked if there was any way that we can move. The blast of cold air coming in each time some brave soul passes through the portal to the next car is going to be tough to sleep through. A kind lady moves us to the rear of the car, the last car on the train.

Here we spread out a bit and use the wee pillows to prop and cling to as we ride through the night. My mind is thinking about *Mr. Toads Wild Ride* at *Disney World* as we twist and turn through the darkness, with a few screams here and there. Hurry morning.

Day 253 September 11, 2007, Tuesday The train lands in Pittsburgh and then car ride to Harrisburg PA

We got so many thrills today they erased all the chills from our evening before spent on the express train. As we were leaving, a lady that had been with us since Portland and I agreed that we could have been there days ago if we would have had this fast engineer at the helm of our other train. We laughed about it, but she said that she heard the one person saying on the slow train that they were playing a game with another train to see which one could get to the station later. Obviously we were on the winning train.

At any rate, I was so glad to be on solid ground. Wobbling until I found my ground legs, I fought the urge to fall to my knees (even the bad one!) and kiss the ground. Stillness on the platform, Morton and I now watched in hopes that our bikes and trailers made it over the four day journey. Joking about our odds for the luggage, we saw the big boxes and trailers taking up an entire tag-along trailer the man was pulling to the baggage claim area. It was going to be a great day.

Sarah was glad to hear the train didn't jump the track and said she was on her way. She also said the rain was about impossible to see through. Morton and I had a few hours to kill in the station and I was overjoyed to get computer connection. I still have to upload pictures and my connection kept letting me down on that. Still, there are so many emails, phone calls (now that I'm off the train and can speak on the phone) and things to take care of, it felt like it was just a few minutes before Sarah arrived.

I was on the phone with her as she was looking for the street to turn on. Making a wrong turn, she was pulled over by a police officer in a tye-die shirt. The lady was nice, knew that she must not be from around here and says it happens all the time. My girl got turned around and was soon arriving with my lovely grandson. This is the good stuff! A great amount of hugging, loving, and kissing was going on here, but mostly just trying to get our gear in the van and heading back in the rain. Our little guy was sleeping most of the way, with just one stop on the four hours back to Harrisburg.

Sarah was just going around a corner on the turnpike in this incredible amount of rain, when her windshield wipers just quit working. Pulling over on an edge so narrow I wouldn't want to park a bike on it, Morton jumped out and set to work under the hood.

This had just been fixed a few weeks ago, but the garage failed to notice that they had the wrong size of wiper blades on. Being a bit too long, they would grab at each other, eventually knocking the motor out of service. Morton, since he does love to dooberize, took about 15 minutes at the most before telling Sarah to try the wipers. They worked and we did the little happy dance, seated in the van in the pouring rain. When he jumped back in, Morton was giving us the full details. We pretended to listen, not understanding a word of it really, but we were so delighted that we were able to SEE again through the river on the windshield. My ears perked up when Morton said that the bicycle tool that Melissa from *Little Capistrano Bike Shop* in Eastham, Massachusetts had given us saved the day.

This tool kit, to replace Morton's' giant bag of found tools from beside the road, proved to be worth it's weight in gold. He keeps it with him, in his pocket and used the torx tool (whatever that is) to tighten whatever needed tightened. He said that I have to be sure to email Melissa and tell her that it is his favorite tool that he's ever had. Then he sort of lost Sarah and I as he kept going on about what all it has on it. We just smiled and listened, nodding our heads and pretending we knew what these things were. He would tire out of talking soon and he was our hero for getting the wipers going again.

Sarah has stairs. Lots of stairs. They aren't easy to go up and I thought they were narrow and steep before, but now they seem even more so. They will do my therapy great though. Show me that I can climb any mountain, one step at a time. The thought of just staying in the area outside the bathroom isn't going to work, so I know that if I climb just one more set of stairs, there is a bed waiting for us. Since we hadn't been in one for four nights, it was worth it. You have heard me talk about million dollar showers, this was a day of one of those, PLUS a million dollar bed! Just incredible. Mix all of this with my little family and shazzam...perfection!

Day 254 September 12, 2007, Wednesday Harrisburg, Pennsylvania

The email today was incredible...so many of you have written wishing me a speedy recovery. I'm healing as we speak and with all the good vibes, well wishes, prayers and positive energy floating around on my behalf, I know it will be fast! Again, I'm not able to really understand all this kindness from strangers, I just know it is the most amazing thing I have ever seen in my life.

Your stories about the little changes that you are making is what really interests me. My favorite emails are when you let us know what is going on in your lives. As I'm smiling through my email, feeling better by the second, Sarah tells me that she has great news. There is a person who has organized to get me a free MRI, courtesy of *Adams Diagnostic Imaging* in Gettysburg, Pennsylvania. This is just overwhelming. Morton and I were really afraid of what we were going to do about the medical bills. We have no insurance and I had no idea WHAT would happen. I was trying not to worry about it, but it was a huge fear of mine. This news stuns me. I feel unworthy of all of this. It is tough to explain, but I think about all the people who are in so much worse shape than we are. Morton is healthy and fit and can get a job. I can get a job too. Push come to shove, we could have done the payment plan and gotten through this. Now, a free MRI is just making me feel like the brightest, prettiest, most fantastic day ever known is waiting for me.

All those dark moments that I felt hopeless from the weight, failure with each failed diet, disappointed in myself worse than any other human being could ever be disappointed in me...all these depressing feelings that have held me for the last three decades are gone. But they die hard sometimes. A thing like a free MRI all puts it into crystal clear view. We can all help ourselves by being honest with ourselves and really looking hard in our own mirrors. Figuring out what we want is a lot tougher than actually getting it. Being able to realize that my dream has just been sitting there waiting on me all these years is the first step. This is true no matter where you are and what you are doing.

Over the next few weeks and months, my big challenges are all going to be shown here. From the MRI to what the training is going to be to get me back on the bicycle will all be part of this journey. It will be fantastic getting to see how my recovery goes this time as opposed to when my knee was injured in 1999. Then I did a whole lot of nothing, sat on my backside, ate a lot more (I WAS depressed!) and gained about 100 pounds in a year. I can say without one little speck of doubt that THIS TIME, it will all be different. Food, movement and honesty with it all will make it a time that I actually do what the doctor says, end up a bit lighter and my knee will be stronger than ever. Instead of being my own worst enemy from now on, I chose to take care of myself in every way that I can. Morton gets his resume out to people. He is also getting registered with a temporary agency that will get him working. We will be fine.

Motivation people....motivation. We all need it and it feels best when you pass it on. I've said it before and will keep saying it, to get motivated, you have to give it.

Sarah, Graeme, Alexander, Morton and I all went to end the perfect day with the perfect evening. We had a great visit with my mom, who was so thrilled to see Alexander come in the door in his little carrier, didn't even say HI to Morton and I. It was really funny! She is madly in love with Alexander as well, I understand fully, but we all had a good laugh after five minutes of being there when I hugged Mom and said "Hello there!" It dawned on us then how this little guy has changed all of our lives.

Children give us all hope. The hope that life goes on. The hope that we have left something behind in this world that might mean we are remembered by family a hundred years from now who look back at a picture and remember their ancestors. Children also hold the promise that anything is possible, right in front of your eyes. They change each and every moment, without even thinking about it. They are indeed, our greatest resource and we all need to remember this. There are many great kids who are watching this journey with their parents or teachers. We get emails from all over telling us that we are being tracked in classrooms, looked at for motivation on personal struggles with obesity and used as an example of the importance of exercise. These are the things that will change the world.

Obesity is a very serious issue that we are not always able to just talk about. Though it is as obvious as the nose on the ends of our faces, it can be uncomfortable to even hear the word obesity when you are the obese person. We have to get over this people. It is a real problem that is killing our country, costing billions of dollars and crippling our medical profession.

Like the lady on the train who occupied the handicapped bathroom, even though she wasn't, obesity is clogging the office visits with sore knees (raising my hand here) back trouble, heart problems, blood pressure, diabetes and so many other issues I would need a medical dictionary and unlimited time to tell you all the things that obesity causes.

My blinders are off. This isn't about me being a super model, it's about me being alive, not being a burden on my family or friends and most of all, about teaching Alexander how to ride a bike in a few years. I want him to ask me the question, "Who is that fat lady holding me in the pictures of me as a baby?" Of course we all know what the answer will be.

Day 255 September 13, 2007, Thursday Harrisburg, Pennsylvania

The weather is getting a bit of autumn in it, especially when the sun goes down. My mind thinks, just for a moment, about the road and I do miss it.

Day 256 September 14, 2007, Friday Harrisburg, Pennsylvania

This day was a LOT like the one before. These next few weeks/months are going to be a challenge. I don't want to slip into any horrible old habits and spend two hours eating each day...or more! Time to find out what it is like to sit in one place and still make incredible things happen with this adventure called life.

The days will be filled with writing at the computer, working with images, working with film footage from the videos and trying to not go crazy, or get depressed.

Day 257 September 15, 2007, Saturday Harrisburg, Pennsylvania

A long time ago, in a life that now seems far away, I made a living selling jewelry that I would make. My kids were smaller, I was a single mom and I needed to do something that would provide me with money and still let me be there when they needed me. My kids were never in day care and I wasn't a welfare mom...it was tough. I did get an incredible amount of help from my parents and we lived with them for about seven years. This morning as Morton and I got up before the sun, I thought about all those times that I would do this with my children, to go sell at a craft fair. We covered a lot of different ones, only on the weekends and it was an adventure for them and for me. It was also a lot of work. We were on the streets today, just with no bicycles. The white tent was up, our one table covered with Scottish Sea Glass pendants, supporter ribbons and free bookmarks we were handing out about the journey. It was a far cry from the elaborate set ups I use to do that would take about three hours to assemble before the shopping could begin.

Today was chilly, but no rain and the people were sort of dotted about the day. We were in a space at the very end of the street that held the festival. This spot can be really bad, when, after trodding along for what seems like an eternity, the shopper stops about twenty stands up, takes a look down and decides they aren't going any further. Something else had stopped some shoppers from coming over to our stall as well. It was our big green banner (that I love) that says *Little Changes - 16,000 miles by bicycle to battle obesity.* It tells the whole story in one line. But it also turns people off. The word OBESITY is something that makes people turn away if they are heavy. Certain people, not all, but a lot. After watching this happen several dozen times, I told Morton that we needed to pull the banner down. Yes, we want to get the word out, but we also needed to make money here. The banner was killing sales. Morton folded the word OBESITY up and under and just like putting out a big neon open sign, suddenly people would come over to the last booth on the left. It was shocking to see and made me want to try something with a camera. Why can't we face the word OBESITY if we are obese? I was sitting under it, chatting to so many people about the journey, while being OBESE...after all, I still am obese, the whole time anyone who cared to look at me could see I am obese. This is something that I can't hide. For years I tried to hide this. Layers of clothing, big baggy things (when I could find them) and I would lie to myself that all these bulges, rolls and bumps under the baggy stuff were hidden. This was a lie that I never believed, but was able to live with for decades.

If we would look for a cure for obesity (p.s., there IS one...it's called MODERATION & MOVEMENT!) like we look for cures for other medical problems, more people might be willing to walk over to a banner that is trying to *BATTLE OBESITY!* But our society isn't ready to handle that yet. It isn't politically correct to put the word OBESITY in the spotlight. It is uncomfortable and we don't want to hurt anyone's feelings. Recently I saw that the obesity problem, at epidemic levels, is going to cost our health care system billions, not to mention all the people that are going to die far earlier than they should. This is a serious crisis people...we are killing our-selves with food and not enough exercise. Wake up and smell the message here! Falling into the days busi-ness, not wanting to hurt anyone's feelings (trust me though, having a knee crumble because of your weight or laying on your back in a hospital bed for two months because you had a stroke...*HURTS*) we hid the word. There needs to be a dialogue about this. We need to help each other with this problem yes, but most impor-tantly, *WE NEED TO HELP OURSELVES!* After years of searching, much money wasted on diets, fads and kicks that just didn't work, I found the secret and this is it. Do something for yourself. You can fix this. It won't happen overnight, but it will happen. Start thinking about all the little changes you can do to make the big ones happen. If you are like me and are/were facing almost 300 pounds to lose, let go of the idea that we will wake up tomorrow svelte! This can happen, but it takes time. We also need to lose the word diet from our dictionary. They don't work and anyone who has ever been on one can tell you this. Get a life and have a fantastic *LIFESTYLE* change! Add things to your daily routine that will bring you pleasure as well as be great for you.

Tonight, we head out to my mom's house and I stop at a little farm stand set up in someone's yard. They are selling various fruits and veg cheap from coolers sitting on top of tables. Potatoes, green peppers, apples and big red tomatoes. My dad would have grown all these things this summer if he would have still been with us, but he's not. I knew that my mom was probably missing them all. We spent $5.00 and had two big bags full of goodness. There is nothing like stands like this. If you have any in your area, use them as much as you can. Better yet, start your own! Let your garden grow people, great exercise and you can't beat what you get out of it.

Mom liked the tomatoes, she said that she *was* missing them and I said that maybe next year she could try her own garden. Smaller in scale than the one my dad kept, just a few plants. They were a real team, my parents. Dad would grow it and mom would freeze it or can it, then cook it. When tomato season was in high swing, many of the meals would just be a huge slab of juicy tomato, warm from the sun, sliced and put between two pieces of bread.

Tonight, at the table I was thankful to be here, missing my dad, but happy for this moment. Sharing food is a long-standing tradition in my family. It also equals love. You don't get to weigh over 400 pounds by hating food, even though I have never really enjoyed it as an adult.

Day 258 September 16, 2007, Sunday Harrisburg, Pennsylvania

Morton put his kilt on for the second day in a row. In Scotland, they were the kilt like the guys over here wear tuxedos. Special occasions only, usually. Since Morton never really gets to wear it on the bike (it is way too heavy to bring along!) I talked him in to putting in on yesterday. It is a real conversation starter and there were quite a few ladies who came by that said they could listen to him forever. I offered to loan him out, but I didn't have any takers. Today we are heading to a Scottish Heritage festival. I have never been to one and a nice man from Australia invited us. We were all up for it, plus, it would be great to hear the bagpipes again. The day was perfect for it, though it was just two hours long, they did an excellent combination of music, dancing and talking. Thinking back to the years I lived in Scotland, I have to confess the dancing was so sub-dued to what I had not only witnessed, but participated in from time to time. This was dancing that I loved. "*Strip the Willow*", "*The Gay Gordons*" and "*Dashing White Sergeants*" are all ones that I had done on many of Hogmany (New Year's Eve) celebrations. Fast and furious, If only I would have taken to the dancing it would have burnt off a million calories. But I didn't. Now today, watching again from the sidelines, I'm reminded of just how important if is. There has to be something out here that I can jump in and do right now. Swim, sit in a chair and do upper body stuff, lie on the floor and do crunches...so many things that we all make excuses as to why we can't do them. Making a mental note that this will not happen to me, I won't sit on the sidelines, the day is over and we are heading home. I wince as I get in to the car. The knee is throbbing, feels like it is falling apart and has a burning in it. When we get back to the house, I un-velcro the straps. My knee feels worse without the brace, but I also can't take the brace a second longer. Propping my leg up, I try to hold it nice and still. It needs elevated. Hopefully the swelling will go down. I did a bit too much walking and I knew I would pay for it later. The laptop works like a heating pad if I put it in just the right spot on my knee. There are pictures to be done, but I get squeamish when I look at the screen. My stomach is turning flips from how my knee feels. Switching the computer off, I stretch out on the couch with a pillow under the end of my left leg. My feet are freezing and I ask Morton to please put my socks on. He does and for just a moment I think about the way things use to be. The days that Morton would put on my shoes because I was too fat to do it. I never will go back to that place again.

Day 259 September 17, 2007, Monday Harrisburg, Pennsylvania

Sometimes I wonder, "Did I write that or think about writing it?" There are many things happening right now, lots of interviews and I'm writing more than I have been able to lately. While at my mom's house, with Morton up on the roof, my phone rang with one of my favorite reporters I have met along the way. This reporter is very understanding and very complete with her story. She digs deeper than almost anyone I have ever met in this field, then really gets to the heart of the story. An hour slid by on the telephone and when we finished talking, I was left with an assignment to pull information together and email her. I just remembered, I forgot to add some pictures she wanted.

The next three hours I spent looking through emails, photos, places we had been and tried to compile a list of highlights that we had along the east coast. This is impossible. I really needed at least three days on this, maybe even three weeks. There are just so many. Each and every day was perfect. Some were tougher than others, some were funnier than others, some were a pure breeze, but they were all perfect. The viewing of these items, sitting in my mom's living room with my leg immobilized seems really odd. Almost as if this isn't happening right now. Fiction and facts blend and memories just pour over me as I keep clicking.

The sound of Morton up on the roof cleaning the chimney and gutters makes me sad. I'm happy he's doing it, just very sad because it was always something my dad would do. He actually had the very same ladder out on the day he died to do that task.

When Morton empties the chimney of all the build up, I wonder if it has been this way since dad left. Time people, like exercise, we never get enough. Enjoy your moments, your family and most of all....MOVE!

Day 265 September 22, 2007, Saturday Harrisburg, Pennsylvania

This has been one tough week. It makes our weeks on the bike, living wild, running out of food, water and shelter sort of pale in comparison. When I say tough, the only really strain on our bodies has been not enough exercise. Working through pain isn't the problem...it's time. Waking up each day with good intentions isn't enough. Now I'm not subject to lack of choice for what to do for exercise, I just don't know what is best for my knee at the moment. But *THIS* is an excuse, dear friends. I could still be doing 30 minutes of upper body stuff, but I'm in an exercise funk. It is tough to explain, but it stops right now. Morton and I got up early to drive an hour to do the craft show in Wrightsville. It was raining when we got there, but we figured if we could ride the bicycle in the rain, we could sell sea glass in the rain. The show cost $35.00 to sell there, we spent $20. on gas and after a day of flogging, we had a $28.00 profit to show for it. This might sound bad, but we had so many great people stop and talk, tell us what they were up to and I met not one, but three writers, all following their dream. It was good inspiration for me to get serious on hitting the keyboard.

While we were tearing down to drive the hour back to my daughter's house, Morton got a migraine. A big, knock him on his backside migraine. I think it might have been standing all day in the heat. When the rain had gone away, the sun came out and got very warm indeed. Whatever the cause, we knew the cure. He had to lay down, in a darkened room and go to sleep.

Day 266 September 23, 2007, Sunday Harrisburg, Pennsylvania

The theme for today was CHANGES. Every time we thought we had a plan for the day, everything changed. Morton and I are not use to having loads of people involved in what we are up to for the day and it showed. We were suppose to get out to visit my mom, but she did have a houseful of people so it was a bit easier to get talked into walking to *WOOFSTOCK*. This was a festival for pooches beside the river in Harrisburg. The day was warm and there were lots of laughs along the way. If you are feeling blue, just look at a dog. Watch how their tails wag when they approach a new dog or person. Some dogs anyway. We have had a few chase us on the bikes that I didn't really want to stop and pet. These dogs today though, were in their element. It took me a lot longer than normal to walk there, but I was so glad I did it under my own steam. Morton kept scolding me for not using crutches, but I was leaning on him and at times, getting to push the stroller to lean on. The plan was, when we got there I would sit and rest my leg up, listen to the live bands, talk to people and then walk back. That all happened except we stopped at tables right in front of the funnel cakes. Before you cringe for me...don't. This is where little changes kicked in. The old me would have had one to myself, the new me had one that I shared with Sarah and Morton.

Ironically, I was wearing a hideous two-toned purple shirt that declared, "SUGAR" in glittery letters across my chest. The shirt was baggy on me now, when just over a year ago it was skin tight. How or why I ever got this shirt escapes me. I think someone bought it for me years ago, but I honestly can't remember. I can't imagine going up to a counter and buying it, but maybe it was on sale. I had on a pair of trousers that had still had the tag on them from about 3 years ago. My sister had given them to me and they never fit.

Morton and I had spent the morning trying to organize our old clothes. We were both so happy with how things fit now, or better still, don't fit. *EVERYTHING* is baggy. I have many things that I had never been able to wear, or couldn't wear for years, that I now snap, zip or button with ease. Deciding that I need to not wear my stretchy waist clothing (except for exercising) I opted for waistbands. After all, I do hope to have a waist before long. My stomach is down to two rolls of fat from four. When I note this to Morton he tells me that I should start doing crunches. Hmmm....do I get angry and tell him he should start doing crunches (along with some other choice comments) or do I take his advice? After all, I did bring the subject up. It's like asking "Does my butt look big in these pants?" We set our poor friends and partners up for a question that has no right answer. It is all based on our mood of the moment if it starts world war three or not.

Today I took onboard what he said about crunches. I really do need to get a routine down and then just do it everyday. It was a lot easier when our bicycling 30 to 50 miles each day was my exercise. Stretching my legs and resting my backside just meant walking and pushing the bike. Easy. Now I have to think about my knee and ankle, how much time I'm spending with my family, how long I'm on the phone or on camera with interviews, how I'm going to get through these next few weeks/months without the bike-life....way too much to juggle. Then we face the reality of money and bills. Morton just needs to get a day job and a night job, period. I need to work. I need to write. As the pages for the book rises in number, my daily journal entries are pathetic.

There was a time in my life when I had my own computer business. It was a good business, not Bill Gates good, but I managed to support myself and my children. This was when I first fell in love with Scotland and managed to take an entire month to go and visit. There was a rental car involved that got over 3,000 miles put on it as I explored Britain, stayed in a few rented houses and got a great source of inspiration from a little village we stayed at in England. When I got to the town, heard a slice of local history, a movie just jumped in my head. I had never attempted to write a screenplay before, but had been keeping a journal, writing songs, poetry, short stories and just mindless thoughts down for ages. On the flight back to New York from London, I worked out all these movie details in my mind.

Even though I had a more than full time job with my business, I would get up early each day and stay awake each night for 22 days. At the end of this time, I had a screenplay in my hands that was nothing like I first imagined on the plane and in that little village. It seems the more I wrote and developed the characters, the more they just took on a life of their own. At the end of the script, even I had no idea what would happen. It was an amazing writing adventure that I practiced with two more screenplays, but my first was still my favorite.

This is where a lot of us fall short of our dreams. I let fear and rejection stand in my way of going for my dream. After sending the script to about 10 sources in Hollywood, I got back a few rejection letters (one or two were actually nice) and I had a few people ask to see other things that I had written and best of all (or worst of all) I had one actually Hollywood agent telephone me. That was where I hit my wall. With that telephone call, in which he asked to see other things I wrote, my dreams came true and unraveled at the same moment. Just getting the call from him was such a thrill. It was enough for the moment to shatter my dream. Even though I did manage to find time to write two more screenplays, I had enough doubts and fears in my head to follow through showing them. *WHAT IF I FAILED?* The age old question that grips us all sometimes if we are honest. The screenplays are still here. Two unread by Hollywood eyes, one that had been around a bit. I waited quietly to see if any movies would come out that were similar to my original, but none has. Sometimes I wonder why I never sent them out. I had a foot in the door with the phone call I had gotten, well, at least a toe or two. But I guess that my mind felt if I didn't try, I couldn't fail. When the truth is, by not trying I had seriously failed. With our journey and my injury at the moment, I feel this fear setting in at times. It is easy walking, even though sore, with my daughter and grandson. It feels so good to be here with them. Let Morton get jobs and we can rent a little place. I could still do things to get the word out that it's time to move. My dream could be shelved, just like the screenplays. But there is something inside me that realizes this is do or die. Stopping is not an option and being in limbo is tough to know what to do next.

My knee has to be the priority in my life right now. It is the key to getting just where I want to go, but not the only way. There are bicycles that you can pedal with your arms. I need to look into this. It might be a great option, Morton and I could switch it up, upper and lower body work outs.

As I type, I'm holding my lovely grandson in my arms. He is sleeping in a little yellow sleep gown that says "Just Duckie" on it. There are two pillows under him, on my lap that wasn't there a year ago. A sleeping baby. So lovely and fragile and the reason life goes on. My arms are stretching out to reach the keyboard and I think about things I had done in the past while holding his mother.

When a child is born, perhaps the mother should grow an extra set of arms. I had thought this often as I held my baby Sarah 26 years ago now. She would sit on my hip as I cooked, kept books, did household chores and in the store. You could say she was spoiled, but she wasn't. She was and is well-loved. Life was simple then, when his mommy was a baby. I was about 220 pounds, felt so much better and was just 19 years old. I had no idea the next few decades would see my weight and life get out of control, to the point that my body was dying from the amount of food I ate.

We have to all work together to break this obesity chain. My grandmother was heavy, my mom was heavy, I am heavy....destiny and in my genes. Why fight it? Pass the funnel cake. But is has to stop here. I never want to have Alexander teased at school when his fat gramma picks him up. But then, look around you. There are more and more people that are obese. It is an epidemic, ask any newspaper.

One out of 3 Americans are too heavy. This little hope of the future I'm holding in my arms right now, might get teased for being normal sized if things don't change. Seats in theaters will become wider to accommodate the big bottoms, clothing stores will all stock size 5XL with the stripes going in the wrong direction, all-you-can-eat-fast-food joints will pop up all over our fair country, then spread to other countries. *NORMAL* will be obese. We will all die younger, live our lives on the sidelines and it will be the new thrill for a 16 year old to get a automatic wheelchair to roll through their lives, rather than a car. Think about it. Things really have to change. The way for us to change the world is to start first with ourselves. Someone must have said that. Why wasn't I listening before? Was it the same inner-failure safe guard voice that kept me from sending the screenplays off? Perhaps. Was it that I had fulfilled my dreams by just getting my thoughts on paper, bound in a way that they could be sent to strangers to be rejected? *What if the best things happened?*

Over the last several months, I have seen the best things every single day of this journey. Every single day! The best things CAN happen when we let them. So on that note, on that very true thought, I will leave you. I'm off to post screenplays, return a few calls, answers email and change the world. Want to come with me?

In The End

Over the next few months many things happened in my life that kept me away from my bicycle. The first being my knee needing rest (three to four months) and the most important being Alexander, my first grandson.

Morton got a regular job which suits him best. He had a wild six and a half months living on a bicycle never knowing what one day to the next was going to hold and he just couldn't stand the thought of any more adventure. He is a creature of habit, has maintained his weight loss and still supports whatever I choose to do. He is also still a great cook who has to be reminded from time to time that I have a real problem with food abuse. If he is left to grocery shop on his own I have to give him explicit instructions to *not* buy the food that will kill me please!

Sarah went back to work and as my knee was healing, I looked after Alexander for four days a week. We rented an apartment near her home, she could come over for lunch with us and I had the pleasure of seeing my grandson learn to walk and talk.

Even though these times with my precious family were sheer bliss, I had a secret I couldn't tell anyone. I was depressed to the point that I would cry in the shower, hiding my gloom from everyone. I felt like after all the riding, the journey would never go again. It was finished and I was a failure that was still fat.

Dirty little habits raised their filthy little heads and I was back to some binge eating, not exercising and actually putting some of my weight back on. This was something that I kept hidden, or tried to, from my family and the world.

For several months I didn't even do anything on the website, which had been such a wonderful source of motivation for me. Again, I was a big fat failure, full of self-hate and loathing about the state that I was in. It was a real sea of emotions because even though the injury took away one dream, it gave me another. Alexander.

To say he is the love of my life is a serious understatement. He is my reason for breathing and the person that makes all the universe seem right to me. He makes me not want to kill myself with food.

Sometime in the spring of 2008 after spending a wonderful day with Alexander, I realized how sore my body was. It was tough getting up and down off the floor and had nothing to do with my knee. I knew what it was. Stepping on to the scale in my apartment kitchen I saw the horrible truth. Almost fifty pounds that I had lost from 440 pounds down to 250 pounds, had came back. The scale was so close to touching 300 and I was terrified.

The answer was right in front of me all the time with LittleChanges.com. I went back to my neglected website, answered emails, updated the website, but kept my secret shame of the weight gain from the world. How could I motivate you and disappoint you all at once?

As the weeks went by, the scale started falling. I started working on making wonderful things happen again. It does take real work after all to get a few miracles going.

Before I knew it the scale was going in the right direction, this book, this story of my wild life on the road was almost finished, there was filming for a television series coming up and even though I should have been close to reaching my total weight loss goal, I was now almost back to where my weight was at the end of the bicycle ride. Working harder than I ever did on the bicycle I tried to focus on helping others with their daily doses of motivation, getting mine as I gave them theirs.

Again there seemed a real destination in my mind with filming at spas to capture the last 100 pounds of my weight to come off at sixteen destinations around the globe. It didn't matter if my knee was still sore and I can't ride the bicycle for more than a mile or two at a time without it hurting, the journey would just have to change. I leave you being a work still in progress. A body that has learned that motivation isn't something you just get one time and are done with it. Like food that we have to eat each day, we all need our daily dose of motivation. Suddenly that magic started happening and things just fell into places that I never expected.

Teaming up with my daughter we set about creating a format for a week long fitness camp that will happen in September 2009. It will be the primary goal to really show people who want to change their health for the better how to make those important lifestyle changes that will lead them down the road to wellness.

My addiction to food is a battle that needs fought almost daily. Hopefully in time it will change and my new good eating habits will erase the bad ones from the past, the same with exercise. Motivate others and move. Honesty is again my *big* little change that I want to make. If I'm having a bad day, I don't have to hide it from those around me, or even those on the internet. After all, I'm not a super human, just a fat lady who decided she wanted to live. Face your worst fears people. Get to know yourselves. Help others. Be the person that you would look up to. If you don't like the way things are, change them. Take care of your own health first. Set good examples and motivate those around you to move towards a healthier way of life.

As long as there is breath in me I pledge to never stop this journey of motivation and trying. Each day is a treasure and I'll treat it like that. Everyday can be the best day of our lives, as long as we are willing to look at life with a positive attitude. Keep watching, the best is yet to come. *Priscilla Houliston* - summer 2008

Trainwrecked

Fifty-three minutes remains on my battery. That is all the time I will have to write about my trauma on the train. In forty-four years I have never ridden a train in the United States. There have been countless train rides in Scotland, England, even a dash in Wales and a super fast train in France. But for whatever reason in the good old US of A, my preferred method of movement has been flight. With a pilot for a father and flying in my families blood, I took to the air like a flying fish. This trip though, this unexpected trip backwards from Portland, Oregon to Pennsylvania, flight didn't seem to be an option. We have the bikes with us, trailers, gear, endless amounts of excess baggage that would have cost about $425,000. on a plane. Maybe I exaggerate a bit, but you get the picture. Flying was too expensive this time. Or was it? After all, time is our most important commodity they tell us. This train that I am on, currently looking at the fields of Montana that go on as big as their famous sky, seems to be frozen in time. Time is just chugging along. The calculations on time is as follows (not a joke) Leave Portland, Oregon at 4:45 pm on Saturday. Arrive in Pittsburgh, Pennsylvania at 5:30 am on Tuesday. Yes, you heard me right. Three days on a train, no time off for good behavior.

Maybe it is because my leg is strapped up from my shin to the top of my fat thigh. Maybe it is the fact that each way I look I'm faced with the fact that my journey of a lifetime is on hold for a few months. Maybe it is because the guy behind that got on sometime during the first night, while I was sleeping (if it can be called that) has taken his shoes off, exposing hot, sweaty and perhaps the smelliest feet on the planet. Then he has been kind enough to wedge them up on the headrest of the seat beside me, just five inches from my nose. It's not going great so far. I should mention that the lovely lady who is riding with Mr. Stinky Feet is thoughtful enough to spray the most obnoxious perfume ever put in a bottle every time Mr. Stinky Feet passes gas. She is averaging 4 to 8 sprays an hour. She isn't content to do it once, she gives it about 4 to 8 squirts, in his direction, but it occasionally floats on the close air up to me. One blast, early this morning, even managed to get into my eyes. Morton wanted mace for the bears and bad people, but I feel we should just ask her what brand it is...trust me, it would stop an attacker. My throat is sore from the fragrance. I call my daughter to hear her voice and feel like I'm doing the right thing by going back to Pennsylvania to recover. This isn't ending the journey, just adding a few months on to it. I repeat this in my head hoping it is true.

Out the window, while my Zen player sings selfishly in my ears, music that Morton doesn't get to hear, I spy two people on bikes. A couple. They have taken a water break. I know that look well. They are pointing at the train, the man is fumbling for the camera and they wave. Minus a few hundred pounds, that was me a few weeks ago. It feels like a million years since I have been on the bicycle. A distant dream now.

It is going to be easy to get depressed right now. I can feel it. I want to burst out in tears, angry at my body for betraying me. I treat it right, for the first time *EVER* and this happens? Then to add insult to injury, I'm on a slow train to China. It feels like we are going that route to get to our final destination of Pittsburgh.

Thirty-two minutes on the battery and I have gotten nothing to show for it. Morton, trying to cheer me up I suppose, feels compelled to keep chatting to me. I have given him all sorts of clues that I'm *WRITING* now, capturing my impressions of the moment. But like Mr. Stinky Feet, Morton won't go away. We had been nice and spread out. He was sitting right across from me. We each had two seats. But then, other people came on board. Our whole car was crammed with people led in by the man in the train hat. He asked Morton to move over to me and my leg, after being rearranged, wasn't too pleased for the squeeze.

There is one handicapped restroom on this train. It's a few cars away, down the stairs. Not a clever arrangement. I haven't made my way there yet. Instead I tried to wedge myself into the tiny regular toilet. Morton is throwing off his normal million watts of heat and I'm sitting in the sun. The train could be solar powered, then maybe I could plug my laptop in. When we asked the man at the station, long ago in Portland if there was power, he said no. He said these trains were built before...then he paused, searching for the word. I wanted to blurt out, "electricity?" but then he found it, "laptop computers!" he announced. No electricity unless you are willing to go to the lounge, ask the man nicely by the coffee urn and even then, the answer might be no. Morton doesn't know it yet, but when I wear the battery out on the lappy, he's going to go charge it.

Twenty-nine minutes. The train is slowing down. I suppose it's time for a smoke break. People jump off at one of the millions of stops we have made so far to walk out on the platform and light 'em up. Sometimes it is for just five minutes, other times it is for a lot longer. As I look at the mental map in my mind I know that after Montana comes North Dakota heading east. Long states and a long way from Pennsylvania. At this rate, I should be home in time to turn around and get back on my bike. Surely my knee and ankle will be healed after this never ending ride.

The guy behind me, Mr. Smelly Feet, has now turned in to Mr. Seat Banger. He is tapping out some sort of evil rhythm on the back of my seat. Why? What did I do to deserve this. Did I mention that when Morton took a walk forward he discovered there are only three people sitting in the whole next car up? We are stuck in the sardine section, they are both coach, but playing with my patience...my dream trip is becoming more and more of a nightmare. Earlier on the phone I joked to Sarah that I would see her in forty-nine days. Right now I feel like calling her and telling her it will be forty-nine years. My stomach is getting sick from the jerking from the jerk behind me.

Morton pulled all our food out of our food bag, after our breakfast of tuna, 1 bag split, 1 can of green beans split, 1 can of red beets split, we realized that we are going to run out of food before this ride is over. We have three cans of veggies left, one green bean, one creamed corn and one mixed veg. We also have a half a bag of melted marshmallows, left over from our carefree toasting at Yellowstone. I can still smell the campfire on the bag. There is a half a bag of prunes, but given the location of the handicapped toilet, I'm afraid they will be only for Morton. This is Sunday, early afternoon and we are going to be on this train until Tuesday morning. You do the math.

Brilliant idea! *The new TRAIN diet.* It would work! Get on the train, don't bring food and just take a trip anywhere. At the end of it you will be well-fasted into a shrunken stomach and quite svelte. Maybe svelte enough to fit into the normal bathroom. And you will suffer no hunger with fellow passengers like Mr. Smelly Gas-Feet, you will have zero appetite.

Sure there is food on this train if you don't mind paying the extortionists prices. A microwaved cheeseburger for $5.50. A bag of chips for $2.50. This isn't going to work. We are going to have to survive on what we have until we hit Chicago, where we switch trains and have a four hour layover. Here, I will be able to limp along while they are transferring our luggage to the train that will take us to Pittsburgh. Morton and I will do a mad dash to somewhere to buy cheap eats to bring on the train.

Perhaps this is my frame of mind that is making the ride so miserable. But let me ponder that a moment. Actually, I can only ponder it for sixteen more minutes. After that, no battery left. There is a cloud of depression I see out the window that is following me to take hold, trying to laugh about this is my only defense against it.

There are a lot of plus marks to be had on my injury. Family, friends, writing, organizing, promoting, interviews all things that need done. But the west coast of America is sitting there just waiting for us to ride down in. The doctor that had performed my knee surgery years ago will be called. Hopefully something can be worked out for payment. Perhaps he will take me under his wing or trade me for Scottish sea glass pendants. After all, that was sort of how we obtained Manhattan. Trade and barter, or was it stealing?

The train rolls on. Out the window the sky is indeed big. Forever really. You can't see the end of it. There are trees, lone houses here and there. A group of three deer running away from the tracks. There is a silver slice of river that is twisting and turning out my south facing window.

Mr. Stinky Feet has quit kicking the back of the chair. Perhaps he read over my shoulder. Hopefully I will shame him enough to put his shoes on.

If I could limp around better, without feeling like I'm going to fall flat on my face each time the train lurches, I would track down whoever has the authority to let us sit in the forbidden, nearly empty car. It would be bliss. Maybe, just maybe, someone could tell us just where we could go to sit and plug in somewhere.

There is always work to be done on my computer. Morton smirks once again, while reading this, telling me that I should have gotten the power generator that he would crank to work, like bike pedals for your hands. For once I have to agree with him. We could charge people on this train to charge their computers. We might even earn enough to afford one of those high-ticket sandwiches from the food car.

Eight minutes. It isn't my style to be bleak. I can't help always looking at the bright side and don't have to look very far to realize that I should be counting all my blessings. We are lucky. My injury could have happened at the hands of a crazy driver and some wild wheels. Instead, it is just a minor set back. A fluke. A somewhat safe accident. There is also the blessing of the lady behind us, spraying that perfume, so right now I'm smelling Mr. Stinky Feets perfume covered gas. This is a different kind of fresh country air. All small blessings that I should count.

Five minutes. My low battery warning just came on. This has been the fastest, almost hour, that has passed on this train. Since Morton is always sleeping, I have this fear he is going to wake up at Chicago and say, "That didn't take long!" at which point we will have to get help in getting my bound leg outta his backside.

Two minutes. Smile, maintain and don't scream. This will be my mantra that I will chant inwardly to myself. Why oh why hasn't someone invented an inward dialogue recorder yet. I could be writing just by thinking, on this never ending track. And the whistle blows, we are slowing down. Must be time to smoke 'em if you got 'em.

Priscilla in Montana - a town called Glasgow is approaching

Monday ramblings on a train

We are still on the train. The difference is now that I have power. Morton has stretched out our green extension cord to reach the only plug in this car. It meant moving our gear forward a car, but that was hardly any bother at all to get power. The day is gloomy out the rain streaked window. It is almost as gloomy as I feel, but not quite that bad. There are various shades of gray that have painted the sky and I think about the next stop that was just called. Wisconsin Dells. My tongue has been bitten so many times that I won't even mentally say the words, "are we there yet?" In a car I would seek out a cheap place to buy food. On the bikes I would have made sure that our food bag was full.

Since we have eaten our last two cans of veggies for breakfast, we buy two personal cheese pizzas for $3.50 each. They are cooked to perfection in a microwave by the man with the lovely voice in the food car located on the bottom deck. Any music producers or *American Idol* people watching, there is a real talent here. He is singing to a song that is playing on a cd player. When I comment on how good his voice is, I'm sure he hears this all the time, he tells me that it is him on the player. He needs to be discovered. He has written and put together this cd, all on his own computer. I offer a few tips, places on the internet that might be beneficial to have his music up and wish him well. Taking my two steaming pizzas I limp up the stairs. The look on Morton's face is priceless when I set the pizzas in his lap and tell him the price. He is too shocked to say anything at first, then tells me how many of them we could buy at a dollar type of store for that. About seven is my guess. Morton chomps his down. I take my time, chewing each bite at least 30 times before swallowing. This is going to be our only food for the next five hours and I want to make the most out of all four inches of it. The grease soaked cardboard looks tempting and I remember a part in the great book, *"Angela's Ashes"* where a young Frank McCourt licks the grease and salt off a newspaper that had held fish and chips back in Ireland. I'm tempted but don't lick grease.

Last night at dinner Morton and I watched in horror as the servers scraped away entire untouched salads into the garbage. What ever happened to waste not want not? It is a question of how hungry you will go before you are forced to do things you never thought you would do. Food from a stranger. Would we get tossed off the train if we offered to bus tables in exchange for eating untouched food?

With my belly full of the cheese, sauce and dough, I focus on the computer. My laptop is telling me that *ROAMING IS NOT AVAILABLE*, so answering emails isn't an option. Must make a mental note to call AT&T and ask them why oh why can't a girl get a signal? My phone is fine, but apparently the computer is different. Sarah and I have spoken. It dawns on me of the real plus side of this setback is getting to enjoy being

Little Changes　　　**299**　　　*Priscilla Houliston*

around my grandson. I also arrive on the third anniversary of Sarah and Graeme meeting. I'm so lucky to have a daughter that is so understanding, supportive and generally wonderful. She is my rock. As the train drives on, there are several bars on my computer that light up. Ever hopeful of a signal, there is still no joy. So you are stuck with me babbling on about my surroundings. Sorry about the misery guts attitude, this is from the soul kind of writing and hopefully therapeutic. The rain is streaming down the windows, still gray outside and very damp. There have been all sorts of landscapes out the window and I wish my mind wouldn't have been as cloudy as this overcast sky for the majority of the trip. An email from my contact at Amtrak tells me that they can't help with the tickets. Le sigh. This isn't a problem. I understand. Some can help, some can't. We will survive! My credit cards (necessary evil) have proved handy and with Morton getting one job or twelve, we will be able to get them paid off before setting off again. I also want to get a bank account with proper funding in it so we won't have to panic when things don't go as planned. After all, they never do!

  Positive vibrations, people. What a wonderful tool we all have within us. Smile, feel better, not reach for a bottle to help the pain, but reach inside. See what the trouble really is and tackle it head on. It is very empowering. It also gives you this blast of energy. I pull all my energy together to try to make myself feel better, but it is a tough thing to do at this moment in my life. At several stations where we have stopped for the smoke breaks and to let people on and off this train, I have managed to get random internet connection off of someone else's signal. Brief, not long enough, but it is still all good. The emails have came in from lots of you reinforcing everything we know and believe in our hearts.

  I get one email, just one, out of the over 20,000 we have gotten since we started this journey, that is a bit heartbreaking. It is from someone we have stayed with. In a private house. She has said that we need to quit begging from people and get to work.

It is really taken Morton and I by surprise and we hope that everything is alright in her world. It really does seem to come from way outfield. I didn't ask her for money, though we did sleep in her spare bed and eat dinner with her. She had only sent us nice emails before, so we think that maybe something in her life is tough right now.   When we had sent the email out to people when I got injured, basically to everyone that has ever emailed us, on Friday, it was to get ideas and feedback. Positive and negative I suppose, though I really didn't expect this. We didn't send a link with it for you to put money into our bank account. We just want people to know that Morton and I are not rolling in the dough. This is something that was adding to our panic, so far from home, limited funds and perhaps...maybe just on a long shot, someone knew someone that might be going our way or able to help. I emailed her back, saying that I was sorry if she got the wrong impression. It is easy when everyone is supportive (and I DON'T mean financially!) to breeze through problems. It was her opinion and of course, we are all entitled to them. The thing I find upsetting is that she says that everyone she invited over to her house to meet us, feels the same way. Then I read on in the emails. There is one from a lovely lady who we did meet that night we spent with our disgruntled hostess. My eyes well up with tears when she simply said she wished me a speedy recovery and safe travels. She said she knew we would be fine and continue to be an inspiration to many. She said she was inspired by what we were doing and was happy to have met us. I guess when we say we speak for everyone, we really can't be sure. Everyone can be a rather large number.   Morton is now dwelling on the negative email and I wish I hadn't showed it to him. Ever the Mr. Doom & Gloom before our journey, he has seen the best of what strangers have to offer, again, NOT money. It is the kindness in the sharing of a moment, it might be just five minutes of conversation beside the road or a bed for the night...it is the real humanity of the world. Now I wonder if that email is going to undo his opinions of the way things REALLY are. He reads over my shoulder to see all the other emails that have came in with well-wishes, ideas, even one lovely lady that had offered to drive out from Michigan to pick us up in Portland, Oregon and drive us back to Pennsylvania. WOW! If we would have been closer to Michigan, that might have been fun. Hopefully we will get to meet her when we go through Michigan. Morton could really read for ages. He doesn't have a clue to how many people write, telling about their own personal struggles and how our journey is giving them the push to get out and live their lives. Take chances. Make changes. Listen to others. Inspire yourself. All wonderful things. Good emails.

  Morton sits back down and leans his head back. I wish I knew what was going on in his mind right now. I know the email will eat at him like a poison, planting doubts in his mind. Maybe what we are doing *IS* wrong. Maybe we shouldn't ask strangers for help. Maybe we should just settle down into a routine and stop trying to get through to people. Not just about weight issues. This is about quality of lives, no matter what your age, station or place is in life. We all have dreams and we are crazy enough to follow ours. I have anyway, Morton has been brought along as a supportive husband. Duty.

Little Changes   **300**   *Priscilla Houliston*

There is a person on the train right now talking about his parents. I feel a million miles away from mine, knowing that I will be seeing my mom tomorrow, another blessing. It would be easy to stay and get on with our lives there, tempting even. After all, I could lose the rest of my weight just walking around in circles. I know this.

There is also a voice deep inside of me, perhaps buried under layers of fat and years of tears. It is telling me to go on. The journey has to go on. There are people on this planet that I know are in the same place I was in just over a year ago. We need to connect. We need to help and inspire each other to go, with whatever our dreams are, as we travel through this beautiful life together. There is a mission that we are all on, whether we know it or not.

My heart will not become hard. My heart will sing with joy and pleasure, even when thinking about this woman that we stayed with. I won't look for negatives or bads anymore, adding them to my long list of problems. Instead I'm taking another direction, one that I never thought I would be on. Motivating people of all shapes, sizes, ages and stations in life feels fantastic. Much better than cheesecake! If I die on this train, *NOT* a slur on how slow it seems to be going, I will die happy. Living a dream and sharing a vision of hope with people, like me, who have felt hopeless.

Keep reading, writing (even the negatives are welcomed) and PLEASE DO NOT think this is money motivated. It has nothing to do with money. Wealth comes and goes, we have learned the hard way that simple things like food, showers, shelter and above all, friends, are what makes the world spin around.

Pick Up Lines From A Train

If you were a pizza topping, what kind would you be? This was the question that was said to have had a 100% pick up success rate when trying to connect to a stranger. Someone should have told the aging man with the long blonde ponytail on the train this line. Instead, his seemed to drag around a picture album that he pulled out of his backpack. He would open it up to the female traveller he was currently "connecting" with, entertaining them with tales of far away places. As we sat on the train, watching, since you really are a captive audience here, it became painful to see. First, he was all smiles and chat lines to a young dark haired woman. She seemed to only want to sleep and didn't want to hear about his rovings in Russia. He tried a little Russian accent on her, speaking just English of course, taking on a character call "Boris" that made me smile and think of my son. This has to be a line from a movie I haven't seen.

Then he moves one car up, about the same time we did in search of power. He was looking for his own source of power, a train romance. This time, his sights were set on a pretty petite blonde who was visiting her son I learned. She didn't seem very impressed as Don Juan was showing her the photos. Morton said something to me and Romeo's ears perked up underneath his long blonde locks. "Where are you from?" he asked. Morton told him that he was from just outside of Edinburgh, Scotland. He announced that he has been there, along with a long list of other places. Then he turned back to the lady he was trying to impress. My laptop called my attention and I tuned them out, him mostly asking her questions, showing her pictures. Smiling. The next thing I heard was him using the Russian accent again. I wanted to change the channel but couldn't. He was just three feet in front of me and not the quiet type. At this point, he rattles off a list of languages he can speak, including Scottish. There were several that I'm sure were only countries that he had seen on a map, not really in his travels. For example, has anyone else heard of speaking Holland?

Remembering that Morton was from Scotland, he turned around and asked him what language he spoke in Scotland. Morton chuckled softly and said, "We speak the Queen's English of course." To this, blondie replied, only to his potential train girlfriend, that they speak another language too. Morton must not know that one. I think he was talking about Gaelic, but since there isn't a country names Gales, he had no clue to what the word was. I wasn't about to pipe up any comments. Half working and half listening, this man showed her a postcard a girl had sent him from South America. It had brightly colored birds on it and said on the back that these were the hottest birds on the beach. He then told her that "birds is what they call women in Britain" jeesh! Oh be still my bitten tongue. This line wasn't working and my knee was throbbing. Switching the computer off I tried to get some sleep while being rocked side to side and back and forth. Each bump was making my knee scream.

Dozing for about an hour, I woke up, thinking I was dreaming. The blonde man was saying the very same pick up lines again. Was this going to be something that my mind would play over and over for me? Was this a dream? Looking forward, I saw the blonde woman asleep, or faking it, on the seat in front of me.

The blonde man had gone just one seat ahead, sat down with a new arrival, a black haired young woman. He was saying the very same things, over and over. Still having no luck. You have to give him high marks for being persistent. He didn't take no or snores for a knock back. He just dug in there, moved ahead and tried again. Something in me told me I should tell him about the pizza topping line, but then I realized he would soon be moving ahead yet another car. There were a group of twenty women, all work mates, that had just boarded. It took blondie about three minutes to realize that nothing was going to be realized with his new companion. He grabbed his backpack and photo album and trotted forward.

The End of This Adventure, The Beginning of Another

www.LittleChanges.com

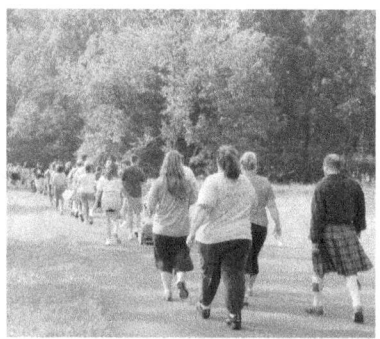 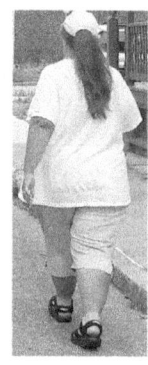 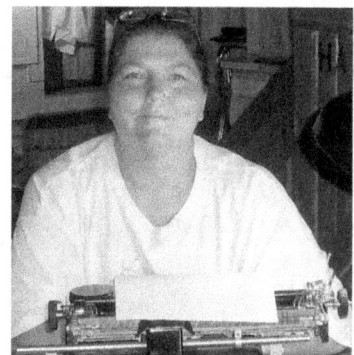

You can do anything that you want in this life if you are willing to work hard and make a few little changes. Never stop trying, get your motivation daily by inspiring others and enjoy this life. It is the only one we get.

Priscilla :)